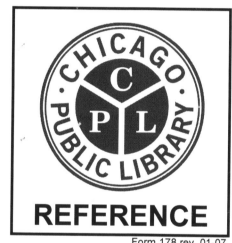

CLINICAL

NEUROLOGY

Second Edition

Frank A. Elliott, M.D., F.R.C.P.

Chief of Neurology,
The Pennsylvania Hospital
Professor of Neurology,
University of Pennsylvania School of Medicine

1971

W. B. SAUNDERS COMPANY   *PHILADELPHIA · LONDON · TORONTO*

W. B. Saunders Company: West Washington Square
Philadelphia, Pa.   19105

12 Dyott Street
London, WC1A 1DB

1835 Yonge Street
Toronto 7, Ontario

Clinical Neurology   ISBN 0-7216-3346-3

Print No.:   9   8   7   6   5   4   3   2   1

To
G. H. E.

Preface to the Second Edition

Like its predecessor, this edition presents a condensed introduction to neurological diseases together with an account of the diagnostic significance of symptoms and signs.

The material has been rearranged by assigning new chapters to hydrocephalus, metabolic disorders, and demyelinating diseases and by combining injuries to the head, spinal cord, and peripheral nerves in a single chapter.

Extensive revision has been necessary to accommodate new information on a variety of topics, including the central modulation of sensory transmission systems, the physiology of pain, the limbic system in relation to violence, the anatomy of aphasia, the biochemistry of mental retardation, the role of slow viruses, the reciprocal relationship between brain damage and electrolyte disturbances, and other matters.

It is pleasant to be able to record advances in the symptomatic treatment of a number of conditions—tic douloureux, cluster headaches, status epilepticus, herpes zoster, syringomyelia, occult hydrocephalus with dementia, paralysis agitans, Huntington's chorea, and elevated intracranial pressure.

The bibliography has been extended and brought up to date. The compilation of almost any list of references to literature must be arbitrary; but in general, priority has been given to review articles, textbooks and monographs with comprehensive bibliographies, which can serve as guides to further reading.

I am grateful to Sir Charles Symonds, Dr. Henry Schutta, Dr. Frederick Simeone, Dr. Michael Sheff, and Dr. Richard T. Johnson for their help. I am also deeply indebted to Mrs. Betty Alexander and Miss Barbara Colvin for their help with the manuscript, and to the staff of the Saunders Company for their forbearance toward a tardy author.

FRANK A. ELLIOTT

Preface to the First Edition

This outline of clinical neurology is intended for students and residents. The first eight chapters are largely concerned with the diagnostic significance of symptoms and signs and the interpretation of clinical phenomena, when possible, in terms of the basic neurological sciences; additional explanatory material is woven into the text of the remaining chapters, which deal with individual diseases. The reason for devoting so much attention to pertinent anatomic and physiologic considerations is to bring a measure of logic and intelligibility to a subject which is admittedly rather complex. Limitations of space have made it necessary to omit discussion on certain contentious issues such as the pathophysiology of extrapyramidal disorders, and to oversimplify others such as aphasia, but a selected bibliography has been supplied as a guide to further reading on these and other topics.

Emphasis on the value of clinical methods is needed at a time when radiological and laboratory procedures are all too often misused as a shortcut to diagnosis. Such procedures are often essential, but should be employed to supplement rather than to supplant the clinical interview, not only because the latter is still the quickest, safest, and cheapest diagnostic tool in the majority of cases, but also because it has furnished and will continue to furnish information as to the form and functions of the nervous system which cannot be obtained in any other way.

The traditional chapter on methods of physical examination has been omitted in the belief that these methods are best learned at the bedside. Common diseases have been given more attention than rare ones, and the eponymous terms and rare syndromes which are at once the delight of the classical neurologist and the despair of the student have been severely restricted.

The brevity of the sections on treatment will do much to sustain the charge of therapeutic nihilism which is so often and so justly leveled at neurologists, but there is nothing to be gained from the continued advocacy of ineffective nostrums; placebos are often necessary, and are justified so long as they are inexpensive and safe, but their choice is best left to the attending physician.

FRANK A. ELLIOTT

Contents

CHAPTER ONE

Disturbances of Somatic Sensation

SENSORY LOSS

The sensory changes which occur as a result of disease depend for their distribution and quality on the site, extent, and nature of the processes responsible for them. It is usually possible to identify the seat of the trouble by determining what sensations are affected and the degree and distribution of the disturbance of each mode, because there are differences in the pattern and quality of sensory loss produced by lesions of the peripheral nerves, sensory roots, spinal cord, thalamus, sensory cortex, and parietal cortex.

Peripheral Nerves. Afferent fibers conducting deep sensibility run in motor nerves, until the latter are joined by cutaneous branches to form mixed nerves. Affections of motor nerves therefore involve deep sensation, whereas lesions of cutaneous nerves leave it intact. The afferent fibers of both deep and cutaneous nerves vary in size and rate of conduction, the large myelinated "A" fibers conducting faster than the small unmyelinated "C" fibers. Pain, cold, and heat are mediated by both fast and slow fibers; lesions which have a selective action on the former, such as tabes and some forms of polyneuritis, sometimes abolish the immediate response to painful and thermal stimuli and spare the late response, but in some cases the delay is so great that some other mechanism must be involved. Delayed sensation can also occur in incomplete lesions of the spinothalamic tracts. A second form of dissociated sensory loss occurs when some sensory modes are lost and others are retained. In some cases of polyneuritis, for instance, there may be impairment of superficial sensation with preservation of proprioception, or vice versa. In leprosy, pain goes before touch, whereas in ischemic neuropathy (including pressure palsies), touch disappears before pain. Dissociated patterns of sensory impairment occurring as a result of disease in the spinal cord and brain will be discussed later in this chapter.

The effects of cutting a sensory nerve are described elsewhere (p. 519), but reference must be made here to certain aspects of the problems of denervation insofar as they bear upon the physiology of sensation. In their classical studies on cutaneous sensibility, Head and Sherren[12] noted that the return of sensation after cutting a cutaneous nerve appeared to occur in two stages, the first of which was marked by return of the capacity to recognize crude stimuli with a high threshold; the response was excessive, diffuse, and ill-localized, and slighter degrees of stimulation were not felt at all. This was followed, after a delay, by

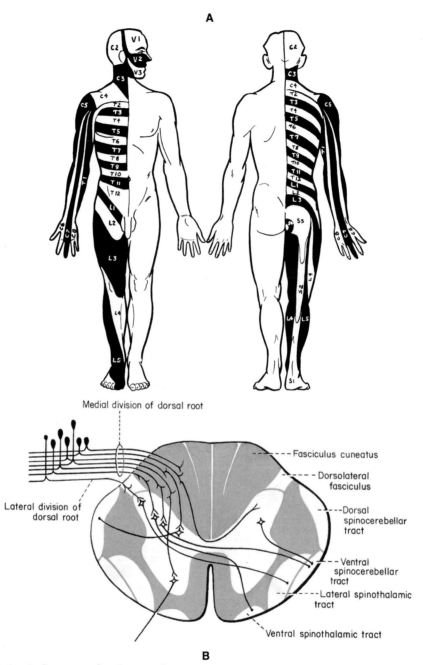

Figure 1–1. A, Cutaneous distribution of sensory roots. Many individuals present minor modifications of this pattern. B, Diagram of the disposition of sensory root fibers entering the spinal cord at the cervical level. (Modified from Ranson, S. W., and Clark, S. L.: *The Anatomy of the Nervous System. Its Development and Function.* 10th Ed. W. B. Saunders Co., Philadelphia, 1959.)

return of the ability to recognize light touch, two-point discrimination, and graduated stimuli; the overreaction was less, and localization became possible.

To explain these findings, Head postulated the existence of two sets of sensory fibers, one subserving crude sensibility, which he called *protopathic*, and the other mediating the more discriminative aspects of sensation, which he termed *epicritic*. This theory is embarrassed by there being no anatomical evidence of a dual system. Furthermore, Trotter and Davies failed to confirm the existence of two completely distinct phases in the recovery process and found it unnecessary to invoke a double mechanism to explain their findings.[36] On the contrary, Weddell and his colleagues [40] found that in every case in which pain of an unpleasant quality could be elicited by a needle prick,

the underlying nerve nets and terminals subserving pain were isolated from their neighbors, and there was a preponderance of small unmyelinated fibers. As will appear below, there is evidence that normal responses to peripheral painful stimuli depend on a balance between A fibers and C fibers.[24, 25]

The Sensory Roots. The sensory roots are composed of the proximal divisions of axons derived from posterior root ganglia. Each root conveys cutaneous sensibility from a strip of skin (the dermatome) and deep sensibility from the corresponding deep tissues, but cutaneous overlap from contiguous roots is so great that in most situations, section of a single root gives rise to a very limited area of *complete* sensory loss, which is most obvious in the periphery of the dermatome. Thus, C6 supplies a

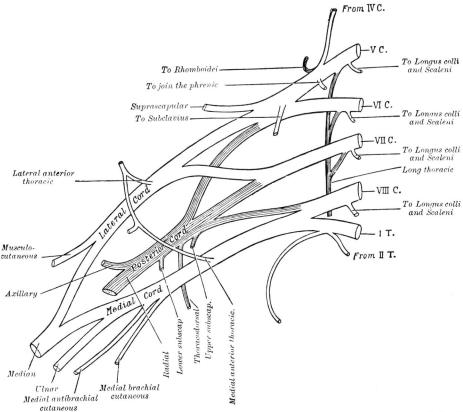

Figure 1–2. Diagram of the brachial plexus. (From Goss, C. M. [ed.]: *Gray's Anatomy of the Human Body.* 27th Ed. Lea & Febiger, Philadelphia, 1959.)

long strip of skin extending from the tip of the thumb to the shoulder, before and behind; but the area of complete sensory loss following section of the sixth root may be limited to the thumb and a thin band of skin along the distal inch or so of the radius, i.e., an area very much smaller than that actually supplied by the root. The total area supplied by each spinal root has been determined by Foerster and others by cutting the roots above and below a given root, thereby eliminating overlap and making it possible to map the area of skin which remains sentient. (Fig. 1–1, A.) Occasionally, cortical sensory loss mimics the radicular type, appearing as a longitudinal strip — resembling, for instance, the impairment caused by a lesion of C5–6 or C8.

The Spinal Sensory Paths. Regrouping of sensory modalities occurs in the spinal cord.

(1) Fibers bearing muscle and joint sense, vibration, and some touch fibers turn upward in the posterior columns of the same side; those from the lower segments of the cord lie medially and those from the upper segments lie laterally. A few touch fibers pass to the opposite ventral spinothalamic tract. The posterior columns end in medullary nuclei (cuneatus and gracilis), whence a fresh relay decussates and ascends to the thalamus in the medial lemniscus. The afferent pathways in the cord contain both monosynaptic and multisynaptic elements, thus providing for both fast and slow conduction.

(2) Fibers conveying temperature, cutaneous and deep pain, and tickle, and a few touch fibers, turn upward and downward for a short distance in the tract of Lissauer at the tip of the posterior horn, and then synapse in the substantia gelatinosa with a new relay which crosses the midline in front of the central canal of the cord, pain and temperature going to the lateral spinothalamic tract and touch to the ventral spinothalamic tract. The former is a laminated structure, sensation from the more caudal roots being mediated by laterally placed fibers and those from rostral roots by medial fibers. Expanding central lesions in the cord,

such as a tumor or syringomyelia, will first of all interrupt the decussating spinothalamic fibers, causing bilateral loss of tickle, temperature, and pain sensibility within the territory of the segments concerned, and will eventually cause a downward extension of sensory loss by encroaching upon the spinothalamic tract on one or both sides, leaving proprioception intact. In such a case, the distribution and dissociative pattern of the sensory loss will indicate that the lesion is probably intramedullary, but it is necessary to stress that in practice many exceptions are encountered.

The sensory loss may be asymmetrical, or unilateral, or it may be limited to the hands, i.e., to the distal portions of the sixth, seventh, and eighth cervical segments, as in Morvan's disease (p. 194 Compression of the cord by an extramedullary tumor or by spondylosis can produce virtually the same pattern of sensory loss as an intramedullary tumor or syrinx. Exceptionally, temperature will be more affected than pain, or vice versa, in a spinothalamic lesion.

The lateral and ventral spinothalamic tracts ascend in the cord, in front of the motor pathways. In the medulla, the touch fibers leave the tract and ascend through the reticular formation to join the medial lemniscus (conveying proprioception and touch). The result of this is that a lesion of the medulla, such as thrombosis of the posterior inferior cerebellar artery, can cause contralateral loss of temperature and pain with retention of touch. The pain and temperature fibers eventually join the medial lemniscus in the pons, and ascend in the ventrolateral portion of the tegmentum of the midbrain behind the substantia nigra to reach the thalamus.

Studies of the brainstem and diencephalon following successful spinal tractotomy for the relief of pain have shown that at the level of the inferior olive many fibers which have traveled in the spinothalamic tract leave it to end in the pontine and medullary nuclei of the bulbar reticular formation. This inflow to the reticular formation is concerned, inter alia, with the alerting func-

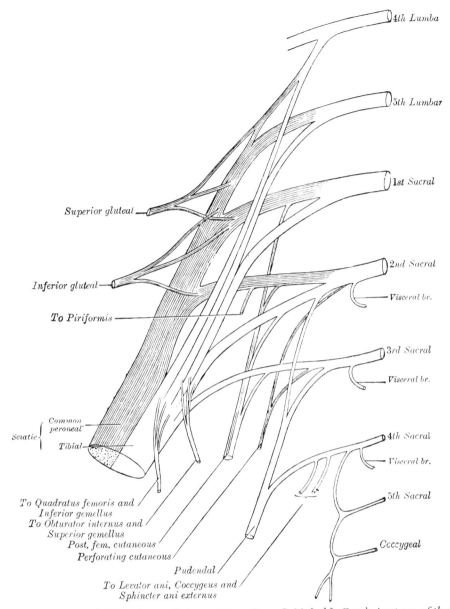

Figure 1–3. Diagram of the lumbosacral plexus. (From Goss, C. M. [ed.]: *Gray's Anatomy of the Human Body.* 27th Ed. Lea & Febiger, Philadelphia, 1959.)

tion of the reticular system, but these fibers may also be concerned with the transmission of pain because the position of the pain pathways in the brainstem correlates poorly with the spinothalamic tract.

Much of the sensory inflow from muscles and joints never reaches consciousness, but is diverted to the cerebellum.

Fibers entering the cord synapse with the cells of Clarke's column in the posterior horns, and a fresh relay passes upward in the spinocerebellar tracts, mainly but not exclusively on the same side. The ventral tract enters the cerebellum through the superior peduncle, and the dorsal tract through the inferior peduncle, thus providing the cerebellum with information as to the position of the limbs, the tone of the muscles, and the progress of movements initiated by the cerebral cortex. Destruction of the spinocerebellar tracts, as in Friedreich's ataxia, can cause ataxia, although conscious proprioception is relatively unaffected.

The Thalamus. Thalamus means an inner room—a suitable name for a collection of nuclei which are concerned with the collection and onward distribution of information from the organs of special and somatic senses, the viscera, the cerebellum, and the corpus striatum. The medial lemniscus ends in the posteroventral nucleus of the thalamus, and the quintothalamic tract from the face terminates medial to it. The anterior part of the lateral nuclear mass receives fibers from the opposite cerebellar hemisphere and from the globus pallidus and relays them onward to the frontal lobe and motor cortex. The internal capsule lies lateral to the thalamus, so that affections of the latter may spread into the former, causing contralateral hemiplegia. The thalamocortical projection system is extensive: Fibers bearing somatic sensibility, taste, and visceral sensations pass upward in the internal capsule and then fan out radially to the sensory cortex proper, which lies in the postcentral gyrus and part of the paracentral lobule on the medial aspect of the hemisphere. Other thalamic projections pass to the frontal, temporal, and parietal lobes.

Certain crude sensations—pain, temperature, deformation of tissue, and gross movements of the limbs—enter consciousness at the thalamic level, but the threshold is high and localization is poor. The more discriminative aspects of sensation depend on the sensory cortex, i.e., light touch, fine graduations of pain and temperature, localization, joint movements of small amplitude, position sense, two-point discrimination, and recognition of weight, size, and texture. Large thalamic lesions give rise to severe contralateral sensory loss, with consequent sensory ataxia.

An overreaction to sensory stimuli can occur in thalamic lesions. It is similar to what is found in partially denervated areas and in some cases of damage to the sensory pathways in the brainstem and spinal cord. It has been variously attributed to (1) loss of cortical inhibition, (2) hypothetical transmission via midline thalamic nuclei which are normally inhibited by the lateral nucleus, or (3) damage to the fast-conducting system, with consequent preponderance of the slow-conducting pathways. In addition to the overreaction to sensory stimuli, there may be attacks of severe and apparently spontaneous pain, referred to a part or to the whole of the contralateral half of the body. The combination of sensory impairment, central pain, and overreaction to crude stimuli (whether pleasant or unpleasant) is spoken of as the *thalamic syndrome of Déjerine and Roussy*,[7] to it there may be added choreoathetosis and hemiataxia. If the thalamus is totally destroyed, there is complete sensory loss on the opposite side of the body, and pain is not usually experienced. Vascular accidents account for most examples of the thalamic syndrome. The thalamus is mainly supplied by (1) perforating branches of the posterior cerebral and posterior communicating arteries to the anterior and medial nuclei; (2) the anterior choroidal, to the posterior part of the pulvinar and superior surface of the thalamus; (3) the thalamogeniculate artery to the lateral nuclei. It is this vessel which is usually involved in the case of thalamic symptoms due to vascular disease.

The Sensory Cortex. Thalamocortical fibers bearing taste, somatic sensation, and visceral sensation end in the postcentral gyrus and the adjacent portion of the paracentral lobule. This is the sensory cortex proper, and the body is represented upside down upon it in the following order from below up: taste, mouth, face, hand, arm, trunk, thigh, leg; the leg below the knee, and the perineum, are represented on the medial aspect of the hemisphere. The lips and tongue are usually bilaterally represented, and so is taste; this explains why the latter is not lost in cortical lesions and why a unilateral cortical lesion often gives rise to bilateral paresthesias of the tongue and lips, for example, during a sensory jacksonian fit. Destruction limited to the true sensory cortex causes contralateral depression of light touch (and therefore of two-point discrimination), vibration, fine degrees of joint movement, sense of position, and the ability to distinguish between degrees of temperature and pain. These defects are most marked in the hands and feet. Occasionally, the sensory impairment is of linear distribution, resembling that of a root lesion — e.g., C5–6 or C8. The appreciation of crude pain, temperature, and large movements of the joints is usually retained. It must be noted, however, that there may be complete sensory loss for a short period immediately after an acute cortical lesion, such as a superficial gunshot wound or a depressed fracture.

Penfield has described a secondary sensory cortical area including the lowest part of the postcentral gyrus and the adjacent portion of the operculum, which covers the insula. Electrical stimulation of this region in conscious man can give rise to sensation on the contralateral side of the body, and localized disease of the area can produce contralateral hypalgesia and severe pain.

Impairment of primary sensations by lesions of the sensory cortex proper also leads to a reduction or loss of the capacity to appreciate complex sensations, such as wetness, dryness, texture, weight, and shape, which are compounded of primary modes of sensibility. Consequently, comparatively mild degrees of sensory deprivation can lead to failure to recognize the nature of familiar objects by handling them, though they may be immediately recognized by the unaffected hand or by vision alone. This is called *astereognosis*. The term "tactile agnosia" is reserved for failure to recognize *familiar* objects by touch alone when ability to distinguish their size, shape, texture, and weight is preserved. Unilateral tactile agnosia is thought to be associated with damage to the postsensory strip of the parietal lobe. It has been said that a left parietal lesion in a right-handed person can give rise to bilateral tactile agnosia, which implies a loss of the patient's tactile memories. This must be very rare. Indeed, some deny the existence of tactile agnosia on the grounds that some form of sensory impairment is always present. The point is, however, that some patients with cortical lesions experience more difficulty in recognizing objects by touch than is justified by the degree of sensory impairment. Moreover, the existence of tactile memories is a fact; they accumulate throughout life, and they must have an anatomical substrate. Such evidence as there is indicates that they are stored bilaterally, posterior to the sensory cortex.

THE PARIETAL LOBE. Lesions of the parietal lobe sometimes cause complex disturbances which are particularly obvious in right-sided lesions in right-handed subjects.[4, 5] In a fully developed case, the patient has a normal appreciation of contralateral tactile, olfactory, auditory, and visual stimuli, but if he is presented with stimuli given simultaneously to the two sides, he will ignore those coming from the side opposite the lesion. This inattention, or "extinction," is thought to be the result of perceptual rivalry. It is apt to vary from hour to hour and from day to day. There may be difficulty in reading a page of print because the patient attends to only one-half of the page, or even to only one-half of each word. Instructed to draw a map of the United States, or a bicycle, he pays little attention to the portion of the drawing in the visual field contralateral to the side of the lesion. The patient may reject the opposite side of the body, forgetting to use it, to wash it, or to clothe it unless reminded to do so, and if the disease has spread to the motor cortex or pyramidal tract with consequent paralysis, he may deny the fact that he is paralyzed (anosognosia). He may ignore events taking place in extrapersonal space on the side contralateral to the lesion so that it is usually easier to take a history when sitting on the "good" side of the patient. There may be difficulty in copying simple figures, or in constructing designs with matches or building blocks; such constructional apraxia seems to be a special feature of lesions of the nondominant hemisphere. The sum total of these disturbances is to impart a bizarre quality to many of the patient's actions, and unless they are recognized for what they are, they may be falsely attributed to psychosis or psychoneurosis.

The effect of cortical sensory loss on motor function is variable. In some cases, there is moderate clumsiness in moving the contralateral limbs, especially if the eyes are shut. Extensive destruction of the parietal lobe of the dominant hemisphere can cause contralateral apraxia; it is usually considered to be due to loss of the sensory motor memories upon which the performance of complicated manual tasks depends. Another and rather uncommon motor effect of a parietal lesion of either hemisphere is the avoiding reaction. If the palm of the patient's hand is lightly stroked, the fingers and hand extend and the whole arm may move away from the contact. According to Denny-Brown, this is a release phenomenon which depends on the integrity of the frontal lobe.

Wasting of the muscles of the contralateral limbs, the hand especially, occurs in some long-standing parietal lesions.

In the presence of a hemiparesis due to a lesion which also involves the parietal lobe, the disorder of motility is somewhat modified. There is greater paucity of movement than can be accounted for on the basis of paralysis, and catatonic-like postures may be adopted by the upper limb. The affected limbs may be flaccid rather than spastic and the plantar response on the sole of the affected foot may be absent.

CENTRAL MODULATION OF SENSORY INPUT

The notion that a sensory stimulus evokes a volley of impulses which inevitably travels unhindered along well defined pathways to the thalamus and cortex is true in the artificial situation which exists under experimental conditions, but it does not explain a number of phenomena encountered in health and disease. It is a matter of common experience that under certain conditions the nervous system appears to be able to shut out unwanted and irrelevant external stimuli. Thus, it is possible to remain seemingly blind and deaf to distracting surroundings when deeply interested in a subject, and a mother, sleeping peacefully in the midst of noise, will be awakened instantly by the cry of a particular child. The pressure of a hard seat, unnoticed during an interesting lecture, becomes intolerable if the discourse is dull. It must also be asked why individuals may fail to feel pain when injured in the excitement of battle, boxing, or automobile accidents, and why surgery can be carried out painlessly under hypnosis. It is not enough to seek an alibi by calling such phenomena "psychological" or to assume — at a more physical level — that they can be explained by transactions limited to the cortex.

Over the past 50 years, and more especially during the past two decades, anatomical and physiological evidence has been accumulating in favor of the concept that sensory input can be modulated by the cortex and subcortical structures via a system of efferent pathways which terminate on sensory nuclei in the brainstem and spinal cord. The evidence, admirably reviewed by Livingston[20] in 1959, has been strengthened by work published since then.[3,10,11,14,15,19,21,25,27,32,37]

In a particularly instructive report, Wall and his colleagues[37] found that in freely moving rats subjected to electrical stimulation from subcutaneous electrodes, there was a decrease in firing frequency and an increase in the threshold of evoked responses in the posterior horns when the animal's *attention* was directed to eating, drinking, or grooming. Hernández–Peón[14] found that in the cat, the potentials evoked in the lateral geniculate body by photic stimulation to the eye were reduced when the animal's attention was distracted by non-visual stimuli. Similarly, auditory-evoked potentials are inhibited when the animal's attention is distracted by visual or olfactory stimuli.

There is also evidence that incoming volleys from the skin can be inhibited at the level of the posterior horns of the spinal cord.[10, 11] In animals, the inhibition seems to be mediated by pathways running down the pyramidal tracts to the posterior column nuclei[3, 15, 32] and to the posterior horn cells.[19, 21, 27] A question still to be resolved by appropriate clinical investigation is whether destruction of the pyramidal tracts in man can cause significant impairment of sensory inhibition.

The existence of an entirely different form of sensory inhibition was foreshadowed by Russell's[30] observation that pain originating from neuromas in amputation stumps could be suppressed by the repeated application to the painful area of mechanical stimuli (tapping with a wooden mallet, or the application of a vibrator). These stimuli activate fast-acting A fibers, and (as judged by the clinical result) this has the effect of inhibiting the slowly conducting C fibers. On the other hand, in a study of postherpetic neuralgia, Weddell[38] found that unmyelinated C fibers predominate in the damaged nerves and posterior roots. Taken together, these two bits of evidence suggest that spontaneous pain and hyperalgesia are due to an imbalance between slow- and fast-conducting fibers. This hypothesis, advanced by Noordenbos[26] in 1959, is supported by the fact that "protopathic" pain is evoked when stimuli are delivered to areas of partly denervated skin, which is supplied exclusively or largely by C fibers.[40]

In order to explain hyperpathia arising from peripheral lesions, Melzack and Wall[24, 25] have suggested that there is a "gate control system" which modulates sensory input. They have shown that when the input to the posterior horns is largely through C fibers, small cells in the substantia gelatinosa inhibit synaptic transmission between the A fibers and the second afferent neuron, and this opens the gate to the type of pain which is carried by C fibers.

PARESTHESIAS

Definition. Affections of the sensory system anywhere from the extreme periphery to the sensory cortex can give rise to sensations variously described as tingling, pins and needles, numbness, cold, heat, tightness, water trickling under the skin, or insects crawling upon it (formication). These are collectively known as paresthesias. They can sometimes be elicited by stimulating the skin of the affected part—as for instance by putting the foot to the ground—and can be removed temporarily by procaine block of the sensory nerve supplying the area in which the unusual sensations are felt. From this, it appears that normal sensory volleys are perverted and magnified when they reach an area of damage in the afferent pathways. Tingling and a sense of numbness arise from implication of fibers and tracts conveying touch and pressure alone; they do not occur, for instance, in pure spinothalamic lesions, which are more likely to be attended by feelings of cold or warmth, or painful pins and needles.

Significance of Paresthesias. Paresthesias *do not accompany pain referred from visceral or somatic structures*, and their presence therefore indicates implication of nerves, roots, central sensory pathways, or the sensory cortex. In the presence of disease of the cervical segments, such as multiple sclerosis, spondylosis, or tumor, paresthesias of the arms, trunk, and legs can sometimes be induced by flexing the neck (Lhermitte's sign); less commonly, the sign is present in cases of disease lower down the spinal cord.

Localizing Value. Paresthesias appear in the areas of skin supplied by the sensory pathways which are affected, and their distribution therefore has localizing value. When they result from disease of the peripheral nerves, they are felt in the peripheral part of the skin supplied by the affected nerve or nerves, and when they result from root irritation, they are felt in the peripheral part of the affected dermatome. Unilateral spinal cord lesions give rise to more diffuse paresthesias: If the posterior columns are affected, the paresthesias are felt on the same side, below the level of the lesion, and when the spinothalamic tract is involved on one side, they are felt contralaterally; in both instances, the sensations may be experienced either over the whole of the area concerned or only in distal parts of the body, such as the hand or foot. If both sides of the cord are implicated, the paresthesias will be felt bilaterally, although not necessarily to the same extent on both sides. Paresthesias limited to one side of the face may occur as a result of lesions involving the gasserian ganglion or the descending trigeminal root, which extends from the lower pons to the second or third segment of the cervical cord. Lesions of the thalamus or sensory cortex can give rise to contralateral paresthesias in the face, arm, and leg; less commonly, they also involve the trunk.

Two special types of paresthesias due to cortical disturbance deserve mention. In sensory jacksonian attacks, the patient experiences a tingling or numbness which spreads rapidly from the leg to hand to face, or vice versa, passing off in reverse order in anywhere from a few seconds to two minutes. This may constitute the entire attack, or the paresthesias may give way to unilateral clonic movements, or even to a generalized convulsion. In migraine, the headache is sometimes preceded by paresthesias which creep either up or down one side of the body, they may last from 10 to 30 minutes, and occasionally the headache does not occur.

Persistent or intermittent paresthesias in the limbs are a common feature of many forms of polyneuropathy. They start in the feet since most forms of polyneuropathy affect the longest neurons first, and as the disease advances they may be felt in the tips of the fingers. Paresthesias which involve the hands but not the lower limbs should not be at-

tributed to a toxic or metabolic polyneuropathy. In mononeuritis multiplex, several peripheral nerves may be involved in a patchy and asymmetrical manner; this is sometimes seen in collagen diseases, and it may occur in the lower limbs as the result of the implication of peripheral sensory nerves by vascular disease, as in diabetes, Buerger's disease, and atherosclerosis. In subacute combined degeneration of the cord (combined system disease), the paresthesias in the feet and hands may antedate signs of pernicious anemia. Paresthesias in the toes and fingers without objective neurological loss are also encountered in association with idiopathic hypochromic anemia of women; in severe cases the tongue is red and smooth, and there may be dysphagia (Plummer-Vinson syndrome).

When the second cervical root is involved by cervical arthritis, paresthesias may be felt together with pain on one-half of the back of the scalp. Paresthesias occupying the *entire* area of the scalp on both sides, not spreading onto the hairless skin, sometimes occur in introspective individuals in the absence of neurological disease. Irritative lesions of the third and fourth cervical roots are rare, but if they cause paresthesias, they are to be found along the ridge of the trapezius and above the clavicle. When the fifth root is implicated, paresthesias may be felt in the thumb or on the lateral aspect of the deltoid. The preferential site of paresthesias from irritation of the sixth cervical root is the index finger, and for the seventh root, the middle finger. If the little and ring fingers are implicated, the trouble may be in the eighth root, the brachial plexus, or the ulnar nerve. Irritation of the thoracic roots gives rise to pain rather than to paresthesias.

Paresthesias from irritation of the second lumbar root are rare, and occur in the groin. In the case of the third lumbar root, they appear in the front of the thigh as far as the knee, and if the fourth lumbar root is involved, they are felt down the shin and on the medial border of the ankle. Paresthesias from fifth lumbar root involvement characteristically occur on the lateral border of the foot and the dorsum of the big toe, and they may also involve the lateral aspect of the leg below the knee. Tinglings in the sole of the foot can indicate involvement of (1) the first sacral root, (2) the posterior tibial nerve, or (3) the plantar nerves. When the abnormal sensations are on the back of the thigh or back of the calf, the second sacral root is affected, while paresthesias in the perianal area usually mean that the third, fourth, or fifth sacral root is involved. It must also be emphasized that paresthesias of segmental or root distribution sometimes occur with lesions of the spinal cord itself; for instance, compression of the cervical cord by spondylosis can give rise to paresthesias in the soles of the feet, or down the back of the legs, or in the buttocks.

A very common source of paresthesias in the thumb, index, and middle fingers is compression of the median nerve in the carpal tunnel, and this may be bilateral. When it has been present some time, there is usually some objective sensory impairment, and there may be wasting of the thenar muscles. Another common condition is paresthesias of the ring and little fingers, and the medial border of the hand, from recurrent small traumata to the ulnar nerve at the elbow. Paresthesias of apparently ulnar distribution are also encountered in the cervical rib and the thoracic outlet syndrome, but the unpleasant sensations usually spread down the ulnar side of the forearm, a distribution which distinguishes them from ulnar neuropathy arising at the elbow itself.

In *meralgia paresthetica*, paresthesias invade a large oval patch of skin on the anterolateral border of the thigh, which may extend from the knee to just below the inguinal ligament. There is objective perversion or impairment of sensation within this area, but there is no weakness of the quadriceps or impairment of the knee jerk. The abnormal sensations are felt in the distribution of the lateral cutaneous nerve of the thigh, and their distribution distinguishes them from the

more localized paresthesias sometimes encountered in irritative lesions of the third lumbar root.

Finally, paresthesias occur around the lips and in the fingers and toes in tetany, and also in emotionally disturbed individuals as a result of overbreathing. It is useful to remember that the patient is often unaware of overbreathing; rarely, hyperventilation of this type leads to unconsciousness.

PHANTOM LIMB

It is usual for a patient to be aware of an absent limb after amputation. Such phantoms are not disagreeable as a rule, and tend to become less prominent as time goes on; the limb appears to shorten and ultimately fades from consciousness. Phantoms have been described in children with congenital absence of one or more limbs.[41] The sensory components of the phantom limb as analyzed by Henderson and Smythe [13] are of three kinds: (1) mild tingling, which is greatest in parts having the largest cortical representation, such as the thumb and index finger or the great toe; (2) sensations of pins and needles induced by touching the stump; and (3) sensations of limb movement, which are accompanied by observable contractions in the muscles of the stump. In a minority of cases, the patient complains of severe spontaneous discomfort in the phantom; it is variously described as a burning feeling, a boring sensation, or a feeling that the limb is being twisted or moved. It may feel as if it is placed in an unusual position—in some cases, the position in which it was at the time of the injury which necessitated amputation. Henderson and Smythe concluded from a survey of some 300 amputations in prisoner-of-war camps that these disagreeable sensations are unrelated to the condition of the stump and are psychophysiological in origin. Operations on the stump, peripheral neurectomies, cordotomies, and even cortical ablations seldom cure the patient *permanently*, though temporary alleviation of symptoms is common following such operations.[30] Russell has found that the pain originating in amputation stumps can be relieved by the repeated application of a vibrator to tender neuromata or by subjecting the area to repeated firm tapping with a wooden mallet. An explanation for this curious phenomenon is discussed on page 9.

PAIN

From the biological point of view, pain differs from other sensations in that it conveys a threat or warning to the organism and evokes a wide spectrum of emotional, somatic, autonomic, and humoral responses. It is true that sight, hearing, heat, cold, and touch may convey warnings of danger, but this occurs as a result of experience; the adult knows that an approaching automobile, or the smell of gas, or the sound of a gunshot may spell danger, but the infant does not. Both infant and adult, however, will respond to a painful pinprick in the same way. This special significance of pain has a physical basis in that painful stimuli are usually accompanied by tissue damage. Whereas the gentle application of a needle to the skin leaves no mark and causes a sense of touch rather than of pain, a painful pinprick causes a small red spot at the site, indicating that the skin has been penetrated. Similarly, the application of a cold or warm object to the skin excites the appropriate sensation, but extreme heat and cold induce not only pain but also local tissue damage. The persistent swelling and tenderness which occur after a painful involuntary muscle cramp further illustrate this principle.

Pain Thresholds. Some people seem to be more sensitive to pain than others. At one end of the scale there are the sensitive, highly-strung individuals of either sex who overreact to the stimulus of a pinprick or to pain caused by disease. They are also apt to overreact to bright lights, sounds, and smells. At the other end of the scale are the individuals who

seem to be more than usually stoical. In both groups, the pain threshold may be lowered as the result of long-continued physical illness, persistent anxiety, or the administration of opiates over long periods.

The term *pain asymbolia*[29, 33] is applied to a situation in which there is no loss of pain sensibility, but the emotional reaction to this sensation is absent. It usually occurs in lesions involving the inferior parietal region of the dominant hemisphere, for which reason the patient may show some degree of aphasia, right-left disorientation, difficulties in calculation, and apraxia. It must be distinguished from the altered emotional response to pain seen as the result of prefrontal leukotomy, in which the patient has a *reduced threshold to pinprick and will withdraw from it sharply,* but ceases to suffer from the emotional accompaniment of pain.

Well beyond the range of what can be considered normal are the individuals who demonstrate *congenital insensitivity to pain.*[16, 22, 28] They can have teeth extracted, fingers crushed, or bones broken without feeling distress, though they are able to distinguish between the head and the point of a pin and between different kinds and degrees of noxious stimuli. It occurs in otherwise normal individuals and is not to be confused with absence of the response to pain and other external stimuli which is seen in congenital idiocy. It can be associated with anhydrosis.[35] The physical basis for insensitivity to pain is not known. As a rule, it is noticed by the beginning of his third or fourth year that the child does not cry when injured, and continues to run about without complaint in the presence of conditions which would incapacitate a normal child. In some cases, the pain of visceral disease is felt and in others it is not. The condition is easily identified because in no other disorder is there complete and universal insensitivity to pain all over the body.

Pain Mechanisms. Pain can be produced by affections involving pain fibers anywhere between the periphery and the thalamus, but in most cases it is the result of the stimulation of peripheral pain endings through the liberation of pain-producing substances, increased tissue tension, or both. Thus, a tooth abscess causes most of its discomfort by increased tension, but pain-producing substances (P) resulting from inflammation are also at work since the pain does not completely disappear after tension has been relieved by extraction of the tooth. The action of P-substances is also seen in inflammation and injuries of the skin and in intermittent claudication and meningitis.

Persistent or intermittent increase of tension, on the other hand, is responsible for irritation of the peripheral nerve endings in pleurisy, muscle cramps, abdominal colic, space-occupying lesions inside the head, glaucoma, osteomyelitis, etc. Affections of the peripheral nerve trunks are more likely to cause paresthesias than pain, but the latter can occur in polyneuritis and leprosy, and in incomplete lesions of large mixed nerves such as the median and the sciatic. Such injuries can give rise to a dull, deep discomfort, or to an intense, burning, superficial pain known as causalgia (p. 531).

The posterior roots, and the sensory roots of the cranial nerves, are extremely sensitive to local pressure, friction, and inflammation. Partial interruption of the spinothalamic tracts and incomplete destruction of the lateral nucleus of the thalamus occasionally give rise to intense pain in the contralateral half of the body; there is no precise information as to how such "central" pain arises, though the fact that it is much aggravated by peripheral stimuli suggests the possibility that incoming sensory volleys are perverted and amplified when they reach the site of the lesion. Affections of the sensory cortex often produce paresthesias, but pain is extremely rare and when it does occur there is always the possibility that the lesion has penetrated to the thalamus.

Referred Pain. In seeking to determine the origin of pain, whether visceral or somatic, attention must be paid to its distribution, quality, and time incidence, and to the factors which aggravate and relieve it. Tic douloureux, lightning pains, causalgia, headaches due to space-occupying lesions, and migraine are examples of pain which can be identified by reference to their situation, quality, and time relationships, as described elsewhere in this book. The same is true of the majority of pains of visceral origin. Nevertheless, there are many examples of somatic pain which are difficult to trace to their source, and for this reason it is necessary to appreciate the mechanisms underlying the reference of pain, so far as they are known.

It is established that both visceral and cutaneous afferent fibers converge upon single neurons in the posterior horns, but the existence of this common pathway does not explain why referred pain usually develops so slowly. Wolff and Hardy[43] suggested that the incoming barrage of pain impulses from the site of disease or injury brings about an increased excitatory state in the spinal cord, and that this gradually causes reference of pain to areas not immediately affected by disease. This would explain why injections of procaine into the area of referred pain sometimes reduce or abolish it.[18]

REFERRED PAIN FROM DEEP LESIONS. In a series of papers, Kellgren[17] showed that whereas superficial lesions cause local pain, more deeply situated lesions give rise to discomfort which is felt not only locally but also in the tissue supplied by the spinal segment which innervates the site of the lesion. The deeper the lesion from the surface, the more likely it is that pain will be referred to a distance. Thus, pain arising from skin supplied by L2 in the upper lumbar area will be felt locally, whereas pain from a lesion of the second lumbar interspinous ligament will radiate outward and downward toward the groin; irritation of the second lumbar root may be felt locally, but pain will also be felt in the peripheral distribution of the root, i.e., around the loin and perhaps in the testis; in renal colic, it will be felt in the same distribution. Thus a distinction between renal pain and root pain is not made on distribution or quality alone, because they can be identical, but by the fact that renal colic comes on in repeated short bouts, whereas root pain is persistent. In many cases they can also be distinguished by the presence of satellite symptoms—disturbances of micturition in the one, and paresthesias or sensory changes in the other.

Pain referred from deep sources is felt as a rule not in the skin, but in deeper tissues. This is of practical importance in areas of the body in which the segmental innervation of the skin and subjacent structures is different. Thus, the pain from an irritative lesion of the sixth or seventh cervical root (as in disc herniation) may be felt below the clavicle because the pectoral muscles are innervated by these roots. This may be mistaken for cardiac pain. Similarly, irritation of the second lumbar root may cause pain in the testis (L2) and not in the overlying scrotum (S3 to S5).

Pain caused by a deep lesion, whether of a nerve root, viscus, or skeletal structure, may not be felt over the site of the disease at all, but only in the area of segmental reference, and it may appear in only a limited portion of that area. Thus pain from a lesion of the fifth lumbar root may be limited to the lateral border of the leg below the knee, just as cardiac pain may be felt in the arm and not in the chest. That pain referred from a viscus, a nerve root, or from a somatic structure can have the same distribution explains the difficulty that sometimes arises in distinguishing between visceral disease on the one hand and affections of the spine and thoracic roots on the other. The risk of error is increased by the fact that pain in the back may be present or absent in both visceral and somatic lesions and that referred pain may be accompanied by muscular rigidity and by cutaneous or deep hyperalgesia within its area of reference. Thus pain, rigidity, and tenderness may be felt in the right iliac fossa as the result of disease affecting the lower dorsal spine, the lower three thoracic roots, the lower half of the pleura, or disease in the right lower quadrant of the abdomen.

In the limbs, the differentiation be-tween pain of neural and skeletal origin is beset by similar difficulties. Discomfort in the buttock and back of the thigh may be due to the irritation of the lower lumbar and sacral roots or to sacroiliac disease. Pain in the front of the thigh can be caused by disease of the hip joint or of the third lumbar root. In such cases we have to rely on symptoms and signs other than the distribution of the pain, and in particular, on the presence of paresthesias, muscular weakness and wasting, sensory loss, and changes in the reflexes. Of these, paresthesias are the most helpful because they usually occur early, before objective neurological signs make their appearance, and they do not occur in association with pain of extra-neural origin. Unfortunately they are sometimes absent in neural lesions. Aggravation of pain by coughing or sneezing, or by flexing the neck while the extended leg is flexed at the hip, is a useful sign of a lumbar root lesion.

An unusual form of erroneous reference of pain is sometimes seen in tabes and after anterolateral cordotomy. The author has also observed the phenomenon in an intelligent and otherwise completely normal adult. A painful stimulus produces pain of low intensity referred to a corresponding site on the opposite side of the body. Some of the collaterals of primary afferent fibers synapse with cells in the posterior horns, which themselves communicate with cells in the posterior horn of the opposite side; this arrangement supplies a theoretical basis for such *allochiria*.

The pain which is sometimes felt in the limbs and trunk in spinothalamic lesions is diffuse and poorly localized. It is usually accompanied by an excessive and unpleasant response to peripheral stimulation, and there is usually some objective impairment of pain and temperature sensibility, but in the early stages of spinal compression it may be difficult or impossible to demonstrate such impairment.

Tenderness. Increased sensibility to cutaneous stimuli can be brought about in four ways: (1) Local injury to the skin causes the liberation of pain-producing substances which sensitize local nerve endings. (2) Severe referred pain from a deeply situated extraneural lesion is sometimes associated with cutaneous hyperalgesia within the area of reference. For example, the cheek may be sensitive in toothache, or the skin of the right iliac fossa in appendicitis. (3) The sensory threshold is raised by affections of peripheral nerves, sensory roots, spinal cord, or thalamus, but stimuli which reach threshold may give rise to an excessive response. (4) The sensory threshold is often lowered in patients who are nervous, frightened, or debilitated by long-continued disease.

Increased sensibility to pressure is seen in muscles as the result of injury, myositis, ischemia, fatigue induced by postural strains and long-continued reflex spasm, and in affections of the sensory nerves, roots, or their central connections. In many cases, the tenderness is of mixed origin. For instance, in sciatica there may be both referred hyperalgesia and tenderness due to reflexly induced spasm in small groups of muscle fibers, which may be felt as distinct nodules.[9] In many painful affections of the brachial plexus and cervical roots, the trapezius and pectoral muscles are painful not only because they fall within the area of referred pain, but also because they are fatigued by guarding the shoulder against movements which aggravate the pain. It is a sound rule to regard muscle tenderness as a manifestation of one or more of the causative factors previously listed, until proved otherwise, and to avoid the diagnosis of "fibrositis," "myalgia," and other vague conditions.

Psychophysiological Aspects of Pain

Attention and Inattention. Attention and inattention play a large part in determining how much pain is felt. Injuries sustained when the individual's attention is distracted by excitement or fear are often painless, and it is a commonplace that the patient with severe pain from physical disorders can have his suffering reduced if his attention is distracted.

Conversely, the individual who dwells upon his symptoms will usually suffer increasingly, as for instance in compensation cases.[2]

The fortitude with which patients bear pain is variable. In some, prolonged pain is accepted with stoicism. In others, it is accompanied by much emotional disturbance, and the total picture is one of great suffering. This is particularly likely to occur in terminal cancer, when the patient is faced not only with pain but also with the knowledge that his illness is terminal. It is in this group that prefrontal leukotomy, which cuts the thalamofrontal projection system, can be helpful. The procedure does not raise the patient's pain threshold; in fact, it may reduce it, yet the effect of the operation in patients with intractable pain and much suffering is remarkable. The pain is still there, but the patient no longer worries about it. Sleep is restored, weight is gained, and analgesics can often be dispensed with. The patient is often apt to display distractability and inattentiveness, and he ceases to bother not only about his pain but also about other matters. If the surgical incision is too extensive, the effect on personality can be catastrophic.[31] Because of the severe dilapidation of the personality which sometimes follows prefrontal leukotomy, many surgeons have turned to stereotaxic thalamotomy, the target area being the region of nucleus medianum, N. parafascicularis, and the intralaminar nuclei. If the lesions are correctly placed, they do not cause sensory impairment, whereas lesions placed in the specific sensory nuclei give rise to contralateral sensory loss without relief of pain. According to White and Sweet,[42] the *mental* suffering which can accompany pain in the terminal stages of malignant disease is best controlled by lesions in the anterior or dorsomedial nuclei and they report that although these patients admit that some pain remains, they are no longer concerned about it. Stereotaxic thalamotomy does not produce the personality changes which often follow prefrontal leukotomy. Foltz and White have also reported favorably on the effects of electrocoagulation of the cingulum, which connects the medial frontal cortex with certain of the thalamic nuclei and with the hippocampal formation. Relief of pain and suffering has been obtained without psychological deterioration.

These operations are best reserved for patients with a limited expectation of life since both the pain and its emotional accompaniment will sometimes return within months, or within a year or two, of the operation. For further information, the reader is directed to White and Sweet.[42]

Suggestibility. Another fact to be taken into consideration in the interpretation of pain is the effect of suggestibility. Some patients with severe angina pectoris may report relief from taking a pharmacologically inert pill. The same phenomenon is seen in the relief of pain following the injection of sterile saline. Consequently, it is unwise to conclude that a patient's pain is imaginary because he is relieved by a placebo. Clearly, some type of suppressor mechanism is at work here, as it is in hypnotic analgesia. To label these phenomena "psychological" does not resolve the problem, for, as pointed out earlier, the brain is the organ of mind and neurophysiological mechanisms must therefore be involved.

Psychological Disorders. Disorders which are primarily psychological or emotional can cause pain. Anxiety causes disorders of motility in the gastrointestinal tract, with consequent dyspepsia or colitis. Tension can cause pain by interfering with relaxation of skeletal muscles, especially in the neck and shoulder girdle. Sustained contraction of the neck and scalp muscles is one cause of tension headaches.

A second and far less common form of psychogenic pain is encountered in persons who display no physical disease whatsoever and who complain for years on end of intolerable pain in the limbs, head, or back. They look well, sleep well, and remain cheerful, but their entire lives are centered around their "pain." Paradoxically, they often con-

tinue to seek relief and are prepared to undergo extensive and even mutilating operations to this end. But the effect of such operations lasts only a short time, and the pain returns. It is inadvisable to try to relieve them by surgical measures, not only because such measures will always fail, but also because the pain is essential to the patient's adjustment to life. For the same reason, psychotherapy is likely to be fruitless. Moreover, if the pain is relieved—by hypnosis, for instance—other and more crippling psychological symptoms may develop.

REFERENCES

1. Angel, A., and Dawson, G. D.: Modification of thalamic transmission by sensory stimulation. *J. Physiol.* 156:23, 1961.
2. Beecher, H. K.: Relationship of significance of wound to pain experienced. *J.A.M.A.* 161:1609, 1956.
3. Chambers, W. W., Liu, C. N., and McCouch, P. C.: Inhibition of the dorsal column nuclei (of the cat). *Exp. Neurol.* 7:13, 1963.
4. Critchley, M.: The phenomenon of tactile inattention with special reference to parietal lesions. *Brain* 72:538, 1949.
5. Critchley, M., Russell, W. R., and Zangwill, O. L.: Discussion on parietal lobe syndromes. *Proc. Roy. Soc. Med.* 44:337, 1951.
6. Davies, H. M.: The peculiarities of sensibility found in cutaneous areas supplied by regenerating nerves. *J. Psychol. Neurol.* 20:102, 1913.
7. Déjerine, J., and Roussy, G.: Le syndrome thalamique. *Rev. Neurol.* 14:521, 1906.
8. Elithorn, A., Glithero, E., and Slater, E.: Leucotomy for pain. *J. Neurol. Neurosurg. Psychiat.* 21:249, 1958.
9. Elliott, F. A.: Tender muscles in sciatica. Electromyographic studies. *Lancet* 1:44, 1944.
10. Fitz, E. E.: Pyramidal tract effects on interneurons in the cat's lumbar dorsal horns. *J. Neurophysiol.* 31:69, 1968.
11. Hagbarth, K. E., and Kerr, D. B.: Central influences on spinal afferent conduction. *J. Neurophysiol.* 17:295, 1954.
12. Head, H., and Sherren, J.: The consequences of injury to the peripheral nerves in man. *Brain* 28:116, 1905.
13. Henderson, W. R., and Smythe, G. E.: Phantom limbs. *J. Neurol. Neurosurg. Psychiat.* 11:88, 1948.
14. Hernandez-Peón, R., Scherrer, H., and Velasco, M.: *Acta. Neurol. Latinoam* 2:8, 1956.
15. Jabbur, S. J., and Towe, A. L.: The influence of the cerebral cortex on the dorsal column

nuclei. *Nervous Inhibition.* Edited by Florey, E., Pergamon Press, London, 1961, p. 419.

16. Jewesbury, E. C. O.: Insensitivity to pain. *Brain* 74:336, 1951.

17. Kellgren, J. H.: On the distribution of pain arising from deep somatic structures, with charts of segmental pain areas. *Clin. Sci.* 4:35, 1939.

18. Kibler, R. F., and Nathan, P. W.: Relief of pain and paresthesiae by nerve block distal to a lesion. *J. Neurol. Neurosurg. Psychiat.* 23:91, 1960.

19. Kuypers, H.: Pericentral cortical projections to motor and sensory nuclei. *Science* 128:662, 1958.

20. Livingston, R. B.: Central control of reception and sensory transmission systems. *Handbook of Physiology,* American Physiological Society, Washington, D. C., 1959, Vol. 1, Section 1, Chap. 31.

21. Lundberg, A., Norrsell, V., and Voorhoeve, I.: Pyramidal effects on lumbosacral interneurons activated by somatic afferents. *Acta Physiol. Scand.* 56:220, 1962.

22. McMurray, G. A.: Experimental study of a case of insensitivity to pain. *Arch. Neurol. Psychiat.* 64:650, 1950.

23. Mehler, W. H., Feferman, M. E., and Nauta, W. J. H.: Ascending axon degeneration following anterolateral cordotomy in the monkey. *Brain* 83:718, 1960.

24. Melzack, R., and Wall, P. D. T.: Pain mechanism: A new theory. *Science* 150:971, 1965.

25. Mendell, L. M., and Wall, P. D. T.: Responses of single dorsal horn cells to peripheral cutaneous unmyelinated fibres. *Nature* (London) 206:97, 1965.

26. Noordenbos, W.: *Problems Pertaining to the Transmission of Nerve Impulses Which Give Rise to Pain.* Elsevier Publishing Co., Amsterdam, 1959.

27. Nyberg–Hansen, R., and Brodal, A.: Sites of termination of cerebrospinal fibres in the cat. *J. Comp. Neurol.* 120:369, 1963.

28. Ogden, T. E., Robert, F., and Carmichael, E. A.: Some sensory syndromes in children: Indifference to pain and sensory neuropathy. *J. Neurol. Neurosurg. Psychiat.* 22:267, 1957.

29. Rubins, J. L., and Friedman, E. D.: Asymbolia for pain. *Arch. Neurol. Psychiat.* 60:554, 1948.

30. Russell, W. R.: Painful amputation stumps and phantom limbs. Treatment by repeated percussion to the stump neuromata. *Brit. Med. J.* 1:1024, 1949.

31. Ryland, R. G.: Personality analysis before and after frontal lobotomy. *Res. Pub. Ass. Res. Nerv. Ment. Dis.* 27:691, 1948.

32. Satterfield, J. H.: Effect of sensorimotor cortical stimulation upon cuneate nuclear output through the medial lemniscus in cat. *J. Nerv. Ment. Dis.* 135:507, 1962.

33. Schilder, P., and Stengel, I.: Asymbolia for pain. *Arch. Neurol. Psychiat.* 25:598, 1931.

34. Stopford, J. S. B.: Disturbance of sensation following section and suture of a peripheral nerve. *Brain* 50:391, 1927.

35. Swanson, A. G.: Congenital insensitivity to pain, with anhydrosis. *Arch. Neurol.* 8:299, 1963.

36. Trotter, W., and Davies, H. M.: Experimental studies in the innervation of the skin. *J. Physiol.* 38:134, 1909.

37. Wall, P. D. T., Freeman, J., and Major, D.: Dorsal horn cells in spinal cord of freely moving rats. *Exp. Neurol.* 19:519, 1967.

38. Weddell, G.: *Neural Physiopathology.* Edited by Grenell, R. G., Paul B. Hoeber, Div. Harper & Row, New York, 1962, Chap. 5.

39. Weddell, G., and Miller, S.: Cutaneous sensibility. *Ann. Rev. Physiol.* 24:199, 1962.

40. Weddell, G., Sinclair, D. C., and Feindel, W. H.: Anatomical basis for alterations in the quality of pain sensibility. *J. Neurophysiol.* 11:99, 1948.

41. Weinstein, S., and Serson, E. A.: Phantoms in cases of congenital absence of limbs. *Neurology.* 11:905, 1961.

42. White, J. C., and Sweet, W. H.: *Pain and the Neurosurgeon: A Forty Year Experience.* Charles C Thomas, Springfield, Ill., 1969.

43. Wolff, H. G., and Hardy, J. D.: On the nature of pain. *Physiol. Rev.* 27:167, 1947.

CHAPTER TWO

Disorders of the Motor System

Motor disabilities resulting from organic disease of the nervous system resolve themselves into five groups: paralysis, disorders of tone, ataxia and disorders of equilibrium, involuntary movements, and apraxia.

PARALYSIS

Loss of power can be caused by disease affecting the corticospinal tract (upper motor neuron), the anterior horn cells and their axons (lower motor neuron), neuromuscular transmission, and the muscles themselves.

Upper Motor Neuron Paralysis

The Motor Cortex and the Upper Motor Neuron. The motor cortex, area 4, occupies the anterior wall of the central sulcus, the posterior half of the precentral gyrus, and part of the paracentral lobule on the medial aspect of the hemisphere (Fig. 2–1). It is characterized histologically by the giant pyramidal cells of Betz and physiologically by the ease with which contralateral movements can be elicited by stimulating this area, and also by the tendency for the excitation produced by an unaltered electrical stimulus to spread throughout its extent.

Anteriorly, the motor cortex merges with area 6, which contains smaller pyramidal cells and appears to be concerned with some aspects of motor integration because, whereas damage to area 4 causes paralysis, lesions of area 6 sometimes interfere with the performance of acts (e.g., writing, turning the head and eyes to one side), without disturbing power or tone. Electrical stimulation of the posterior part of the second frontal convolution in front of the motor cortex can cause turning of the head and eyes to the opposite side, a movement sometimes seen at the start of an epileptic seizure resulting from an irritative lesion in this area. Contraversive movements of this sort can also be obtained, albeit with greater difficulty and less consistency, by stimulating the temporal and parietal lobes. There is evidence, in both animals and man,[22] of the existence of a supplementary motor cortex, which is situated mainly on the medial aspect of the hemisphere, anterior to area 4. Its threshold for effective stimulation is higher than that of the primary motor area, and the responses are more in the nature of an assumption of a posture rather than the quick movements induced by stimulation of the precentral area; moreover, the posture tends to be held after the stimulus has ceased. The supplementary motor cortex does not appear to contribute to the pyramidal

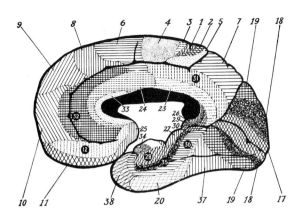

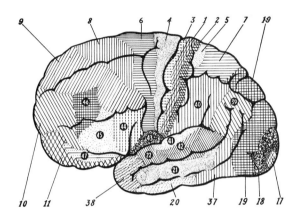

Figure 2–1. Architectonic areas of the brain. (After Brodmann.)

tract, but it has connections with the extrapyramidal motor system.

FUNCTION OF THE MOTOR CORTEX. In the motor cortex proper, the body is represented upside down, owing to the ventral flexion of the forebrain, which occurs in the early stages of fetal development. The feet and perineum are represented in the paracentral lobule (along with autonomic centers concerned with control of the bladder), and the thigh at the top of the precentral gyrus; below this, in the order given, are the areas concerned with the trunk, forearm, hand, face, tongue, swallowing, and mastication (Fig. 2–2). The area for the hand is larger than that for the lower limb.

The motor cortex receives afferents from (1) area 6, the sensory cortex, and the temporal lobe; (2) the opposite hemisphere via the corpus callosum; (3) the corpus striatum via the thalamus; (4) the mesencephalic reticular formation;

and (5) the contralateral cerebellar hemisphere. The motor cortex serves, in Fulton's words, as "a funnel through which highly organized movement patterns are ultimately discharged." The stem of this funnel is the corticospinal tract, which is derived from the giant pyramidal cells and a large number of smaller cells in the motor cortex, the premotor cortex, the post-Rolandic sensory cortex, and the temporal lobe. The pyramidal tract derives its name from the medullary pyramids and not from the pyramidal cells of Betz, from which only about one in 20 of its fibers originates. The alternative term, corticospinal tract, is not entirely accurate because some of its fibers end in the nuclei of the motor cranial nerves and in the reticular formation.

The pyramidal tract occupies a small area in the posterior limb of the internal capsule. The tract converges downward

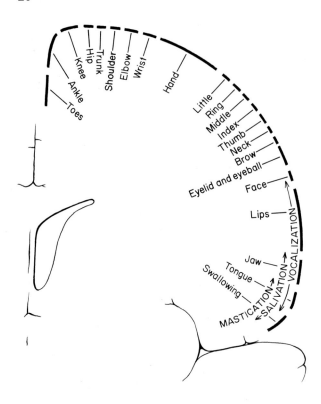

Figure 2–2. Representation of motor function in the pre-Rolandic gyrus of man. (After Penfield, W., and Jasper, H.: *Epilepsy and the Functional Anatomy of the Human Brain.* Little, Brown & Co., Boston, 1954.)

and medially on the internal capsule, between the thalamus medially and the corpus striatum laterally (Fig. 2–3). The anterior limb and genu of the capsule contain efferent fibers from the frontal and temporal lobes (destined for the nuclei of the brainstem), and fibers of the thalamofrontal projection system. The capsule also contains a large number of autonomic fibers from the frontal, premotor, and motor cortex, which explains the frequent occurrence of sudomotor and vasomotor disturbances in limbs paralyzed by a capsular lesion. The projection of sensory fibers from the thalamus to the sensory cortex lies immediately behind the corticospinal fibers, and the optic radiation lies behind them. Consequently, a large capsular lesion will usually cause contralateral hemiplegia, hemianesthesia, and homonymous hemianopia.

The pyramidal tract[3] occupies the middle three-fifths of the cerebral peduncle on each side, but curiously enough, sectioning of the tract at this site in monkeys or in man does not give rise to complete or permanent hemiplegia, whereas capsular lesions do. In the pons, the tract splits into several bundles, which pass between the cellular masses of the pontine nuclei, in which the corticopontine fibers end. About three-quarters of the tract decussates in the lower part of the medulla and descends in the lateral column of the cord as the crossed corticospinal tract. Most of the fibers terminate on internuncial neurons, which in their turn connect with the dendrites of the anterior horn cells. A few corticospinal fibers end directly on motor neurons. Others, derived from the sensory cortex, terminate in the posterior horns, and may be concerned with the modulation of sensory input (Chap. 1).

The proportion of pyramidal fibers which do not cross varies from case to case. These take two routes: A small number from the lower portion of area 4 lie in the ventral part of the cervical and upper thoracic segments, and a large group runs in the lateral column of the cord to terminate on internuncial neurons, which link them with the ipsilat-

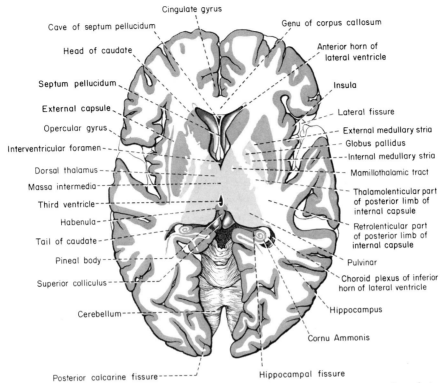

Figure 2–3. Diagram of a horizontal section through the human brain, illustrating the relationships of the internal capsule to the thalamus and globus pallidus. (From Crosby, E. C., Humphrey, T., and Lauer, E. W.: *Correlative Anatomy of the Nervous System.* Macmillan Co., New York, 1962.)

eral anterior horn cells. These uncrossed tracts serve the bilaterally acting muscles of the trunk and (perhaps) the limb girdle muscles, and their presence helps to explain the persistence of clumsy group movement in the proximal portions of the limbs after complete unilateral destruction of the motor cortex or internal capsule. It is probable that the reticulospinal tracts play a part in the preservation of these movements.[3, 7]

The clinical signs of interruption of the corticospinal tracts vary with the site and acuteness of the lesion. The earliest sign of *slowly developing* disease is slowness and lack of dexterity of fine movements of the hand and foot. *Acute* total sectioning of the tract gives rise to flaccid paralysis of the contralateral limbs and the lower half of the face; these signs may be accompanied by transient disturbances of bilateral acting mechanisms, so that there may be difficulty in turning the head and

the eyes to the opposite side, dysarthria, and weakness of the contralateral trunk muscles and diaphragm. These features soon pass off, leaving the classic signs of disease affecting the corticospinal tracts: The affected limbs are weak and become spastic, the tendon reflexes are exaggerated, knee and ankle clonus may be present, and the abdominal and cremasteric reflexes are absent on the affected side. The plantar responses are extensor if the fibers to the leg are involved.

Wasting is not conspicuous except as a result of prolonged disuse, though atrophy of the hand muscles is sometimes seen—for some obscure reason—in parietal lesions.[5] The increase of tone affects all muscles, but it is greater in the extensors than in the flexors of the leg, which is therefore extended at the hip, knee, and ankle. The arm is adducted, flexed at the elbows and wrist,

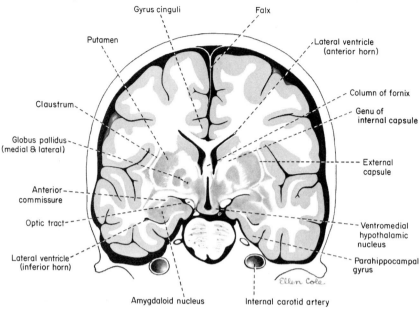

Figure 2–4. Coronal section of the skull and brain behind the chiasm. (Adapted from Delmas, A., and Pertuiset, B.: *Craniocerebral Topometry.* Charles C Thomas, Springfield, Ill., 1959.)

and the fingers are flexed. The degree of spasticity varies greatly from case to case, and is the "clasp-knife" variety, i.e., attempts to overcome it evoke an increase of tone, but the resistance suddenly gives way when greater force is used. In some cases, spasticity is a greater handicap than weakness; the explanation for this is by no means certain, but it appears likely that in such cases the impact of the disease has been on extrapyramidal fibers arising from the cortex, or on the reticulospinal system, rather than on the fibers derived from the giant cells of Betz. Occasionally, wounds limited to the motor strip of the cortex give rise to hemiplegia which remains flaccid throughout its course, although the tendon reflexes are exaggerated. This circumstance strengthens the view that the spasticity of the conventional hemiplegic results in some measure from an involvement of the nonpyramidal fibers which are so numerous in the corticospinal tract.

The Plantar Reflex. In health, a noxious stimulus to the sole of the foot causes plantar flexion of the foot, adduction and flexion of the toes, and short-

ening of the quadriceps. Babinski pointed out that with damage to the pyramidal tract or to the cells from which it springs, the response changes: The foot and the big toes retract, the toes abduct, and the hip and the knee flex. This reflex occurs in normal infants up to the age of about 18 months, and it may be mimicked in normal adults with ticklish feet, but in this case the toes seldom abduct, and the dorsiflexion of the foot and toes is abrupt, lacking the slow and deliberate motion of a true extensor response. The reflex is abolished by interruption of the afferent path from the sole of the foot to the spinal cord, and by lower motor neuron paralysis of the limb. The field from which the reflex can be elicited varies from case to case. In complete transection of the cord, it can sometimes be obtained by stimuli applied to the foot, leg, thigh, and lower abdomen. It is best applied to the lateral border of the sole.

If plantar stimulation is impracticable for any reason, the reflex may be obtained, albeit with greater difficulty, by noxious stimuli applied elsewhere, e.g., by squeezing the tibia between the finger and thumb with a stroking movement toward the ankle (Oppenheim), by squeezing the calf muscles (Gordon), or by pricking the dorsum of the foot with a pin (Bing). Hyperactivity of the stretch reflexes can be demonstrated by a host of tests. Though these tests are part of the tradition of classical neurology, few of them are used today. Hoffmann's sign is an exception in that it provides a method of demonstrating hyperreflexia in the hand. The distal phalanx of the middle finger is fully flexed by the examiner and is then released abruptly. As it springs back to the extended position, the thumb and index finger flex and adduct. In Rossolimo's hand sign, flexion of the fingers follows percussion of the volar aspect of the fingertips; this occurs in some normal individuals and is significant only when there is a gross disparity between the responses of the two hands.

Lower Motor Neuron Paralysis. Destruction of the anterior horn cells or of their axons causes flaccid paralysis of individual muscles, with loss of the deep tendon reflexes, atrophy, fasciculation, and changes in electrical excitability. Weakness and paralysis of lower motor neuron origin also differs from that of corticospinal tract origin in that the weakness affects muscles or portions of a muscle rather than group movements. Although absence of a tendon reflex usually indicates the presence of a lower motor neuron lesion, it should be noted that injury to a joint such as the knee or the ankle can permanently abolish the reflex at that site. Another practical point deserving of notice is the fact that a tendon reflex which has been suppressed as a result of an incomplete lower motor neuron lesion can return if the limb in question is affected at a later date by an upper motor neuron lesion.

Denervated muscles waste rapidly and develop characteristic histological changes, which differ in important respects from the pathological effects of disuse on the one hand and of diseases of muscle on the other.

Electrodiagnostic Aids

STUDIES OF EXCITABILITY. Electrodiagnostic aids include electromyography and studies of neural and muscular excitability. After severance of a nerve, the distal portion remains excitable until the axis cylinders begin to break up, in from two to three days, but the region of the motor end-plate retains its excitability for an additional five to 10 days, after which its excitability changes abruptly to approximately that of muscle. A faradic current now fails to excite the muscle, while the galvanic current still produces a contraction. This is the reaction of degeneration, which can be measured in terms of chronaxie, but for practical purposes, the absence of response to the faradic current remains a useful test.

ELECTROMYOGRAPHY. The more refined technique of electromyography can yield more information (and more artefacts) than earlier methods. It records the brief action potential of muscle fibers. It will be recalled that a single spinal motor neuron supplies anything from a dozen to hundreds of muscle fibers, which lie in separate fascicles. These are not necessarily contiguous to each other, so that the muscle fibers supplied by a single anterior horn cell may be scattered over a considerable area. The motor fiber, together with the muscle fibers it supplies, is called a motor unit. When the electromyogram needle is inserted into a normal muscle, it often produces a burst of large potentials, which range in duration from 1 to 25 milliseconds and have an amplitude of a few millivolts. Normal insertional activity may last for as much as a second. Once the needle is in place, the resting muscle is silent if the patient is truly relaxed. Voluntary contraction produces repetitive action potentials of a fixed pattern: The discharge rate builds up rapidly to a maximum of 50 to 80 per second, and eventually the discharge of individual units is lost in the asynchronous activity of full contraction. Normal motor unit potentials vary in amplitude from a few microvolts to 3 millivolts, and their duration ranges from 2 to 10 milliseconds. The configuration of the patterns varies considerably, depending on the site of the tip of the needle. Fibrillation represents repetitive activity in single muscle fibers and appears as very brief spikes of low amplitude; it is found in partly or wholly denervated muscles, but it may be impossible to demonstrate fibrillation in the early stages of degeneration and in muscles that have undergone fibrosis. If denervation is incomplete, motor unit potentials are present, and since the muscle is hyperirritable to mechanical stimuli, insertional activity is increased.

Estimation of motor conduction times can be of value. In adults, the ulnar, median, and peroneal nerves have conduction times which vary from 42 to 74 meters/sec., but in children under the age of five or six years, the rates are often considerably slower. The conduction time is slowed in polyneuropathy; in diabetics, low conduction times may precede the clinical evidence of neuropathy. Another application of the technique serves to enable the clinician to identify the site of a nerve lesion—e.g., to decide whether the lesion responsible for weakness of the ulnar intrinsic muscles in the hand is at the wrist or at the elbow; a normal conduction time between elbow and wrist points to a distal lesion.

Electromyography helps to distinguish between weakness resulting from muscle disease, peripheral nerve lesions, and anterior horn cell lesions. It should be emphasized, however, that valuable as it is in special cases, electromyography is usually less useful than a careful history and a meticulous physical examination.

Disorders of Neuromuscular Transmission

The Myoneural Junction. The only diseases in which weakness or paralysis comes on as the result of a disorder of neuromuscular transmission are myasthenia gravis and botulism. In myasthenia, the power of the affected muscles declines progressively during exertion, but can be restored by an injection of neostigmine or Tensilon. In botulism, the exotoxin secreted by the organism blocks neuromuscular transmission at the motor end-plates; botulism is easily identified because it usually occurs in a group of people who have partaken of the same food, and there are severe gastrointestinal symptoms prior to the occurrence of cranial nerve palsies and weakness of the trunk and limbs.

Weakness Due to Disorders of the Muscles

Episodic weakness of muscular origin occurs in familial periodic paralysis, adynamia episodica hereditaria, paroxysmal myoglobinuria, McArdle's disease (Chap. 19), and hypo- and hyperkalemia (Chap. 21).

Persistent muscular weakness is seen in the heredofamilial muscular dystrophies, various forms of myositis, and a number of noninfective myopathies (Chap. 19). Although most of the individual conditions in this group are rare, together they account for a considerable number of cases, and can cause much difficulty in diagnosis. The episodic disorders referred to above are easily identified, and the same applies to muscular weakness supervening in a member of a family known to suffer from heredofamilial dystrophy, but difficulty arises when the patient in question happens to be the first member of the family to be affected by muscular dystrophy and in the many cases of myopathy in which the early symptoms are vague and the physical signs elusive. Such patients are apt to be dubbed "psychoneurotic," or their symptoms are attributed to "rheumatism" or fatigue. For this reason, it is useful to remember the existence of this group of disorders when confronted with a patient complaining of muscular weakness in the absence of objective signs of neurological disease. Diseases of muscle are described in Chapter 19.

Disturbances of Tone

All muscular activity, whether reflex, automatic, or purposive, depends for its efficiency upon the existence of a background of tone, by which is meant the resistance of muscle to passive elongation or stretch. Reflex tone depends mainly on afferent impulses coming from sensory receptors in muscle, notably the muscle spindles; it is lost if the reflex arc is cut, but it is increased in lesions of suprasegmental structures which involve the corticospinal, reticulospinal, or extrapyramidal systems, and it is reduced in some cerebellar lesions. In normal man, tone is influenced by emotional factors, and is subject to modification as the result of labyrinthine, visual, auditory, and cutaneous stimuli.[7,17]

Ever since the role of the stretch reflexes in posture was first delineated by Sherrington in 1893, there has been an increasing volume of research in this field, and it received an additional impetus from the fortuitous discovery by Cooper that a destructive lesion of the pallidus could obliterate parkinsonian tremor and rigidity on the side opposite the lesion, and by the demonstration by Magoun and Rhines [17] in 1946 that stimulation of the reticular formation lying ventromedially in the caudal part of the bulb could inhibit the knee jerk, decerebrate rigidity, and movements resulting from stimulation of the motor area of the cerebral cortex. At present, there is no agreement as to the mechanisms involved in the production of extrapyramidal rigidity, and no good purpose would be served by attempting to summarize the abundant but often conflicting evidence bearing on this problem.[7,16,19]

Affections of the Upper Motor Neuron. The increase of tone which occurs as a result of lesions in the upper motor neuron is conventionally called spasticity, to distinguish it from the rigidity of striatal disease. In the leg, spasticity is greatest in the extensors, while in the arm, the flexors are most affected. If a muscle is stretched, a reflex contraction is evoked with undue ease, and the resistance to stretching increases; but, if further pressure is exerted, the resistance suddenly gives way, whence the term "clasp-knife spasticity." It is associ-

ated with increased tendon reflexes, loss of the abdominal and cremasteric reflexes, and an extensor plantar response on the affected side if the corticospinal pathway to the leg is affected.

Affections of the Extrapyramidal System. Although there are good physiological reasons for including the cerebellum and its connections in the extrapyramidal system, clinicians commonly use this term to refer to the corpus striatum, the subthalamic nucleus, the substantia nigra, and the red nucleus, together with their interconnecting tracts and their projection systems to the reticular formation, thalamus, and cerebral cortex.

Extrapyramidal rigidity is most commonly seen in paralysis agitans. It is unaccompanied by paralysis, affects extensors and flexors equally, is present throughout the whole range of any passive movement, and involves the trunk as well as the limbs *if the lesions are bilateral.* The stretch reflexes are not exaggerated, and the plantar responses remain flexor. When a muscle is passively stretched, the rigidity gives way in a series of little jerks (cogwheel rigidity); this is not always present, and when it is absent, the rigidity is described as plastic. Extrapyramidal rigidity is often, but not invariably, accompanied by a parkinsonian tremor. Paralysis agitans is the most common cause of striatal rigidity, but it is often seen in phenothiazine intoxication and also occurs in arteriosclerotic cerebral degeneration, Wilson's disease, chronic manganese poisoning, some cases of Huntington's chorea, the juvenile form of cerebromacular degeneration, juvenile paralysis agitans of Hunt, and occasionally as a result of tumors and vascular accidents involving the corpus striatum.

Many patients with parkinsonism exhibit akinesia, a peculiar stillness which is not necessarily associated with, or due to, rigidity. They fidget little and blink infrequently. Paradoxically, this stillness may be associated with a desire to move or to be moved.

A different and more dramatic form of

akinesia is seen in the syndrome known as *akinetic mutism.* The patient appears to be conscious but is speechless and lies in bed, without movement, staring into space with little or no response to noise or other stimuli. The tendon reflexes are within normal limits, and the plantar responses are flexor. This condition, originally described by Cairns in a patient with a benign cyst of the third ventricle, has also been seen in the course of encephalitis lethargica, in anterior communicating aneurysms, and following bilateral destruction of the cingulate gyri. In experimental animals, an analogous condition has been produced by placing a lesion in the periaqueductal gray matter and in the caudal hypothalamus and tegmentum of the midbrain. Akinetic mutism must be differentiated from the *"locked-in syndrome,"* a term coined by Plum and Posner to describe the condition of patients with bilateral infarction of the basis pontis. In these cases, the patient is quadriplegic and mute but remains alert and can communicate by vertical eye movement which, with elevation of the lids, are the only voluntary movements that are preserved. In these cases, the patient is conscious, and—in contradistinction to the situation in akinetic mutism—the limbs are paralyzed and display the usual signs of bilateral interruption of the corticospinal tracts.

Hypotonia. Affections of the lower motor neuron invariably cause hypotonia of the affected muscles, since the final common pathway of the reflex arc is cut. This contributes to the hypotonia of severe polyneuropathy, subacute combined degeneration of the cord associated with peripheral neuropathy, and some cases of amyotonia congenita. In tabes dorsalis, hypotonia results from disease of the posterior (sensory) roots. Hypotonia is also seen in Friedreich's ataxia, in which there is degeneration of the spinocerebellar tracts and posterior columns, and in disease of the cerebellum. Destruction of one labyrinth, or of the vestibular component of the eighth nerve, also causes transient ipsilateral hypotonia.

Decerebrate Rigidity. Decerebrate rigidity corresponds to the decerebrate posture produced in animals by a transverse lesion between the superior colliculi and the vestibular nuclei. It can occur in man as a result of lesions in the upper part of the brainstem. The patient lies in rigid extension. The upper limbs are internally rotated at the shoulder, extended at the elbow, and pronated, with the fingers extended at the metacarpophalangeal joints and flexed at the interphalangeal joints. The lower limbs are extended at the hip and knee, and the ankles and toes are flexed. As Sherrington showed long ago, decerebrate rigidity results not from damage to the corticospinal tracts, but from interruption of descending systems from the cortex, the basal ganglion, and the cerebellum, which converge on the reticular formation of the lower brainstem. The removal of predominantly inhibitory effects from above releases the reticulospinal tracts, and this in turn greatly heightens the activity of the stretch reflexes of extensor muscles.

The localizing significance of decerebrate rigidity is discussed in Chapter 16.

The Stiff Man Syndrome. This rare condition of adult life is characterized by recurrent episodes of severe rigidity and tonic muscular spasms.[15, 21] Despite the name, it can occur in both sexes. Both rigidity and spasm involve the proximal and trunk muscles more than the periphery. Trismus does not occur. The rigidity may be boardlike, so that in standing the patient is unable to stoop or bend. The tonic spasms may be either mild and brief, or they may be severe and continue intermittently for days. They may be precipitated by loud noises and fright. Sudden movements induced by the spasm may cause fractures.

Apart from the severe rigidity during the attacks, neurological findings are normal. Electromyographic studies fail to demonstrate any consistent pattern other than that of prolonged contraction of muscles. It has been suggested that the motor discharges are due to some process which interferes with the inhibiting mechanism of the anterior horn cells, which was first described by Renshaw.

An abnormal glucose tolerance curve has been found in some cases, and there is sometimes a reducing substance in the urine.

The condition is easily mistaken for a manifestation of hysteria, and a first attack, with no previous history of similar attacks, may suggest tetanus. The fact that Diazepam in oral doses of 10 to 15 mg. four times a day can control the symptoms suggests that they are of spinal origin. The drug can also be given intravenously or intramuscularly in doses of 5 to 10 mg.

Ataxia

The term *ataxia* is applied to incoordination occurring in the absence of apraxia, paresis, rigidity, spasticity, or involuntary movements. It commonly arises in diseases of the cerebellar system, but it may also occur as a result of proprioceptive sensory loss — sensory ataxia — and episodically in the course of acute labyrinthine vertigo.

Cerebellar Ataxia. The movements mediated by the corticospinal system depend for their efficiency on a background of postural contraction or tone, which changes with and during each act. Experimental work on animals has established that the anterior lobe of the cerebellum can either augment or inhibit tone, but although this is perhaps true for healthy man, cerebellar disease always produces hypotonia, provided the brainstem is not involved. It has been argued that all the features of cerebellar ataxia can be traced to hypotonia, but this is too extreme a view, because experimental and clinical studies show that suitably placed lesions of the cerebellum can disturb the direction and reduce the rate of movement without alteration of tone.

There is some degree of localization of function in the cerebellum.[4] This is well developed in animals, and in man it is implied by remarkable case-to-case differences in the distribution of ataxia. It can be severe in the legs and slight in the arms, or it may be limited to the upper limbs; nystagmus may be present or absent in cases with severe ataxia of the limbs, and the same is true of dysarthria.

Each cerebellar hemisphere receives afferents from (1) the opposite frontal and temporal lobes via frontopontine and temporopontine tracts, which lie in the anterior limb of the internal capsule and are relayed onward via the pontine nuclei; (2) the spinocerebellar tracts and posterior columns, which convey proprioception from the ipsilateral limbs and trunk; (3) the vestibular nuclei; (4) the opposite olivary nucleus; (5) the opposite cerebellar hemisphere. Efferent pathways from each cerebellar hemisphere pass to (1) the opposite red nucleus; (2) the opposite thalamus, and thence to the frontal, motor, and temporal cortex; (3) the reticular formation; (4) the homolateral nucleus of Deiters; (5) the opposite olive; (6) pontine nuclei on both sides; and (7) the third, fourth, and sixth cranial nuclei.[3]

These arrangements endow each cerebellar hemisphere with the power to influence tone and coordination on its own side of the body, and they explain why ataxia can occur with lesions of the afferent and efferent cerebellar connections as well as in affections of the cerebellum itself. Thus, disease of the thalamus and frontal lobe can cause moderate ataxia of the contralateral limbs (this is often obscured by weakness or sensory loss), and disease of the spinocerebellar tracts and posterior columns is responsible for much of the "cerebellar" incoordination of Friedreich's ataxia.

Clinical Features. Cerebellar ataxia[8] appears in the eyes as nystagmus, in speech as one form of dysarthria, and in the limbs as a specific type of incoordination. It is best seen in acute cerebellar lesions because of the considerable capacity for adaptation and adjustment manifested by the corticospinal system in cases of chronic cerebellar disease. With an *acute* unilateral lesion, there is marked unilateral hypotonia, which allows the limbs on the affected side to be thrown about and placed in unnatural positions. The imbalance between the two sides of the body leads to the adoption of a cerebellar posture. The head is tilted slightly to the affected side and rotated so that the chin points slightly away from it; the shoulder is advanced, and the trunk is concave to the affected side. On attempting to stand, the patient falls to the side of the lesion, and when recumbent, he tends to keep the cheek corresponding to the side of the lesion pressed into the pillow. The eyes may be deviated to the opposite side. Speech is slurred. There is no actual paralysis of the limbs, but the muscles fatigue readily, and movement is further embarrassed by hypotonia and asynergia.

HYPOTONIA. Hypotonia imparts a flabbiness to the muscles on the affected sde. If the arm is held out, it tends to droop and may rotate on its long axis in such a way that the palm faces downward and outward, while the wrist flexes and the fingers hyperextend at the metacarpophalangeal joints. The arm tends to sway when passively displaced. Hypotonia interferes with the delicate balance between agonists and antagonists which is necessary for the smooth execution of movement, so that the limb oscillates during purposive movement; while attempting to touch the nose with the forefinger, for example, the hand approaches its objective in jerky fashion and the oscillations become increasingly marked as the end-point is reached. This intention tremor or action tremor is the result of incoordination plus voluntary attempts at correction. Unlike the irregular movements encountered in sensory ataxia, it is not much aggravated by closing the eyes. A further effect of hypotonia is inability to control the force required to touch an object—the hand either overshoots or falls short (dysmetria). In the legs, dysmetria gives rise to an erratic gait, in which the feet meet the floor with a force which varies from step to step.

ASYNERGIA. The term *asynergia* (or *dyssynergia*) signifies failure of the cooperation between prime movers and other muscle groups which is necessary for the effective execution of movement. For instance, the efficiency of the long flexors of the fingers in grasping an object is increased by extension of the wrist; in cerebellar ataxia, the wrist on the affected side will either flex or fail to extend, thus impairing the strength of the grip. Again, rapid pronation-supination of the forearm requires fixation of the shoulder and elbow, and failure of this synergic action in cerebellar cases leads to clumsy, slow, imperfectly coordinated movements of the whole limb, a sign dignified by the term *dysdiadochokinesia*. When the head is thrown back, vestibular volleys to the cerebellum and brainstem lead to flexion of the knees and forward flexion of the pelvis, thus maintaining the center of gravity in the correct position; failure of this synergistic response of distant groups is responsible for some of the falls which occur in cerebellar disease.

DECOMPOSITION OF MOVEMENT. Voluntary attempts to correct the disturbances of movements caused by a cerebellar lesion are responsible for some of the features of the ataxia. This has already been referred to as a factor in intention tremor, and it is also seen in the phenomenon described as decomposition of movement. The patient attempts to circumvent his difficulties by breaking up complicated movements into single components, which are easier to perform. For instance, when the recumbent patient is asked to place the heel of the ataxic leg on the opposite knee, he learns to break down this movement into its constituent parts and does each separately: The thigh is flexed, the heel is lifted off the bed, the leg is adducted, and the heel is allowed to fall on the knee. Similarly, slurring of speech is decreased by breaking up words into syllables and enunciating each separately, thus giving rise to scanning speech—a feature of long-standing severe cerebellar dysarthria, and therefore especially common in multiple sclerosis.

NYSTAGMUS. The quick movement of cerebellar nystagmus is subcortical in origin; in acute lesions, the eyes deviate conjugately to a rest point from 10 to 20 degrees to the opposite side. On looking to the affected side, there is a coarse oscillation of wide amplitude, consisting of a quick movement away from, and a slow return to, the rest point. On looking away from the side of the lesion, the nystagmus is quicker, but the quick component is still away from the rest point. In *chronic* cases, there is no deviation of the eyes, but the characteristics of the nystagmus are the same: The eye tends to deviate away from what the patient is looking at, and reflex correction brings it back to its objective. It is necessary to emphasize that nystagmus may be absent in cerebellar disease and that, conversely, it may be present with lesions in the upper cervical cord, the brainstem, or the cerebral hemispheres.

GAIT. Cerebellar gait is caused by a mixture of hypotonia, asynergia, dysmetria, and cortical correction. The patient tends to deviate to the affected side, and if the arm is affected, it will not swing with a natural rhythm. The base is wide and the feet may be put down with irregular force. Voluntary attempts to overcome lateral deviation lead to a zig-zag course. The patient may find it impossible to stand still with the feet together, but unsteadiness is not as profoundly increased by shutting the eyes as is the case in sensory ataxia. Inability to stand on one leg or to walk in tandem fashion is an early sign of cerebellar ataxia.

Lesions of the flocculonodular lobe impair the equilibrium of the body when standing or, less commonly, when sitting.[8] If the lesion is limited to this area, there is no nystagmus or dysarthria, and there is no incoordination of the limbs when the patient is lying in bed. When the patient sits up unsupported, swaying movements of the trunk may occur, especially if the eyes are closed. The patient has difficulty in standing and walking because of the lack of balance. Unless the examiner is aware that this type of dysequilibrium can occur in the absence of the other features of cerebellar ataxia, he may conclude that the disorder of gait is hysterical in origin; indeed, at one time, the term *astasia abasia* was applied to dysequilibrium of functional origin. If this term is to be used at all, it should refer to inability to stand or walk, without implying either organic or psychological causation.

Sensory Ataxia

Both the motor cortex and the cerebellum depend for their efficiency on a continuous stream of sensory information as to the position of the head and limbs in space, the attitude of joints, and the evolution of movements. The sensory inflow to the cerebellum comes via the posterior columns and the spinocerebellar tracts and does not reach consciousness, so that in some cases of Friedreich's ataxia, for instance, there may be considerable ataxia from involvement of the spinocerebellar tracts, despite the integrity of conscious proprioception— but this is not what is meant by sensory ataxia.

In the presence of sensory loss, the motor cortex loses contact with the periphery, and ataxia occurs. The range, power, and direction of movement is ill-judged, and incoordination is much aggravated if the eyes are shut or if the patient is in the dark. Thus, he may be able to stand still with the feet together and the eyes open, but he will sway if the eyes are closed (rombergism). The gait is broad-based and clumsy. When the upper limbs are held out, with the eyes shut, they fall away from this position, and the fingers may execute slow pianoplaying movements of which the patient is unaware.

Sensory ataxia can occur in disease of the peripheral nerves, such as polyneuritis, but coincident weakness usually complicates the picture. A comparatively pure form occurs in tabes dorsalis, in which there is degeneration of the sensory roots and posterior columns; in rare cases, there is little or no loss of the conscious sense of position or passive movement, but incoordination occurs because of degeneration of the spinocerebellar tracts. Severe sensory ataxia in one limb is occasionally seen as the result of a lesion of the root entry zone of the spinal cord, such as a plaque of multiple sclerosis or a tumor. Ataxia of the legs is a feature of subacute combined degeneration of the cord, but here again it is often complicated by weakness from peripheral neuritis and degeneration of the corticospinal tracts.

A special example of sensory ataxia is seen in Bell's palsy; muscle sense, as well as power, is impaired, with the result that during the period of recovery, voluntary movements of the face can be facilitated by using a mirror, in this way providing visual aid to a motor cortex which is bereft of sensory guidance as to what the facial muscles are doing.

Ataxia in Lesions of the Cerebral Hemispheres

Incoordination can occur in the arm and leg as a result of disease of the contralateral thalamus. This usually results from sensory impairment, but sometimes the ataxia is out of proportion to the sensory loss, and in such cases it may be due to interruption of the pathway which links one cerebellar hemisphere with the opposite motor cortex.

The question whether lesions of the frontal lobe can give rise to contralateral ataxia has been debated for a long time. The history of this controversy is well set forth by Dow and Moruzzi.[8] The subject is summarized on page 410.

Labyrinthine Ataxia

Equilibrium is disturbed by thermal or rotational stimulation of the labyrinth and by acute disease of the internal ear.

An acute irritative lesion of the labyrinth gives rise to intense vertigo, vomiting, nystagmus, and past-pointing. On attempting to touch an object, the finger deviates to the affected side. On trying to stand with the eyes shut, the patient deviates to the affected side, and his attempts to avoid this produce a staggering gait. Nystagmus is present and differs from the cerebellar form in that the slow phase is toward the side of the lesion and the quick movement is in the opposite direction.

Labyrinthine ataxia is seen in acute labyrinthitis, hemorrhage into the internal ear, acute lesions of the vestibular nuclei (as in transient ischemic attacks), and during the attacks of vertigo caused by Meniere's disease. Similar ataxia occurs in the episodes of vertigo caused by *chronic* disease of the internal ear and eighth nerve. There is no ataxia between the attacks except in the case of large cerebellopontine angle tumors which compress the cerebellum.

INVOLUNTARY MOVEMENTS

Involuntary movements fall into seven classes: tremors, athetosis, choreiform movements, clonic spasms, tonic spasms, fasciculation, and the tics or habit spasms.

Tremors

Tremor is seen in many diseases, neurological and otherwise. It is produced by fast, rhythmic, alternating contractions of agonists and antagonists. It occurs as a physiological response to fatigue and anxiety, and is a familiar feature of thyrotoxicosis, hypoglycemia, convalescence from exhausting illness, and exogenous intoxicants, such as alcohol, heavy metals, barbiturates, and the hydantoinates. Cocaine and morphine addicts, like alcoholics, develop a tremor when the drug is withheld.

Of greater neurological interest are the tremors which develop in the course of disease of the frontal lobe, corpus striatum, red nucleus, and cerebellum. Frontal lesions are occasionally accompanied by a tremor of the contralateral hand, which is aggravated by using the limb and can be mistaken for a cerebellar tremor. In general paresis, there is often an irregular "frontal" tremor of the outstretched hands, the lips, and the tongue. In some cases, the movement of the tongue consists of vigorous alternating retraction and protrusion—the trombone tongue.

PARKINSONIAN TREMOR. This is marked by a coarse, rhythmic oscillation, with a frequency of 3 to 6 oscillations per second and is usually best seen during the maintenance of a fixed posture. It is temporarily inhibited by voluntary movement, but returns with the assumption of a new posture. Sometimes this tremor is accompanied by an action tremor. It is aggravated by excitement and abolished by sleep. The movements may involve the head, jaw, arm, or leg. In the upper limbs, they consist of alternating flexion-extension of the fingers, adduction-abduction of the thumb or other fingers, flexion-extension of the wrist, and pronation-supination of the forearm; these can occur alone or in combination. Parkinsonian tremor is best seen in paralysis agitans, but also occurs following encephalitis lethargica, and in hepatolenticular degeneration, vascular accidents and neoplasms involving the corpus striatum, chronic manganese poisoning, and chronic arteriosclerotic cerebral degeneration. Exceptionally, parkinsonian tremor is seen following severe head injuries and carbon monoxide poisoning.

CEREBELLAR TREMOR. A coarse, irregular oscillation of the limb during voluntary movement occurs in many diseases of the cerebellum and its peduncles. It is present in the limbs on the side of the lesion, and is brought out by voluntary movement, such as the finger-nose and heel-knee tests; oscillation becomes progressively intensified as the finger or heel approaches its goal. This "intention tremor" is not an invariable feature of cerebellar disease. It is a familiar feature of multiple sclerosis and occurs in other acute and chronic lesions of the cerebellum, in-

cluding alcoholic cerebellar degeneration and some cases of heredofamilial ataxia.

HEREDOFAMILIAL TREMOR. This is a common affection, which usually involves the upper limb but may also affect the head. The tremor is precipitated by using the hand, but it is unassociated with other signs of cerebellar disease. It may start in childhood, middle age, or advanced life. The tremor is not only a source of considerable embarrassment, but it can also interfere with the performance of fine movements. Like most other involuntary movements, it is aggravated by nervousness and is improved, temporarily, by alcohol. It can be treated, if severe, by stereotaxic thalamotomy.

OTHER TYPES OF TREMOR. A slow, coarse tremor is sometimes seen in the acute phase of encephalomyelitis following the specific fevers of childhood, vaccination, and inoculation against rabies. A lesion of the red nucleus can give rise to a third nerve palsy on the side of the lesion and a coarse intention tremor of the contralateral hand (Benedikt's syndrome); the tremor is explained by the fact that the lesion interrupts the cerebellar fibers running to the red nucleus through the brachium conjunctivum.

Athetosis

Athetosis is well described as mobile spasm. The movements consist of slow, sinuous, writhing contortions, which are usually seen in the upper limbs and less often in the face and legs. The spasm invades opposing muscle groups alternately. The fingers are hyperextended and either abducted or adducted; the wrist flexes slowly or extends; the forearm pronates or supinates, and the arm is adducted to the chest or retracted. If the face is involved, it undergoes a series of grimaces, which may interfere with speech. The toes are extended and the feet plantar-flexed and extended; rarely, the knees are drawn up and adducted. The movements occur intermittently and are much aggravated by excitement. They cease during sleep.

Severe athetosis interferes with speech and swallowing and with ordinary manual tasks, and it is often complicated by concurrent pyramidal and extrapyramidal rigidity. It is almost entirely confined to congenital, neonatal, and infantile affections of the extrapyramidal system, e.g., congenital diplegia, infantile hemiplegia, and kernicterus, but occasionally it occurs as the result of vascular or neoplastic affections of the basal ganglia in adults, or as a feature of chronic hepatic encephalopathy. Athetoid movements can also be induced by phenothiazine drugs (p. 581).

In torsion spasm (dystonia musculorum deformans), the movements have the same writhing quality as those of athetosis, but the muscles of the neck and trunk and the proximal segments of the limbs are chiefly affected, the hands and face being either spared or but slightly involved. It can occur as a symptom of hepatolenticular degeneration and encephalitis lethargica, and as a familial disorder sui generis. It is discussed in Chapter 12.

Choreiform Movements

Choreiform movements are quick, jerky, and irregular, involving the muscles in a nonsequential and disorderly manner, without reference to segmental or cortical patterns of movement. Swift grimaces, flickering twitches of the limbs, brief contractions of the abdominal or respiratory muscles, sudden movements of the head, tongue, and pharynx — such are the elements which make up the picture of chorea. They interfere with voluntary movement, which becomes inaccurate, jerky, and exaggerated. Manual tasks, speech, deglutition, and gait are affected. In mild or early cases, the diagnosis depends on the detection of slight occasional clumsiness of the hands, grimacing, apparently causeless falls, and general restlessness.

Choreiform movements occur as the result of lesions of the corpus striatum, substantia nigra, and subthalamic nucleus. The movements are seen in (1) congenital chorea, (2) Sydenham's chorea, (3) Huntington's chorea, (4) epidemic encephalitis, and (5) senile chorea. The first four of these diseases are described elsewhere in this book.

SENILE CHOREA. This is a disease of the seventh and later decades, characterized by mild choreiform twitches of the legs, less often of the upper limbs, which are unassociated with other signs of disease.

HEMIBALLISMUS. The name is given to a particularly violent type of choreiform movement, often limited to one side of the body or to one limb, which usually occurs as the result of a vascular accident but does not necessarily result from a lesion of the subthalamic nucleus (of Luys), as is commonly stated.[24] The movements are of large amplitude and great violence; the limb thrashes about until it is captured and held. In one case, the patient had to give up playing cards and visiting the hospital movies because of the violence of the movements when he was excited.

CHOREOATHETOSIS. Chorea is sometimes associated with athetosis; if the movements are more rapid than those of athetosis and slower than those of chorea, they are referred to as "choreoathetosis." This is usually seen in congenital and neonatal affections, and may also occur in hepatic disease and intoxication by tranquilizers and L-dopa.

Exaggerated Startle Reactions

A startle or surprise reaction following an unexpected stimulus is an everyday experience, but it can be somewhat excessive in neurotic persons. It is also seen as a pathological phenomenon in some children with cerebal palsy and in Tay-Sachs disease. In addition, there are two conditions in which the startle reaction is sufficiently severe and frequent to bring the patient to the doctor.[10] The first is a hereditary syndrome transmitted by a dominant autosomal gene. There is hypertonia and hypokinesia at birth, and the cerebral bulbar reflexes are very brisk. The infants exhibit exaggerated startle reactions. Violent jerks may also occur as the patient drifts into sleep. The EEG is normal, and the condition does not respond to the drugs which are effective in epilepsy. Suhren and his associates named this condition *familial hyperexplexia*. A somewhat similar condition, which Gastaut and Villeneuve called *essential hyperexplexia*,[10] can occur sporadically. Violent "jumps" occur in response to sudden noise or other stimuli which surprise the patient. The head and upper limbs are always involved. The eyes close, the head bends forward towards the chest, the shoulders are elevated, and there is a symmetrical flexion of the arms and clenching of the fists. There is no impairment of consciousness, but the tongue may be bitten if it is outside the mouth at the time of the "jump." Sometimes the movement also involves the lower limbs, causing repeated falls. The resting electroencephalogram is normal, but during a "jump," there is a vertex spike followed by general desynchronization of the cortical rhythms. These EEG features help to distinguish hyperexplexia from myoclonic epilepsy.

Restless Legs
(Ekbom's Syndrome)

This is a disorder of adult life which can affect both sexes. The patient complains of unpleasant feelings in the legs which impel him to move them about. It usually comes on during the night, disrupting sleep, but in some cases it also plagues the patient even when sitting down. There are vague complaints of irritating sensations in the legs, which tend to be relieved by walking about. Sometimes the legs kick out spontaneously. There are no signs of organic disease in the blood vessels, nervous system, peripheral nerves, or muscles.[13] Even heavy sedation may fail to improve

matters, but some patients appear to benefit from Diazepam in doses of 10 mg. three times a day.

Tonic Spasm

Tonic spasm is the clinical term for physiological tetanus—a sustained contraction of a muscle or group of muscles. It occurs in the tonic phase of an epileptic seizure and in decerebrate rigidity, the flexor and extensor spasms of spastic paraplegia, oculogyric crises, phenothiazine intoxication, tetanus, tetany, strychnine poisoning, and the preparalytic phase of rabies.

Myoclonus

Myoclonus occurs in a wide variety of diseases.[27, 28] It consists of shock-like contractions of a portion of a muscle, an entire muscle, or a group of muscles. It may be restricted to one region of the body or may appear synchronously or asynchronously in several areas. Hiccup is a familiar and almost physiological example of localized myoclonus (i.e., of the diaphragm). Each myoclonic jerk is exceedingly brief, and appears to be caused by a brief discharge of a small group of motor cells; experimental and clinical evidence[27] indicates that such discharges can arise at the level of the anterior horn cells of the spinal cord (e.g., spinal tumor or myelitis), in the brainstem (e.g., palatal myoclonus, encephalitis, etc.), and in subcortical structures of the cerebral hemisphere (myoclonic petit mal, Unverricht's myoclonic epilepsy, metachromatic leukodystrophy, etc.).

Etiology. Myoclonus[1, 11, 18, 25, 27, 28] is found in certain infections, degenerative diseases, the lipidoses, and intoxications of the nervous system. It also occurs in some types of epilepsy. The infections include many forms of acute encephalitis and encephalomyelitis. Myoclonus was a common symptom of epidemic encephalitis lethargica, and is prominent in subacute sclerosing encephalitis. It has been seen in polioencephalitis, Jakob-Creutzfeldt disease, and cat-scratch disease. The intoxications in which myoclonus can occur include uremia, hepatic failure, anoxic encephalopathy, hypoglycemia, and phenothiazine intoxication. Myoclonus triggered by voluntary use of a limb may be a disabling sequel of acute cerebral anoxia, as in survivors of cardiac standstill. It is usually accompanied by some degree of cerebellar ataxia. The myoclonus can be controlled by Diazepam in doses of 10 mg. four times a day. Degenerative diseases in which it may occur include metachromatic leukodystrophy, Schilder's disease, juvenile cerebromacular degeneration, hepatolenticular degeneration, and Unverricht's myoclonic epilepsy. In epilepsy, myoclonic jerks occur in myoclonic petit mal and in some patients suffering from grand mal; paramyoclonus multiplex is described below. Myoclonic jerks occasionally occur in otherwise normal persons when they are drifting off to sleep.[28]

Hiccup usually occurs as the result of gastric or abdominal distention, but it is also seen in uremia and encephalitis. Facial hemispasm, described in Chapter 6, takes the form of repeated synchronous unilateral twitches of the muscles supplied by the facial nerve.

PALATAL MYOCLONUS. Sometimes called palatal nystagmus, palatal myoclonus [12, 14] is set apart from other forms of myoclonus by the fact that the jerks are rhythmic and persistent; they continue during sleep and even in coma. It is characterized by a rapid, rhythmic, up-and-down movement of one side of the palate, sometimes accompanied by ipsilateral synchronous clonic movements of the face, tongue, pharynx, and diaphragm. Palatal myoclonus is usually caused by disease of the olive and its connections. The commonest cause is basilar artery disease, but it has also been described in multiple sclerosis, severe head injury, tumor, angioma of the brainstem, progressive bulbar palsy, encephalitis, and syringobulbia.

Understandably, with this pathologi-

cal background, palatal nystagmus is usually associated with other neurological symptoms. Occasionally the patient complains of a rhythmic clicking sound in the ear, caused by the myoclonic contractions of the muscles around the eustachian tube. In one case, a woman was for long deemed eccentric because she said that she heard a clock ticking in her left ear.

PARAMYOCLONUS MULTIPLEX. This rare syndrome, first described by Friedreich in 1881, is characterized by myoclonic contractions, and is unassociated with any pathological changes in the brain so far as is known at the present time.

The disease is found more often in males than in females, and although it is usually sporadic, occasional examples of familial incidence have been reported.[23] It usually starts in middle age, but may begin in infancy or adolescence. The myoclonus consists of sudden shock-like contractions of muscles or portions of muscles. At first, the proximal muscles of the arms and the shoulder girdles are affected, but eventually any muscle of the limbs or trunk may be involved. The face and bulbar muscles are the last to be affected. The movements are often induced by active or passive stretching of the muscles, and are abolished by sleep. In some cases, the movements are almost constant, but intermissions can occur. The cerebrospinal fluid and electroencephalogram are normal.

The course of the disease is very slow; some patients continue to live an active life until old age.

Familial Myoclonus and Ataxia

This rare condition is inherited as an autosomal dominant trait with incomplete penetrance.[11] The child exhibits myoclonic jerks which affect the proximal muscles of the limbs and the neck, together with nystagmus, intention tremor, and ataxia of gait. There is no muscular weakness, sensory loss, or impairment of the reflexes. In some cases, a progressive loss of hearing starts in early adult life. The spinal fluid and electroencephalogram are normal. Familial myoclonus with ataxia was included by Hunt in the syndrome of dyssynergia cerebellaris myoclonica.[23]

APRAXIA

The term *apraxia* refers to inability to perform familiar, purposeful physical tasks despite normal mobility, coordination, tone, sensation, and comprehension.[2, 5, 9, 10a, b] By definition, the patient understands what is required of him, and if he is asked to use a tool or instrument, he must be able to recognize it.

Apraxia is a symptom that is seldom complained of and can only be demonstrated by special, though simple, tests. Clinicians who do not look for it will not see it.

In a series of papers published from 1900 onwards, Liepmann subdivided the apraxias into three varieties: (1) ideational, (2) ideokinetic, and (3) limb-kinetic apraxia. In ideational apraxia, the patient cannot conceive how to carry out the desired action. In the ideokinetic form, he knows what he wants to do but he cannot do it on command. In limb-kinetic apraxia, he carries out the task clumsily. Liepmann's ideas are considered by many to oversimplify the problem, and Bay and others have questioned the very existence of pure apraxia. Nevertheless, ideokinetic apraxia is a not uncommon result of focal lesions.[2,10a,b] For instance, a left-sided apraxia is often seen in right-handed patients with motor aphasia and right hemiplegia. In its simplest form, the patient cannot protrude the tongue or smile to order, although he may carry out both actions involuntarily. This facioglossal apraxia is sometimes accompanied by difficulty in swallowing. In other cases of motor aphasia with right hemiplegia, the left upper limb is affected: The patient cannot comb his hair, make a fist, or carry out the motions of using a hammer to drive in a nail, and he will have more than the ordinary difficulty in using the left hand (if he is right-handed) to write, print, or draw. The face and upper limbs are more often affected than the legs, but a lesion of the premotor cortex can cause difficulty in walking; one foot will not move after the other. This may be associated with difficulty in carrying out other complex movements of the feet, such as imitating the action of kicking an imaginary ball. The patient can envisage what is required, but his feet will not do what is needed.

To understand how these symptoms come about, it is convenient to consider the manner in which motor skills are acquired. A child's first attempts to use a knife and fork are not conspicuously successful, but in time the problem is mastered to such an extent that he can feed himself automatically while his attention is otherwise engaged. This process of learning depends on visual, kinesthetic, and tactile memories, which somehow come to be fused into a composite memory, which subsequently serves to control and direct a succession of precise movements in the correct sequence. The process is analogous to computer-controlled manufacturing, packaging, and sealing of a commercial product.

The information required for the programming of purposeful movements appears to be stored in the premotor frontal cortex and in the inferior portion of the parietal lobe of the dominant hemisphere. These two areas receive inputs from all the major sensory association areas of the cortex, and they are connected to each other by subcortical association tracts, and to the contralateral motor cortex by fibers that cross the midline in the corpus callosum. It is thought that the dominant hemisphere can control the opposite motor cortex because lesions of the left hemisphere can cause left-sided apraxia, and because disease of the anterior part of the corpus callosum sometimes produces the same effect. On the other hand, complete surgical division of the corpus callosum in man does not produce apraxia,[10a,b] while tumors or infarction of the anterior part of the corpus callosum seldom do so. On present evidence, these discrepancies suggest that in many cases the right hemisphere contains its own programming system for the left side of the body and does not depend wholly on the dominant hemisphere.

Lesions involving the inferior parietal region of the dominant hemisphere can cause bilateral apraxia,[5] but it is apt to be obscured and compounded by other symptoms, including sensory aphasia from involvement of the temporal lobe. Similarly, apraxic features can often be discerned in the behavior of patients suffering from intoxications and diffuse diseases of the brain, but comprehension is usually depressed in such cases, and it is difficult to know whether the patient is suffering from a true apraxia or whether he is unable to understand what is required of him. Also, inability to use a familiar instrument can be caused by failure to recognize its nature; this is sometimes known as *agnostic apraxia.*

Two special varieties of apraxia require special mention. In *dressing apraxia,*[5] the patient recognizes his garments but cannot put them on, or puts them on in the wrong order, or back to front. This usually occurs in parietal lesions and is rather more common when the minor hemisphere is involved. It seems to be the result of impairment of the body image and the relationship of the body to external objects. *Constructional apraxia*[5] refers to inability to copy drawings or to reproduce patterns in matchsticks or building blocks. It often is associated with defects of writing; lines may be directed obliquely across the paper or they may intersect or overlie each other. A woman patient may find herself unable to lay a table or—as in a case seen by the author—to arrange a vase of flowers.

Parietal lesions of either hemisphere can also give rise to so-called trunk apraxia (Rumpsapraxie), which is characterized by difficulty in sitting down or lying down. The patient exhibits a hesitancy and misdirection in opposing the seat of his body to that of the chair, which is reminiscent of the clumsiness of toddlers when faced with the same task, and he may find difficulty in arranging his body along the long axis of a bed. The underlying difficulty seems to be the same as that which causes dressing apraxia.

TICS AND HABIT SPASMS

A *tic* is a rapid coordinated movement, originally purposeful in character, which is always carried out in the same manner and in the same part of the body, and which is especially apt to appear in moments of emotional stress. Tics commonly appear in individuals who are obsessional and compulsive and the tic usually has its origin in some past experience: for instance, repeated shrugging of one shoulder may date from an uncomfortable collar; a tic of sniffing from a cold in the head; blepharospasm may follow conjunctivitis. The author has seen a patient in whom spasmodic torticollis began as a slight turning of the head to the left as the patient put down a telephone receiver with her right hand after receiving a telephone message to the effect that her brother intended to commit suicide—the third member of her family to do so. A man with a severe obsessive-compulsive neurosis traced the onset of his torticollis to an occasion during early adolescence when he awoke at night to find his mother engaged in bizarre sexual activities with a stranger in a bed which lay to the left of his. In both these cases, the torticollis seems to have started as a movement of aversion. Examples such as these weaken the case of those who regard spasmodic torticollis as entirely organic in origin.

Spasmodic Torticollis. This comparatively rare condition usually starts late in adolescence or early in adult life and is marked by tonic or clonic movements of the sternomastoids, trapezius, and other muscles of the neck, which turn the face to one side, pull the head backwards or to one side, and elevate the shoulder. The movements are intermittent and increase with emotion and fatigue; they cease during sleep. In the early stages, they can be inhibited easily by laying the hand lightly against the face or lower jaw. The spasm may give rise to aching pain, and there may be hypertrophy of the affected muscles. The condition waxes and wanes, and remissions may occur, but it resists all forms of treatment and is entirely unresponsive to psychotherapy. Despite the fact that a somewhat similar condition has been known to follow encephalitis lethargica, and that in other cases torticollis has been the presenting symptom of dystonia musculorum deformans,[29] it seems likely that spasmodic torticollis is usually psychogenic.

Drug therapy has been disappointing. In mild cases, the wearing of a plastic collar may be effective while the collar is in position. Bilateral anterior rhizotomy of the eleventh cranial nerve and the upper three cervical nerves gives variable and at times disastrous results.[26] The effects of bilateral stereotaxic lesions in the ventrolateral thalamic nuclei are unpredictable.

Generalized Convulsive Tic (Gilles de la Tourette's Disease). This condition is characterized by complicated and widespread tics. The movements are violent and can involve any part of the body. They include sudden retraction of the head, spasms of the abdominal muscles, opisthotonos, and abrupt movements of the limbs. The movements may be accompanied by grunting noises or obscene and abusive language. Intermissions may occur, as in a woman who had suffered from this disorder for 10 years in early adult life, only to have it recur with great violence at the age of 46.

OCCUPATIONAL CRAMP

Persons whose occupation entails the persistent use of finely coordinated movements of the hand sometimes develop spasms of the muscles of the hand and forearm. The most common example is writer's cramp, but similar symptoms have been encountered in telegraphers, gold beaters, piano players, and violinists. Generally speaking, the "cramp" is not induced by using the hand for other purposes. There is often a background of tension caused by the need to carry out accurate work at high speed. In some cases, the patient harbors a conscious or subconscious dislike of the occupation in which he finds himself.

In *writer's cramp*, the patient holds the pen or pencil too firmly and this induces fatigue, with or without mild pain. Calligraphy becomes irregular, and in an effort to circumvent this, the pen is gripped even more firmly, which in turn increases the irregularity of the script. Eventually there is a spasm of the muscles of the hand and the forearm; sometimes the entire upper limb is involved. The nib may be driven into the paper, and in some cases either a tremor or a sudden spasmodic movement may occur from time to time. Examination discloses no weakness, atrophy, sensory impairment, or change in the reflexes.

Occasionally, writer's cramp proves to be an early symptom of paralysis agitans or Wilson's disease. In the majority of cases, however, there is no organic disease of the nervous system, and none develops subsequently.

Neither psychotherapy nor drugs are of any avail. A change of occupation is often necessary, but occasionally a new form of cramp is developed in the new occupation—for instance, the patient may take to a typewriter instead of writing and then proceeds to develop stiffness and inaccuracy of the fingers in tapping the keys.

REFERENCES

1. Aigner, B. R., and Mulder, D. W.: Myoclonus. *Arch. Neurol.* 2:600, 1960.
2. Brain, R.: The apraxias. *Speech Disorders.* Butterworth and Co., Washington, D.C., 1961, Chap. 13.
3. Brodal, A.: *Neurological Anatomy in Relation to Clinical Medicine.* Oxford University Press, London, 1969.
4. Chambers, W. W., and Sprague, J. M.: Functional localization in the cerebellum. II.

Somatotopic organization in cortex and nuclei. *Arch. Neurol. Psychiat.* 74:6, 1955.

5. Critchley, M.: *The Parietal Lobe.* Edward Arnold Publishers, Ltd., London, 1953.

6. Denny-Brown, D.: *The Cerebral Control of Movement.* Charles C Thomas, Publisher, Springfield, Ill., 1966.

7. Denny-Brown, D.: The general principles of motor integration. *Handbook of Physiology.* American Physiological Society, Washington, D.C., 1960, Vol. 2, Section 1, pp. 781–797.

8. Dow, R. S., and Moruzzi, G.: *The Physiology and Pathology of the Cerebellum.* University of Minnesota Press, Minneapolis, 1958.

9. Elliott, F. A.: The corpus callosum, cingulate gyrus, septum pellucidum, septal area and fornix. *Handbook of Clinical Neurology.* Vol. 2, Chap. 24. Edited by Vinken, P. J., and Bruyn, G. W., North Holland Publishing Company, Amsterdam, 1969.

10. Gastaut, H. and Villeneuve, A.: The startle disease or hyperexplexia: Pathological surprise reaction. *J. Neurol. Sci.* 5:523, 1967.

10a. Geschwind, N.: Disconnection syndromes in animals and man. I. *Brain* 88:237, 1965.

10b. Geschwind, N.: Disconnection syndromes in animals and man. II. *Brain* 88:585, 1965.

11. Gilbert, G. J., McEntee, W. J., and Glaser, G. H.: Familial myoclonus and ataxia: Pathophysiologic implications. *Neurology* 13: 365, 1963.

12. Guillain, G.: The syndrome of synchronous and rhythmic palato-pharyngo-laryngo-oculodiaphragmatic myoclonus. *Proc. Roy. Soc. Med.* 31:1031, 1957.

13. Harriman, D. G. F., Taverner, D., and Woolf, A. L.: Ekbom's syndrome and burning paraesthesias. A biopsy study by vital staining and electronmicroscopy of the intramuscular innervation with note on age changes in motor nerve endings in distal muscles. *Brain* 93:393, 1970.

14. Hermann, C., and Brown, J. W.: Palatal myoclonus: A re-appraisal. *J. Neurol. Sci.* 5:473, 1967.

15. Howard, F. M.: A new and effective drug in the treatment of stiff-man syndrome. *Proc. Mayo Clin.* 38:203, 1963.

16. Jung, R., and Hassler, R.: The extrapyramidal motor system. *Handbook of Physiology.* American Physiological Society, Washington, D.C., 1960, Vol. 2, Section 1.

17. Magoun, H., and Rhines, R.: *Spasticity.* Charles C Thomas, Publisher, Springfield, Ill., 1947.

18. Mahloudji, M., and Pikielny, R. T.: Hereditary essential myoclonus. *Brain* 90:669, 1967.

19. Martin, J. P.: *The Basal Ganglia and Posture.* J. B. Lippincott Co., Philadelphia, 1967.

20. McFie, J., and Zangwill, O. L.: Constructional apraxia. *Brain* 83:243, 1960.

21. Olafson, R. A., Mulder, D. W., and Howard, F. M.: "Stiff man" syndrome. *Proc. Mayo Clin.* 39:131, 1964.

22. Penfield, W., and Jasper, H.: *Epilepsy and the Functional Anatomy of the Human Brain.* Little, Brown and Co., Boston, 1954.

23. Pratt, R. T. C.: *The Genetics of Neurological Disorders.* Oxford University Press, London, 1967.

24. Schwartz, G. A., and Barrows, L. J.: Hemiballism without involvement of Luys' body. *Arch. Neurol.* 2:420, 1960.

25. Sherwin, I., and Redmon, W.: Successful treatment in action myoclonus. *Neurology* 19:846, 1969.

26. Sorensen, B. F., and Hamby, W. B.: Spasmodic torticollis. Results in surgically treated patients. *Neurology* 16:867, 1966.

27. Swanson, P. D., Luttrell, C. N., and Magladery, J. W.: Myoclonus—a report of 67 cases and review of the literature. *Medicine* 41: 339, 1962.

28. Symonds, C. P.: Myoclonus. *Med. J. Austral.* 22:765, 1956.

29. Tarlov, E.: On the problem of the pathology of spasmodic torticollis in man. *J. Neurol. Neurosurg. Psychiat.* 33:457, 1970.

CHAPTER THREE

Disorders of Speech and Language

Disturbances of speech fall into three main categories: disorders of vocalization (hoarseness, aphonia, and mutism); of enunciation (dysarthria and stammering); and of language (aphasia).

DISORDERS OF VOCALIZATION

Hoarseness. Hoarseness is usually due to disease affecting the larynx itself—overuse of the voice, acute or chronic laryngitis (including tuberculosis, syphilis, and leprosy), neoplasm, myxedema, and acromegaly—but may also be caused by affections of the tenth cranial nerve. Paralysis of the cricothyroid muscles, which act as tensors of the vocal cords and are supplied by the external branch of the superior laryngeal nerve, gives rise to hoarseness and loss of high notes. The other intrinsic muscles of the larynx are supplied by the recurrent laryngeal nerves, and the first sign of paralysis is weakness of abduction on the affected side. If unilateral, the voice is often unaffected, but if the condition progresses to total paralysis the adductors are also involved so that the vocal cord is motionless during phonation and inspiration, and the voice is weak and hoarse.

Aphonia. In bilateral recurrent laryngeal paralysis, the cords cannot be abducted, the voice is weak, and there is stridor on deep inspiration. Bilateral *adductor* "paralysis" by itself is usually hysterical in origin; in such cases, the patient speaks not at all or in a whisper, but will cough normally. Difficulty in bringing the cords together is not infrequent in bulbar palsy; the rima glottidis does not completely close during phonation, and speaking is an effort. The lesions responsible for complete bilateral paralysis of the superior laryngeal and recurrent laryngeal veins lie above the inferior ganglion of the vagus, and therefore the palate and pharynx are usually paralyzed as well.

Mutism. Mutism, in which the patient is completely silent, can be a symptom of hysterical conversion or schizophrenia. It is also encountered in severe Broca's aphasia and in akinetic mutism. The latter is an organically determined condition in which the patient lies completely silent and still, except for random movements of the eyes. There is no response to auditory or visual stimuli or to pain. Yet the patient looks as if he is awake. It has been seen in bilateral lesions of the cingulate gyri, ruptured anterior communicating aneurysm, bilateral thalamic lesions, tumors involving the floor of the third ventricle, and in disease involving the upper part of the midbrain, such as epidemic encephalitis and infarcts.

39

DISORDERS OF ENUNCIATION

Stammering. Stammering (stuttering) usually starts in early childhood and tends to grow less as life advances, but is apt to reappear during emotional crises. The flow of speech is broken by pauses, during which the patient may stay silent or may repeat sounds or syllables. Attempts to get the word out may be accompanied by facial grimaces. There is a close association between stammering and left-handedness; the association is likely to be seen especially in children who have been slow to develop distinctive handedness. Stammerers may show psychoneurotic traits, but these may well be the result rather than the cause of the disorder, for child stammerers exhibit no more psychological abnormalities than other children. The case for an organic basis is strengthened by the occasional appearance of stammering for the first time in the early stage of an organically determined aphasia, or when it is passing off.

Travis suggested that stammering might have a neurophysiological basis in the form of bilateral cerebral representation of speech. This theory is supported by Jones,[19] who reported four patients who had recent lesions in the vicinity of the presumed "speech" areas and who had been stammerers since childhood. After surgical correction of these lesions, the patients ceased to stammer. He concluded that stammering is associated with an interference by one hemisphere with the speech performance of the other.

Lalling and Lisping. Lalling speech consists of a want of precision in pronouncing consonants, e.g., the substitution of letters V, TH, or W for the letter R. The corresponding difficulty with the letter S is known as lisping. Lalling and lisping occur frequently in feeble-minded children, but are also found in normal persons who have not outgrown a childish habit. It can also be an affectation. In some cases the substitution of consonants is on so vast a scale that the subject speaks what is virtually a new language peculiar to himself—idioglossia. This is normal in infancy, but may occur in adults as a result of hysterical conversion. Idioglossia must not be confused with neologisms, new words coined by schizophrenics and severe obsessionals to represent a condensation of some sentence or idea which is of particular significance to the patient.

Palilalia. Palilalia is a condition in which a phrase or word is repeated with increasing rapidity. It is sometimes seen in pseudobulbar palsy and in the parkinsonian syndrome following encephalitis lethargica. The rapidly increasing tempo of the utterance distinguishes this condition from verbal perseveration in which the patient repeats the last word of a sentence and finds it difficult to switch to a new one, a symptom found in association with dysphasia, and also in frontal lobe disease without dysphasia.

Dysarthria. The term is applied to defects of enunciation caused by organic disease. The correct words are used, but they are distorted and slurred. Dysarthria may result from local disease of the lips, tongue, or fauces, but the diagnosis is obvious in such cases, and it is with the neurological variety that we are concerned. Neurogenic dysarthria may be classified according to the situation of the lesion—muscles, myoneural junction, lower motor neuron, upper motor neuron, extrapyramidal system, cerebellum, and (rarely) the sensory pathways. When dysarthria is due to disease in the posterior fossa, several of these mechanisms can be impaired simultaneously.

DISEASES OF MUSCLES. Weakness of the lips, e.g., in familial muscular dystrophy with facial involvement, interferes with the pronunciation of labial consonants. Myotonia and weakness combine to cause dysarthria in dystrophia myotonica, and transient myotonia may obscure enunciation in myotonia congenita and paramyotonia. Stiffness of articulatory muscles can impair speech in dermatomyositis. The myoneural junction is the site of the disorder in myasthenia gravis, and weakness of the lips, tongue, palate, and respiratory muscles is induced by using the voice; improvement follows rest or the administration of neostigmine or Tensilon.

DISORDERS OF THE LOWER MOTOR NEURON. These are a common cause of dysarthria. Disease of the facial nerve causes difficulty with labial consonants, as in Bell's palsy and congenital facial diplegia. Affections of the tenth and twelfth nerves or their nuclei give rise to slurred speech and a nasal intonation, a combination seen in the bulbar palsy of motor neuron disease, syringobulbia, bulbar poliomyelitis, severe generalized polyneuritis, and neoplastic conditions in the posterior fossa. The movements required for precise articulation are extremely refined, and it is therefore not surprising that in the early phases of bulbar dysarthria speech may be considerably disturbed, though inspection of the lips, tongue, and palate fails to reveal any obvious paralysis.

THE PYRAMIDAL CORTICOBULBAR SYSTEM. A unilateral pyramidal lesion does not as a rule cause dysarthria except in the earliest and most severe phase of a vascular accident, but bilateral affections produce slow, slurred speech, in which an element of spasticity can be discerned. This is well seen in the spastic bulbar palsy of motor neuron disease, spastic diplegia, double hemiplegia, and occasionally in multiple sclerosis. In general paresis, the dysarthria is accompanied by tremor of the lips and tongue which imparts a tremulous quality to the voice. In lesions of the dominant hemisphere which produce aphasia and hemiplegia, dysarthria may complicate the aphasia; such dysarthria should probably be regarded as an apraxia of enunciation. Occasionally dysarthria occurs without aphasia in prefrontal lesions, and following stereotaxic thalamotomy for Parkinson's disease.

THE EXTRAPYRAMIDAL SYSTEM. Extrapyramidal rigidity, whether due to paralysis agitans or to other diseases of the extrapyramidal system, gives rise to a slow, monotonous, slurring dysarthria. In advanced cases, fixity of the thoracic and laryngeal muscles interferes with the fine adjustments of airflow through the larynx, and the patient finds it convenient to concentrate as many words as possible into a single expiration; words are abbreviated and telescoped, and come out with a rush, with a pause before the next effort.

Involuntary movements of the face, tongue, palate, and muscles of respiration can interfere with the smoothness of articulation in rheumatic chorea, athetosis, hepatolenticular degeneration, and Huntington's chorea.

THE CEREBELLUM. The degree of dysarthria caused by cerebellar disease varies from case to case. It may be absent or may amount to little more than a thickening of enunciation. In other cases, it is so severe that speech becomes almost unintelligible. In multiple sclerosis it may take the form of slurring dysarthria, or the patient may circumvent his difficulty by breaking down words into their constituent syllables and enunciating each separately—scanning speech. Cerebellar dysarthria occurs in intoxication by alcohol, barbiturates, and hydantoinates. It is also seen with tumors, abscesses, and vascular lesions of the posterior fossa and in heredofamilial ataxias.

SENSORY ATAXIA OF SPEECH. This condition is very rare; it is probable that loss of kinesthetic feedback contributes to the dysarthria caused by lesions of the fifth, tenth, and twelfth cranial nerves.

DISORDERS OF LANGUAGE

Aphasia

Any discussion of aphasia must of necessity involve some degree of oversimplification if it is to be brief. The following account offers no more than a practical guide to the clinician who is in search of approximate definitions and a working hypothesis. The bibliography should be consulted for more detailed expositions of this complex subject.

Definition. The term *aphasia* is used to denote inability to understand and use the symbols of language, both written and spoken, and although incapacity short of complete loss is more properly referred to as dysphasia, it is convenient for descriptive purposes to employ the word aphasia for both total and incomplete deficiencies in this field. It embraces inability to communicate by speaking or by writing, and inability to understand what is said or written. The executive aspect of aphasia—loss of the ability to speak and write—has affinities with apraxia in that there is inability to carry out a special motor skill in the absence of paralysis, rigidity, or ataxia. In the same way, incapacity to understand the significance of spoken or written words in the presence of normal hearing and vision is closely related to agnosia, in which there is failure to recognize familiar sensory patterns.

The Anatomy of Language. Immediately behind the sensory strip of the postcentral gyrus there is an area which seems to be concerned, inter alia, with the storage of tactile memories because lesions of this region can give rise to tactile agnosia (an inability to recognize the identity of a familiar object by touch alone). This implies loss of tactile memories formed over the years and stored in the cortical gray matter. Similarly, whereas unilateral destruction of the calcarine cortex produces homonymous hemianopia, bilateral destruction of the adjacent area 19 on the lateral aspect of the occipital lobes can produce visual agnosia (inability to recognize the identity of things that the patient can see (p. 84). Here again there is a loss of visual memory, so that incoming visual impressions are no longer recognized. In the same way, the cortex of the middle third of the upper temporal convolution, adjacent to Heschl's gyrus (the cortical area for hearing), acts as a storehouse for auditory memories; *bilateral* destruction of this area, a rare event, can produce auditory agnosia (the patient hears but fails to recognize familiar sounds). These examples illustrate the fact that areas of cortex adjacent to the primary cortical end stations for touch, vision, and hearing appear to be concerned with the storage of memories.

It will be readily appreciated that the acquisition of speech may depend upon a similar mechanism. There is ample clinicopathological evidence that auditory memories for words are stored in the posterior half of the upper temporal gyrus, usually in the dominant hemisphere. Destruction of this area produces auditory aphasia: The patient hears words but fails to understand what they mean (an auditory agnosia for the symbols used in speech). This loss of verbal memories may have wider effects, however. In many instances, there is also difficulty with expression because if verbal memories are lost, the patient's vocabulary will suffer, as will grammar and syntax, giving rise to jargon aphasia. The patient may use wrong or nonexistent words and will not recognize his mistakes if the verbal memories which act as a monitor to speech are damaged or destroyed. If the lesion has spread still further back to the parieto-occipital lobe, as is often the case, it will involve the area concerned with the visual symbols of speech, so that the patient will also have difficulty in reading (dyslexia) and this, in its turn, may interfere with writing (dysgraphia) because the patient will fail to recognize the meaning of the marks that his pen makes on the paper. In fact, he returns to the childish state in this respect, being unable to read or write. A further result of the loss of the auditory and visual memories of the symbols of speech is interference with thinking. Much of our thinking is done in words, and if there is any considerable loss of verbal memories, this will necessarily embarrass "internal speech."

Intonation, gestures, and facial expression can convey information and can modify the meaning of what is spoken, and these visual and auditory clues may or may not be appreciated by the patient with receptive aphasia.

The *classification of aphasia* is a subject which has given rise to a large literature and a chaotic nomenclature.[4, 6, 18, 34] In general, there have been two major schools of thought. The first (exemplified by Head[17, 18]) attempts to classify the dysphasias in psychological terms and asserts that there is no such thing as an isolated loss of one part of speech function; instead, all functions are affected together, though not necessarily to the same degree. The second school of thought, to which the author of this text subscribes, is that language is composed of a mosaic of physiological functions, each with a specific anatomical substrate; this is based on the fact that individual pieces of the mosaic may be lost, while the others remain intact, e.g., pure expressive aphasia, pure word blindness, and pure word deafness. Such cases are necessarily rare because most cases of aphasia result from vascular disease or tumor, neither of which is a respecter of physiological or anatomical boundaries. Thus, the entire area of the cortex concerned with speech functions lies in the territory of the middle cerebral artery, and it is to be expected that in occlusive disease of this vessel, several cortical areas concerned with speech will be affected. Small infarctions limited to territory supplied by a minor cortical vessel are rare, but when they do occur, they can give rise to a sharply defined defect.[29]

The distinction between cortical and subcortical aphasia is beset with practical difficulties, but it is well to remember that the cortex does not function in isolation from subcortical structures. Thus, aphasia can develop as a result of vascular lesions limited to the thalamus, especially those involving the pulvinar.[5] Moreover, transient dysphasia with or without dysarthria is a frequent though temporary result of stereotaxic operations on the thalamus[1] or globus pallidus of the dominant hemisphere. This phenomenon has yet to be explained, but the extensive projections from the pulvinar to the parietotemporal cortex[31] provide an anatomical substrate for interaction between the speech area and the thalamus.

CEREBRAL DOMINANCE

Right handedness commonly implies that the left hemisphere is dominant for speech, but in a small percentage of cases, this does not apply. In some of these, the handedness has been imposed by training and the patient will admit that he prefers the left foot for kicking and the left hand for activities other than eating and writing. In left-handed patients, the dominant hemisphere for speech is more often the left than the right, and in more than half of all left-handers, language is disturbed by lesions of the left hemisphere. In most cases, it is possible to establish which hemisphere is dominant for language, irrespective of a patient's handedness, by comparing the results of an intracarotid injection of sodium amytal on the two sides; when the injection is made on the nondominant side, consciousness and the capacity to speak are recovered almost simultaneously, whereas when the injection is made on the dominant side, the patient remains partially aphasic for some minutes after the recovery of consciousness.[25]

It is well to recognize that the term "cerebral dominance" does not represent an absolute value as regards speech. Zangwill[35] has observed that, like handedness, "cerebral dominance is in all probability a graded characteristic varying in scope and completeness from individual to individual." Hughlings-Jackson recognized that occasionally a patient with expressive aphasia from a lesion of the dominant hemisphere may be able to sing or recite poetry with little hesitation and few errors in articulation. This has been seen following hemispherectomy of the dominant hemisphere; thus, in a man aged 47, described by Smith and Burkland,[27] there was not only ability to recall and sing familiar songs, but in the fifth postoperative month there was also some capacity for propositional speech and for comprehension of the spoken word. Transfer of language to the nondominant hemisphere is of course not uncommon up to the age of 15, but it is very rare in adults.

On the other hand, patients whose cerebral hemispheres have been disconnected by cutting the corpus callosum, the anterior commissure, the hippocampal commissure, and the massa intermedia do not suffer from aphasia and do not display any capacity for vocal ex-

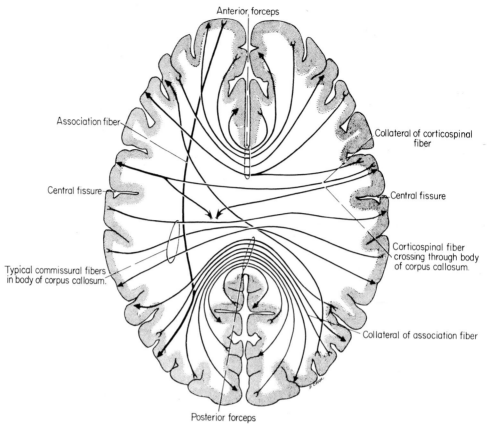

Figure 3–1. Diagram illustrating some of the components of the corpus callosum. (From Crosby, E. C., Humphrey, T., and Lauer, E. W.: *Correlative Anatomy of the Nervous System.* The Macmillan Co., New York, 1962.)

pression via the minor hemisphere.[13, 28] This applies, at any rate, to the comparatively few cases studied thus far. After recovery from surgery, speech is unaffected and the patient can write with either hand. Printed words flashed on a screen in the right visual field are recognized and can be read, but printed words seen in the left visual field cannot be repeated. That is to say, the patient cannot read, in the ordinary sense of the word, because the visual symbols of speech recorded by the right occipital cortex cannot be decoded by the speech area of the opposite hemisphere since the corpus callosum has been cut. However, it is not quite so simple as that. Gazzaniga and Sperry[13] have found that if a word such as "pen" is flashed on the left-hand side of the screen, the patient is able to pick out a pen from a collection of objects placed before his view. From this it appears that though the minor hemisphere is dumb, it is not really word-blind, even if the patient has no conscious sense of reading or understanding the word placed on the screen.

CLINICAL TYPES OF APHASIA

The definitions which follow are approximate only. It takes only a small increase in the size of a lesion to alter the clinical characteristics of the speech defect. It is generally agreed that temporoparietal lesions are associated with a predominantly receptive form of aphasia, whereas more anteriorly placed disease produces a mainly expressive aphasia. In practice, it is found that most cases of aphasia are mixed, exhibiting impairment of both receptive and expressive capacities in varied proportions.

Expressive Aphasia (Broca's Aphasia, Cortical Motor Aphasia). When the lesion damages the posterior part of the inferior frontal gyrus and the lowest portion of the precentral convolution, the patient understands what he hears and reads but he cannot express himself. He knows what he wants to say because his verbal memories are intact, but he cannot say it. It is often associated with right-sided hemiplegia and apraxia of the left hand. If improvement occurs, words such as yes or no, or even a phrase or two, become possible but are often used inappropriately. In the early stages, there is usually some mental confusion. In another type of case, motor aphasia is accompanied by paralysis of the face on the side opposite to the cerebral lesion, and Symonds[29] has pointed out that in this type there is no mental confusion, and as soon as recovery starts to occur, words and phrases used are appropriate and grammatical. The responsible lesion is thought to be subcortical. This is known as *pure word dumbness* or *aphemia.*

Nominal Aphasia (Amnestic Aphasia). In the author's opinion, this term should be reserved for inability to name objects, qualities, or conditions. It is a familiar and almost commonplace experience of the aging brain and can occur in otherwise normal persons as a result of mental fatigue. It is also an early symptom of central aphasia (caused for instance by a cerebral tumor) and can be the last symptom to disappear during recovery from central aphasia. Internal speech is not affected since the patient has a clear concept of what he is talking or thinking about, even if he cannot name the objects, conditions, or qualities.

Central Aphasia (Wernicke's Aphasia). This condition is caused by a posterior temporoparietal lesion of the dominant hemisphere and is marked by difficulty in the understanding *and* expression of speech. The patient's vocabulary is limited by nominal aphasia. Grammar and syntax are impaired, and the comprehension of speech is so affected that the patient not only fails to understand what is said to him but also fails to notice some of his own mistakes and may use wrong or nonexistent words, so producing a jargon aphasia. Reading may or may not be impaired, depending on whether the responsible lesion has spread to the occipital lobe; if dyslexia is present, it is usually accompanied by some degree of dysgraphia and dyscalculia. The use of nonexistent or incorrect words is spoken of as paraphasia.

Pure Word Deafness. This is very rare. The patient can distinguish words from other sounds but cannot understand them and his own speech sounds like gibberish to him, though it may be intelligible to others. He cannot repeat words or take dictation but can read and write spontaneously. Since spontaneous speech is possible, verbal memories have not been destroyed and it is assumed that the condition is due to interruption of the pathway between the cortical area for hearing and the adjacent area of the temporal lobe in which verbal memories are stored, i.e., the middle part of the superior temporal gyrus of the dominant hemisphere.

Pure Word Blindness. In this condition the patient suffers from an inability to read because he fails to recognize the visual symbols of speech, but he can still write spontaneously[9] and take dictation, and other speech functions are normal. This usually results from a vascular lesion within the territory of the posterior cerebral artery and may range from an inability to recognize certain letters to incapacity for reading words. In either case, there is a difficulty in reading. There may be alexia for letters but not for figures. Though earlier writers recognized this syndrome,[4] it was Déjerine[10] who first established its anatomical basis. He described dyslexia in a case of infarction of the dominant occipital lobe and the splenium of the corpus callosum as a result of thrombosis of the posterior cerebral artery. The callosal lesion isolated the right occipital lobe from the speech area of the dominant hemisphere. Therefore, visual information reaching the right occipital lobe from the left visual fields could not be decoded by the speech area of the left hemisphere, but the patient was able to read letters traced on the palm of his left hand because the right sensory cortex was still connected with the speech areas of the left hemisphere via the undamaged portion of the anterior corpus callosum. Had Déjerine applied the tests used by Gazzaniga and Sperry,[13] he might have found that the right hemisphere was still able to appreciate visual symbols though unable to repeat them. In other cases quoted in the literature, the lesion has interrupted the pathways between the left occipital cortex and area 19.

Impairment in the use of Braille owing to constructional apraxia has been recorded following a right parietal lesion.[21] This is not an aphasic defect; the loss of ability to read is due to loss of the capacity to appreciate the spatial relationships of the dots. The author has encountered a young adult with cortical blindness as a result of cardiac arrest. Speech was unaffected. Although sensibility in the fingers was unimpaired, he failed to learn Braille and there was impairment of graphesthesia in both hands.

Agraphia. A lesion at the posterior end of the middle frontal gyrus may produce an apraxia of the contralateral hand, and the patient may be able to write with the other hand or by holding a pen in his teeth.[4] This is not a true agraphia; the term is more properly limited to inability to express meanings in writing or print in the absence of motor deficits. It is usually associated with alexia, and this combination (referred to as *visual asymbolia*) is due to loss or isolation of the storehouse of visual memories of the symbols of speech which is usually situated in or near the angular gyrus of the dominant hemisphere. It is more usual, however, for visual asymbolia to be part of a severe central aphasia. Pure agraphia, without word blindness, can also result

from a lesion in the neighborhood of the left angular gyrus in right-handed persons; since there is no dyslexia, copying is more successful than spontaneous writing or writing from dictation.

Difficulties in writing are also experienced by some patients with a lesion of the parietal lobe of the nondominant hemisphere.[7, 8] The lines are irregular and often obliquely written and may intersect one another. There may be a very wide margin on one side and none on the other. The calligraphy resembles that of a person writing in the dark or with the eyes closed. If the lesion is in the dominant hemisphere the difficulty with calligraphy may be compounded by the errors of a true semantic dysgraphia.

Acalculia. Mental arithmetic involves words which are symbols for numerals, and words referring to the manipulation of such symbols, e.g., division, subtraction, etc.[16] Therefore, calculation is often impaired as part of a central aphasia and paraphasia,[2] and it is also depressed in any generalized loss of cortical function, as in dementia. Sometimes acalculia occurs from a lesion of the left angular gyrus, and it is then often associated with finger agnosia, dysgraphia, and inability to distinguish between left and right (Gerstmann's syndrome).[14]

Amusia. Failure to recognize familiar music is known as sensory amusia; inability to sing or whistle a tune is motor amusia. These may occur in the absence of aphasia and in lesions of the minor hemisphere. Inability to read musical notations is a special form of dyslexia and is usually associated with inability to read printed or written words. Needless to say, inability to play a familiar musical instrument may be an expression of manual dyspraxia and it is not necessarily associated with amusia.

DEVELOPMENTAL DISORDERS OF SPEECH

Developmental Motor Aphasia. This term is applied to otherwise normal children who cannot learn to articulate clearly but understand the spoken word.

There is more difficulty with consonants than with vowels. In the most severe cases, the child is almost mute. In mild cases, improvement occurs spontaneously and this can be accelerated by special training.

Specific   Developmental   Dyslexia
This condition is characterized by inability to read with normal facility despite normal sight and hearing, normal intelligence, adequate motivation, and conventional instruction.[7, 22, 26] It is about four times more common in boys than in girls and is often familial. Reading disabilities are said to occur in some 10 per cent of all schoolchildren, but this figure is almost certainly too high for specific developmental dyslexia, as defined above.

The cause, in terms of anatomy and physiology, is unknown. No pathological studies are available. There is no consistent relationship to handedness. It has been ascribed to lag in the development of cortical maturity, but this is doubtful since it is occasionally encountered in adult life in individuals who are mature in all other respects.

Speech is normal, but there is difficulty in reading, either silently or aloud. There is a tendency to read words from right to left or from the middle of the word to the left; small words are reversed (e.g., "dog" becomes "god") and there is failure to discriminate between words which are somewhat similar in spelling or sound. Difficulty is experienced in switching from one line to the next. Some vowels and consonants are ignored. Phonemes may be interpolated incorrectly, or dropped entirely, and there may be perseveration. In some cases, there is additional difficulty in the recognition of numerical symbols, with consequent dyscalculia. Calligraphy is usually untidy and malaligned, and spelling and punctuation may be bizzarre.

Understandably, neurotic patterns of behavior are apt to develop, especially if the child is unjustly accused of being stupid or lazy, and disciplined accordingly. Inability to read, from any cause, predisposes to juvenile delinquency.

With appropriate tuition, the dyslexic can be helped to read simple material and can have a successful career if the correct niche is found for him or her.[26]

Developmental   Auditory   Imperception. This is a specific speech disability which cannot be ascribed to mental deficiency, deafness, motor disability, or severe personality disorder. As in developmental dyslexia, males are more often affected than females, and the condition is frequently familial and hereditary.

Although these children are not deaf, as judged by audiometric findings, they may exhibit difficulty in localizing the source of a sound, have a lower level of functional hearing than is to be expected from audiometric findings, and show an inconsistency of responses to sound.[11] Moreover, there may be loss of the arousal reaction to sound even when the stimulus is known to be within the child's hearing range, and there is marked oscillation of auditory threshold. The child's capacity to hear is better than his ability to listen.

There is no information as to the pathologic nature of the condition, but several studies have revealed a higher than average incidence of electroencephalographic abnormalities in children with developmental aphasia. Thus, Forrest and his colleagues [12] found that 36 of 73 such children had abnormal EEG recordings. In 22, the EEG abnormalities were localized, and 19 of these were in the left hemisphere.

The defect is usually not noticed until the child reaches an age at which speech is to be expected. Then it is discovered that the child takes no notice when spoken to and does not learn to repeat words. Later on, a defect in appreciating written and printed symbols may also become apparent. Many develop a language of their own, which is comprehensible only to those closely associated with them.

Most of these children can be taught lip-reading and to speak more or less intelligibly.

MIRROR WRITING

Some normal individuals can write backwards with the left hand, the script being a mirror image of normal writing. Some children go through a phase of mirror writing. It can also be found in right-handed individuals who develop right hemiplegia. In patients suffering from developmental dyslexia, both mirror reading and mirror writing may occur. They tend to read words from right to left and to pronounce some of them accordingly.

REFERENCES

1. Bell, D. S.: Speech functions of the thalamus inferred from the effect of thalamotomy. *Brain* 91:619, 1968.
2. Benson, D. F., and Denckla, M. B.: Verbal paraphasia as a source of calculation disturbance. *Arch. Neurol.* 21:96, 1969.
3. Benton, A. L.: Developmental aphasia and brain damage. *Cortex* 1:40, 1961.
4. Brain, W. R.: *Speech Disorders*, Butterworth and Co., Washington, D.C., 1961.
5. Ciemins, V. A.: Localized thalamic hemorrhage: A cause of aphasia. *Neurology* 20:776, 1970.
6. Critchley, M.: Aphasiological nomenclature and definition. *Cortex*, 3:2, 1967.
7. Critchley, M.: *Developmental Dyslexia*. Charles C Thomas, Springfield, Ill., 1964.
8. Critchley, M.: *The Parietal Lobes*. Edward Arnold, London, 1953.
9. Cumming, W. J. K., Horwitz, L. J., and Perl, N. J.: A study of a patient who had alexia without agraphia. *J. Neurol. Neurosurg. Psychiat.* 33:34, 1970.
10. Déjerine, M. J.: Contribution à l'étude anatomo-pathologique et clinique des différentes variétés de cécité verbale. *C. R. Soc. Biol. (Paris)* 4:61, 1891.
11. Eisenson, J.: Developmental patterns of nonverbal children and some therapeutic implications. *J. Neurol. Sci.* 3:313, 1966.
12. Forrest, T., Eisenson, J., and Slink, J.: EEG findings in 113 nonverbal children. *Electroenceph. Clin. Neurophysiol.* 22:291, 1967.
13. Gazzaniga, M. S., and Sperry, R. W.: Language after section of the cerebral commissures. *Brain* 90:131, 1967.
14. Gerstmann, J.: Syndrome of finger agnosia, disorientation for right and left, agraphia, acalculia. *Arch. Neurol. Psychiat.* 44:398, 1940.
15. Granich, L.: *Aphasia: A Guide to Retraining.* Grune and Stratton, Inc., New York, 1947.
16. Grewel, F.: Acalculia. *Brain* 75:397, 1952.
17. Head, H.: Speech and cerebral localization. *Brain* 46:355, 1923.
18. Head, H.: *Aphasia and Kindred Disorders of Speech.* The Macmillan Co., New York, 1926.
19. Jones, R. K.: Observations on stammering after localized cerebral injury. *J. Neurol. Neurosurg. Psychiat.* 29:192, 1966.
20. Luria, A. R.: *The Higher Cortical Function in Man.* Basic Books, New York, 1966.
21. Meckler, R. J., and Horenstein, S.: Paralexia for Braille following a right parietal lesion. *Neurology*, 20:378, 1970.
22. Money, J.: *Reading Disability: Progress and Research Needs in Dyslexia.* Johns Hopkins Press, Baltimore, 1962.
23. Nielsen, J. M.: *Agnosia, Apraxia, Aphasia. Their Value in Cerebral Localization.* 2nd Ed. Harper & Brothers, New York, 1946.
24. Penfield, W., and Roberts, L.: *Speech and Brain Mechanisms.* Princeton University Press, Princeton, 1959.
25. Perria, L., Rosadini, G., and Rossi, G. F.: Determination of side of cerebral dominance with amobarbital. *Arch. Neurol.* 4:173, 1961.
26. Schonell, F. J.: *Backwardness in the Basic Subjects.* Oliver and Boyd, Edinburgh, 1948.
27. Smith, A., and Burkland, C. W.: Dominant hemispherectomy: Preliminary report on neuropsychological sequelae. *Science* 153:1280, 1966.
28. Sperry, R. W., Gazzaniga, M. S., and Bogen, J. E.: Interhemispheric relationships: Syndromes of hemisphere disconnection. *Handbook of Clinical Neurology*, North Holland Publishing Co., Amsterdam, 1967, Vol. 4, p. 273.
29. Symonds, C. P.: Aphasia. *J. Neurol. Neurosurg. Psychiat.* 16:1, 1953.
30. Van Buren, J. M., and Borke, R. C.: Alterations in speech and the pulvinar. *Brain* 92:255, 1969.
31. Walker, A. E.: Internal structure and afferent-efferent relations of the thalamus, *The Thalamus.* Edited by Purpura, D. P., and Yahr, M. D., Columbia University Press, New York, 1966.
32. Weisenberg, T. H., and McBride, K. E.: *Aphasia, a Clinical and Psychological Study.* Oxford University Press, London, 1935.
33. White, J. C., and Sweet, W. H.: *Pain and the Neurosurgeon: A Forty Year Experience.* Charles C Thomas, Springfield, Ill., 1969.
34. Wilson, S. A. K.: *Aphasia.* Kegan Paul, London, 1926.
35. Zangwill, O. L.: *Cerebral Dominance and Its Relation to Psychological Function.* Charles C Thomas, Springfield, Ill., 1960.

CHAPTER FOUR

Mental Disorders in Organic Disease

Psychoses caused by intoxications, structural disease of the brain, head injuries, vitamin B deficiency, and other physical disorders are commonly referred to as the organic psychoses or the organic brain syndrome, in contradistinction to the primary psychoses, notably schizophrenia and manic depressive psychosis, in which there is (as yet) no evidence of structural disease or biochemical disturbance. These two groups, in their turn, have to be distinguished from the psychoneuroses and from built-in character disorders.[19]

The relationships between mental disorders and physical diseases can be classified under eight headings. (1) Congenital mental retardation is commonly due to developmental defects, inborn metabolic disorders, or damage to the brain at or shortly after birth; psychotic and neurotic patterns of behavior may be superimposed on this background.[34] (2) Acquired disease of the brain and head injury are the common causes of the organic brain syndrome. (3) Metabolic disorders and exogenous and endogenous intoxications arising *outside* the brain can give rise to organic psychoses. (4) Latent primary psychoses can be uncovered by physical disease inside or outside the brain. (5) Physical disease outside the nervous system can evoke reactive depression and anxiety. (6) Emotional tensions can cause headache, tachycardia, dyspepsia, asthma, rheumatoid arthritis, and other stress diseases; psychosomatic disorders can also occur in mental defectives and in the course of primary psychoses. (7) Epilepsy can give rise to episodic disturbances of mind, mood, and behavior in the form of temporal lobe seizures and postictal automatism. (8) Hypochondriacal delusions of disease can occur as a symptom of a psychosis or a neurosis.

FACTORS INFLUENCING THE SYMPTOMATOLOGY OF THE ORGANIC PSYCHOSES

Since the brain is the organ of thought and emotion, it is not surprising that intellectual impairment and emotional disturbances, with consequent aberrations of overt behavior, frequently accompany disease which affects the structure of the brain or influences its functions via metabolic pathways.[23] The symptoms which result from such disorders are by no means uniform, for they are influenced by several factors. In the first place, they depend to some extent on the acuteness of the disease; a slowly growing tumor of the frontal lobe may produce no psychological disturbances, whereas a rapidly growing tumor of comparable size and in the same site may interfere considerably with the level of consciousness and with behavior.

Secondly, diffuse or global disease (including intoxications) will usually have a far greater effect on mental processes than focal disease. Consequently, we expect to see a more severe degree of dementia in general paresis or Alzheimer's disease than from a cerebral tumor or an infarction of a large portion of one cerebral hemisphere from thrombosis of the internal carotid artery. An exception to this rule is that small midline tumors adjacent to the lateral and third ventricles can cause psychological symptoms early in their course, before there is any rise of intracranial pressure, perhaps because the limbic system is involved.[6]

A third point of practical importance is the influence on symptoms of the patient's premorbid personality, social training, and mental endowments, for it is not only the nature and distribution of the disease which determines the clinical picture, but also the type of person in whom it has occurred.[29, 39] Repressed memories and desires, for instance, influence behavior in disease as they do in health, and play a considerable role in the emotional and behavioral responses of the patient with an organic psychosis. This can be illustrated by the case of a maiden lady of 65 who, as the result of a stroke, refused to wear clothes, used obscene language, and made inappropriate suggestions to her gardener. Organic disease of the brain and intoxications may uncover latent schizophrenia, manic depressive psychosis, or paranoia.[49] The influence of premorbid social training and conditioning is also seen in the extent to which social graces are maintained, in some cases, despite advancing intellectual loss, and the façade may be so convincingly preserved that the dementia may escape detection for some time. This is especially likely to occur in individuals whose work and domestic circumstances do not tax their capacity to the full, so that there is a margin between their mental endowment and the demands made upon it. The nature of the initial mental impairment also influences

the situation; for example, difficulty in calculation will become obvious at an early stage in an accountant but not in an individual whose duties do not include arithmetical tasks; dyslexia would more seriously inconvenience a student than a laborer, and would bring him to seek medical advice at an earlier date.

The fourth point to which attention must be drawn is the variability of individual defects from hour to hour or from day to day. This is particularly well seen in the acute organic brain syndrome, in which lucid intervals can interrupt gross confusion, and it is a commonplace that if aphasia is incomplete, it fluctuates in degree from time to time. Similarly, disorders of perception such as difficulty in recognizing faces or places are seldom static and unchanging during the course of an organic psychosis. The explanation for this lack of consistency is not known.

It is useful to recognize that the symptoms fall into three groups—symptoms resulting from impairment or loss of mental capacity, those resulting from the release of limbic centers from cortical control, and those which represent the patient's conscious or unconscious attempt to meet or circumvent his difficulties.[29] An example of release of limbic structures from control is the explosions of violent rage, comparable in some ways to the sham rage induced in experimental animals by a lesion of the hypothalamus, which sometimes occur with lesions of the temporal lobe, septal area, and cingulate gyrus. Circumvention of symptoms is illustrated by the manner in which the patient may withdraw from professional or social life with which he cannot cope; again, he may become excessively orderly in the disposition of his possessions because this makes it easier for him to know where they are. A more dramatic example is the violence which a mentally disordered patient may exhibit as a result of faulty perception or hallucinations. Thus, it is natural and appropriate for a patient either to run away, or to attack, if the nurse bearing a hypodermic syringe appears to be a threat to him. It is equally natural for the hallucinating patient to seek to rid his bed of the snakes and insects which he sees crawling upon it.

NEUROPSYCHOLOGY OF THE ORGANIC PSYCHOSES

It would be easier to relate the symptoms of the organic psychoses to normal neuropsychology if there were unanimity on mind-brain relationships, which there is not. There is, for instance, a continuing though unnecessary conflict between those who insist that the brain works as a whole, and those who emphasize the anatomical localization of some mental functions, and there is an even deeper gulf between upholders of the psychoanalytic school and the more physically oriented exponents of Pavlovian reflexology. To some, a more eclectic view appears to be not only preferable but essential, for there is no doubt that conditioning plays an important part in our lives, or that buried memories influence behavior, or that some tools of the intellect are related to particular portions of the brain while others are not.

In the interests of simplicity, it is convenient to consider the mental symptoms of the organic psychoses under three headings: disorders of intellect, disorders of affect, and disorders of biological drives. Obviously, these three categories are to some extent interdependent; for instance, affect is influenced by the satisfaction or thwarting of biological drives [19] and intellectual frustrations or incapacity can induce anger, depression, or anxiety. Likewise, some forms of intellectual activity (e.g., judgment) are much influenced by affective attitudes. The net effect of disturbances of mind, mood, and biological drives is to produce changes of behavior and personality which are often the first thing to be noticed by relatives and colleagues, and which may appear before there is any evidence of intellectual or affective disorder as judged by the results of clinical investigation. An individual's capacity to cope with the vicissitudes of professional and domestic life in sophisticated communities is often a better yardstick of normality than are the results of psychometric tests, in the early stages of an organic psychosis.

Intellectual Activity. Intellectual activity depends primarily on five physiological mechanisms: (1) perception,[1, 51] (2) the capacity to form and recall memories,[45] (3) association, (4) attention, (5) awareness or consciousness. The first four of these capacities are sometimes referred to as the instrumentalities or tools of the mind, but such terms are of dubious validity, for they imply that they are used by some superior organization to serve certain ends. It is preferable to regard these physiological mechanisms not as instruments, but as elements which contribute to man's adaptive responses to his environment. They are all necessary for abstract thought, which constitutes the highest form of integrated mental activity.[10, 29] For instance, in carrying out an operation, the surgeon must perceive the physical situation which has to be corrected; he must be capable of sustained attention to the task; and he must be able to draw upon memories of his previous experience and knowledge derived from books if he is to carry out his task successfully. The housewife doing her marketing for a large family has to keep in mind a dozen domestic and financial factors if she is to make the correct purchases.

Abstract thought and the activities to which it may lead are influenced by the patient's attitude of mind which, in its turn, is dependent on both conscious and subconscious factors. This is particularly true of memory, for some of our memories may be falsified or actually suppressed so that our conscious judgments may be based at times on faulty or incomplete memories. Perceptions, too, may be influenced by the subconscious. The man who thinks that he can believe the evidence of his eyes and ears fails to recognize that in emotionally charged situations his perceptions may not be entirely reliable —a truth enshrined in the German proverb, "He lies like an eyewitness."

Perception. The term "perception" is used here to indicate the conscious mental registration of a sensory stimulus. Perception usually involves some degree of recognition, but of course it is quite possible to perceive something without knowing what it is. Disorders of perception include the faulty recognition of sensory impressions (illusions), hallucinations, difficulty in distinguishing between figure and background,[29, 53] and imperception of bodily illness or incapacity.[5] All these can occur in organic psychoses. Misinterpretation of sensory impressions is well illustrated by the delirious patient who thinks that his hospital room is a ship's cabin, or that his wife is his mother, or that his left arm belongs to somebody else (as in right parietal lesions); in these cases, the sensory input does not elicit the appropriate sensory memory. Hallucinations are sensory experiences occurring without an external stimulus. They can be evoked in conscious man by electrical stimulation of the cortex, especially of the temporal lobe, and also occur as the result of epileptic discharges arising within this and other areas of the brain. Such hallucinations probably represent fragmentary and disordered activation of olfactory, visual, kinesthetic, or auditory memories. Visual and auditory hallucinations are seen in delirious states (e.g., delirium tremens, bacterial intoxications), but also occur in focal disease of the brain and in the primary psychoses.

A more subtle disorder of perception is the inability to distinguish between figure and background.[29, 53] For instance, a musician with a parieto-occipital glioma found himself unable to distinguish the sounds made by individual instruments in a concerto, and another patient complained that if he looked at a table it seemed to be "all mixed up with the background." This can give rise to difficulty in the appreciation of topographical relationships and of photographs and paintings. In the psychological sphere, there is an analogous difficulty in distinguishing between the important and the irrelevant, and this may perhaps play a part in the extreme circumstantiality

displayed by patients in the early stages of organic dementia and also by normal persons of limited mental endowment whose prolixity can be a sore trial to the examiner who wishes to get to the point of the story. Inability to get to the heart of a matter, to grasp the essential point of a problem, is often an early feature of an organic dementia and contributes to the inefficiency in business or social affairs which often precedes more easily recognizable features of mental dilapidation.

Imperception of bodily incapacity is sometimes seen in parietal lesions.[33] Thus, a patient with a lesion of the right parietal lobe extending forward to the motor cortex may not perceive that he has hemiplegia and will deny it when the idea is suggested to him. He may even get out of bed and attempt to walk. In one case of this type, the patient, when asked why he had come into hospital, replied that he had trouble with his right ear. This and other manifestations of imperception in parietal lobe lesions are described more fully in Chapter 16. Denial of illness (anosognosia) is sometimes seen in general intoxications and global disease of the brain, probably because the parietal lobe suffers in the general process.

Delusions, in contrast to hallucinations, are not sensory experiences, but false beliefs. When they are due to organic disease, they are usually changeable and fleeting, lacking the systematization seen in the delusions of the primary psychoses, and they usually occur in a setting of disturbed consciousness, as in delirium tremens, senile psychoses, and general paralysis. In the senile psychoses, delusions of poverty are common and are often linked with a fixed idea that the patient's relatives are after his money; the latter is not always a delusion. In general paresis, delusions of grandeur are sometimes seen, accompanied by an appropriate expansiveness of mood.

Memory. It seems possible that the physical mechanism underlying the coding or imprinting of memory is a physiochemical change in cell proteins, analogous to the storage of the spoken word on a recording tape.[15, 18, 35] Unlike the tape recorder, however, human memories do not remain unchanged. Decay sets in with the progressive degeneration of neurons which occurs in advancing life, though not all impairment of memory is due to decay, for under hypnosis it is possible to retrieve memories which for one reason or another have been buried in the subconscious. Furthermore, our memories are subject to distortion at the hands of conscious or subconscious likes and dislikes, so that falsification of past memories- is not necessarily a result of physical disease.

Memory is not a function of a single center, for the capacity to encode and store information is widely spread through the parietal, occipital, and temporal lobes; moreover, the same process is probably involved in the formation and retention of conditioned reflexes in the visceral nervous system.[35]

FORMS OF MEMORY FAILURE. Clinicopathological observations on patients with localized cortical and subcortical lesions [56] indicate that sensory memories are stored in the area of cortex adjacent to the appropriate sensory end-stations. Thus, visual memories are grouped in area 19 immediately anterior to the occipital pole, auditory memories around Heschl's gyrus in the temporal lobe, olfactory memories in the uncus of the hippocampal gyrus, and tactile and kinesthetic memories in the postcentral region of the parietal lobe. Lesions limited to any one of these areas can impair the patient's capacity to recognize the nature of appropriate sensory stimuli, but since sensory memories (with the exception of those concerned with the written and spoken symbols of speech) appear to be stored bilaterally, diffuse diseases and intoxications are more likely to cause disturbances of recognition than are unilateral focal lesions. Defective capacity to recognize the familiar must necessarily contribute to some of the confusion of mind and disorders of behavior which appear in the presence of intoxications or diffuse cerebral disease.

A second form of memory failure, amnesia for life's experiences, occurs in the presence of bilateral disease of the hippocampus.[22, 36, 40, 44, 54] The patient is able to recognize what he sees, feels, hears, and smells, and he retains the capacity to read, calculate, recognize familiar objects, dress himself, and so on, but he is unable to recall the personal events of his life for months or even years prior to the illness. He may therefore lose his sense of personal identity and not know whether or not he is married, the nature of his former occupation, or where he lives. This form of amnesia has been reported in bilateral temporal lobe infarctions, following head injuries and encephalitis,[44] and after bilateral temporal lobectomy.[47]

A third type of memory defect is seen in Korsakoff's psychosis,[36, 42] which occurs in alcoholism (from thiamine deficiency), and less often as a result of head injury, meningitis, and subarachnoid hemorrhage. In alcoholic cases, lesions have been found in the mamillary bodies, the fornix, and the medial nucleus of the thalamus; the memory defect correlates most closely with the thalamic lesions. The patient not only appears unable to learn, in the sense of forming immediate memories, but he also confabulates, filling in the blanks in his memory with fictitious accounts of his activities and current events. The incapacity to remember is not total, for with perseverance the patient may be able to learn simple figures and words with concrete meanings, and he will sometimes recall events, or things he heard, during the illness. The confabulation has many interesting features, not the least of which is that it occurs at all, for in other types of amnesia the patient admits that he cannot remember, and does not attempt to fill in the blanks with confabulation. Some of the confabulated material represents fragments of past events which have been dislocated from their proper temporal sequence and context.[36] Analytical studies in patients with organically determined amnesia have revealed that what is remembered and what is forgotten are influenced to some extent by emotional factors, the amnesia being most marked for matters which have an unpleasant significance for the patient.[50]

Inability to remember data over a short period of time occurs in all the organic psychoses. If the patient is given the name of a flower, a street address, and the name of a person and asked to repeat them five minutes later, he will often fail to do so. In some cases, this is due to inability to form a memory, and in others to difficulty in bringing it back into consciousness.

EFFECTS OF MEMORY FAILURE. Defects of memory formation and recall can have a profound effect on mentation because memory enters into so many of our mental processes. For instance, amnesia for words and syntax interferes not only with speaking and understanding what is said, but also with internal speech or thinking in words. Again, correct orientation in time depends partly on immediate past memories; the patient who cannot remember what has transpired during the morning will have difficulty in realizing what time it is, and if the amnesia extends still further back, he may not be able to identify the day of the week, or the month. Similarly, disorientation for place depends partly on the recognition of surroundings, itself a function of memory; a normal individual knows where he is, either because he recognizes his surroundings or, if in a totally new place, because he knows where he planned to get to. Disorientation for place may also be caused by faulty perceptions. Disorientation for person is rare, but as noted above, it occasionally occurs as the result of bilateral hippocampal lesions which have obliterated the patient's memory of his past life, with the result that he has no sense of personal identity. Another form of disorientation is seen in patients who, as a result of a lesion in the region of the angular gyrus of the dominant hemisphere, are unable to distinguish between left and right, something which is learned and remembered from childhood. There is no need to emphasize the aberrations of behavior

that can result from this and other forms of memory loss.

Loss of the motor memories which enable us to carry out learned skills is one cause of apraxia, a disability which sometimes contributes to the behavioral disturbance of patients with global cerebral disease or damage to the parietal lobe of the dominant hemisphere.[5] In the presence of any considerable degree of organic dementia, it is often difficult to decide whether loss of motor skills (e.g., use of a cigarette lighter or pen) occurs because the patient fails to recognize the object, or because of a true apraxia; in either case, a defect of memory is involved.

Memory plays a part in insight—the capacity for correct assessment of one's own condition. In the early stage of organic dementia, the patient may realize that all is not well because he is able to compare his present state with his recollection of what his condition used to be, but as the disease progresses, insight is lost. Judgment of external situations is similarly affected, partly through faulty perception, partly from inability to draw upon memories of similar situations in the past, and partly because the process of reasoning which precedes judgment requires a capacity for correct association and abstract thought.

Calculation is another faculty which can be interfered with by a disturbance of memory, for if there is amnesia for numbers, mathematical symbols, multiplication tables, and mathematical procedures, dyscalculia must necessarily result.[24, 30] Moreover, when the power to form new memories is grossly disordered, the patient may have forgotten the nature of the problem by the time he is halfway through it. Calculation can also be disturbed by inattention (as in some frontal lobe lesions) and by perseveration or inability to alter the mental "set" as calculation proceeds.

The dilapidation of social graces, manners, and morality which sometimes occurs in the dementing subject has multiple origins. Politeness, consideration for others, cleanliness, and the containment of sexual impulses are things that we are taught, and impairment of memory sometimes plays a part in the loss of these virtues. In other cases the patient knows quite well what he should or should not do, but either does not care (in frontal lesions, for instance), or—in the case of sexual activity—has lost control of the biological drive.

Attention. The capacity to attend or concentrate involves two physiological mechanisms. First, the mind is focused on the chosen object or idea; secondly, irrelevant ideas and distracting sensory stimuli are excluded. For instance, the commuter returning home by train and concentrating on the stock market quotations may be unconscious of the hardness of his seat, the noise of the train, and the arthritis in his knee, but were he not engrossed in his subject he would notice these things. Current experimental work in man and animals suggests that the suppression of unwanted stimuli is made possible by the existence of a neuronal network extending from the sensory-motor cortex to the thalamus and more distant sensory relay stations in the brainstem and spinal cord, and that it is through this system that the brain can modulate sensory inflow in accordance with the needs of the situation (Chap. 1). Whether or not this explanation is correct, the fact remains that attention to a single subject can be achieved in the fullest degree only if distractions are excluded from consciousness. Weakening of attention reduces the patient's capacity to persist with mental or physical tasks and interferes with the formation of memories, because attention, whether from interest, curiosity, fear, or a sense of duty, is essential to the process of memorizing. Another abnormality of attention sometimes seen in organic disease of the brain is the inability to switch from one subject to another, with consequent perseveration of ideas or repetitive activity. Distractibility, which is not the same as inattention, is also seen in lesions of the frontal lobe; the patient's attention is caught and momentarily held by every passing stimulus, and concentration on any one subject is difficult or impossible.

Association. The smell of an orange, received and recognized in the olfactory cortex, conjures up a round yellow object of a particular size and weight, and with a characteristic odor, taste, and texture. Thus, a single olfactory stimulus conjures up a series of related memories, and even just thinking about an orange can have the same effect. The anatomical substrate of this psychological mechanism is presumed to be the association pathways of the brain, which pass from side to side and from end to end. At a higher level of integration, the words "income tax," heard and recognized in the temporal lobe of the dominant hemisphere, are competent to evoke a complex of thoughts and emotions appropriate to the individual's knowledge (i.e., memory) of his own fiscal situation.

Impaired powers of association seriously impede mental processes, contributing to mental slowing, dearth of ideas, and impairment of abstract thought. Their impact on abstract thought is particularly marked, since abstraction requires the mobilization of memories of diverse experiences which must be brought to bear on the subject at hand.[29] Thus, the driver of an automobile slows down when he sees a child standing on the curb because he knows from previous experience that the child may be about to run across the road; in organic dementia (as well as in persons of limited intellect), this capacity to foresee the implications of a situation is often lacking.

Consciousness and Awareness. Full consciousness implies that the patient is fully in touch with his surroundings. In organic psychoses, the level of consciousness can range from normal to coma, but there may be focal disturbances of awareness against a background of general alertness, as in the case of the conscious patient with a parietal lobe lesion of the minor hemisphere, who is unaware that he has a contralateral hemiplegia, ignores visual, auditory, and tactile stimulation on the left side of the body, and may ignore all events occurring on the left-hand side of his immediate surroundings.[5, 33]

The conscious state is thought to be largely dependent on the integrity of the reticular formation and the cerebral cortex. Impairment of consciousness can develop as the result of either generalized cortical depression or localized lesions at various points in the ascending reticular formation in the brainstem and diencephalon. There are certain modifications of full consciousness for which there is no completely satisfactory terminology; for instance, in psychomotor seizures and in postepileptic automatism, the patient is capable of complicated activities which are, however, irrelevant to the needs of the moment and are not remembered afterward. Similarly, following a head injury, there may be a prolonged period of automatism during which the patient appears conscious but may not behave rationally.

Two symptoms which do not fit easily into any single category of intellectual defect are loss of creativity and curiosity. Creativity is eventually impaired by the organic psychoses, though there have been examples of heightened imagination in the early stages, perhaps due to an emotional release comparable to that which is afforded, transiently, by alcohol. Capacity for curiosity is also reduced. Little notice has been taken of this faculty, so important in the history of man's partial conquest of his surroundings. It is seen in its simplest form in children who explore their surroundings, pick up unfamiliar objects, and ask innumerable questions. At a higher level of integration, curiosity asks not only "What?" but also "Why?" A child seeing an apple fall from a tree runs to see what it is, but Isaac Newton asked himself why apples always fall downward. Loss of curiosity is often conspicuous in progressive dementia. Confronted with an unusual situation or an unfamiliar object, the patient ignores it. This lack of interest may sometimes have its roots in faulty perception, defective association, or impairment of memory, but it probably goes deeper, signifying impairment of something which is the psychological equivalent of the biological drives. Whatever its origin, lack of curiosity

contributes to the loss of interest in his surroundings exhibited by the dementing subject.

Disturbances of Affect. Alterations of mood often occur in the course of intoxications and organic disease of the brain. The form of such disturbance is influenced to some extent by the basic character or personality of the individual; the cheerful extrovert may become more cheerful, and the depressed individual become more pessimistic. Sometimes, however, there is a reversal of affect. In old age there is often a physiological flattening of mood, and care must be taken not to read too much into this symptom when it is present in aging persons. It is also necessary to distinguish between emotional disturbances caused by the disease and reactive depression or anxiety. Thus, a patient who has insight into his declining mental powers may become apprehensive and depressed, but since this response requires some capacity for abstract thought (which enables him to see the full implications of his predicament) reactive anxiety tends to diminish as insight is lost, and the patient ultimately becomes apathetic or fatuous and euphoric. Euphoria can occur in the absence of severe dementia. For instance, it is not uncommon in multiple sclerosis, even in patients who realize the severity of their incapacity: "I know my legs are paralyzed, but I feel as if I could run a mile." Euphoria is also seen in some patients with frontal lobe lesions, and takes the form of an unwonted jocularity. Following severe bilateral frontal lesions and after bifrontal lobotomy, facetiousness may be accompanied by a variety of other symptoms, including incessant activity, distractibility, irritability, disregard for social niceties, lack of affection, severe inertia, gluttony — symptoms referred to by Freeman as "the Boy Scout virtues in reverse."

A commonly seen emotional response is the catastrophic reaction, which occurs in patients with moderate incapacity.[10] When confronted with a task or situation which appears to the patient to be beyond his capacity, he becomes agitated and anxious. For example, a brain-injured soldier, while carrying out an intelligence test, suddenly started to tremble, swept the papers and ink to the floor, and rushed out of the room—an attempt to escape from unbearable tension. Another patient, also brain injured, rushed out of his house because the noise made by his small children caused him such extreme tension that he felt himself in danger of assaulting them. Mild catastrophic reactions are also seen in otherwise normal people under conditions of fatigue and severe strain.

When aggressive behavior occurs in a setting of acute delirium, drug intoxication, or chronic brain syndrome, there is no question as to its organic origin, but it is more difficult to determine the causes of habitual aggression in otherwise normal people. The violent temper tantrums of childhood often pass off with advancing maturity, but in some individuals they continue throughout life and are a burden to the individual and to those around him. Psychological studies have linked such episodic aggression with heredity, and in the author's experience this is certainly true in some cases. In other cases, adverse home and social factors may be responsible, but the question still remains as to why certain individuals survive such an environment and others do not. The cause of the outburst is often trivial, or seems so to the outsider, and things said and done during the attack may not be remembered afterwards. The episodes are often triggered by alcohol, a cortical depressant. In some cases, the electroencephalogram reveals diffuse abnormalities of a nonspecific type, but the attacks last too long to be considered epileptic. It is pertinent that Williams[57] found abnormal EEG recordings in 57 per cent of a large group of habitually aggressive delinquents; the abnormalities almost invariably involved the anterior part of the cerebrum, and the anterior temporal lobes were involved in all cases.

Attacks of rage are sometimes encountered for the first time following brain damage from disease or trauma. They are not uncommon in children as a result of encephalitis lethargica, a disease with a particular impact on the diencephalon. The author has seen episodic rage in a boy of 5 years following the removal of an interparietal meningioma which involved both cingulate gyri. Attacks of rage have also been seen in cases of tumors of the pellucidum and septal area. Such attacks are akin to the sham rage produced in experimental animals by lesions in the anterior hypothalamus and by electrical stimulation of various points in the limbic system. Heath and his colleagues[31] produced episodes of rage in a conscious schizophrenic patient by electrical stimulation of the amygdaloid nucleus. In some cases, aggressive outbursts have been reduced or abolished by surgical attack on the amygdala or the posteromedial hypothalamus. Mark and Ervin[37] provide a bibliography of work in this important field.

These clinical and laboratory observations sustain the view of Cannon and of Papez that the limbic system is the anatomical substrate for the expression of emotional responses, and that such responses can be excessive and inappropriate when the limbic system is partly removed from cortical control.

Emotional responses depend on a variety of factors, including perception, bodily comfort, the satisfaction or frustration of biological drives, a sense of security, social conditioning, powers of association, etc. Thus, perceptual misinterpretation may lead to fear or anger, as in the delirious patient who thinks that his nurse with a syringe constitutes a threat to him. Pain and other forms of physical discomfort provoke anxiety, depression, or anger. Frustration of biological drives—thirst, hunger, sex—have effects which are known to all. Threats to security, either real or imaginary, give rise to anxiety and fear. Failure to recognize the implications of a situation can influence emotional responses, as for instance in the patient who inadvertently sets a match to his bed, but exhibits no fear and takes no avoiding action until he experiences the pain of a burn.

It would be a mistake to attribute all the emotional explosions encountered in the organic psychoses to liberation of diencephalic structures from cortical control, however, because the patient with hallucinations, delusions, or illusions may be reacting appropriately when he evinces fear, pleasure, or aggressive tendencies.

In the final stages of dementia, the patient is entirely lacking in emotional responses, but in some cases bursts of apparently causeless laughter, weeping, or both, may occur. Such pathological laughter or weeping is accompanied by all the physical signs of emotion and is usually attributed to loss of cortical control. When these reactions occur in persons who are not demented, or are only mildly so (as in pseudobulbar palsy), the nature of the response is often appropriate to the quality of the stimulus but is excessive: A funny remark or even just smiling at the patient will set off a gale of laughter, while reference to some only mildly unpleasant matter may induce tears. In one case, the patient, who was suffering from bilateral pyramidal disease, said in reference to an attack of weeping that he didn't feel "all that sad," but in severely demented individuals, it is often impossible to identify the stimulus which elicits this curious response.

CLINICAL FEATURES OF THE ACUTE ORGANIC BRAIN SYNDROME (DELIRIUM)

Mental symptoms arising suddenly in a person who has previously been psychologically normal constitute a medical emergency in which great care must be exercised to avoid missing an organic disorder. When organic disease is present, the symptoms can be due either to a severe intoxication or to cerebral disease in a previously normal individual, or to a comparatively minor affection in a person who is vulnerable by reason of old age, general enfeeblement, or preexisting cerebral disease; the latter is particularly true of the liability to delirium in elderly people suffering from infections such as pneumonia and gram-negative septicemia from infection of the urinary tract.

Etiology. The causes of the acute organic brain syndrome cover so wide a spectrum that only the more common can be mentioned here. They include (1) head injuries and cerebral fat embolism from injuries to long bones and subcutaneous tissue; (2) intracranial infections, e.g., meningitis, encephalitis (notably herpes simplex encephalitis), brain abscess, cerebral malaria, rabies; (3) parainfectious conditions, such as Sydenham's chorea and postinfectious encephalomyelitis; (4) intoxications from generalized infections, e.g., pneumonia, acute pyelonephritis, septicemia, typhoid fever, etc.; (5) endogenous intoxications, e.g., hepatic failure, uremia, hypoglycemia, hypoxia, carbon dioxide narcosis,[48] hypocalcemia, hypernatremia, water intoxication, acute porphyria, thyrotoxicosis, addisonian crises; (6) exogenous intoxications, e.g., alcohol, carbon monoxide, LSD, encephalopathy due to heavy metals such as lead, arsenic, gold, etc.; idiosyncrasy to drugs; overdosage with bromides, barbiturates, tranquilizers, opium and its derivatives, Dilantin, mescaline, cannabis indica, belladonna, etc.; (7) drug and alcohol withdrawal in addicts; (8) cerebrovascular accidents; (9) postepileptic automatism; (10) nutritional deficiency, as in Wernicke's disease, Korsakoff's psychosis, and severe pellagra; (11) heat stroke and heat exhaustion; (12) acute episodes of confusion and amnesia in tumors of the third ventricle[58] and neoplasms undergoing rapid cystic degeneration; (13) acute exacerbations of mental symptoms in patients with chronic degenerative diseases of the brain, such as Huntington's chorea, multiple sclerosis, and the diffuse scleroses; (14) puerperal psychoses, some of which appear to be due to exhaustion and toxemia; (15) recurrent pancreatitis, usually in chronic alcoholics.

Symptoms. The acute organic psychoses are characterized by delirium or by confusion short of delirium.[21, 23, 38] There is disorientation for time and place, based on faulty perception and defective memory,[59] together with distractibility, restlessness, excitement, and (sometimes) aggressive activity. Illusions and hallucinations are common. In short, virtually any of the symptoms described above as characteristic of the organic brain syndrome may appear, albeit in variable combinations and degrees of severity. In encephalitis, bizarre disorders of behavior may occur without headache, meningism, or significant fever; the psychosis can resemble an episode of schizophrenia.

Delirium tremens is described in Chapter 21. It differs in many ways from the delirium of acute infections. The characteristics of the latter deserve mention, although it has become rare since the introduction of chemotherapy.

The intensity of febrile delirium is usually proportional to the intensity of the infection, though not necessarily to the height of the temperature, since pyrexia may be slight in elderly individuals and in persons with an overwhelming infection. In the mildest cases, the delirium occurs only at night and consists of a mild wandering of the mind, a kind of half-dreamy condition from which the patient can be temporarily recalled by conversation. When it is more severe, there is more or less continuous clouding of consciousness, well seen in typhoid fever. The name *typhoid* is derived from Greek for "cloud." The patient often talks to himself in a quiet, rambling fashion, is disoriented for time and place, and his attention is poor. Illusions and hallucinations may occur, with appropriate reactions on the part of the patient. Delusions may appear, but are usually changeable rather than fixed. The patient tugs at his sheets, or keeps picking up imaginary objects from his bed coverings. His mental experiences are usually unpleasant and frightening, but occasionally there are intervals of happiness and jocularity. If the underlying infection is brought under control, the delirium gradually passes off; if not, the patient passes into stupor and coma. During recovery from febrile delirium, he may show impairment of memory for recent events, and some degree of inattention and mental fatigability, but complete recovery is usual when the delirium has been due to an extracerebral infection. On the other hand, when it results from severe meningitis or encephalitis, mental impairment may persist.

Differential Diagnosis. It is important to be able to distinguish promptly between acute organic brain syndromes and other acute psychological illness, notably schizophrenia, hypomania, and depression. In the acute primary psychoses, orientation for time and place is usually unaffected and there is no neurological or systemic sign of disease, injury, or intoxication. In hysterical amnesia, the memory defect is usually either too gross or too spotty to be consistent with an organic origin; in the spotty type, there is complete clarity for some things and complete amnesia for others. In the functional neuroses and psychoses, the electroencephalogram will not show the diffuse slowing usually seen in the acute organic brain syndrome.

CLINICAL FEATURES OF THE CHRONIC ORGANIC BRAIN SYNDROME

Neurological interest in the organic reaction type of mental disease centers mainly around chronic forms, whether stationary or progressive, for these are the cases the neurologist is most likely to encounter. The clinical features appear in a variety of combinations and degrees of severity, depending on the nature, situation, and extent of the disease and upon the previous personality and attainments of the patient, but common to them all is some degree of intellectual loss, together with affective disturbances and consequent changes of personality and disorders of behavior.

Etiology. In countries with high standards of personal, public, and industrial hygiene, the most common causes of the organic psychoses are cerebrovascular disease, senility, tumors of the brain, and severe head injuries. General paresis, at one time the most important single cause of organic dementia, is now relatively uncommon, and in general, other infections do not play a considerable role in the production of the organic psychoses (African trypanosomiasis excepted). Progressive cerebral degenerations, both familial and sporadic, have to be kept in mind, notably the presenile dementias of Pick and Alzheimer, "normal pressure" hydrocephalus, hepatolenticular degeneration, Huntington's chorea, amaurotic familial idiocy and other cerebral lipidoses, the progressive leukodystrophies, and occasional cases of multiple sclerosis. Endocrine disorders in the form of myxedema, thyrotoxicosis, and hyperparathyroidism yield occasional cases of the organic brain syndrome. The mental disorders associated with untreated pellagra and subacute combined disease have become uncommon in recent years, but unhappily the thiamine-deficiency syndromes induced by chronic alcoholism are still common. Chronic deterioration from exogenous and endogenous intoxications (bromides, opium, manganese, hepatic disease, etc.), is not common. The mental and behavioral changes seen in some severe chronic epileptics are usually due to multiple factors, some of which are functional and some organic (Chap. 7).

Insufficient attention has been given to the fact that lesions of deep midline structures, which involve the limbic system, can cause mental dilapidation.[6] Mental symptoms are sometimes the first to appear in tumors involving the corpus callosum and cingulate gyri, the septal area, the third ventricle, and the inframedial aspect of the temporal lobes. Apathy is a prominent early sign in such cases. Severe memory impairment is a prominent feature of bilateral hippocampal lesions, commonly as a result of

vascular disease. Goldberg and Norton[9] have described two patients with bronchial carcinoma who had a gross memory defect and were demented, and in whom the pathological findings consisted of both inflammatory and degenerative changes concentrated mainly in the temporal parts of the limbic gray matter. Friedman and Allen[8] reported a case of complete limbic destruction following acute encephalitis in an adult male who displayed gross memory failure, excessive motor activity, loss of sustained goal-directed activity, uninhibited verbal sexuality, impotence, and docility. The confusion and memory defects which occur in the early stages of Wernicke's syndrome provide an example of the impact on mental processes of diffuse lesions in the hypothalamus and thalamus.[54] Mental symptoms can be an early feature of tumors of the brainstem (Chap. 16).

Clinical Features. The pattern of symptoms varies from case to case, and any or all of the features of organic dementia may contribute to the ultimate mosaic, but common to them all there is an ultimate failure of intellect, disturbances of mood, disorders of biological drives, and consequent aberrations of overt behavior.

In most cases, the symptoms develop very slowly and a considerable time may elapse before they reach a degree of severity sufficient to bring the patient to the doctor. In many instances, it is the family or the patient's colleagues who first realize that all is not well. There is a loss of spontaneity, lack of drive and initiative, and slowness in decision-making. Social activities are avoided and creative activity dwindles. The capacity to concentrate and to persist in uncongenial tasks is diminished. There is a lessening of interest in new ideas. Affect is not blunted at this stage; on the contrary, since the patient has insight, he may become anxious and irritable. Tolerance for alcohol and sedatives is decreased.

As the condition continues, there is progressive slowing in thought, speech, and action. Abstract thought, including judgment, is obviously impaired. There is difficulty in initiating plans, with consequent procrastination. All the tools of the intellect are blunted, and there is often a conspicuous slowness of comprehension. The patient becomes careless in dress and personal hygiene. The defect of memory interferes to an increasing degree with normal efficiency in the conduct of daily tasks. Some patients are hyperactive and others just sit quietly. Gross errors of judgment occur both domestically and in business activities. Explosions of irritability may occur, and unreasonable likes and dislikes appear; this can lead the individual to change his will inappropriately. There is sometimes difficulty in switching the mind from one subject to another, and this disability may cause perseveration in speech. When the frontal lobe is involved, there may also be perseveration of movement —for instance, when the patient is asked to draw a single circle, he will continue drawing circles. This is usually associated with a grasp reflex. As a rule, sexual vigor is much diminished, but in some cases there is a loss of life-long reticence in sexual matters. The symptoms are often aggravated by surgical operations, intercurrent infections, changes of domicile, or domestic troubles.

Ultimately, the patient becomes mindless, incontinent of urine and feces, unable to talk or to comprehend what is said, and unable to walk.

The speed of this process depends upon the underlying disease; it may take several years, as in Alzheimer's disease, or it may be compressed into a few weeks or months; again, in some diseases, such as general paresis, the process of deterioration can be stopped by appropriate treatment.

DISORDERS OF CONSCIOUSNESS

Somnolence, stupor, and coma may be considered as different degrees of the same thing. In somnolence, the patient is sleepy but can be aroused to make appropriate verbal and motor responses. In stupor, there may be occasional spontaneous movements, and the patient can be aroused by vigorous stimuli to make avoidance movements. In coma, he is totally unresponsive. In akinetic mutism, the patient lies with his eyes open and with an appearance of wakefulness, which is belied by mutism and by a total disregard for environmental and painful stimuli. All these conditions can result from either structural lesions or biochemical disorders involving the reticular formation of the upper brainstem or its projection to the thalamus. Akinetic mutism (p. 39) can also be produced by bilateral destruction of the cingulate gyri. Widespread disease *limited* to the cortex can give rise to dementia and reduced awareness to particular stimuli, but not to coma. There is, of course, early and severe cortical depression in general intoxications, hypoxia, hypoglycemia, and head injury, but it is thought that in such cases the level of consciousness is determined by the effect of these conditions on the reticular formation rather than on cortical function per se.

THE DIFFERENTIAL DIAGNOSIS OF COMA

When unconsciousness occurs as an intercurrent or terminal event in the course of an illness, the nature of which is understood, there is seldom any difficulty in coming to a conclusion as to the cause of the coma, but it is more difficult to identify the cause when coma is the presenting sign, as for instance in the case of a patient who is found unconscious in bed.[7, 43] Under these circumstances, a large number of possibilities has to be kept in mind, and since prompt diagnosis can be a matter of life or death, it is desirable to follow a scheme which gives priority to the identification of conditions which are amenable to immediate treatment. The order of priority varies to some extent with geography and circumstances. Thus, cerebral malaria and heat stroke must be accorded a higher priority in the tropics than in temperate climates, and in West Africa, trypanosomiasis deserves a higher place than it does in New York. Treatable conditions include diabetic coma, hypoglycemia, extradural and subdural hemorrhage, poisoning (drugs, alcohol, carbon monoxide), bacterial meningitis, cerebral abscess, cerebral malaria, heat stroke, long exposure to cold, vitamin B deficiency, myxedema,[41] hyper- and hyponatremia, hypercalcemia, carbon dioxide narcosis,[48] uremia, the apoplectic type of general paresis, pituitary apoplexy, Addison's disease, some cases of hepatic coma, hypertensive encephalopathy and eclampsia, and (rarely) colloid cysts of the third ventricle.[58] Treatment seldom avails when coma is due to intercerebral or subarachnoid hemorrhage.

In some cases there is a dual pathology —for instance, alcoholic intoxication plus head injury, hepatic failure plus subdural hematoma, concussion plus hypoxia from internal hemorrhage.

A second pitfall is to be misled by circumstantial evidence; for instance, a seaman taken from the engine room of a ship in the tropics may be suffering from cerebral malaria or a stroke and not from heat stroke. Alcohol on the breath does not necessarily indicate alcoholic coma. The fact that the patient is a known diabetic does not necessarily mean that the coma is due to diabetic ketosis or hyperinsulinism. A head injury sustained in a fall may not be the whole answer to the patient's condition, for he may have fallen as the result of a seizure, stroke, or subarachnoid hemorrhage. An empty medicine bottle by the bedside may suggest attempted suicide, but other conditions should be looked for as well. In accidental electrocution, unconsciousness may be due not to the electric shock but to a head injury sustained when the victim was hurled to the ground.

IRREVERSIBLE COMA

Improvements in methods of resuscitation sometimes result in an individual whose heart continues to beat but whose brain is irretrievably damaged. A brain that no longer functions and has no possibility of functioning again is for all practical purposes dead. The continued survival of the remainder of the body, in such instances, depends on procedures which are costly in terms of manpower, money, and the occupancy of beds sorely needed for patients for whom something effective can be done. The Ad Hoc Committee of the Harvard Medical School, which was formed to examine the definition of brain death, has suggested four criteria for the determination of this state of affairs: (1) The patient is totally unaware of externally applied stimuli and of his inner needs, and is totally unresponsive. (2) There is no spontaneous breathing and there are no muscular movements. (3) Reflex activity is in abeyance: The pupil is fixed, dilated, and unresponsive to bright light, and there is no ocular movement in response to head turning or irrigating of the ears with ice water; in addition, there is no evidence of postural activity, such as decerebrate rigidity. Swallowing, yawning, and vocalization are in abeyance; corneal and pharyngeal reflexes are absent; the tendon reflexes cannot be elicited; noxious stimulation to the sole of the foot produces no response. (4) The electroencephalogram is entirely flat; one channel should be used as a noncephalic lead to pick up and identify space-borne and vibration-borne artifacts.

If all these criteria are satisfied over a period of 24 hours, the brain may be deemed to be dead *except* in the presence of hypothermia (below 32.2°C.) or when the coma is the result of barbiturate intoxication.

PSYCHOLOGICAL TESTS

A great deal of ingenuity has gone into devising means of quantitating intellectual endowment, knowledge acquired by education, and personality traits. By the application of a battery of such tests, and by careful observation of the manner in which the patient performs them, much helpful information may be derived, provided that the tests are carried out by an experienced psychologist and that it is recognized that the test situation itself introduces a factor to which not all patients react in the same way. In the present context—the organic psychoses—such tests have several uses: (1) The detection of organically determined impairment in patients who have developed psychotic symptoms, as, for instance, a schizophrenia-like picture uncovered by a cerebral tumor or head injury; (2) the measurement of the organic factors involved in patients with known brain damage who have developed neurotic or psychotic patterns of behavior—especially compensation cases and other situations in which the fact of secondary gain has to be considered; (3) the evaluation of progress, i.e., improvement or deterioration, in organic psychoses; (4) a guide to the best type of employment in nonprogressive cases of brain injury, e.g., after head injury, meningitis, encephalitis, etc., and to the educational possibilities of children with focal disabilities such as word blindness; (5) to assist the physician in deciding whether psychological treatment is needed to enable the patient to adjust to his incapacity; (6) research on brain-mind relationships.

However, facilities for skilled and comprehensive psychometric tests are not available everywhere, so physicians are often faced with the necessity of deciding from their own observations whether or not mental symptoms are organic. Fortunately, a reasonably accurate assessment can be made at the bedside or in the office, without recourse to formal testing devices, by means of a few simple tests of memory, calculation, orientation, insight, sustained attention, comprehension, and abstract thinking.[20, 26] Observations as to mood, the presence or absence of hallucinations, illusions, delusions, tics and mannerisms, and general behavior are helpful, but on the whole they are less useful than intellectual tests in distinguishing between organic and nonorganic psychoses. Focal neurological defects, such as aphasia, agnosia, apraxia, hemianopia, etc., or impairment of the level of consciousness, imply that at least some of the mental symptoms are organic in origin.

Defects often become apparent during history-taking and physical examination. It is also desirable to interview friends, relatives, or colleagues, because they are often able to supply facts which the patient may not himself realize, such as a recent change of personality, inefficiency in domestic or professional affairs, disturbance of mood, etc. This is particularly important in the early stage of an organic dementia since the patient may retain sufficient social graces and intellectual flexibility to hide his incapacity. In these early cases, it is often difficult to apply psychometric tests because the patient may be apt to become hostile unless the interrogation is suitably camouflaged. It may be quite appropriate to ask a dementing patient, "Who is buried in Grant's tomb?" but the question is unlikely to be well received by an intelligent banker with a mild disability. Emotional lability and irritability are features of many cases of early dementia, and the chances of eliciting useful information from an antagonized patient are slim.

Tests of mental capacity are best carried out at the end of the neurologic examination, not only because defects are more apparent when the patient is tired, but also because his responses during physical examination may have disclosed inattention, defective comprehension, aphasia, slowing of the stream of thought, or affective disturbances. Furthermore, observation of his behavior will sometimes suggest the presence of hallucinations: He may suddenly break off the conversation and appear to be listening, or he may appear to be watching the progress of an invisible something across the room. Similarly, an attitude of fear or suspicion may betoken delusions.

In the carrying out of psychometry, it is desirable to take into consideration the intellectual, educational, social, and national background of the patient and to modify the testing procedure in accordance with this background. It is also necessary to remember that the results of an examination will not necessarily be reduplicated on later occasions; on the contrary, the level of performance often varies from day to day and from hour to hour, and for this reason it is desirable to repeat the tests, especially in patients who are suspected to be suffering from an organic psychosis but in whom the initial examination has failed to reveal that anything is amiss.

Mental testing can be satisfactorily carried out only if the patient is fully alert; somnolence and stupor vitiate results, as does any considerable degree of sensory or motor aphasia. It is therefore necessary to start by determining the presence or absence of aphasia, minor degrees of which are easy to miss unless speech function is specifically tested. Another organic sign is apraxia, which will occasionally become obvious during the course of physical examination: e.g., in ideational apraxia the patient is unable to see how to set about performing a skilled task. Constructional apraxia is elicited by asking him to copy a simple design with matchsticks or with a child's building blocks. The examiner can then proceed to test for agnosia: Can the patient recognize a book, a face, a picture, letters, words, figures, familiar sounds? Can he recognize objects by touch alone?

Memory is important: Can the patient give an accurate account of events during the preceding hour or two? Can he give his personal history, with dates? Is his fund of general information appropriate to his educational background? Can he repeat a man's name, a flower, and a street address after five minutes? Can he repeat seven digits forward? How often must a test sentence be repeated before he is word perfect (e.g., One thing a nation must have to become rich and great is a large and secure supply of wood)?

Orientation for place and time is easily disposed of by asking the patient where he thinks he is and what time, day, and week it is. Disorientation for person is uncommon, depending as it does on an obliteration of the patient's personal life memories, as in some bilateral temporal lobe lesions. A special form of disorientation is inability to distinguish between left and right, which is found in some cases with a lesion in the region of the angular gyrus of the dominant hemisphere.

Attention—the patient's capacity to concentrate on one subject—is often weakened in the organic psychoses, and this is usually obvious by the time the history has been taken. Sometimes the converse is seen, it being difficult to get the patient to switch his attention from one subject to the next one—a form of perseveration.

Insight is determined by the patient's view of his present condition and his ideas as to what he will do when he leaves hospital. Judgment is more difficult to assess. It depends on the capacity for abstract thought as well as accurate perception, memory, and powers of association. Impairment of judgment in the course of a man's work or domestic affairs is often an early symptom, so that the earliest and best evidence may come from the patient's associates or family. He can be asked whether he thinks that the President of the United States should be a temporary or a lifelong appointment, or whether farmers are more useful than bankers, or whether $20,000 a year is a suitable salary for a stenographer, or whether expensive books are better than cheap ones.

Capacity for arithmetical calculation is often disturbed in the organic psychoses. The patient is asked to do serial subtractions of 7 from 100, to multiply or divide simple figures, to state what the annual interest would be on a thousand dollars at $4\frac{1}{2}$ per cent, or to calculate what change should be received after tendering a five dollar bill for something which costs one dollar and twenty-three cents. Obviously the level of test should be appropriate to the educational background of the patient.

Affect, or mood, can be observed and described but cannot be measured. Is the patient's affect appropriate to his condition, or is it unduly elevated or significantly depressed? Is there evidence of emotional lability or excessive irritability? Is there any evidence of pathological laughter or weeping?

The patient's motor behavior can be revealing. Reference has already been made to apraxia. Perseveration, wherein the patient continues with a given activity, and finds difficulty in switching to a new task, is sometimes seen in organic psychoses. Excessive and painstaking orderliness and its converse, slovenliness, can give a clue to the presence of an organic defect. A sign of parietal lobe involvement which will escape notice unless special tests are conducted is the result of spatial disorientation. If he is asked to draw a clock face or a flower, the left-hand side of these objects may be poorly represented or left out, in the case of a right parietal lesion; when he is instructed to draw a map of the United States, the western half of the country may receive scant attention. When writing a letter, the patient may cram it into the right-hand side of the paper, leaving the left untouched.[5, 33] Again, the patient may ignore sounds and sights in the left-hand side of extrapersonal space, and may fail to recognize his left arm and leg as his own. These and other features of the parietal lobe syndrome are discussed in Chapter 16.

Expanded accounts of these and other clinical tests, some of which do not require the services of a skilled psychologist, can be obtained from the texts recorded in the bibliography.[3, 4, 26, 34]

GENERAL REFERENCES

1. Bender, M. B.: *Disorders in Perception.* Charles C Thomas, Springfield, Ill., 1952.
2. Brain, R.: *Speech Disorders, Aphasia, Apraxia, and Agnosia.* Butterworth and Co., Washington, D. C., 1961.
3. Catell, R. B.: *A Guide to Mental Testing.* University of London Press, London, 1948.
4. *Clinical Examinations in Neurology.* Mayo Clinic and Mayo Foundation. W. B. Saunders Co., Philadelphia, 1963.
5. Critchley, M.: *The Parietal Lobes.* Edward Arnold, London, 1953.
6. Elliott, F. A.: The corpus callosum, cingulate gyrus, septum pellucidum, septal area and fornix. *Handbook of Clinical Neurology,* Edited by Vinken, P. J., and Bruyn, G. W., North Holland Publishing Company, Amsterdam, 1969, Vol. 2, pp. 758–775.
7. Fazekas, J. F., and Alman, R. W.: *Coma.* Charles C Thomas, Springfield, Ill., 1962.
8. Friedman, H. M., and Allen, N.: Chronic effects of complete limbic lobe destruction in man. *Neurology* 19:679, 1969.
9. Goldberg, G. J., and Norton, A. R.: "Limbic encephalitis" and its association with carcinoma. *Brain* 91:481, 1968.
10. Goldstein, K.: Functional disturbances in brain damage. *American Handbook of Psychiatry.* Basic Books, Inc., New York, 1959, Chap. 39.
11. Halstead, W. C.: *Brain and Intelligence: A Quantitative Study of the Frontal Lobes.* University of Chicago Press, Chicago, 1947.
12. Hebb, D. O.: *The Organization of Behavior.* John Wiley and Sons, Inc., New York, 1949.
13. Herrick, C. J.: *The Evolution of Human Nature.* University of Texas Press, Austin, 1956.
14. Herrick, C. J.: The nature and origins of human mentation. *World Neurol.* 2:1027, 1961.
15. Humphrey, G., and Coxon, R. V.: *The Chemistry of Thinking.* Charles C Thomas, Springfield, Ill., 1963.
16. McIlwain, H.: *Biochemistry and the Cerebral Nervous System.* Little, Brown and Co., Boston, 1959.
17. Russell, W. R.: *Brain, Memory and Learning.* Clarendon Press, Oxford, 1959.
18. Schmitt, F. O.: *Macromolecular Specificity and Biological Memory.* Massachusetts Institute of Technology Press, Cambridge, 1962.
19. Waelder, R.: *Basic Theory of Psychoanalysis.* International Universities Press, Inc., New York, 1960.
20. Wells, F. L., and Ruesch, J.: *The Mental Examiner's Handbook.* The Psychological Corporation, New York, 1942.

SPECIAL REFERENCES

21. Bleuler, M.: Psychiatry of cerebral diseases. *Brit. Med. J.* 2:1233, 1951.
22. Brierley, J. B.: Clinico-pathological correlations in amnesia. *Gerontol. Clin.* 3:97, 1961.
23. Cobb, S.: Neurology. *American Handbook of Psychiatry.* Basic Books, Inc., New York, 1959, Chap. 81.
24. Cohn, R.: Dyscalculia. *Arch. Neurol.* 4:301, 1961.
25. Denny–Brown, D.: The frontal lobes and their function. *Modern Trends in Neurology.* Edited by Feiling, A., Paul B. Hoeber Div., Harper and Row, New York, 1951, Chap. 2.
26. Denny–Brown, D.: *Handbook of Neurological Examination and Case Recording.* Harvard University Press, Cambridge, 1960.
27. Gerard, R. W.: Brain and behavior. *American*

Handbook of Psychiatry. Basic Books, Inc., New York, 1959, Chap. 80.

28. Goldstein, K.: Significance of frontal lobes for mental performances. *J. Neurol. Psychopath.* 17:27, 1936.

29. Goldstein, K.: *The Organism.* American Book, New York, 1939.

30. Grewel, F.: Acalculia. *Brain* 75:397, 1952.

31. Heath, R. G., Monroe, R. R., and Mickle, W. A.: Stimulation of the amygdaloid nucleus in a schizophrenic. *Amer. J. Psychiat.* 111:862, 1955.

32. Himwich, H. E.: *Brain Metabolism and Cerebral Disorders.* The Williams & Wilkins Co., Baltimore, 1951.

33. Horenstein, S.: Parietal lobe disorders. *Med. Sci.* 13:35, 1963.

34. Jervis, G. A.: The mental deficiencies. *American Handbook of Psychiatry.* Basic Books, Inc., New York, 1959, Chap. 63.

35. Kety, S. S.: Contribution of biochemistry to psychiatry. *Trans. Stud. Coll. Phys. Phila.* 29:101, 1962.

36. Lewis, A.: Amnesic syndromes; the psychopathological aspect. *Proc. Roy. Soc. Med.* 54:955, 1961.

37. Mark, V. H., and Ervin, F. R.: *Violence and the Brain.* Harper and Row, Inc., New York, 1970.

38. Mayer–Gross, W., Slater, E., and Roth, M.: *Clinical Psychiatry.* The Williams & Wilkins Co., Baltimore, 1960, pp. 15–36, 419–543.

39. Mulder, D.: Psychoses with brain tumors and other chronic neurological disorders. *American Handbook of Psychiatry.* Basic Books, Inc., New York, 1959, Chap. 55.

40. Nielsen, J. M.: Amnesia for life experiences. *Bull. Los Angeles Neurol. Soc.* 23:143, 1958.

41. Nordquist, P., Dhuner, K. G., Stenberg, K., and Orndahl, G.: Myxoedema coma and CO_2 retention. *Acta Med. Scand.* 166:189, 1960.

42. Nyssen, R.: Contribution experimentale à l'étude de l'amnésie de fixation dans la maladie de Korsakow d'origine alcoolique. *Acta Neurol. Psychiat. Belg.* 57:639, 1957.

43. Plum, F., Posner, J. B.: Diagnosis of Stupor and Coma. F. A. Davis Co., Philadelphia, 1966.

44. Rose, F. C., and Symonds, C. P.: Persistent memory defect following encephalitis. *Brain* 83:195, 1960.

45. Russell, W. R.: The physiology of memory. *Proc. Roy. Soc. Med.* 51:9, 1958.

46. Russell, W. R., and Nathan, P. W.: Traumatic amnesia. *Brain* 69:280, 1946.

47. Scoville, W. B., and Milner, B.: Loss of recent memory after bilateral hippocampal lesions. *J. Neurol. Neurosurg. Psychiat.* 20:11, 1957.

48. Sieker, H. O., and Hickam, J. B.: Carbon dioxide intoxication: The clinical syndrome, its etiology and management. *Medicine* 35:389, 1956.

49. Symonds, C. P.: Disease of mind and disorder of brain. *Brit. Med. J.* 2:1, 1960.

50. Talland, G. A., and Ekdahl, M.: Psychological studies of Korsakoff's psychosis: IV. The rate and mode of forgetting narrative material. *J. Nerv. Ment. Dis.* 129:391, 1959.

51. Teuber, H.-L.: Perception. *Handbook of Physiology.* American Physiological Society, Washington, D.C., 1960, Vol. 3, Chap. 65.

52. Teuber, H.-L.: The riddle of frontal lobe function in man. *Frontal Granular Cortex and Behavior.* Edited by Akert, J., and Warren, J. M., McGraw-Hill Book Co., Inc., New York, 1963.

53. Teuber, H.-L., and Weinstein, C.: Ability to discover hidden figures after cerebral lesions. *Arch. Neurol. Psychiat.* 76:369, 1956.

54. Victor, M., Angevine, J. B., Mancall, E. L., and Fischer, C. M.: Memory loss with lesions of the hippocampal formation. *Arch. Neurol.* 5:244, 1961.

55. Wechsler, I. S.: *Clinical Neurology.* 9th Ed. W. B. Saunders Co., Philadelphia, 1963.

56. Whitty, C. W. M.: Mental changes as a presenting feature in subcortical cerebral lesions. *J. Ment. Sci.* 102:719, 1956.

57. Williams, D.: Neural factors related to habitual aggression. *Brain* 92:503, 1969.

58. Williams, M., and Pennybacker, J.: Memory disturbances in third ventricle tumors. *J. Neurol. Neurosurg. Psychiat.* 17:115, 1954.

59. Williams, M., and Zangwill, O. L.: Disorders of temporal judgment associated with amnesic states. *J. Ment. Sci.* 96:484, 1950.

CHAPTER FIVE

Disorders of the Hypothalamus and Vegetative Nervous System

Although the hypothalamus is small, accounting for only about 0.3 per cent of the total brain weight, it is the chief center for the maintenance of the internal milieu of the body, exercising its metabolic and visceral functions through the pituitary gland and the autonomic nervous system. There is no organ or system of the body which wholly escapes its influence. Furthermore, the hypothalamus serves as a link between mind and body in that the physical manifestations of emotion, such as fear and anger, are mediated via the parasympathetic-sympathetic-hypothalamic complex, as are the visceral disturbances resulting from emotional conflicts. The word "center" is misleading if it is taken to imply central control, for in health there is nothing autonomous about this or any other portion of the brain. The hypothalamus is itself influenced by inputs from the cortex,[25] subcortical gray matter, and sensory pathways, by the osmolarity of the blood, and by the plasma levels of certain hormones and glucose (Fig. 5–1). For instance, the amount of ACTH secreted by the anterior pituitary in response to electrical stimulation of the lateral hypothalamic nuclei depends to some extent on the existing blood level of the hormone. Again, the hypothalamus controls the body temperature only in the sense that it adjusts the several factors concerned in the maintenance of normal temperature in response to sensory input from the surface of the body (e.g., cold or heat) and the temperature of its own blood supply.

Anatomy. The hypothalamus occupies the floor and walls of the third ventricle and extends from the optic chiasm in front to the interpeduncular region behind; its upper limit is the sulcus hypothalamicus, which separates it from the thalamus.[17] This traditional anatomical definition leaves out the medial and lateral preoptic nuclei in front of the chiasm, although they are linked both functionally and anatomically with the anterior group of hypothalamic nuclei.

THE NUCLEI. The nuclei of the hypothalamus (Fig. 5–2) fall into three broad functional groups: those largely concerned with the parasympathetic nervous system; those which have a predominantly sympathetic function; and a group which link the nervous system to the endocrine system via the pituitary gland.[15, 17, 23] It is often stated that the anterior portion of the hypothalamus is predominantly parasympathetic in function, while the posterior portion represents the head ganglion of the sympathetic nervous system, but this is only an approximation; sympathetic effects can be derived from stimulation of the

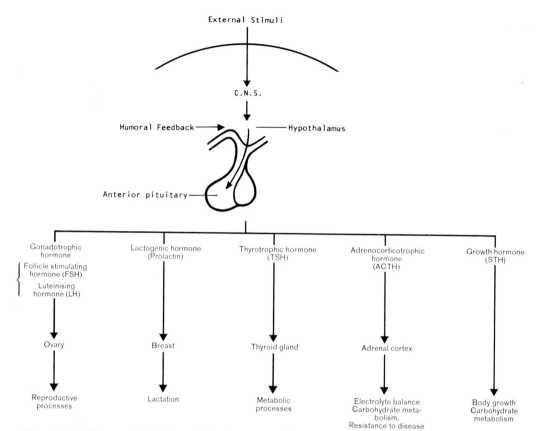

Figure 5–1.   Diagram illustrating relationships among the central nervous system, anterior pituitary gland, and the peripheral effects exerted by the anterior pituitary hormones. (Adapted from Harris, G. W.: Triangle 4:242, 1964.)

anterior portion, and parasympathetic effects from stimulation of the posterior portion.

The preoptic nuclei, two on each side, extend above and in front of the optic recess. Their functions in man are not known, but in animals, electrical stimulation in this area causes contraction of the bladder.

The lateral hypothalamic nucleus is an ill-defined collection of cells which lies in the wall of the third ventricle and is continuous in front with the lateral preoptic nucleus and behind with the gray matter of the midbrain tegmentum. Stimulation of this nucleus causes inhibition of peristalsis, loss of tone in the stomach and small intestine, and dilatation of the pupil.

The supraoptic, paraventricular, and tuberal nuclei are intimately concerned with the pituitary gland, with which they have both vascular and neural connections of a unique type.[16, 17, 23] The supraoptic nucleus straddles the dorsal aspect of the chiasm and gives rise to the supraoptico-hypophyseal tract. Some fibers from the paraventricular nucleus join the tract, which ends on blood vessels amid the cells of the neural hypophysis. The antidiuretic hormone (ADH) is formed in the cells of the supraoptic nucleus and carried down the tract to the neurohypophysis. Oxytocin, on the other hand, is thought to be liberated within the neural hypophysis itself. Sectioning of the hypophyseal stalk does not necessarily produce diabetes insipidus, because ADH is secreted into the blood from the proximal end of the

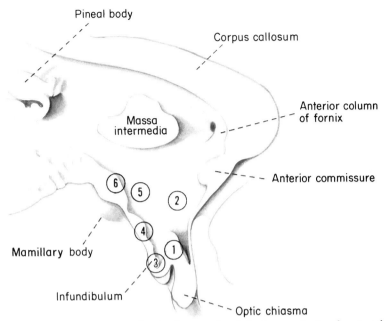

Figure 5–2. Median section through the third ventricle of the human brain, showing the approximate positions of some hypothalamic nuclei. 1, Supraoptic; 2, paraventricular; 3, tubero-infundibular group; 4, ventromedial; 5, dorsomedial; 6, posterior hypothalamic. (Adapted from LeGros Clark, W. E.: *The Hypothalamus.* Oliver & Boyd, Edinburgh, 1938.)

stalk, whereas oxytocin is not secreted, because the efferent nerve fibers required for its production have been interrupted.

The tuberal nuclei are grouped around the tuber cinereum, from which the infundibulum or pituitary stalk descends to the hypophysis. Fibers from these nuclei end on the tufts of the capillaries found in the infundibulum. These tufts are part of the portal system,[17] which consists of two sets of capillaries, one in the hypothalamus and the other in the hypophysis, joined by a venous plexus. This system is not connected with the exceptionally well developed vascular supply to the supraoptic and paraventricular nuclei, which have almost twice as many capillaries per unit volume as the rest of the brain, a circumstance which suggests that they have chemoreceptor and osmoreceptor functions. The nerve fibers from the tuberal nuclei liberate hormonal substances into the capillaries of the infun-

dibulum and these substances are carried by the portal vessels to the anterior pituitary, where they excite or inhibit the secretion of hormones (ACTH, gonadotropins, growth hormones, and thyrotrophin). The sympathetic nerve supply to the adrenal medulla provides a second link between the hypothalamus and the endocrine system.

The tuberal nuclei project to the brainstem as well as to the portal capillaries. Both in animals and in man, lesions confined to the tuberal region give rise to obesity and gonadal failure (as in the Frölich syndrome), and animal experiments suggest that this area of the hypothalamus contains centers for thirst, hunger, and satiety.

Caudal to the tuberal area lies the posterior hypothalamic nucleus, which is continuous posteriorly with the gray matter of the midbrain tegmentum, and is intimately linked by the efferent outflow from the hypothalamus to the brainstem.

THE MAMILLARY BODIES. Behind the posterior hypothalamic nucleus lie the large and well defined mamillary bodies, which receive: (1) afferent fibers from the hippocampus via the fornix; (2) an important input via the mamillary peduncle from the medial lemniscus in the brainstem, so bringing the hypothalamus into relation with somatic sensory pathways; and (3) fibers from the cingulate gyrus by way of the mamillothalamic tract. This tract is largely efferent, however, and serves to connect the mamillary bodies with the anterior nucleus of the thalamus and thereby with the cingulate gyrus and frontal lobe. A second significant efferent system is the mamillotegmental tract, part of which passes to the third nerve nucleus. Lesions in the region of the mamillary bodies induce somnolence and cataplexy in animals.

Although the efferent and afferent pathways of the hypothalamus are not as yet fully understood, in general it may be said that the hypothalamus receives inputs from the cortex (especially the cingulate gyrus, the orbital portion of the frontal lobe, and the hippocampal gyrus), from subcortical gray matter, including the amygdaloid nucleus, corpus striatum, and thalamus, and from the medial lemniscus in the brainstem. It is also influenced by the chemical and hormonal constituents, and the temperature, of its own blood supply.

The complex of hypothalamic nuclei serves as the "head ganglion" of the parasympathetic and sympathetic nervous systems, which pass down through the brainstem to the vagus nerve and the cord. In animal experiments,[1, 17] stimulation of appropriate areas in the anterior portion of the hypothalamus can effect a reduction of heart rate, peripheral vasodilatation, and a fall of blood pressure. It can also either increase or decrease the tonus and motility of the gastrointestinal tract, and it increases the secretion of hydrochloric acid, saliva, and tears. Blood flow to the splanchnic area is also influenced. The tone and motility of the bladder can be increased, and evacuation may occur. The rate and depth of respiration is reduced, and the pupil is constricted. A destructive lesion in this area can produce hyperpyrexia.

Stimulation of the posterior and ventromedial hypothalamic nuclei[1, 15, 17] usually produces peripheral vasoconstriction, increased blood flow to the heart, lungs, and skeletal muscle, acceleration of heart rate, and increased arterial blood pressure. Respiration is increased in rate and depth, and the motility and tone of the gastrointestinal tract and bladder are inhibited. The posterior hypothalamus also possesses a temperature regulating function which controls the response of the body to ambient low temperatures by bringing about shivering, piloerection, and peripheral vasoconstriction. The effects of experimental hypothalamic lesions on appetite and thirst are discussed later in this chapter. Many of the visceral effects produced by stimulation of the hypothalamus can also be induced by stimulating the sensory-motor cortex, the cingulate gyrus, the orbital cortex, and the temporal lobe.[15, 25]

CLINICAL ASPECTS OF HYPOTHALAMIC LESIONS

In general, acute lesions are more likely to produce symptoms than a slowly progressive disease. It is remarkable how few visceral or metabolic effects are encountered in large tumors of this region so long as they grow slowly; consequently, the absence of signs of hypothalamic disorder does not exclude the possibility of disease in this region. A second point of practical importance is that disease affecting the hypothalamus may also interfere with neighboring structures, notably the pituitary gland and the hippocampal gyrus, and care must be exercised to distinguish between symptoms of hypothalamic origin and those resulting from the effects of disease on these structures. Third, it is important to remember that posterior fossa tumors can affect hypothalamic function by producing internal hydrocephalus, with consequent pressure on the floor and walls of the third ventricle.

Hunger and Thirst. There is evidence that the hypothalamus exerts direct control on the sensations of hunger, thirst, and satiety. [1, 6, 14, 26, 29, 31] Destruction of the ventromedial nucleus in the rat or cat causes voracious eating and a rapid gain in weight for a few days; the animal does not realize when he has had enough, and this area of the hypothalamus has therefore been referred to as "the satiety center." Stimulation of the hypothalamus lateral to the tuberal nuclei produces overeating and overdrinking in cats, and destruction of this area causes abrupt cessation of eating. The parallel between these behavioral disturbances in the experimental animal and the psychogenic alterations in appetite that occur in man is striking.[11]

DIABETES INSIPIDUS. Diabetes insipidus, characterized by thirst and the production of large quantities of urine with a low specific gravity, is one of the commonest symptoms of damage to the tuberal region of the hypothalamus.[6,7,16,17] In some cases, however, it occurs without any known etiological basis. When it results from injury or progressive disease, it may exist on its own or in association with obesity, hypersomnia, amenorrhea, impotence and serum electrolyte disturbances. A rare cause of polyuria and polydipsia is failure of the renal tubules to respond to the antidiuretic hormone, which is produced in normal amount. This usually occurs as a hereditary defect in male infants (Chap. 11).

Etiology. Vasopressin is produced in the bodies of the neurons of the supraoptic nuclei and is transported down the axons of these neurons to be stored in axon terminals in the posterior pituitary gland. The fact that diabetes insipidus does not necessarily develop in patients after sectioning of the pituitary stalk or in disease of the posterior pituitary indicates that the hormone can be released into the bloodstream from the hypothalamus. Vasopressin is secreted (1) when blood osmolarity is increased, or (2) when extracellular fluid volume is depleted. It alters the permeability of the distal portion of the renal tubules.

Diabetes insipidus is likely to arise as the result of any condition which damages the hypothalamus or the stalk of the pituitary. It can occur as a result of head injury, subarachnoid hemorrhage, meningitis, pituitary tumors (when they erupt out of the sella) and other tumors in this region.

Diagnosis. Polyuria can also be the result of compulsive water drinking,[11] in which event the plasma osmolarity is somewhat reduced, in contrast to the elevated osmolarity of diabetes insipidus. Second, polyuria occurs in nephrogenic diabetes insipidus, which is rare. Third, mild polyuria can occur in association with hypercalcemia and hyperkalemia. Fourth, polyuria is associated with chronic renal insufficiency and uncontrolled diabetes mellitus. The diagnosis of diabetes insipidus can be established by giving the patient 0.1 to 0.2 I.U. of aqueous vasopressin intravenously; in the patient with diabetes insipidus there will usually be a prompt reduction of urine volume, whereas a patient with nephrogenic diabetes insipidus does not respond to this treatment. However, it should be noted that *in diabetes insipidus the response to the initial administration of vasopressin may be poor, but it improves after repeated medication.*

Treatment. If polyuria and thirst are not severe, the patient can be allowed to drink his fill, and specific therapy is not required. If this does not suffice, the patient should be given an intramuscular injection of 4 to 5 I.U. of vasopressin tannate in oil. This will give relief for from three to five days. The administration of thiazide diuretics can reduce polyuria in patients with diabetes insipidus, and the same is true of chlorpropamide, an oral hypoglycemic agent, in doses of 500 mg. daily. For patients with nephrogenic diabetes insipidus, thiazide diuretics are the only form of therapy available. Snuff-containing pitressin, repeated two or three times per day, can control diabetes insipidus, but it can give rise to a troublesome rhinitis, and it is less effective than intramuscular pitressin tannate in oil.

Bulimia. Excessive hunger is less common than polydipsia in hypothalamic lesions. It is also seen in bilateral lesions of the frontal lobe, including diffuse diseases of the cortex, such as Alzheimer's or Pick's disease and following bilateral prefrontal leukotomy and bilateral temporal lobectomy. A mild form can occur during treatment with cortisone and ACTH, and it is seen in lymphoblastic leukemia. The patient, like the experimental animal, fails to appreciate a sense of satiety. In the Kleine-Levin syndrome,[20] excessive hunger is associated with periodic attacks of hypersomnia, motor unrest, and mental confusion; it is usually attributed, on theoretical grounds, to a lesion in the region of the hypothalamus. Voracious eating of both food and inedible objects is a feature of the Kluver-Bucy syndrome, first reported in Rhesus monkeys following bilateral temporal lobectomy, but also seen occasionally as the result of bilateral temporal lobe lesions in man.[29] The bulimia is associated with visual agnosia (including inability to recognize natural enemies), extreme visual distractibility, loss of aggressive behavior, and heightened sexual activity. Human patients will eat meal after meal and may even attempt to eat things other than food; with recovery, there is complete amnesia for the events of the illness.[29]

Obesity and Wasting. Extreme obesity can result from hypothalamic lesions. If the disease responsible for it occurs before adolescence, there is no stunting of growth, unlike the situation with pituitary obesity. Most cases of hypothalamic obesity also show other disturbances such as polyuria, sexual dystrophy, or hypersomnia. The commonest cause of obesity is, of course, compulsive overeating.

Wasting can occur in infants as the result of a tumor or other disease involving the hypothalamus.[31] In adults, there may be slight loss of weight and strength, but extreme cachexia always suggests damage to the pituitary. This occurs in Simmonds' syndrome, which is characterized by loss of weight, anorexia, atrophy of the skin, loss of hair, muscular weak-

ness, sensitivity to cold, bradycardia, and a lowered metabolic rate. First described as a result of infarction of the pituitary in a case of postpartum hemorrhage, this type of wasting is also seen in other acute lesions of the pituitary, including head injuries and rapidly growing tumors, and following hypophysectomy. Pituitary cachexia reflects the effect of a loss of anterior pituitary hormones on the thyroid, suprarenal cortex, and gonads. It can be imitated by anorexia nervosa, which usually occurs in neurotic young women who abstain from eating.

The treatment of emaciation—whether from hypothalamic or pituitary disorders—is by administration of steroids, thyroid extract, testosterone, and a high protein diet. Extra salt may be required.

Sexual Disorders. Gonadal disturbances are common in hypothalamic lesions. Children may show either sexual retardation or (rarely) precocity.[7] When the damage to the hypothalamus occurs after puberty, there may be impotence or amenorrhea. Amenorrhea and persistent galactorrhea (the Chiari-Frommel syndrome) can occur when the hypothalamus is encroached upon by tumors such as a craniopharyngioma or pituitary tumor.[3]

Precocious puberty has long been known to occur with tumors in the region of the pineal and has also been seen in gliomas infiltrating the mammillary bodies. It usually occurs in males, but a few cases have been seen in young female children, who exhibit both the physical and the mental features of sexual maturity. This precocity may exist on its own for a year or two before other evidence of hypothalamic tumor appears. Episodic or persistent eroticism is occasionally seen in adults in the presence of lesions of the septal area, below the genu of the corpus callosum. It also occurs when the hypothalamus is "released" by bilateral removal of the temporal lobes in man.

Disturbances of Sleep. The waking state is the normal response of man to his external and internal milieu and seems to be maintained by the play of sensory inputs upon the activating mechanisms of the reticular formation, reinforced by mental and emotional factors. Both the tegmental and lower brainstem elements of the reticular formation receive contributions from the medial lemniscus, the special senses, the caudal part of the hypothalamus, the cortex, the thalamus, the amygdala, the hippocampus, the septal nuclei, and the caudate nucleus. Reduction of sensory inputs doubtless plays a part in the production of normal sleep, which is facilitated by a dark room, a comfortable bed, and a quiet mind. A reduction of input to the reticular formation as the result of a lesion of the posterior end of the hypothalamus is one cause of pathological somnolence and of the deep sleep which can occur in animals after interruption of the projection of the tegmental reticular formation to the thalamus, hypothalamus, and cortex. Low-frequency stimulation of the zone between the thalamus and the hypothalamus can also produce somnolence in animals, presumably by blocking the activating system of the reticular formation.[17]

Hypersomnia is a feature of some diseases affecting the caudal portion of the hypothalamus. It was seen in the epidemic of encephalitis lethargica in 1918; in some cases, pathological changes were conspicuous in this area and in the upper part of the brainstem. Somnolence may also be seen in Wernicke's encephalopathy, midbrain tumors, and inflammatory or neoplastic lesions of the posterior hypothalamus. Periodic attacks of hypersomnia during the day are also a feature of the Kleine-Levin[14, 20] syndrome, which is usually encountered in adolescence. In addition to episodic hypersomnia, the patient becomes withdrawn and timid, eats and drinks too much, and gains weight. Aberrant sexual behavior has been described in males. The attacks may occur at intervals of months in otherwise apparently healthy individuals but they have also been seen following head injuries and in some cases of intracranial tumor and encephalitis.

Bilateral lesions of the anterior portion of the cingulate gyrus can cause hypersomnia, coma, or akinetic mutism in man and experimental animals.[4] Stimulation of this area can give rise to excitement and sympathetic effects.

Thermal Regulation. Moderate pyrexia can occur during the course of diseases affecting the hypothalamus.[28] Fatal hyperpyrexia sometimes follows head injuries and surgical operations in this neighborhood and also occurs in acute vascular lesions of the pons. The author has seen recurrent, brief attacks of hyperpyrexia without other evidence of hypothalamic disturbance in a woman suffering from multiple sclerosis. Pyrexia of hypothalamic origin is easily identified because it does not give rise to malaise or to the appearance of severe illness which accompanies similar degrees of fever from infections, and it is not affected by antipyretic agents. It is often accompanied by coldness of the extremities and can be controlled by the administration of chlorpromazine and by cold sponging and other physical methods used to induce hypothermia.

Hypothermia is sometimes caused by diseases of the hypothalamus, such as tumors and angiomas, and both hypothermia and poikilothermia have been reported following acute trauma to the upper cervical spinal cord,[18] presumably as a result of damage to the sympathetics, since complete removal of the sympathetic in animals renders them poikilothermic. Duff has reported two cases of idiopathic hypothermia,[12] in one of which the attacks were preceded by sweating. In a patient seen by the author, a girl of 18, several attacks of hypersomnia lasting two or three days occurred, and these were accompanied by fluid retention, a fall of temperature to 96° F., bradycardia, and extreme slowness of thought and speech when aroused. Ten years later, the attacks have disappeared and no evidence of progressive hypothalamic disease has appeared. Fox and his colleagues have reported the case of a young man who suffered from repeated episodes of hypothermia, which were demonstrably the result of defects in the heat conserving mechanism—i.e., peripheral vasoconstriction and shivering. Autopsy revealed a localized but severe degenerative lesion in the anterior hypothalamus. On one occasion, the patient developed transient cardiac arrest associated with hypokalemia.

Miscellaneous Disorders. The *blood cytology* can be disturbed by hypothalamic lesions. An increased red cell count amounting to true polycythemia can occur in the absence of hemoconcentration, and polymorph leukocytosis has been recorded from time to time in the absence of infection.[7]

The *blood sugar*[1,7] may be raised in acute lesions of the hypothalamus, as for instance in head injuries, subarachnoid hemorrhage, and acute meningitis. The presence of high blood sugar in a comatose patient may suggest a diagnosis of diabetic coma, but the absence of ketones in the serum and urine will clarify the situation.

Gastric and duodenal ulceration with consequent bleeding may accompany acute hypothalamic lesions in man and in animals, and similar ulceration can be produced by prolonged electrical stimulation of the anterior portion of the hypothalamus, so long as the vagi are intact. Lesions can also be induced by stimulation of the vagi alone. Severe melena has occurred from time to time in tumors of the third and fourth ventricles, and in acute lesions of the upper thoracic spinal cord.[7]

Cardiovascular effects are sometimes seen.[15,25] They include paroxysmal hypertension, periodic hypotension, paroxysmal tachycardia, sinus tachycardia, bradycardia, and changes in the electrocardiogram. Intermittent attacks of orthostatic hypotension can be the first symptom of a craniopharyngioma,[30] antedating the appearance of other symptoms by months or even years. The EKG changes found following strokes, subarachnoid hemorrhage, and acute lesions of the brainstem and hypothalamus bear a superficial resemblance to the effects of myocardial infarction.[9] After intracerebral or subarachnoid hemorrhage, the typical pattern in the limb leads is one of flat or negative T waves and prolongation of the QT interval. There may be a prominent U wave. These changes are not results of variations of body temperature, abnormalities of the serum electrolytes, or the blood pressure. The cause is not known, but similar abnormalities have been recorded following electrical stimulation of the vagus in the region of the carotid body and of area 13 of the orbital cortex.

Alterations in serum electrolytes and fluid balance sometimes occur after head injuries, subarachnoid hemorrhage, and neurosurgical operations in the vicinity of the hypothalamus. Diabetes insipidus has already been referred to. Brisman and Chertorian[5] have recorded the case of a child with a hypothalamic glioma, in whom there was discontinuous inappropriate secretion of antidiuretic hormone and a persistent hyponatremia. Reeves and Plum[26] report the case of a 20-year-old woman who developed hyperphagia and obesity, aggressive behavior, dementia with hallucinations, diabetes insipidus, diabetes mellitus, pyrexia, and hypofunctioning of the adrenal, thyroid, and gonads. She was found to have a circumscribed hamartoma, which had destroyed the ventromedial hypothalamus bilaterally as well as the median eminence. Killeffer and Stern[19] described a case of a female child who died six years after the removal of a craniopharyngioma. She had displayed deficiencies in the regulation of body fluid, endocrine deficiencies, behavioral abnormalities, hyperphagia, disturbance of sleep pattern, and abnormalities of body temperature. There was destruction of the anterior and middle portions of the hypothalamus, with partial preservation of the more caudal hypothalamus and the pituitary gland.

Psychological symptoms are sometimes seen in acute lesions of the hypothalamus. They include excitement, pathological weeping and laughter, disorientation, hallucinations, uncontrollable rage, and the emotional accompaniments of diencephalic epilepsy. It will be recalled that attacks of sham rage can be caused by a lesion in front of the preoptic nucleus.

Micturition and Defecation

MICTURITION. The bladder is innervated by parasympathetic and sympathetic fibers, of which the former are the more important. The preganglionic parasympathetic fibers leave the spinal cord at S3, with small contributions from S2 and S4, and pass to the bladder via the pelvic nerves (nervi erigentes) and the inferior hypogastric plexus, to synapse with postganglionic neurons in ganglia in the bladder wall. These parasympathetic fibers are the efferents for the detrusor muscle and the internal sphincter.

The sympathetic supply seems to be relatively unimportant. The preganglionic fibers are from the upper lumbar and lower thoracic segments of the spinal cord. The postganglionic fibers from the lumbar prevertebral ganglia and preaortic nerve plexus descend along the abdominal aorta to form the presacral "nerve" (the superior hypogastric plexus), which divides into the hypogastric nerves. These pass downwards over the anterior surface of the sacrum to join the inferior hypogastric plexus.

Efferent fibers, conveying the sense of bladder fullness, traverse the pelvic nerves. Pain from the trigone is conveyed by the pelvic nerve, and from the remainder of the bladder by the hypogastric nerves. According to Nathan and Smith,[21, 22] efferent fibers conveying pain, thermal sensations, and the awareness of fullness, are located near the surface of the cord at the junction of the pyramidal and spinothalamic tracts, opposite the central canal, while axons subserving the muscular control of urination lie more medially.

After unilateral percutaneous spinothalamic cordotomy, micturition may be temporarily impaired, but it soon recovers. After a bilateral operation, about 20 per cent of the patients remain unaware that the bladder is full and may lose voluntary control of the sphincter. When the spinothalamic tracts are cut on both sides by open operation, the incidence of bladder symptoms is greater.

Fairly effective emptying of the bladder can usually be reestablished by local sacral reflex arcs, but evacuation is seldom complete. A similar situation exists with disease of the cauda equina, conus, and spinal cord.

The cerebral influence on the bladder is best illustrated by the urgent need to evacuate a full bladder at the sound of running water. In disease states, it is exemplified by the bladder disturbances which can occur early, as the first symptom of organic cerebral lesions. These are usually situated in or near the midline—the paracentral lobule on the medial aspect of the hemispheres, the anterior portion of the cingulate gyrus, the posterior portion of the first frontal convolution,[2] the septal area, the septum pellucidum, and the anterior part of the hypothalamus. Parasagittal tumors, aneurysms of the anterior cerebral artery and the anterior communicating artery, and gliomas of midline structures are to be thought of. Symptoms of the same type may occur for a brief period following frontal leukotomy.[2] The earliest disturbances of micturition are urgency and increased frequency, and *distention of the bladder is not felt.* Retention may occur. There is also impairment of the ability to suppress micturition, which must be distinguished from the "incontinence" which arises from indifference to social niceties in the course of diseases involving the frontal lobes.

Disturbances of micturition occur in disease of the brainstem. To the author's knowledge, most of the information on this topic comes from animal experiments. Micturition, a stretch reflex of the bladder, is subject to facilitation and inhibition from several levels of the nervous system, including the cerebrum, hypothalamus, the brainstem, and the spinal cord. This work, summarized by Ruch,[27] may or may not be applicable to man. It would be interesting to learn, for instance, whether bladder disturbances are ever the *presenting* symptom of disease limited to the brainstem.

In neurological practice, the majority of cases with disorder of micturition are found to have disease of the spinal cord, the cauda equina, the posterior nerve roots (tabes dorsalis), and the peripheral autonomic nerves (diabetes). Retention with overflow *may precede* all other clinical symptoms and signs of diabetes.

Nocturnal enuresis in highly strung but otherwise normal children is probably the result of delayed development of the adult capacity to inhibit reflex bladder evacuation. The habit may persist into adolescence for psychological reasons and is best treated by encouraging the patient to resist the temptation to evacuate the bladder during daytime, thereby raising the stretch threshold of the bladder.

Treatment. Stimulation of the parasympathetic fibers by a subcutaneous injection of an acetylcholine preparation, such as urechol, is useful on a short-term basis, but if retention continues for more than 4 hours, a Foley catheter should be inserted and the urine should be released every two hours. The bladder should be irrigated with antibiotics in solution (neomycin, 100 mg.; polymyxin, 25 mg. in 1 liter of water) twice daily during the first few weeks. A wide-spectrum antibiotic can also be given orally. If the bladder shows signs of returning function, the patient can be trained to encourage reflex evacuation by bending forward and pressing upon the lower abdominal wall.

The irritable bladder, manifested by frequency and precipitancy of micturition, can be helped by belladonna, or by propantheline bromide in doses of 15 mg. four times per day.

A sheath attached by a tube to a polyethylene bag which is strapped to the thigh can be used to protect male patients from occasional incontinence, especially at night, but no apparatus is available for women.

DEFECATION. The physiology of defecation is identical with that of micturition, but the spinal parasympathetic "center" lies in the second, third, fourth, and fifth sacral segments. There is a reciprocal relationship between the rectum and the anal sphincters; distention of the former leads to reflex relaxation of the latter. Acute lesions of the spinal cord above the sacral segments are followed by atony of both the rectum and the sphincters. If the feces are solid, constipation results, and if they are liquid, there is dribbling incontinence. Later on, tone returns to the sphincter, with consequent constipation, and still later, reflex

evacuation may occur from time to time as it does in the bladder. When the sacral segments or their roots are destroyed, both the rectum and the sphincter remain relaxed, and *reflex evacuation does not occur;* there is then obstinate constipation if the feces are solid, and intractable incontinence if they are loose.

The effects of acute lesions of the spinal cord and brain on defecation follow the same general pattern exhibited by the bladder, but the rectum and anal sphincter usually recover more quickly and more completely than the bladder. Disturbances of defecation can occur as an isolated symptom of early disease of the spinal cord or brain.[25]

Disturbances of Sweating. The hypothalamus is connected by efferent and afferent tracts to subsidiary nuclei in the brainstem and spinal cord, which give rise to two sets of efferent fibers, the sympathetic and the parasympathetic. The latter emerge in the third, seventh, ninth, and tenth cranial nerves and the second, third, and fourth sacral roots, and pass to minute ganglia situated in or near the viscera to which they are directed.

The sympathetic system is anatomically more distinct and more compact; the efferent tracts traverse the reticular formation of the brainstem and the lateral columns of the cord. The preganglionic neurons lie in the intermediolateral and intermediomedial cell columns in the thoracic and upper lumbar segments (T1 to L2 or L3) of the spinal cord. From there, a fresh relay passes out in the corresponding ventral roots to the sympathetic chain of ganglia, whence they are distributed to the same viscera as the parasympathetic and also, via somatic nerves and around major blood vessels, to the sweat glands and to the blood vessels throughout the body. Those destined for the sweat glands of the face and head come from T1 and T2, those for the upper limb from T4 through T8, those for the trunk from T5 to T12, and those for the leg from T10 to L3.

Sweat glands are of two types, exocrine and apocrine. Both are innervated by sympathetic nerves. In man, the postganglionic fibers to the exocrine glands are usually considered to be cholinergic in type, and they control thermoregulatory sweating. The apocrine glands in the axilla, on the other hand, respond to adrenergic stimulation, which explains axillary sweating in response to fear and anxiety. Emotion can also give rise to "cold sweat" (i.e., without vasodilation) on the palms of the hands, the soles of the feet, the forehead, and the axilla.

Generalized hyperhidrosis occurs in fever, shock, and emotional disturbances, and as a response to external heat. It can occur, intermittently, as a result of a lesion of the hypothalamus. Excessive sweating of the hands and feet is an embarrassing congenital condition which is devoid of neurological significance and which can be cured by bilateral sympathectomy. Localized sweating of the face on one or both sides sometimes occurs as a response to highly seasoned foods (gustatory sweating) in otherwise normal subjects.

Flushing and profuse sweating of the skin of the temple induced by mastication—the auriculotemporal syndrome—sometimes follows injury to the auriculotemporal nerve in the neck or as the result of parotitis with local scarring; occasionally it occurs without antecedent disease or injury.

Hyperhidrosis of the face, arm, and leg is sometimes seen in hemiplegia as the result of a cortical or capsular lesion. Anhidrosis on one side of the face and on the opposite side of the body can occur in lesions of the pons or medulla. Acute transection of the spinal cord is followed by transient dryness of the skin below the level of the lesion; this can be a useful localizing sign in an unconscious patient. As reflex activity returns to the isolated section of the cord, sweating returns and is much increased during mass reflexes. A transverse lesion of the neuraxis at any point between the upper part of the midbrain and the first thoracic segment renders an animal poikilothermic, and the same thing has been seen in man as the result of acute lesions of the upper cervical cord, though hypothermia is more usual.[18]

Interruption of the cervical sympathetic below the level of the bifurcation of the common carotid artery causes anhidrosis of the face, ptosis, and miosis on the affected side (Horner's syndrome). It is occasionally seen in syringomyelia and other lesions of the cervical and upper thoracic segments of the cord. Destruction of the upper two or three lumbar roots causes anhidrosis in the lower limb.

Hyperhidrosis is seen in familial dysautonomia (the Riley-Day syndrome). This rare disorder occurs mainly in Jewish children and is attributed to an autosomal recessive gene. Some of the symptoms appear to be the result of an inborn error of catecholamine metabolism which results in an increased excretion of homovanillic acid in the urine, but this does not explain all the clinical features. The condition usually is recognized shortly after birth. The infant has episodes of cyanosis and vomiting, unexplained fever, and difficulty in sucking. Convulsions may occur. There is decreased lacrimation, marked hyperhidrosis, and intermittent hypertension. These symptoms may be associated with relative insensitivity to pain, which can lead to corneal laceration and lesions of the skin. There may be hypotonia, arreflexia, dysarthria, and dysphagia. Increased susceptibility to infection often leads to early death, but those who survive may show some improvement. The pathological basis of the disorder is not fully understood. Abnormalities have been found in the peripheral autonomic ganglia, the posterior columns of the cord, and the reticular formation of the brainstem, but such changes have not always been present in the few cases that have come to autopsy.

The effect of peripheral nerve lesions on sweating is discussed in Chapter 18.

REFERENCES

1. Anderson, F., and Haymaker, W.: Disorders of the hypothalamus and pituitary gland. *Clinical Neurology.* 2nd Ed. Edited by Baker, A. B., Paul B. Hoeber Div., Harper and Row, New York, 1962, Chap. 27.

2. Anderson, J., and Nathan, P. W.: Lesions of

the anterior frontal lobes and disturbances of micturition and defecation. *Brain* 87:233, 1964.

3. Anderson, M. S., Erickson, L. S., and Luse, S. A.: Chiari-Frommel syndrome associated with a craniopharyngioma in a woman of 28. *Neurology* 12:583, 1962.

4. Barris, R. W., and Schuman, H. R.: Bilateral anterior cingulate gyrus lesions. *Neurology* 3:44, 1953.

5. Brisman, R., and Chertorian, A. M.: Inappropriate antidiuretic hormone secretion. *Arch. Neurol.* 23:63, 1970.

6. Brobeck, J. R.: Regulation of feeding and drinking. *Handbook of Physiology.* American Physiological Society, Washington, D.C., 1960, Vol. 2, Chap. 47.

7. Clarke, W. E. LeG., Beattie, J., Riddoch, G., and Dott, N.: *The Hypothalamus.* Oliver and Boyd, London, 1938.

8. Crompton, M. R.: Hypothalamic lesion following the rupture of a cerebral berry aneurysm. *Brain* 86:301, 1963.

9. Cropp, J. G., and Manning, G. W.: Electrocardiographic changes simulating myocardial ischemia and infarction associated with spontaneous intracranial hemorrhage. *Circulation* 22:25, 1960.

10. Dercum, F.: Three cases of a hitherto unclassified affection resembling in its grosser aspect obesity but associated with special nervous system symptoms: Adiposis dolorosa. *Amer. J. Med. Sci.* 104:521, 1892.

11. DeWardener, H. E., and Barlow, E. D.: Compulsive water drinking. *Quart. J. Med.* 27:567, 1958.

12. Duff, R. S., Farrant, P. C., Leveaux, V. M., and Wray, S. M.: Spontaneous periodic hypothermia. *Quart. J. Med.* 30:329, 1961.

13. Fox, R. H., Davies, T. W., Marsh, F. P., and Urich, H.: Hypothermia in a young man with an anterior hypothalamic lesion. *Lancet* 2:185, 1970.

14. Gallinek, A.: Syndrome of episodes of hypersomnia, bulimia, and abnormal mental states. *J.A.M.A.* 154:1081, 1954.

15. Gillilan, L. A.: *Clinical Aspects of the Autonomic Nervous System.* Little, Brown and Co., Boston, 1954.

16. Harris, G. W.: *Neural Control of the Pituitary Gland.* Edward Arnold Publishers, Ltd. London, 1955.

17. Haymaker, W., Anderson, E., and Nanta, W. J. H.: *The Hypothalamus.* Charles C Thomas Springfield, Ill., 1969.

18. Holmes, G.: Spinal injuries of warfare. *Brit. Med. J.* 2:815, 1915.

19. Killeffer, F. A., and Stern, W. E.: Chronic effects of hypothalamic injury. *Arch. Neurol.* 22:419, 1970.

20. Levin, M.: Periodic somnolence and morbid hunger: A new syndrome. *Brain* 59:494, 1936.

21. Nathan, P. W., and Smith, M.: The centripetal pathway from the bladder and urethra within the spinal cord. *J. Neurol. Neurosurg. Psychiat.* 14:262, 1951.

22. Nathan, P. W., and Smith, M.: The centrifugal pathway for micturition within the spinal cord. *J. Neurol. Neurosurg. Psychiat.* 21:177, 1958.

23. Ortmann, R.: Neurosecretion. *Handbook of Physiology.* American Physiological Society, Washington, D. C., 1960, Vol. 2, Chap. 40.

24. Payne, R. W., and DeWardener, H. E.: Reversal of urinary diurnal rhythm following head injury. *Lancet* 1:1098, 1958.

25. Pool, J. L.: The visceral brain of man. *J. Neurosurg.* 11:45, 1959.

26. Reeves, A. G., and Plum, F.: Hyperphagia, rage, and dementia accompanying a ventromedial hypothalamic neoplasm. *Arch. Neurol.* 20:616, 1969.

27. Ruch, T. C., and Patton, H. D.: *Physiology and Biophysics.* W. B. Saunders Co., Philadelphia, 1965.

28. Strom, G.: Central nervous regulation of body temperature. *Handbook of Physiology.* American Physiological Society, Washington, D.C., 1960, Vol. 2, Section 1, Chap. 46.

29. Terzian, H., and Ore, G. D.: Syndromes of Kluver and Bucy reproduced in man by bilateral removal of temporal lobes. *Neurology* 5:373, 1955.

30. Thomas, J. E., Schirger, A., Love, J. G., and Hoffman, D. L.: Orthostatic hypotension as the presenting sign in craniopharyngioma. *Neurology* 11:418, 1961.

31. White, P. T., and Ross, A. T.: Inanition syndrome in infants with anterior hypothalamic neoplasms. *Neurology* 13:974, 1963.

CHAPTER SIX

Disorders of the Cranial Nerves

THE OLFACTORY NERVE

Unmyelinated fibers from nerve cells embedded in the mucosa of the upper part of the nose pierce the cribriform plate and turn backward along the olfactory groove in the floor of the anterior fossa to terminate in the olfactory bulb, beneath the frontal lobe. A fresh relay passes to the cortical olfactory center in the uncus of the hippocampal gyrus,[4] anterolateral to the optic chiasm and the pituitary fossa. These relationships explain the occurrence of anosmia in diseases of the nasal mucosa, severe head injuries (which tear the delicate olfactory fibers as they thread the cribriform plate), meningioma arising from the olfactory groove, tumors of the frontal lobe, and meningitis.

The relationship of the hippocampus to the pituitary and to the optic chiasm is emphasized by the uncinate attacks which sometimes occur when the uncus is involved by a pituitary tumor, suprasellar cyst, or glioma of the chiasm. Tumors, vascular malformations, and traumatic scars of the temporal lobe are also sources of uncinate attacks which are characterized by a sudden hallucination of smell or taste, followed by a peculiar dreamy state, during which there may be smacking of the lips, champing of the jaws, and swallowing movements; these may or may not develop into a generalized convulsion.

Increased sensitivity of smell and taste is seen in cases of cystic fibrosis and adrenal insufficiency.[26]

VISION

The majority of all complaints of visual disturbance are due to refractive errors, opacities of the conducting media, glaucoma, or disease of the retina—that is to say, the symptoms are ophthalmic rather than neurological in origin. It is therefore necessary to assess the efficiency of the eye as an optical instrument before looking for a neurological basis for visual defects. If no ocular abnormality is found, or if any abnormality which is present fails to account for all the visual symptoms, attention must be directed toward four possibilities. (1) There may be interference with nerve conduction between the retina and the occipital cortex, in which event there will be defects in the visual fields. (2) There may be a lesion of the parieto-occipital cortex, which is concerned with the interpretation of what is seen; the fields may or may not be grossly normal, depending on whether the underlying optic radiation is damaged, but the patient cannot recognize the nature or significance of what he sees (visual agnosia). (3) The visual fields are normal and recognition is intact, but movement of the eyes is interfered with. The usual disturbance under this head-ing is diplopia. (4) Vision may be disturbed as a symptom of neurosis or psychosis.

The detection of visual impairment in cooperative patients is satisfactorily accomplished by measuring corrected visual acuity and charting the visual fields by the perimeter and tangent screen. These methods cannot be applied to babies and very young children, to retarded children and adults, or to stuporous or comatose patients of any age. Harden and Pampiglioni [23] have applied a neurophysiological approach to such cases. They combine electroretinography, visually evoked responses, and electroencephalography. With this technique, it is often possible to detect a visual impairment, and to determine whether the disease is in the retina, the optic nerves, or the brain.

The Visual Pathways

THE OPTIC NERVES

Impulses generated by light in the rods and cones of the retina are relayed through a layer of bipolar cells to the dendrites of the ganglion cells of the retina. Axons from the lateral part of the retina do not run through the macula, but circle it. The macula represents the area of maximum visual acuity, and is used when we look directly at an object. Consequently, this is the portion of the visual field which is involved in tests for visual acuity by test-types. A small hemorrhage at this point will impair central vision, as for instance in hypertensive retinopathy, or thrombosis of the central vein of the retina, whereas hemorrhages and exudates of comparable size situated peripherally cause scotomas which are seldom noticed by the patient.

At the optic disc, the nerve fibers bend sharply backward to form the optic nerve, and it is at this point that they are vulnerable to the increase of intraocular pressure which occurs in glaucoma; nerve fiber bundles are involved, with a corresponding loss of vision in the retinal seg-

ments which they supply. Nerve fiber bundles can also be destroyed by the proliferation of glial connective tissue which follows the resolution of papilledema, with consequent constriction of the peripheral fields. The optic nerve, clothed in an extension of the meninges, is frequently involved by retrobulbar neuritis and occasionally by disease in the orbit.[7] It traverses the orbit on its way to the optic foramen through which it accompanies the ophthalmic artery into the cranial cavity. In the "foramen," which is more a canal, it may be affected by closed head injuries,[31, 49] tumors, and Paget's disease. The intracranial portion of the nerve, seldom more than 10 mm. long, is related to the frontal lobe above, the sphenoid sinus beneath, and the carotid and ophthalmic arteries laterally. The anterior communicating artery may cross it transversely. A saccular aneurysm on one of these vessels can reduce vision by pressure on the nerve, but a more common event is diplopia from involvement of the third, fourth, or sixth cranial nerves, which lie lateral to the nerve. A tumor of the frontal lobe pressing down upon the nerve may cause optic atrophy on that side, with papilledema in the opposite eye (the rare Foster–Kennedy syndrome).

The *optic chiasm* lies about 1 cm. above the pituitary gland, and the hypophyseal stalk curves upward behind it to join the infundibulum of the third ventricle. Sometimes the chiasm is placed further forward or further back: Its position will determine whether a tumor arising out of the pituitary fossa will impinge upon the optic nerves or the chiasm itself. Fibers from the temporal half of each retina pass backward through the lateral part of the chiasm into the optic tract of the same side, while the nasal fibers, representing the temporal fields of vision, cross to enter the opposite optic tract. Some of the nasal fibers appear to loop into the opposite optic nerve before continuing backward, because a lesion of the optic nerve as it joins the chiasm may cause complete blindness in one eye, and a defect in the temporal field of the opposite eye. Fibers from the upper halves

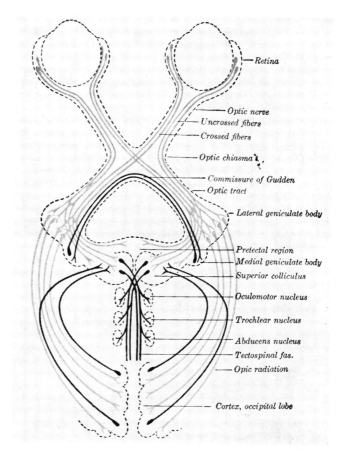

Figure 6–1. Diagram of central connections of the optic nerves. (From Goss, C. M. [ed.]: *Gray's Anatomy of the Human Body.* 27th Ed. Lea & Febiger, Philadelphia, 1959.)

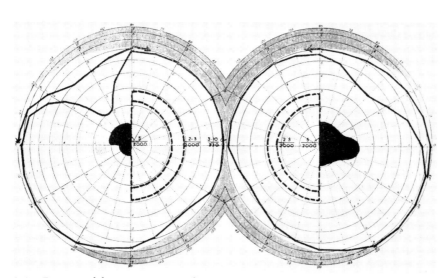

Figure 6–2. Bitemporal hemianopic central scotomas, with some depression of the upper field, in a case of pituitary adenoma. (Courtesy of Dr. Brodie Hughes.)

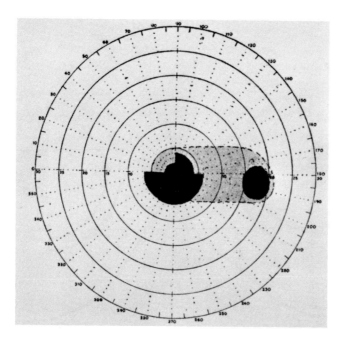

Figure 6–3. A case of compression of the optic nerve, producing quadrantic centrocecal scotoma. (Courtesy of Dr. Brodie Hughes.)

of the retina maintain their superior position in the optic nerve and chiasm.

The chiasm is liable to compression from below when a tumor of the pituitary gland breaks out of the sella turcica and invades the space between the optic tracts, or—if the chiasm is postfixed—the space between the optic nerves. In either event, the nasal fibers are involved first and the result is an upper quadrantic bi-temporal hemianopia which eventually progresses to complete loss of both temporal fields. In the early stages, bitemporal field defects can be detected only by careful use of the perimeter and the tangent screen.[27, 47] In some cases, the peripheral field is affected first but often the initial contraction is seen in the intermediate isopters, and these defects will be missed unless a screen is used in

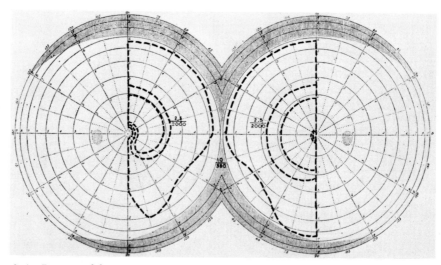

Figure 6–4. Bitemporal hemianopia, with depression in the lower nasal fields in a case of pituitary adenoma. (Courtesy of Dr. Brodie Hughes.)

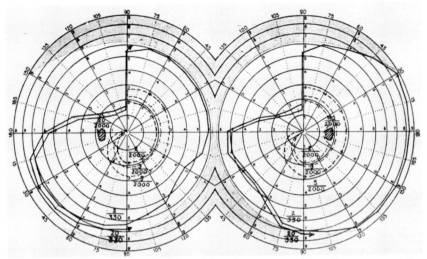

Figure 6–5. Generalized depression of the left homonymous fields, affecting especially the upper quadrants in a case of right temporoparietal glioma. (Courtesy of Dr. Brodie Hughes.)

addition to a perimeter.[27] The chiasm can be compressed from behind by a meningioma or a craniopharyngioma, and from above by an aneurysm of the anterior communicating artery, a hypothalamic tumor, or a distended third ventricle in internal hydrocephalus. This last can occur as a result of posterior fossa tumors, and the pressure on the chiasm gives rise to bitemporal hemianopia, a false localizing sign. The chiasm may itself be the seat of a glioma. It is a curious fact that bitemporal field changes—whether peripheral or in the internal isopters—are the usual response of the chiasm to factors as diverse as pressure from above, pressure from below, malignant infiltration, and a plaque of multiple sclerosis.

THE OPTIC TRACTS

The optic tracts diverge backward from the chiasm and proceed laterally, skirting first the tuber cinereum and then curving around the posterolateral surface of the cerebral peduncles in the form of narrow, flattened bands. The fibers subserving vision enter the lateral geniculate body, a nucleus of the thalamus, and in this body there is a point-to-point representation of the retina serving the contralateral half fields of vision. Consequently, a lesion in the lateral geniculate body can cause hemianopic field defects comparable in all respects to those resulting from a lesion of the geniculocalcarine pathway or the calcarine cortex itself. Other fibers of the tract form a small fasciculus which extends backward between the lateral and medial geniculate bodies to the pretectal nucleus; they transmit the retinal impulses which are concerned with the pupillary light reflex, and fibers from each eye pass to both the ipsilateral and contralateral nuclei. A second relay from the pretectal nucleus passes to the oculomotor nuclei. Consequently, a single midline lesion at the decussation of this pathway will abolish the direct and consensual reactions to light bilaterally. Fibers from the optic tract also end in the superior colliculus of the corpora quadrigemina; they are concerned with reflex movements of the head and eyes in response to visual stimuli.

Lesions of the optic tract are uncommon but are occasionally seen in multiple sclerosis, pituitary and temporal lobe tumors, and vascular lesions. They are rare after penetrating head injuries, presumably because such injuries in this region may be fatal. A complete lesion of one tract produces homonymous hemianopia with absence of the light reflex if the light is directed onto the blind side of the retina. If the lesion is incomplete, the hemianopia is often incongruous, i.e., the field defect is not quite the same either in extent or in density in the two eyes, in contrast to the congruity of the defects usually seen in lesions of the geniculocalcarine pathway. Incongruous field cuts have been found, however, in cases of traumatic lesions *apparently* limited to the anterior portion of the geniculocalcarine pathway.

THE GENICULOCALCARINE TRACT. Clinicians commonly refer to this tract as the optic radiation. At their commencement, the fibers lie in the posterior limb of the internal capsule behind the fibers conveying common sensation. They then spread out in such a way that those conveying visual impulses from the inferior retinal quadrants fan out into the temporal lobe and turn backward around the tip of the temporal horn [17, 50] of the lateral ventricle to reach the inferior lip of the calcarine fissure. The fibers from the upper quadrants pass back to the upper lip of the fissure. As a result of this arrangement, a lesion of the temporal lobe can give rise to a sharply cut quadrantic hemianopia limited to the contralateral upper quarters of the visual fields, while a lesion deep within the occipitoparietal lobe causes a lower quadrantic hemianopia. The visual field defects found after surgical removal of the anterior portion of the temporal lobe are often incongruous.[36]

The optic radiations also contain efferent fibers leading from the occipital cortex to the superior colliculus, whence a fresh relay passes to the third, fourth, and sixth cranial nuclei and to the tectospinal tract. This efferent system is intimately concerned with reflex movements of the eyes, neck, and limbs in response to visual stimuli. It also serves the fixation reflex, whereby the eye can quickly follow moving objects. This reflex is normally subservient to the will but it becomes paramount when disease interrupts both pyramidal pathways to the third, fourth, and sixth cranial nuclei, as in double hemiplegia and pseudobulbar palsy. In this event, gaze tends to be glued to any object which excites interest and cannot easily be moved from it—a "spasm" of fixation—unless the patient momentarily shuts his eyes. There is usually an associated impairment of conjugate movement of the eyes.

THE VISUAL CORTEX

The macula is represented at the tip of the occipital pole, while the rest of the retina is arranged along the calcarine fissure, the extreme periphery of the retina being represented at its anterior end. The upper retinal quadrants are represented above the fissure and the lower quadrants below it. A lesion limited to the tip of one occipital pole will give rise to a homonymous hemiscotoma, whereas if it is placed further forward there will be a homonymous loss in the peripheral half fields. Many lesions of the geniculocalcarine pathway produce contralateral homonymous hemianopia with sparing of macular vision; sometimes this sparing is due to incomplete interruption of the tract, but at other times it seems to be caused by faulty fixation, especially in large lesions involving areas 18 and 19 of Brodmann, in addition to the calcarine cortex itself.

The visual cortex is the end station for sight as such, but the interpretation and recognition of what is seen is a function of the inferior part of the parietal cortex in the region of the angular gyrus, which is connected with the visual cortex by subcortical association fibers. This is certainly the case as regards recognition of the written symbols of speech since lesions in this area of the dominant hemisphere give rise to dyslexia, but there is less agreement as to the existence of visual agnosia for other objects. Indeed, Bay, Luria, and others have attacked the very concept of visual agnosia. In the opinion of the author, this is going too far. It is obvious that the identification of objects by sight is something that is learned, and that such visual memories have to be stored somewhere. Secondly, in dementia, such as Alzheimer's disease, and in conditions of delirium with widespread depression of cortical function, patients frequently fail to recognize familiar faces and objects. Thirdly, although clinical examples of visual agnosia are very rare, they do occur from time to time. Presumably, the condition is rare because it requires bilateral lesions in the posterior portion of the parietotemporal region to abolish visual memories (other than those of the written word). In the only convincing case seen by the author, one of the earliest symptoms caused by bilateral bronchogenic metastases in the posterior parietotemporal areas was inability not only to read but also to recognize faces and familiar objects, although the visual fields were full and corrected visual acuity was 20/20. The patient could recognize his wife's voice, but not her face, and he recognized a pen by touch but not by sight. That the non-dominant hemisphere can recognize objects is well attested by the study of individuals whose hemispheres have been disconnected by section of the corpus callosum, anterior commissure, massa intermedia, and hippocampal commissure.

The occipital lobes and the visual cortex are supplied by the posterior cerebral artery, branches of which also supply the lateral geniculate body and the geniculocalcarine pathway; consequently, insufficiency within the vertebral-basilar system frequently gives rise to visual disturbances, and may even cause complete blindness with preservation of pupillary reactions (cortical blindness).

Optic Atrophy

Optic atrophy is the result of degeneration of the nerve fibers which run from the retinal ganglion cells through the optic nerve and optic tracts to the external geniculate body. It is recognized clinically by pallor of the optic discs in the presence of visual impairment or a past history of such impairment. In *primary optic atrophy*, the margin of the disc is clear-cut and the retina is normal in appearance; this is seen in tabes and following acute lesions of the optic nerve behind the eye. In *secondary optic atrophy*, the disc is white and its margins are blurred owing to gliosis of the nerve head, which spreads into the adjacent retina. This follows papilledema from any cause. The term *consecutive atrophy* is used for pallor of the disc associated with severe and visible disease of the retina such as choroiditis, retinitis pigmentosa, thrombosis of the central artery of the retina, etc.

It is convenient to classify the cause of optic atrophy on an anatomical basis by considering factors operating (1) in the retina, (2) at the optic disc, (3) in the optic nerve, (4) at the chiasm, (5) in the optic tracts. Disease of the optic radiation involves a new set of neurons and does not give rise to pallor of the discs except in a few long-standing cases, in which some degree of transneuronal atrophy may have occurred.

Disease of the Choroid and Retina. Diseases of the choroid and retina include diffuse choroidoretinitis, occlusion of the central artery of the retina by thrombus or embolus, retinal vasculitis,[51] retinal detachment, retinitis pigmentosa, and retinal anoxia following intoxication by quinine and carbon monoxide and as a result of massive hemorrhage from the uterus or elsewhere. Degeneration of retinal ganglion cells is probably responsible for the optic atrophy seen in the heredofamilial spinocerebellar ataxias, Leber's disease, and Tay-Sachs disease.

Diseases Affecting the Optic Disc. *Glaucoma*, a very common cause of blindness and optic atrophy in persons over 50, leads to deep cupping of the disc with disruption of nerve fibers as they bend backward into the optic nerve. This gives rise to a highly characteristic central scotoma and a depression of the peripheral field of vision. *The intraocular pressure should be tested in every case of impaired vision in adults.*

Papilledema is a common cause of secondary atrophy. During the period of edema there is engorgement of the retinal veins and edema of the disc and adjacent portion of the retina; when the papilledema subsides, the disc is pale and its margins blurred, and the cup is filled with glial scar tissue.[40]

Diseases Affecting the Optic Nerve. The most common cause of optic atrophy *affecting one eye* is retrobulbar neuritis, which is usually a symptom of multiple sclerosis (Fig. 6–6). If the patch of demyelination is adjacent to the globe, there is pain on movement of the eye and there may be moderate unilateral papilledema; owing to the supposed inflammatory origin of such edema, it is sometimes referred to as "optic neuritis." However, in most cases of retrobulbar neuritis, there is no visible edema and the patient complains of loss of central vision, for which no cause can be found on retinoscopy. Later, as vision improves, atrophy becomes obvious on the temporal side of the disc. Retrobulbar neuritis occurs in other demyelinating conditions, including neuromyelitis optica, Schilder's disease, Leber's disease, and encephalomyelitis following the specific fevers

of childhood and after vaccination against rabies and smallpox.

Bilateral retrobulbar optic neuritis occasionally occurs in otherwise healthy children under the age of 10, with severe loss of central vision progressing to almost complete blindness but with full recovery of vision within a few weeks. So far as is known at the present time, the great majority of these cases do not develop multiple sclerosis.

The optic atrophy of tabes is discussed in Chapter 14.

Bilateral failure of vision with varying degrees of optic atrophy is also seen in *toxic amblyopia* (Fig. 6–7). As a result of idiosyncrasy or overdosage, a proportion of persons exposed to certain medications and poisons suffer visual loss. Carroll's list[7] of 50 causes includes aniline dyes, arsenic in trivalent or pentavalent forms (notably tryparsamide, used for sleeping sickness in Africa), Felix mas, Atabrine, benzine and its many industrial derivatives, carbon bisulphide, carbon tetrachloride, Chloromycetin, Dilantin, ergot derivatives, methyl alcohol, lead, methyl bromide, methyl chloride, methyl iodide, para-aminosalicylic acid, antifreeze preparations used

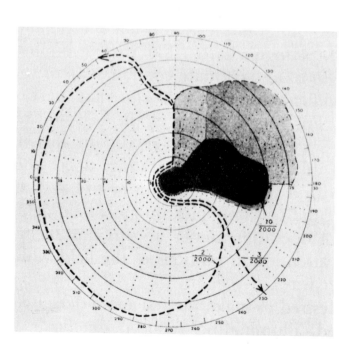

Figure 6–6. Retrobulbar neuritis in multiple sclerosis. There is a dense central scotoma and an additional depression of acuity in the temporal field. (Courtesy of Dr. Brodie Hughes.)

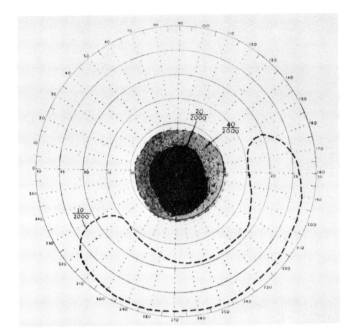

Figure 6–7. Pericentral scotoma with dense central visual loss and depression of the rest of the field, except for a peripheral crescent, in a case of toxic amblyopia. (Courtesy of Dr. Brodie Hughes.)

in radiators, quinine, salicylates, santonin, streptomycin, sulfonamides, thallium, tobacco (Fig. 6–8), toluene, and trichlorethylene.

Optic atrophy following abuse of *ethyl* alcohol is regarded as *nutritional* in origin. Atrophy with bilateral central scotomas is seen in other *deficiency* diseases, e.g., malnutrition, and in occasional cases of pernicious anemia.

Neoplasm of the optic nerve or its dural sheath is an occasional cause of unilateral optic atrophy with loss of vision, while primary and secondary new growths of the orbit and other space-occupying lesions such as gummas and parasitic cysts can involve the optic nerves secondarily. In advanced cases of exophthalmic ophthalmoplegia there is gross proptosis with edema of the lids and conjunctiva, diplopia from paresis of one or more muscles, and visual loss due to papilledema, which can progress to secondary atrophy with blindness.

Disease of the blood vessels serving the optic nerves is a common cause of optic atrophy in an aging population. Abrupt decrease of vision in one eye can be caused by infarction of the optic nerve. There is transient swelling of the optic disc and the field loss is of the altitudinal fiber-bundle type, which may be either in the upper or the lower fields. In advanced atherosclerosis, incomplete binasal hemianopic defects are occasionally seen. Hemorrhage into one of the optic nerves is a rare event in hypertensive subjects, and in patients suffering from a bleeding diathesis; it is characterized by sudden pain behind the eye and immediate impairment of vision on that side. Sudden loss of vision in one or both eyes with subsequent optic atrophy can occur in the course of temporal arteritis.

As the nerve passes through the optic canal it can be damaged by *head injuries* with or without fracture of the bony walls of the canal.[49] Visual loss, whether it be complete or incomplete, is immediate, but pallor of the disc usually takes about three weeks to appear. Primary atrophy is occasionally seen as a result of compression of the optic nerve in the canal by a meningioma and by Paget's disease.

Unilateral atrophy is sometimes seen when the optic nerve is involved by tumor of the overlying frontal lobe, by a meningioma of the olfactory groove, or by an aneurysm of the carotid or anterior communicating artery. If intracranial

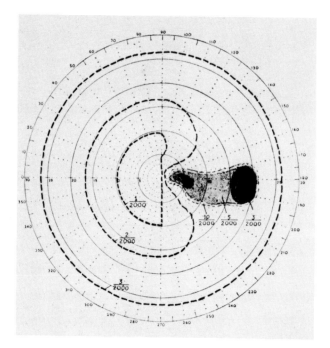

Figure 6–8. Tobacco-alcohol amblyopia. The scotoma lies between the blind spot and the macula area and is particularly dense at the macula. (Courtesy of Dr. Brodie Hughes.)

pressure is raised by a frontal tumor, there may be primary optic atrophy on the side of the lesion and contralateral papilledema (the Foster–Kennedy syndrome), but this is very rare.

Diseases of the Chiasm. Visual loss from chiasmal lesions [27, 47] usually takes the form of complete or incomplete bitemporal hemianopia which can start as a localized or generalized depression of the peripheral temporal fields, or as bitemporal scotomas. The resulting atrophy of the nerve fibers usually takes weeks or months to become visible on retinoscopy. Pituitary neoplasm, craniopharyngioma, meningioma, glioma of the chiasm itself, and gummatous meningitis have to be remembered. Multiple sclerosis can involve the chiasm, giving rise to bitemporal scotomas, and chronic arachnoiditis is a rare cause of bilateral visual defects with optic atrophy (p. 340).

Affections of the optic tract rarely cause optic atrophy because the tract is seldom involved by disease; the resulting pallor is slow to appear and mild in degree. It is associated with partial or complete homonymous hemianopia, and the field loss is usually incongruous if the lesion is incomplete.

Pallor of the optic disc is occasionally seen in persons who are totally blind as a result of damage to the occipital cortex in early life. In such cases, the preservation of the light reflex serves to indicate that the blindness is suprageniculate in origin; the most likely reason for the pallor of the disc would appear to be vascular regression in an organ which is never used.

Papilledema

Nineteenth century ophthalmologists coined the term "optic neuritis" for the reddening and swelling of the optic discs seen in intracranial tumor and in some cases of retrobulbar neuritis. In both cases the cause of the swelling is an obstruction to the venous return to the retina, which passes by the central vein to the ophthalmic vein and thus to the cavernous sinus.

The term *papilledema* was introduced by Parsons in 1908 for cases of raised intracranial pressure with at least two diopters of swelling. In 1911, Paton and Holmes [40] defined it as passive edema of the disc due to raised intracranial pressure without primary inflammatory changes and often without disturbance of vision, whereas optic neuritis was defined as swelling of the disc caused by inflammation and accompanied by impairment of vision. Since unilateral papilledema can also be produced by obstruction of the retinal venous return by a mass in the orbit, Traquair[47] introduced the term "plerocephalic edema" to indicate edema of the disc due to raised intracranial pressure only, but this term has not been widely adopted.

Clinical Features. The disc becomes reddened and its margins ill-defined, and the retinal veins swell. At this stage, vision is normal but as the condition advances, the physiological cup fills, the disc bulges forward, and small perivascular hemorrhages appear. The patient may complain of transient obscuration of vision now and again (amaurosis fugax), and perimetry will reveal enlargement of the blind spot. Edema spreads and visual acuity is reduced when the macula is involved either by edema or by perivascular hemorrhage. Ultimately there is progressive depression of central vision and constriction of the peripheral fields, and unless the situation is speedily relieved, permanent blindness will occur as a result of gliosis of the nerve head.

Differential Diagnosis. In hypertensive retinopathy, swelling of the discs is accompanied by constriction of the arterioles and the veins are not much engorged; hemorrhages are characteristically widespread rather than confined to the area of the optic nerve as in papilledema. In thrombosis of the central retinal vein, the veins are distended and tortuous, and edema and profuse hemorrhages are generalized. In posterior uveitis and juxtapapillary choroiditis, there are signs of inflammation accompanied by vitreous opacities. In retrobulbar neuritis, there is immediate impairment of central vision, and if the lesion is placed in the anterior portion of the optic nerve, there may be a modest amount of swelling of the disc.

In pseudopapilledema, a congenital abnormality, the disc contains excess neuroglial tissue, which causes it to bulge forward, but there is no edema or hemorrhage, the veins are not distended, and vision is normal. Extreme tortuosity of the veins limited to one eye or to a segment of the affected retina is an uncommon congenital anomaly. Drüsen bodies can cause confusion; they are discrete, shiny, white, beadlike bodies on the disc; there is no swelling of the nerve head, and hemorrhage is rare.

Papilledema can occur, without a rise of intracranial pressure, in tumors of the spinal cord,[42] and also in some cases of acute infective polyneuritis; in neither case is the explanation known. It can also occur in chronic pulmonary disease associated with acute heart failure, as a result of hypoxia, hypercapnia, and heightened venous pressure. It is seen in the superior mediastinal syndrome, in which the superior vena cava is partially occluded, but in this condition the papilledema is accompanied by cyanotic edema of the face and edema of the eyelids and conjunctiva. The papilledema which is sometimes encountered as a complication of drug therapy (oral contraceptives, steroids, vitamin A, tetracyclines) is caused by benign intracranial hypertension.

OCULAR MOVEMENTS

The Control of Ocular Movements. The main cortical "center" for ocular movements[10] is situated in area 8 (Brodmann) in the second frontal convolution. When this area is stimulated electrically or irritated by local disease, the eyes move conjugately to the opposite side. Deviation, usually accompanied by turning of the head in the same direction, is sometimes seen at the start of a seizure arising from this part of the brain. Vertical movements of the eyes can also be obtained by electrical stimulation, but with greater difficulty. The fibers from this center pass downward anterior to the pyramidal tract proper, in the anterior part of the internal capsule, and undergo incomplete decussation in the brainstem

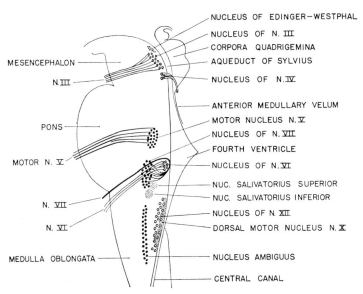

Figure 6-9.   Diagram of the nuclei of the motor cranial nerves, lateral view.

en route to the nuclei of the third, fourth, and sixth nerves (Figs. 6–9, 6–10). Because the decussation is incomplete, each nucleus receives cortical control from both sides, which explains why paralysis of conjugate ocular movement does not usually occur in a lesion of one hemisphere alone; transient inability to turn the eyes to the diseased side is sometimes seen after an acute lesion of the motor or premotor area, or of the internal capsule, but it does not persist.

Bilateral disease, on the other hand, can cause paralysis of voluntary conjugate movements of the eyes (laterally, vertically, or both), whether the lesions are in the cerebral hemispheres, the midbrain, or (in the case of lateral movement) the pons. Loss of vertical movement (Parinaud's syndrome) is the most common and is frequently seen in lesions in the neighborhood of the pineal.

Supranuclear palsies may be recognized by three characteristics: (1) There is no diplopia; (2) both eyes are affected; (3) there is persistence of reflex movements of the paralyzed muscles: A patient who cannot voluntarily move his eyes to the left may nevertheless do so in response to a sudden unexpected noise on

that side; the anatomical basis of this reflex is a pathway from the temporal lobe to the third, fourth, and sixth nuclei. Similarly, the eyes will deviate to one side on caloric stimulation of the labyrinth, though voluntary movement in that direction is impossible.

Some of these cases also exhibit a spasm of fixation; the patient's gaze becomes glued to an object and the eyes cannot easily be moved away from it. However, if the object is slowly moved, the head remaining still, the eyes will move together in the direction for which voluntary movement is impossible. This spasm of fixation is thought to result from the release of the fixation reflex which is normally dominated by the anterior oculomotor center in the second frontal convolution.

Supranuclear palsies are seen in some cases of double hemiplegia, in tumors in the region of the pineal, in tentorial pressure cones, and occasionally as a result of multiple sclerosis and encephalitis.

Progressive supranuclear palsy, with restriction of conjugate movements, is sometimes found in late adult life in association with slowly progressive pseu-

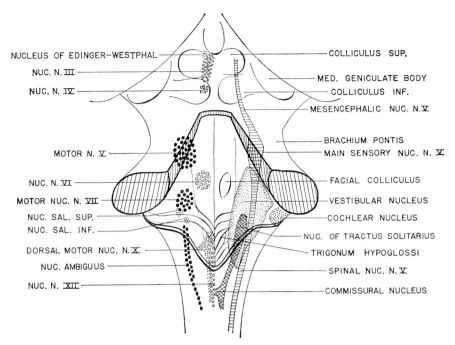

Figure 6–10. Diagrammatic scheme of the cranial nerve nuclei in the brainstem. The cerebellum and roof of the fourth ventricle have been removed. (After Ranson, S. W., and Clark, S. L.: *The Anatomy of the Nervous System. Its Development and Function.* 10th Ed. W. B. Saunders Co., Philadelphia, 1959.)

dobulbar palsy, dysequilibrium in standing and walking, and a tendency to keep the neck extended. In four such cases reported by Behrman and his colleagues,[2] the pathological changes were largely confined to the brainstem and cerebellum. There was swelling and degeneration of the nerve cells, many of which contained neurofibrillary tangles, and severe loss of nerve cells in the dentate nuclei of the cerebellum without any significant abnormality of the cerebellar cortex. The etiology is unknown.

The third, fourth, and sixth nuclei are interconnected by the medial longitudinal bundle, which extends on either side of the midline from the optic thalamus to the anterior horn cells of the spinal cord. It is especially well developed in the region between the nuclei of the oculomotor and the vestibular nerves and contains many fibers from the vestibular nuclei. It provides the anatomical pathway for relaying impulses for conjugate *lateral* gaze from the pontine centers to the oculomotor nuclei, for the coordination of eye movements, and for vestibular control. A small lesion of the medial longitudinal fasciculus on one side produces a selective paralysis of the ipsilateral medial rectus on attempted conjugate lateral gaze; the lateral rectus which is innervated by fibers coming directly from the pontine centers without traversing the medial longitudinal fasciculus, is not affected by such a lesion. This is known as internuclear ophthalmoplegia. It is often bilateral, as in multiple sclerosis, thrombosis of small branches of the basilar artery, tumors, and Wernicke's encephalopathy.

When the lesion is in the caudal part of the tract, internuclear ophthalmoplegia is often associated with nystagmus, and convergence is retained.[10] With more rostrally placed lesions in the midbrain, nystagmus may or may not be present, but convergence is either decreased or abolished. The nystagmus may be vertical, horizontal, or rotary. When it is horizontal, it is more marked in the abducted eye than in the adducted eye, owing to the weakness of the medial rectus.

Paralysis of lateral gaze, involving the lateral rectus of one eye and the internal rectus of the other, is sometimes seen in lesions of the pons, suggesting the presence of an accessory "para-abducens" center, which is probably in the vicinity of the abducens nucleus.

Disease affecting the nuclei of the third, fourth, and sixth nerves causes paralysis of individual muscles and not of conjugate movement. Rarely, bilateral nuclear lesions cause symmetrical paralysis of upward or downward movement but—unlike what happens in supranuclear palsies—the paralysis involves both reflex and voluntary movements, and diplopia is invariable unless one eye happens to be blind.

DIPLOPIA

Weakness or paralysis of ocular muscles is accompanied by diplopia and strabismus. In persistent cases, a patient may tilt or rotate the head in such a way as to obviate the need for using the faulty muscle (ocular torticollis). Thus, the diplopia caused by paralysis of a muscle which elevates the eyeball can be avoided by tilting the head backward.

Certain anatomical facts relevant to the interpretation of diplopia may be mentioned.[10] The medial wall of the orbit runs in the sagittal plane, while the lateral wall is at an angle of about 23 degrees to it. With the exception of the inferior oblique, which arises from the anteromedial part of the floor of the orbit, all the extrinsic ocular muscles arise from the tendon of Zinn around the optic nerve at the apex of the orbit. Therefore, with the eye looking directly forward, the superior and inferior rectus run forward and slightly laterally to their insertion on the eyeball. The superior oblique is reflected over the trochlea and thus approaches the eye from the anteromedial part of the orbit to be inserted into the upper and outer quadrant of the eye, behind the insertion of the recti. The inferior oblique also approaches the eye from the anteromedial part of the orbit and is inserted into the lower and outer quadrant of the eye. The action of the lateral and medial recti is in the horizontal plane. The action of the superior and inferior recti and the obliques is complicated because in the primary position of the eye, contraction of each of these muscles not only moves it horizontally and vertically but also rotates it. However, the superior rectus becomes a pure elevator when the eye is turned outward about 23 degrees, and the inferior rectus becomes a pure depressor in the same position. When the eye is turned medially to its fullest extent, the superior oblique becomes largely a depressor and the inferior oblique an elevator.

The identification of the muscle or nerve at fault can usually be carried out at the chair side without special apparatus.[10] The patient is asked to hold his head steady and to look at a linear object, such as a pencil, which is held at least 30 inches away from him. The object is then placed in various positions both above and below the horizontal meridian. Diplopia will occur when the object is held in the position requiring contraction of the affected muscle, and separation of the two images increases when the object is moved in its direction of action. Palsy of the lateral or medial rectus muscle will produce horizontal diplopia, the images being side by side, while palsy of the superior or inferior rectus or of an oblique muscle produces a predominantly vertical separation of images. The more peripheral of the two images comes from the lagging eye. The peripheral image is usually relatively indistinct, but this is an unreliable guide if visual acuity is unequal in the two eyes because the patient will sometimes fix with the better of the two. Therefore, to establish which eye the peripheral image comes from, one eye is covered and the patient is asked which of the two images disappears. Thus, if diplopia occurs on looking down and the images are found to be separated maximally when looking down and to the right, and the peripheral image disappears when covering the right eye, we are dealing with palsy of the right inferior rectus. Covering one eye with a red glass and the other with a green one helps to identify the origin of the images.

Analysis of Diplopia.[10, 51]   In paralysis of the right lateral rectus, the right eye does not move to the right, and there is horizontal homonymous diplopia which increases on looking further to the right.

In paralysis of the right medial rectus, the right eye does not move to the left, and there is horizontal crossed diplopia which increases on looking to the left.

In paralysis of the right inferior rectus, the right eye does not move downward when the patient looks to the right, and there is vertical diplopia on looking down and to the right. The image from the right eye is below that from the left.

In paralysis of the right superior rectus, the eye does not move upward when the eyes are turned to the right, and there is vertical diplopia, which is increased by looking to the right and up. The image from the right eye is uppermost.

In paralysis of the right superior oblique, the right eye does not move downward when the eyes are turned to the left, and there is vertical diplopia on looking to the left and down. The image of the right eye is below that of the left.

In paralysis of the right inferior oblique, the right eye does not move upward when the eyes are turned to the left, and there is vertical diplopia which is increased on looking up and to the left. The image of the right eye is uppermost.

When the entire oculomotor nerve is paralyzed, there is ptosis and dilatation of the pupil.

In some cases, the nature of the diplopia will be found to vary on successive examinations, as for instance in myasthenia gravis and in the presence of a tentorial pressure cone. Marked variations during a single examination suggest hysteria or malingering. Diplopia may

also be due to mechanical displacement of one eye as in proptosis from any cause, and in fractures of the orbital floor.

THE THIRD CRANIAL NERVE

The oculomotor nerve supplies the levator of the upper lid, and all the extrinsic ocular muscles except the lateral rectus and the superior oblique. Its vegetative components supply the sphincter pupillae and the ciliary muscle. In complete paralysis there is ptosis, lateral deviation of the eye, moderate dilatation of the pupil, loss of the direct and consensual light reflexes, paralysis of accommodation, and paralysis of all ocular movement except laterally and inferomedially.

THE NUCLEUS.   The nucleus of the third nerve is composed of five elements in the gray matter in front of the sylvian aqueduct and extending for a short distance in the floor of the third ventricle. The medial longitudinal bundle lies on its ventromedial aspect. The Edinger–Westphal nucleus, the most rostral portion, supplies fibers for the sphincter of the pupil and the ciliary muscle. Below it is a column of cells, the more proximal of which are concerned with upward movements and the more distal with downward movements. Fibers destined for the internal rectus arise medial to these. There is doubt as to the existence in man of the nucleus of Perlia, which was once thought to control convergence.[54] Nuclear lesions may affect all the functions of the third nerve on the affected side, or only some of them, but such lesions are far less common than affections of the third nerve itself. Tumors, multiple sclerosis, encephalitis, Wernicke's encephalopathy, and vascular lesions are the least rare. It is likely that at least some of the impairment of oculomotor function seen in tentorial pressure cones is due to pressure on the oculomotor nucleus itself. Diplopia from barbiturate or alcoholic intoxication is probably nuclear in origin. The condition formerly known as progressive

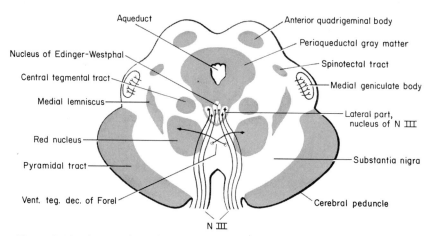

Aqueduct

Nucleus of Edinger-Westphal

Central tegmental tract

Medial lemniscus

Red nucleus

Pyramidal tract

Vent. teg. dec. of Forel

Anterior quadrigeminal body

Periaqueductal gray matter

Spinotectal tract

Medial geniculate body

Lateral part, nucleus of N III

Substantia nigra

Cerebral peduncle

N III

Figure 6–11. Section through the midbrain at the level of the third cranial nerve.

nuclear ophthalmoplegia is now known to be due to muscular dystrophy (p. 538).

THE EFFERENT FIBERS. The efferent fibers of the third nerve pass through the midbrain and the red nucleus to emerge from the medial side of the cerebral peduncle (Fig. 6–11). A lesion involving the red nucleus and the third nerve gives rise to Benedikt's syndrome—ocular palsy on one side and tremor of the contralateral arm. A lesion a little further forward and lateral can cause oculomotor palsy and contralateral hemiplegia—Weber's syndrome. Infiltrating tumors of the brainstem may produce combinations of

nuclear and infranuclear palsies of both the third and the trochlear nerves; there is occasionally a remarkable sparing of the long motor and sensory tracts in the early stages of such cases.

NERVE PATHWAY. The third nerve runs forward through the interpeduncular cistern beneath the posterior cerebral artery, and in this part of its course it is liable to be involved by inflammatory conditions of the meninges and by saccular aneurysms of the posterior cerebral artery. It perforates the dura lateral to the posterior clinoid process and then lies in the roof of the cavernous sinus,

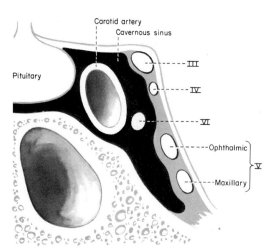

Carotid artery
Cavernous sinus

Pituitary

III

IV

VI

Ophthalmic

Maxillary

V

Figure 6–12. Oblique section through the right cavernous sinus.

above the trochlear nerve and lateral to the intracavernous portion of the internal carotid artery (Fig. 6–12). In this situation it can be involved by aneurysm of the artery, and rarely by thrombosis of the sinus itself. It may also be involved by a granulomatous condition within the cavernous sinus described by Tolosa.[46]

The nerve enters the orbit through the superior orbital fissure, at which point it may be involved by a meningioma, fracture of the skull, periostitis, and orbital lesions of various types. Proptosis, pain in and about the eye, and paralysis of the abducens, trochlear, oculomotor, and first division of the fifth nerve constitute the *syndrome of the superior orbital fissure*,[33] and periostitis should be invoked only when all other explanations fail. It usually follows inflammatory disease of the paranasal sinuses.

Other Conditions Involving the Third Nerve. Partial or complete paralysis of external ocular movement can be seen in acute infective polyneuritis. Temporary paralysis of the third nerve occurs sometimes in diabetes, probably due to ischemia of the nerve trunk induced by disease of the vasa nervorum.[12, 15]

Congenital *oculomotor apraxia*[1] is a very rare condition, first noticed in infancy, and characterized by absent or defective voluntary horizontal eye movements, normal random movements, absence of the quick phase of optokinetic nystagmus, and jerking movements of the head. Later on, there may be difficulty in learning to read because although vertical eye movements are normal, horizontal following movements are poorly performed.

Intermittent diplopia and ptosis is seen in myasthenia gravis; in this case there is usually a clear relationship between paresis and fatigue, and the symptoms usually respond to neostigmine and Tensilon. In ophthalmoplegic migraine,[19] diplopia and ptosis occur briefly, in association with other features of a migrainous attack. However, if the oculomotor paresis lasts for days or longer in association with a unilateral headache, it is more likely to be due to an intracranial aneurysm or some other disease.

Widening of the palpebral fissure occurs in lower motor neuron facial paralysis, irritation of the cervical sympathetic, thyrotoxicosis, and exophthalmic ophthalmoplegia. Active retraction of the upper lid is sometimes seen in supranuclear and nuclear paralysis of upward movement of the eye, as for instance in lesions of the midbrain. It can also occur during regeneration of the third nerve, lid retraction occurring when the eye is directed downward as a result of misdirected growth of nerve fibers.

Ptosis can result from disease of muscle (ocular myopathy), disease of the myoneural junctions (myasthenia gravis), affections of the third nerve (intracranial aneurysm, etc.), and lesions of the cervical sympathetic. Horner's syndrome produces a mild degree of ptosis, together with miosis on the affected side. In addition, there is loss of sweating on one side of the face when the sympathetic is interrupted below the carotid bifurcation. Ptosis can be congenital, and in some such cases it is associated with jaw-winking, in which the lid elevates when the mouth is opened, so that mastication or even speech may be attended by constant winking. The only method of escape from this embarrassing situation is to carry out a tenotomy on the levator and to correct the resulting ptosis by a plastic operation.

THE PUPILS

The pupillary sphincter is innervated by parasympathetic fibers from the third nerve, and the dilator by the sympathetic. The sympathetic pathway starts in the premotor cortex and passes through the hypothalamus, the cerebral peduncles, the tegmentum of the pons, the medulla, and the lateral horn of gray matter in the spinal cord. Preganglionic fibers pass out through the eighth cervical and upper two thoracic anterior roots and so reach the cervical sympathetic. Postganglionic fibers enter the skull around the internal carotid artery, ultimately passing from the carotid plexus to the ophthalmic division of the trigeminal nerve and thence to the pupil via the nasociliary and long ciliary nerves.

Miosis (constriction of the pupil) can be congenital; it can also occur as a result of iritis, in which event the pupil is irregular in outline and close examination may reveal adhesions between its free border and the anterior surface of the lens. Unilateral miosis is more often the result of paralysis of the sympathetic. It is rarely, if ever, seen in disease above the level of the hypothalamus unless such disease has produced a pressure cone.

Lesions of the brainstem can produce unilateral or bilateral miosis, and the same is true of lesions in the cervical cord (syringomyelia, tumors), but the commonest causes of unilateral miosis involve the ascending cervical sympathetic trunk and its prolongation through the head to the eye. Injuries to or diseases of the lower cervical and upper two dorsal roots must be remembered in this connection. Thrombosis of the internal carotid artery in the neck can cause miosis and ptosis. A lesion of the stellate ganglion will produce unilateral miosis and ptosis with loss of sweating on the ipsilateral face, neck, and upper limb (Horner's syndrome); the pupil fails to dilate when cocaine is instilled into the eye.

The constrictor fibers of the pupil originate in the Edinger–Westphal nucleus. They enter the third nerve and terminate in the ciliary ganglion, from which postganglionic fibers pass to the eye via the short ciliary nerves. Unilateral dilatation or constriction of the pupils sometimes occurs in acute lesions of one hemisphere, as at the commencement of a stroke, but in general, pupillary inequality associated with expanding lesions in the cerebral hemispheres is more often the result of a tentorial pressure cone. Affections of the third nerve from the region of the nucleus to its termination in the eye give rise to dilatation of the pupil on the side of the lesion. The pupil can become fixed and dilated following a blow on the eye.

The Pupillary Reflexes

The *light reflex* can be lost through a lesion of the afferent or efferent pathway: (1) If one eye is blind, neither pupil will contract when that eye is illuminated, but both pupils will react to light shone into the good eye. (2) In hemianopia due to a lesion in one optic tract, illumination of the blind half of the retina will evoke no pupillary reaction, but there will be a normal response if the light is thrown onto the seeing half (Wernicke's reaction). In hemianopia due to disease of the optic radiation, on the other hand, the pupillary reflexes are normal. (3) A lesion in the midline of the pretectal region will involve the afferent fibers on their way to the Edinger–Westphal nucleus, with consequent bilateral loss of the light reflex and retention of the convergence reaction. This is not to be confused with the Argyll Robertson pupil, in which similar reactions to light are associated with miosis. (4) Destruction of the Edinger–Westphal nucleus, the third nerve, or the ciliary ganglion paralyzes both direct and consensual reactions on the affected side, and the pupil dilates. Midline lesions of the Edinger–Westphal nuclear complex can give rise to loss of pupillary constriction on convergence, the light reflex remaining intact.

The classic Argyll Robertson pupil [37] occurs in some 20 per cent of all cases of tabes dorsalis, and in less than 10 per cent of general paresis. The pupil is small, does not contract to light, contracts normally on convergence, and dilates slowly and incompletely with belladonna or atropine. The term is sometimes used (incorrectly) to include pupils of normal size which react feebly or not at all to light, but which contract briskly on convergence. The Argyll Robertson pupil as originally described is pathognomonic of neurosyphilis, but large nonreacting pupils are seen in brain tumors, postencephalitic parkinsonism, head injuries, and unilaterally after herpes zoster ophthalmicus and injuries involving the oculomotor nerve.

The *tonic pupil* is a benign disorder

which occurs predominantly in females aged 20 to 40 years. It is suddenly discovered that one pupil is larger than the other; in a few cases, failure of the pupil to constrict rapidly on coming into bright light can cause complaints of dazzle or photophobia, but usually there are no symptoms at all. The affected pupil is larger than its fellow at first, but with the passage of time the difference becomes less marked. Reactions to light and darkness are so slow that they may be deemed to be absent on hasty examination. The reaction to convergence is slow and sluggish, and occasionally there is loss of accommodation. The pupil dilates with atropine and contracts briskly if a few drops of 2.5 per cent mecholyl are instilled into the conjunctival sac; normal and syphilitic pupils do not react to this dilution. In about 10 per cent of all cases, the condition is bilateral. There is often an associated depression or absence of one or more of the peripheral tendon reflexes, notably in the legs (the Adie-syndrome), and the combination of a poorly reacting pupil and absent reflexes can lead to an unjustified suspicion of neurosyphilis.

The cause of the tonic pupil is unknown. Harriman and Garland[24] found degeneration in the ciliary ganglion of the affected eye in a single case. Hedges has reported a family in which both parents and three of their seven offspring were affected.[25]

In juvenile taboparesis, the pupils are commonly large and fail to react to light, but respond to convergence. Bilateral dilated and fixed pupils which react to convergence are also seen in tumors of the region of the pineal, in which case there is sometimes paresis of conjugate upward movement of the eyes.

Disturbances of accommodation do not figure prominently in neurological disease. Though the Edinger–Westphal nucleus contains cells which control accommodation, the frequency of defective accommodation after cervical sympathectomy suggests that the sympathetic system also plays a role. Paralysis of accommodation is seen in diphtheria and occasionally occurs as a result of other infections, such as influenza, measles, encephalitis lethargica, and neurosyphilis. It can occur after a blow on the eye. Weakness of accommodation is a common complaint among patients who are receiving belladonna or ganglion-blocking agents for the treatment of asthma, parkinsonism, or hypertension. Spasm of accommodation is not uncommon in subjects with uncorrected errors of refraction, and also occurs as a manifestation of neurosis; it causes poor distant vision and asthenopia for close work.

Dilatation of the pupil can be caused by accidental or willful instillation of belladonna or cocaine. Morphine causes constriction of the pupils through its central action.

THE FOURTH CRANIAL NERVE (TROCHLEAR NERVE)

The trochlear nucleus is situated below the third nucleus in the midbrain. It receives connections through the medial longitudinal bundle from the third and sixth nuclei, the vestibular nucleus, and the cerebellum, and is under the control of the pyramidal tracts.

After leaving the nucleus, the nerve fibers decussate to the opposite side, emerge behind the brainstem below the inferior quadrigeminal body, wind round the cerebral peduncle, traverse the interpeduncular cistern, and pierce the dura below the third nerve. The nerve enters the lateral wall of the cavernous sinus, lying above the first division of the trigeminal nerve, and passes into the orbit through the superior orbital fissure to supply the superior oblique muscle.

Conditions Involving the Fourth Cranial Nerve

Paralysis of the nerve is infrequent; it causes diplopia, which is greatest when the patient looks downward and medially. Because of the decussation, a lesion of the nucleus will cause paralysis of the superior oblique muscle of the opposite eye, whereas the paralysis will be on the same side as the lesion if the nerve is involved after it leaves the midbrain. A large lesion involving the fourth nucleus may spread upward to involve the oculomotor nucleus as well, giving rise to third nerve palsy on the side of the lesion and trochlear paralysis on the opposite side. A single lesion situated in the midline, at the point where both trochlear nerves decussate, could cause paralysis of both superior oblique muscles.

Vascular lesions, tumors, a tentorial pressure cone, and Wernicke's encephalopathy are the common lesions in this area. As the nerve crosses the subarachnoid space it can be involved by any form of meningitis, by meningioma, and by aneurysm of the posterior cerebral artery. Inside the cavernous sinus it can be paralyzed by a carotid aneurysm (the third nerve is commonly affected as well) and by cavernous sinus thrombosis.

After leaving the sinus, the nerve is liable to the same hazards as the third cranial nerve. In the presence of complete third nerve paralysis, it is easy to miss the presence of a simultaneous fourth nerve palsy.[10] To identify this, the patient is asked to turn the affected eye about 40 degrees laterally, which he accomplishes by contracting the external rectus. If he is now asked to look downward, the eye will rotate slightly if the fourth nerve is intact.

THE SIXTH CRANIAL NERVE (ABDUCENS NERVE)

The sixth cranial nerve supplies the lateral rectus muscle of the eye. When paralyzed, diplopia is experienced on turning the eyes to the affected side, the false image lying lateral and parallel to the true image. The nerve arises from a nucleus situated immediately behind the nucleus of the facial nerve in the lower part of the pons. Consequently, nuclear affections of the sixth nerve are sometimes associated with facial paralysis, and this association is seen in congeni-

tal bilateral aplasia of the sixth and seventh nuclei, a condition known as congenital facial diplegia. The sixth nucleus is linked with the opposite motor and premotor cortex by the pyramidal tract, and it is connected with the third and fourth nuclei by the medial longitudinal bundle, which also conveys information from the visual cortex, the temporal lobe, the vestibular nucleus, and the cerebellum.

Etiology. Supranuclear affections are relatively rare. Irritative lesions of the posterior end of the first and second frontal convolutions—the contraversive field—can cause tonic deviation of the eyes to the opposite side with or without rotation of the head. Inability to turn the eyes to the side of the lesion may be seen as a transient symptom following an acute destructive lesion of the prefrontal cortex or the underlying white matter.

There is probably a subsidiary "center" for lateral deviation of the eyes in the lower pons, because damage in this area can paralyze conjugate movement to the opposite side. Interruption of the medial longitudinal bundle causes internuclear paralysis (p. 91).

Nuclear paralysis of the sixth nerve is indistinguishable from infranuclear paralysis of the nerve, unless there are satellite signs to indicate the situation of the lesion. The nucleus may be involved by poliomyelitis, encephalitis, encephalomyelitis, herpes zoster, tumor of the pons, and vascular lesions. The ocular palsies of botulism are peripheral in origin. The nerve fibers may be involved, as they traverse the pons, by multiple sclerosis, tumor, and vascular lesions.

The greatest number of abducens palsies are due to affections of the nerve after it leaves the pons. It runs upward and forward between the pons and the anterior inferior cerebellar artery, and it has been thought that it may be nipped by this vessel in arteriosclerotic subjects, who sometimes present partial or complete abducens palsy for which no other cause can be found. Infarction appears to be a more reasonable explanation.

On its way across the subarachnoid

space, it is liable to be involved by meningitis, meningovascular syphilis, arachnoiditis, subarachnoid hemorrhage, polyneuritis, tumors, and tabes. An isolated sixth nerve palsy sometimes follows spinal anesthesia. After piercing the dura, the nerve crosses the inferior petrosal sinus, and thrombosis of this sinus is one of the causes of abducens paralysis in infections of the ear and mastoid. It then crosses the upper border of the petrous temporal bone, and a lesion at this point can cause pain of trigeminal distribution and sixth nerve palsy — Gradenigo's syndrome, usually seen in children with otitis and attributed to periostitis of the petrous bone.

The nerve enters the cavernous sinus, where it may be involved by sinus thrombosis and intracavernous aneurysm of the carotid, and passes into the orbit through the superior orbital fissure.

Abducens palsy is a common false localizing sign in the presence of raised intracranial pressure, because any expanding lesion situated above the tentorium — tumor, abscess, hemorrhage, acute internal hydrocephalus — can displace the brainstem downward toward the foramen magnum, thereby stretching the sixth nerve. Finally, the possibility of myasthenia gravis must always be kept in mind in considering the cause of abducens palsy, especially if it is incomplete and remittent.

NYSTAGMUS

Nystagmus [10, 14, 18, 21] is an involuntary to-and-fro movement of the eyeballs. It can be horizontal, vertical, or rotary, and is composed of fast and slow phases (jerk nystagmus), or of two movements of equal speed (pendular nystagmus).

Degrees of nystagmus can be graded as follows: In Grade I, there is nystagmus on gaze to one side only; in Grade II, there is nystagmus on gaze to one side and also straight ahead; in Grade III, nystagmus occurs on gaze to both sides and straight ahead.

Under normal conditions, the extrinsic muscles of the two eyes are in a state of balanced tonic innervation, so that in looking at an object a constant direction of gaze can be sustained. Disease of the labyrinth and brainstem interfere with this tonic innervation, with the result that the eyes tend to drift away from the object of fixation and are brought back to it by a quick corrective movement which is probably cortical in origin.

Nystagmus is usually assessed by direct observation of the eyes but can be studied in greater detail by means of the electronystagmograph, which utilizes the fact that the cornea is electropositive with respect to the retina; consequently, when the eye rotates in its socket the positive charge carried by the cornea is picked up by nearest periorbital electrode. It is thus possible to study spontaneous or induced nystagmus when the eyes are shut, or in the dark. Nystagmography can supplement clinical observation but cannot supplant it because it cannot record the rotary component of nystagmus. Moreover, gaze-evoked nystagmus and muscle paretic nystagmus will be missed by routine electronystagmographic tests.

Optokinetic nystagmus occurs in normal individuals when looking at a continuously moving panorama, as from a car or train. The slow phase is a following movement mediated through the visual centers, and the fast phase is a corrective movement which brings the eyes back to their original position. It can be induced by asking the subject to look fixedly at a slowly revolving drum on which alternate colored and white stripes are painted longitudinally, or by having him look at a strip of cloth about three inches wide and one yard long, on which similar stripes are printed, while it is moved first from left to right and then from right to left in the horizontal plane. In lesions of the occipital lobe and posterior thalamus there is absence or easy fatigability of the nystagmus caused by rotating the drum, or moving the cloth, towards the side of the lesion. In brainstem lesions, the defect is apt to be bilateral. For obvious reasons, optokinetic nystagmus is absent in the blind, so if it is found in somebody who professes complete bilateral loss of vision, malingering or conversion hysteria is to be suspected.

Nystagmus can be induced by thermal stimuli (the caloric test). The patient lies on a couch with the head raised to 30 degrees above the horizontal, thus bringing the horizontal canal into the vertical plane, which is its position of maximum sensitivity to thermal stimuli. Water at 30°C. is run into one ear continuously for 40 seconds. At least 250 ml. should be used. There is a slow movement of the eyes toward the side which has been stimulated and a rapid return to the opposite side. When the test is repeated with water at 44°C., the direction of nystagmus is reversed. The duration of nystagmus is carefully timed.[6, 14, 21]

This test may show suppression of activity on one side (canal paresis) or the nystagmus in one direction may be stronger than in the other direction (directional preponderance).[21] In labyrinthine lesions, acoustic neuroma, and vestibular neuronitis, canal paresis is the commonest abnormality, but directional preponderance can also occur. In brainstem lesions, canal paresis is less common than directional preponderance away from the side of the lesion. In cerebral lesions, particularly those involving the posterior part of the temporal lobe, there may be directional preponderance towards the side of the lesion.[18] The localizing significance of directional preponderance, as described by Hallpike and his associates, has been questioned by other workers in this field. Arguments for and against have been summarized by McNally and Stuart.[35] Many otologists content themselves with running a small quantity of ice water into each ear in turn and find it fairly reliable for the demonstration of a disorder of the labyrinth or eighth nerve. Others combine the Hallpike technique with electronystagmography and claim that the results are more informative.

Jerk Nystagmus. The direction of nystagmus is named according to the direction of the fast component, which is inappropriate since the slow component is the primary abnormality. Jerk nystagmus occurs as a result of disease, injury,[20] or intoxication involving the labyrinth, the vestibular nerve, and the vestibular nuclei and their connections in the brainstem. It can also be induced in normal subjects by stimulating the labyrinth with thermal or galvanic stimuli, by spinning the patient, and by the optokinetic test.

Nystagmus of labyrinthine origin may be horizontal, vertical, or rotary. It depends on imbalance between the impulses from the two labyrinths. Thus, while stimulation of one labyrinth causes conjugate deviation of the eyes to the opposite side, with a quick corrective movement toward the stimulated side, removal of the opposite labyrinth will have the same effect. Rotary nystagmus is usually due to disease affecting the vestibular nuclei but it can also occur in affections of the internal ear. Vertical nystagmus is not produced by stimulation or destruction of the labyrinths but occurs in lesions of the brainstem.

Nystagmus originating in disease of the internal ear can usually be differentiated from the nystagmus caused by disorders of the vestibular nuclei. The presence of severe vertigo, tinnitus, and deafness usually indicates a lesion of the internal ear or eighth nerve. The abolition of visual fixation enhances labyrinthine nystagmus but depresses or abolishes the central variety. Changing the position of the head can change the direction and degree of central nystagmus but has little or no effect upon the nystagmus produced by disease of the semicircular canals. If spontaneous nystagmus is present without vertigo, it is unlikely to be labyrinthine in origin. Spontaneous vertical nystagmus is always due to brainstem disease, whereas lateral or rotary nystagmus can be peripheral or central in origin. Nystagmus from peripheral lesions is greatest at the outset of the disease and seldom lasts more than a few weeks, whereas central nystagmus lasts longer and may worsen as time goes by.

The common causes of labyrinthine or

canal nystagmus are Meniere's disease and labyrinthitis. Intoxications (streptomycin, barbiturates, Dilantin, alcohol) probably act both on the end-organs and on the central nuclei. Nystagmus from involvement of the eighth nerve is seen in cerebello-pontine tumors and vestibular neuronitis. Sudden loss of hearing with vertigo and nystagmus can occur from occlusion of the internal auditory artery.

Jerk nystagmus of central origin occurs in multiple sclerosis and other demyelinating diseases, vascular lesions of the brainstem, Wernicke's encephalopathy, tumors of the brainstem and cerebellum, encephalitis involving the brainstem, basal head injuries, tentorial and medullary pressure cones, heredofamilial cerebellar ataxias and other heredofamilial diseases, platybasia, and syringobulbia. Occasionally, jerk nystagmus is seen in tumors of the upper part of the cervical cord; this is yet to be explained.

Disease limited to the cerebral hemispheres does not produce nystagmus unless, as in the case of an expanding mass, a tentorial or medullary pressure cone is present. On the other hand, nystagmus induced by caloric stimulation may be modified by unilateral cerebral lesions (notably but not exclusively in the posterior portion of the temporal lobe), with loss of the fast component. Optokinetic nystagmus is abolished by lesions involving the occipital lobe and thalamus and is sometimes transiently disturbed by acute lesions involving the anterior oculogyric "center" in the second frontal convolution.

Vertical nystagmus with a quick upward phase occurs in lesions of the vestibular nuclei and the cerebellar vermis. It also occurs in association with lateral nystagmus as a result of intoxication by Dilantin, barbiturates, and alcohol. "Downbeat" nystagmus, i.e., with a quick phase downward, is uncommon but is sometimes seen in diseases affecting the cerebellum and the lower end of the brainstem.

Positional Nystagmus. This term refers to nystagmus which can be induced by certain positions of the head, and it occurs in two forms. The first, known as benign paroxysmal positional nystagmus, is caused by disease of the labyrinth, including the otolith organ. The patient complains of vertigo when he places his head in a certain position, provided the head is moved *rapidly* into that position. The vertigo does not come on immediately, but only after a delay of from one to five seconds. Rotary nystagmus toward the affected ear accompanies the vertigo. If the patient has the fortitude to maintain the critical position, both the nystagmus and the vertigo rapidly pass off, but if the head movement is repeated within minutes, the symptoms recur in a less acute degree; a third trial may fail to produce either the vertigo or nystagmus. In other words, adaptation occurs. In some cases, there is a mild upper respiratory infection or a history of middle ear disease, but the precise cause of the degenerative changes in the ear is not known. In most cases, the condition passes off within weeks or months.

The second type of positional nystagmus occurs with intrinsic lesions of the lower part of the brainstem and can also occur when the pons and medulla are compressed by an extramedullary tumor. Vertigo is slight and may be absent, but the nystagmus is more prolonged since adaptation does not occur. In contrast to positional nystagmus arising in the ear, abolition of visual fixation tends to reduce or abolish the nystagmus.

PENDULAR NYSTAGMUS

Congenital nystagmus consists of a rapid, fine nystagmus of pendular type on looking forward and a coarse, jerk nystagmus on looking to either side. Vision is not impaired. The head is often turned so that the eyes are in the position of least nystagmus. The lateral optokinetic response may be absent or defective, but the vertical response is normal. The labyrinthine caloric responses are often hyperactive. In a minority, the condition is hereditary; in most other cases, there is no obvious cause for the disorder.

Pendular nystagmus also occurs as a result of loss of central vision early in infancy, before the fixation reflex develops. It can be caused by congenital or acquired cataracts, failure of the macula to develop, complete color blindness, and chorioretinal disease involving both eyes. It is characterized by oscillations of approximately equal rate, which may be fine or coarse. On conjugate gaze to either side, jerk nystagmus appears, with a fast component to the side of gaze. It is sometimes accompanied by head nodding, the movement of the head being opposite to that of the eyes. If the head is held firmly, the nystagmus is increased.

In *spasmus nutans*, pendular nystagmus is associated with head nodding. It may be monocular or binocular. It comes on during the first two years of life and lasts weeks or months. There is no impairment of central vision, and the cause of the condition is unknown.

Miner's nystagmus occurs in persons who work in poorly lighted mines. There is a fine, rapid, pendular nystagmus. Symptoms may be present or absent. Sometimes the nystagmus is associated with blepharospasm and other features of an anxiety neurosis, in which event the patient complains that outside objects appear to move in time with the movements of the eyes. Such awareness of movement is also experienced by persons who have the gift of producing nystagmus voluntarily. Since many individuals with miner's nystagmus have no ocular symptoms, it is possible that those patients who do complain are interested in the benefits of Workmen's Compensation.

OTHER FORMS OF NYSTAGMUS

In *latent nystagmus*, a jerk nystagmus is induced by covering one eye; the uncovered eye drifts towards the side of the covered eye, with a fast corrective phase in the opposite direction. It has no pathological significance, but loss of one eye will result in nystagmus in the other.

Paretic nystagmus, due to muscular weakness, is sometimes seen in otherwise normal persons at the extreme limits of conjugate gaze. It is commonly encountered in association with a defect of the ocular muscles or of the nerves which control them. The nystagmus is always horizontal or vertical, and the fast component is in the direction of the paresis of gaze. The movement is most marked in the affected eye.

In *dissociated nystagmus*, due to a lesion of the brainstem, the nystagmus may be confined to or more evident in the abducted eye and absent or less evident in the adducted eye. It is often associated with internuclear ophthalmoplegia.

A rare form of involuntary eye movement on conjugate gaze is "*nystagmus retractorius*," which consists of irregular jerks of the eye backward into the orbit, when the patient looks in one or another direction. It is usually associated with paralysis of upward gaze caused by a lesion in the midbrain, and it is thought that the retraction of the eyes is caused by simultaneous contraction of the rectus muscles and relaxation of the oblique muscles.

In *see-saw nystagmus*, one eye moves up while the other moves down. The up-and-down movements are accompanied by a slight torsion of each eyeball. It is usually encountered in patients with bitemporal hemianopia from lesions in the region of the optic chiasm or third ventricle, but can also occur on a congenital basis without any defect of visual fields.

The term *opsoclonus* is applied to chaotic, nonrhythmic oscillations of the eyes in horizontal and vertical directions. It usually occurs in patients who are unconscious as a result of disease in the posterior fossa and has also been described in subacute parenchymatous degeneration of the cerebellum associated with carcinoma of the breast. It is not to be confused with nystagmus.

In "*ocular bobbing*," regular, bilaterally synchronous, up-and-down bobbing movements of the eyes occur in association with palatal myoclonus; the movements of the eyes are synchronous with those of the soft palate.

Voluntary nystagmus is a special variety of pendular nystagmus in which the subject can produce fine, rapid, horizontal oscillations of the eyes for two or three minutes at a time. It has no clinical significance. Other diverting tricks, rarely encountered, are the ability to protrude one or both eyes at will, and a capacity to rotate both eyes, either clockwise or counterclockwise, at great speed.

PROPTOSIS (EXOPHTHALMOS)

Proptosis is often associated with diplopia, which can be due either to displacement of the eye or to involvement of the nerves and muscles by whatever is causing the protrusion of the eye.

A modest degree of proptosis without diplopia is common in thyrotoxicosis. A more severe condition, exophthalmic ophthalmoplegia is described below.

Trauma to the bony walls of the orbit can produce an orbital hematoma, with or without emphysema, while crushing injuries to the chest which interfere with venous return from the head can cause proptosis and widespread ecchymoses of the skin of the face and neck, together with gross edema of the conjunctivae.

Vascular causes of exophthalmos include angiomatous malformations of the orbit, cavernous sinus thrombosis, carotid-cavernous fistula (in which event the eye pulsates), and compression of the superior vena cava by a mass in the superior mediastinum. Intracranial saccular aneurysms do not as a rule cause protrusion of the eye.

Primary tumors of the orbit may arise from the optic nerve or its meningeal investment, from the walls of the orbit, from the lacrimal glands, or from the lymphatic tissue. Invasion of the orbit by neoplasms from the paranasal sinuses is not infrequent. Proptosis can also be caused by metastases from the suprarenal, and occurs in chloroma and Hodgkin's disease. Retro-orbital intracranial

tumors occasionally cause a modest degree of unilateral exophthalmos.

In pseudotumor of the orbit,[29] there is unilateral proptosis with paralysis of external ocular muscles of varying degree. The proptosis is painful, and the patient looks ill. The sedimentation rate is elevated. The soft tissues of the orbit are infiltrated by lymphocytes, plasma cells, and occasional giant cells. The blood vessels are involved with mural and perivascular cell infiltration. Unlike endocrine exopthalmos, the condition is unilateral and painful, visual loss is apt to occur early and rapidly, and there may be evidence of collagen disease elsewhere in the body.

Parasitic cysts, notably hydatid cysts and onchocerciasis, are an occasional cause of unilateral proptosis. Paget's disease of bone, whether generalized or in the form of leontiasis ossea, is a rare cause. Periostitis of the superior orbital fissure associated with ethmoiditis can cause protrusion of the eye and diplopia.[33] Craniostenosis (p. 195) and Hand–Schüller–Christian disease are rare causes of exophthalmos.

Unilateral or bilateral angioneurotic edema can cause a considerable degree of swelling of the lids, exophthalmos, and diplopia; in rare instances, it is associated with transient neurological signs, which can include hemiparesis, cortical blindness, loss of vision in one eye, bulbar symptoms, and seizures.

Voluntary protrusion of one or both eyes has been recorded in individuals who appear to have the ability to contract the oblique muscles and relax the recti at the same time.

EXOPHTHALMIC OPHTHALMOPLEGIA

(Malignant Exophthalmos, Thyrotrophic Exophthalmos, Endocrine Exophthalmos)

Progressive exophthalmos with impaired movement of the eyeballs occurs in a small number of patients with thyrotoxicosis; in the majority of the patients, the general symptoms of the disease are slight, and in others the condition occurs following partial thyroidectomy or treatment by thiouracil.

The condition is not due to an excess of thyroid hormone, as it may occur following thyroidectomy when the basal metabolism is normal or subnormal. It has been suggested that exophthalmos results from excess secretion of the thyrotrophic hormone of the anterior pituitary because exophthalmos and changes in the orbital tissues similar to those of exophthalmic ophthalmoplegia can be produced in guinea pigs by injections of this hormone.

Pathology. There is considerable increase in size of the external ocular muscles, which are edematous and infiltrated with lymphocytes. In the late stages, they may become fibrotic. The tension in the orbit is increased.

Clinical Features. Exophthalmic ophthalmoplegia is rather more common in men than in women and rarely occurs before the age of 40. In many cases the condition is bilateral, but one eye is usually more affected than the other. There is progressive exophthalmos associated with double vision due to paresis of one or more of the extraocular muscles. Diplopia occasionally occurs early, before proptosis is evident. The pupillary reactions are not affected. The ocular movements most frequently involved are elevation and abduction of the eyeball. There is edema of the conjunctiva and eyelids. If the exophthalmos is extreme, there is danger of corneal laceration because the lids cannot close over the eye. Occasionally, papilledema with consecutive optic atrophy and impaired visual acuity have occurred.

In the majority of patients, the condition progresses for some months and then becomes stationary; in a few cases, spontaneous improvement may then occur.

Treatment. If the degree of proptosis is such as to interfere with closure of the lids, or if papilledema appears, the orbit should be decompressed. The results of treatment with a variety of endocrine extracts have been unconvincing, as has x-ray therapy to the orbit or pituitary gland or both.

FUNCTIONAL DISTURBANCES OF VISION

Visual symptoms are common in psychoneuroses and psychoses. The nature of the complaints varies widely from case to case, but common to them all is a background of psychological or emotional aberration and an absence of organic changes sufficient to account for the symptoms. They occur in hysteria, hypochondriasis, anxiety states, obsessional neurosis, the psychoses, and malingering.

Conditions Causing Functional Disturbances

Perhaps the most common complaint is of "spots before the eyes." The patient sees floating specks, which are sometimes due to vitreous bodies. They are ignored by normal persons, but become a source of preoccupation to the anxious. Similarly, patients may become preoccupied with the normal after-images which are seen when an object is moved about, especially in rooms illuminated by alternating current. Concentric contraction of the visual fields occurs as a manifestation of hysteria, and sudden blindness in one or both eyes may have the same basis. When complete blindness is professed, diagnostic assistance can be obtained from the normality of the optic discs, brisk pupillary reflexes, the presence of optokinetic nystagmus, and the fact that the electroencephalogram responds normally to photic stimulation of the eye. Care must be taken not to confuse hysterical fugues (during which familiar objects and people are not recognized) with true visual agnosia due to disease of the temporoparietal lobes. The latter is usually, but not always, associated with homonymous field defects and is seldom total; some objects are recognized, others are not.

Visual hallucinations may be organic or psychogenic in origin. The former group includes intoxications, Wernicke's encephalopathy, fevers, acute head injuries, and focal disease situated anywhere between the retina itself and the cerebral cortex. The hallucinations caused by organic disease may be either formed or unformed, i.e., the patient may "see" persons, animals, or other complex forms which bear some resemblance to normal visual experiences, or he may observe flashes of light, amorphous objects, colored spectra, and so on. In general, formed hallucinations are more common in affections of the temporoparietal lobes than elsewhere in the brain, while the unformed type is more typical of disease involving the retina and the calcarine area. The hallucinations experienced by patients suffering from psychoses, such as schizophrenia, depression, and paranoia, are usually of the formed variety. Patients are seldom eager to admit to visual hallucinations, but sometimes their presence can be deduced from the fact that the patient appears to be watching things which are not visible to the bystander.

Double vision is rarely functional, but it can be. Monocular diplopia sometimes occurs in individuals with congenital or traumatic "double" pupil, dislocation of the lens, or lesions of the parieto-occipital region.[45] Binocular diplopia should never be regarded as functional until every other possibility has been excluded. It sometimes happens that somebody who normally neglects the image from one eye because of a refractive error or a squint, suddenly ceases to suppress this image, and thereupon sees double. This can occur in anxiety states. Another strange condition, apparently functional, is double vision occurring as a result of willed dissociation of ocular movement: When asked to follow a moving object, the patient follows now with one eye, now with the other, appearing to be able to move each eye independently. In yet others,

diplopia is induced by active convergence of the eyes.

Blepharospasm is a relatively common functional complaint, which is often seen following conjunctivitis, but it may occur without antecedent disease in anxiety states and obsessional neuroses. Excessive or defective convergence and spasm of accommodation can occur, leading to ocular fatigue and headache—a form of asthenopia. This is to be suspected when a patient develops ocular fatigue when carrying out uncongenial tasks, but not when using the eyes for more acceptable work.

THE FIFTH CRANIAL NERVE

The trigeminal nerve consists of a small motor portion and a larger sensory element (Fig. 6–13). The motor nucleus lies in the lateral part of the tegmental portion of the pons, and its fibers pass forward, emerging from the ventral aspect of the pons with the sensory root and passing below the gasserian ganglion to join the mandibular division of the nerve. The motor nucleus receives fibers from both pyramidal tracts. Paralysis of the motor root paralyzes the muscles of mastication on that side; on opening the jaw, the mandible is pulled to the side of the lesion by the unopposed action of the pterygoid muscles on the normal side. Lesions of the peripheral fibers are rare, whereas nuclear palsies are not uncommon in poliomyelitis and the bulbar form of amyotrophic lateral sclerosis. Inability to open the mouth through spasm of the masseters (trismus) occurs in tetanus and in acute inflammatory disease of the tonsillar region, teeth, jaws, and temporo-mandibular joint. Unilateral pyramidal lesions seldom interfere with mastication.

The sensory fibers of the trigeminal originate in cells situated in the gasserian ganglion, the equivalent of the dorsal root ganglia, which lies in a dural recess at the apex of the petrous bone, lateral to the internal carotid artery and behind

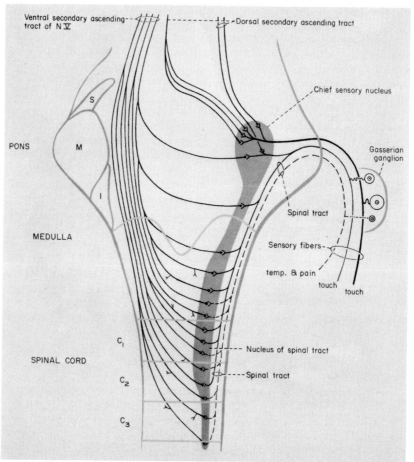

Figure 6–13. Projection of the somatic sensory branches of the trigeminal nerve. (Modified from Crosby, E. C., Humphrey, T., and Lauer, E. W.: *Correlative Anatomy of the Nervous System.* The Macmillan Co., New York, 1962.)

the cavernous sinus. The axons divide into central and peripheral branches. The latter form three bundles, the ophthalmic, maxillary, and mandibular divisions of the nerve.

OPHTHALMIC DIVISION. The ophthalmic division passes forward in the lateral wall of the cavernous sinus, lying lateral to the carotid artery and below the oculomotor and trochlear nerves, and the maxillary branch lies below it. These relationships explain why pain in the eye and forehead is a feature of some aneurysms of the intracavernous portion of the carotid artery and why sensory impairment occurs in the distribution of the ophthalmic division in thrombosis of the cavernous sinus. The ophthalmic

division furnishes the main sensory supply of the intracranial dura mater above the tentorium. It enters the orbit through the superior orbital fissure and supplies the skin of the anterior half of the scalp, the forehead, the ridge of the nose, the upper eyelid, the eye, the upper part of the nasal cavity, and the frontal sinus. It carries sympathetic fibers to the iris and sends a twig to the lachrymal gland. Loss of the corneal reflex is an early feature of a lesion of the ophthalmic division or of its sensory root, and is an important sign in *large* tumors of the cerebellopontine angle, such as an acoustic neurinoma. The first division is also liable to be involved in fractures of the orbit and in inflammatory lesions of the superior orbital fissure.[33] Because of its widespread dural distribution, many intracranial lesions involving the dura and the venous sinuses cause referred pain in the forehead.

MAXILLARY DIVISION. The maxillary division leaves the skull through the foramen rotundum, crosses the pterygopalatine fossa (where it may be involved by a growth of the nasopharynx, with pain and paresthesias in the cheek), traverses the floor of the orbit in the infraorbital groove, and emerges onto the face through the infraorbital foramen. It supplies the skin of the temple, the cheek, and the upper lip, together with the upper teeth and gum, the hard and soft palate, the anterior part of the tonsillar fossa, the lower part of the nasal cavity, part of the middle ear, the maxillary antrum, and the nasopharynx. It is occasionally injured in fractures of the maxilla, and during recovery there may be troublesome paresthesias in the cheek. The distribution to the temple explains the occasional reference of pain from the upper teeth or hard palate to the side of the head; this may occur without much local discomfort at the site of the disease.

MANDIBULAR DIVISION. The mandibular division is formed by fusion of the third division with the motor root. It leaves the skull through the foramen ovale to supply the skin over the lower jaw (excluding the angle of the jaw, which is innervated by C2–C3), the anterior two-thirds of the tongue, the floor of the mouth, the lower teeth and gums, and the external auditory meatus and the ear drum. This last explains why earache can occur with painful lesions of the tongue and lower jaw. The chorda tympani runs with the lingual nerve to supply taste in the anterior two-thirds of the tongue; unilateral impairment of taste sometimes occurs temporarily during degeneration of the mandibular branch after section of the sensory root of the trigeminal nerve. Injuries to the auriculotemporal branch of the third division can give rise to the *auriculotemporal syndrome*, characterized by flushing and profuse sweating of the skin of the temple during mastication.

The Sensory Root and Its Connections

The central fibers from the gasserian ganglion pass to the pons in the sensory root, in which the three divisions of the nerve remain distinct, so that it is possible for the surgeon to cut fibers representing the upper, middle, or lower face in the treatment of trigeminal pain.

After the sensory root enters the pons, a rearrangement takes place. Fibers for touch and proprioception end in both the mesencephalic nucleus and the principal sensory nucleus in the lateral part of the tegmentum of the pons, whence a fresh relay crosses to the opposite side to form the quintothalamic tract, lying on the inner side of the medial lemniscus. Fibers conveying pain and temperature turn downward to end in the spinal nucleus of the trigeminal nerve, which runs through the medulla and into the upper three segments of the cervical cord. This nucleus also receives sensory fibers from the seventh, ninth, tenth, eleventh, and twelfth cranial nerves. Fibers from the ophthalmic division end in the lower part of the spinal nucleus, those from the mandibular division in the highest part, and those in the maxillary division have an intermediate termination. From the nucleus, a fresh relay sweeps upward, crosses the midline, and joins the medial lemniscus (Fig. 6–13).

The presence of pain fibers from the trigeminal nerve in the upper cervical cord explains why pain from lesions in the upper part of the neck can be referred to the forehead; sensory fibers entering the cord through the upper three or four cervical roots synapse with cells in the spinal trigeminal nucleus. Lesions of the lower part of the brainstem and upper portions of the cervical cord can cause dissociated sensory loss in the face; a lesion in the pons, involving the principal sensory nucleus, causes impairment to light touch with preservation of pain and temperature sensibility, whereas lesions involving the medulla and upper cervical segments of the cord cause impairment to pain and temperature, with preservation of the corneal reflex and sensibility to light touch. Lesions in this region can produce pain in the face, which can simulate idiopathic tic douloureux. When syringobulbia involves the descending nucleus, sensory loss usually occurs in the peripheral parts of the face first, and gradually converges down toward the mouth and tip of the nose. Occlusion of the posterior inferior cerebellar artery causes loss of pain and temperature sensibility on the face, with relative sparing of light touch; this is part of a far wider clinical picture, which includes ipsilateral cerebellar ataxia, paralysis of the ipsilateral bulbar nuclei, and contralateral weakness and sensory loss below the level of the lesion.

TRIGEMINAL NEUROPATHY

This term has been applied to cases displaying persistent sensory impairment on one side of the face, without other neurological signs, and a chronic course which sometimes ends in recovery after months or years.[25, 44] Occasionally it is bilateral.

Little is known about the pathology. Hughes [28] reported three patients in whom sudden pain was followed by sensory deficit on one side of the face; at operation, all showed gross atrophy of the sensory root, and the histology suggested a mild chronic inflammatory process. It has been reported in collagen disease—systemic lupus erythematosus, Sjögren's syndrome, and progressive systemic sclerosis. For the time being, it would be prudent to regard isolated trigeminal neuropathy as a syndrome rather than as a single disease.

In one group of cases, the onset is slow, with tingling and progressive loss of sensation on one side of the face. There is often a sense of burning on the affected side of the tongue. Sensory loss usually starts around the upper lip and nostril and extends slowly to involve the cheek, lower jaw, and the inside of the mouth on the affected side. Pain sensibility may be more depressed than touch.

The second and third divisions are involved with about equal frequency, the first division being less often affected. Indolent ulceration of the nostril and upper lip may occur.

In other cases, the onset is acute, with or without pain in the face. Of 16 cases reported by Spillane and Wells,[44] seven were painful and 10 had an acute onset. The muscles of mastication were seldom involved. Ptosis or Horner's syndrome may be present. In 10 further cases reported by Blau and his colleagues, the neuropathy developed rapidly, was painless, and did not affect motor function. The first division was affected in only one patient. Five of their patients recovered completely within four and a half months, but two showed no recovery after two years.

Differential diagnosis should take into consideration multiple sclerosis, nasopharyngeal carcinoma, neurinoma of the trigeminal ganglion or root, meningioma, and tumors and small infarcts of the pons.

FACIAL HEMIATROPHY
(PARRY–ROMBERG SYNDROME)

This very rare condition is characterized by gradual atrophy of the bone and subcutaneous tissue on one side of the face, without sensory loss or paralysis. It can come on at any age and is commoner in women than in men. It usually starts over the cheek, where the skin and subcutaneous tissues become thin, leaving a small depression. Ultimately, the bone atrophies and the zone of shrinkage may extend to the forehead, eye, mandible, tongue, and pinna. Sometimes it extends to the side of the neck, and, in a case described by Martin, it also involved the breast on the same side. Dull pain may be present over the face. There is some loss of hair near the midline on the affected side of the face and scalp, with either increase or decrease of sweating on the affected side. Pupillary abnormalities have been described, and in some cases Horner's syndrome has been present. In a case described by

Brain, there was marked atrophy of the *ipsilateral* cerebral hemisphere. Jacksonian seizures on the side opposite to the atrophy have occurred in some cases.

The cause is unknown, but it is possible that facial hemiatrophy is related to progressive hemiatrophy of the whole body.

No successful treatment for the condition is known. Subcutaneous injections of liquid silicone are used for cosmetic reasons, but further time is needed to assess the long-term effects of this procedure.

THE FACIAL NERVE

The facial nerve supplies the muscles of facial expression and the platysma. It arises from the motor nucleus in the lower pons, runs backward to hook round the nucleus of the sixth nerve, and then turns forward through the pons to emerge at its lower border, close to the eighth nerve. Its sensory root (nervus intermedius of Wrisberg) contains fibers conveying deep sensation from the face and also taste fibers from the anterior two-thirds of the tongue. The latter fibers pass to the nucleus solitarius in the medulla, where they are joined by taste fibers from the glossopharyngeal nerve. The facial nerve also conveys secretory fibers destined for the lachrymal, sublingual, and submandibular glands (the parotid gland receives autonomic fibers from the auriculotemporal branch of the mandibular division of the fifth nerve). The facial nerve crosses the subarachnoid space and passes into the internal auditory canal immediately above the eighth nerve. It first runs laterally, then turns downward, and at this point traverses the geniculate ganglion, which is the nucleus of the sensory root. It arches through the wall of the aditus to the tympanic antrum, where it is exposed to the danger of being cut during radical mastoidectomy, and emerges through the stylomastoid foramen. The taste fibers leave the nerve before it reaches the foramen, passing between the layers of the

tympanic membrane (whence the name chorda tympani) and leave the skull to join the lingual nerve en route to the tongue.

Conditions Involving the Facial Nerve

Paralysis of the muscles of expression is most commonly seen in Bell's palsy, which is described later in this chapter. The facial nerve can also be damaged in lesions of the parotid region—birth injuries from forceps, war wounds, operations on the parotid gland itself, parotid tumors, and sarcoidosis of the gland. Injury or disease in the region of the stylomastoid foramen likewise causes facial paralysis, without loss of taste on the anterior two-thirds of the tongue. If the lesion is just below the geniculate ganglion (fracture of the petrous temporal bone, disease of the inner ear), there is loss of taste as well as facial palsy. Deafness is usually present in lesions at this point; if hearing is not lost, there may be hyperacusis from paralysis of the stapedius muscle. Geniculate herpes is an occasional cause of facial paralysis. A lesion between the auditory meatus and the pons (acoustic neuroma, meningitis) sometimes spares taste and deep sensation from the facial muscles.

Gross disease of the motor nucleus is likely to involve the adjacent sixth nerve as well, but this may not occur when the lesion is very small, as in poliomyelitis. Congenital aplasia of the seventh nucleus may be unilateral or bilateral; when bilateral, the resultant facial paralysis is known as facial diplegia, and is often associated with bilateral abducens paralysis.[51]

Supranuclear facial paralysis, the result of a unilateral pyramidal lesion, affects the lower half of the face more than the upper, whereas the upper and lower halves are equally involved in nuclear and peripheral lesions. Disease in or near the motor cortex sometimes causes loss of emotional movements of the lower face with retention of voluntary movements. Bilateral supranuclear paralysis causes complete paralysis of the face, both upper and lower, and affects both volitional movements and emotional expression. It is very rare and is usually part of a double hemiplegia.

BELL'S PALSY

Bell's palsy is a common disease characterized by the rapid onset of facial palsy of peripheral type, usually followed by recovery in a matter of weeks or months (Fig. 6–14). It occurs sporadically and, at times, in small localized epidemics.

Pathology. Bell's palsy is considered to be the result of an inflammatory condition of the fibrous sheath of the nerve as it lies in its bony canal proximal to the stylomastoid foramen; in some cases, the inflammation spreads up the canal to involve the chorda tympani, causing impairment of taste on the affected side a day or two after the onset of the paralysis.

Clinical Features. Bell's palsy is predominantly a disease of adult life, with an equal sex incidence. Pain behind the ear is sometimes present at onset, and at this stage there may be

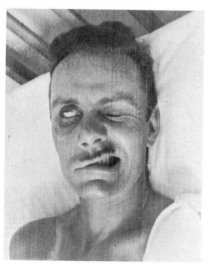

Figure 6–14. Bell's palsy on right side. (Courtesy of Dr. A. Ornsteen.)

deep tenderness behind the angle of the jaw. The affected side of the face feels stiff and numb, and paralysis comes on rapidly. Indeed, the patient may awaken one morning to find one side of the face paralyzed without any antecedent symptoms. In other cases, it takes a day or two to become complete. The affected muscles fail to respond to volitional or emotional stimuli, and the unopposed muscles of the sound side may pull the mouth over. Though the patient often complains that the face feels numb, there is no superficial sensory loss; deep pressure pain and vibration may be slightly impaired, and there is sometimes loss of taste over the anterior two-thirds of the tongue on the affected side. In a few cases, hyperacusis occurs, probably from involvement of the nerve to the stapedius. The lower lid is apt to fall away from the eye, allowing tears to escape onto the cheek.

In about 70 per cent of all cases there is no fibrillation to be found on electromyography, and no reaction of degeneration; such cases recover quickly and completely. In the remainder, degeneration of the nerve occurs, as determined by electrophysiological tests,[48] and recovery may not start for three months or more. It has been claimed that prognostic information can be obtained by measuring the conduction time in the facial nerve between the front of the ear and the angle of the mouth. In normal subjects and in patients with facial paralysis who will recover fully, conduction time is always less than 4.0 milliseconds. Partial denervation is indicated by slowing beyond 4.0 milliseconds, and when complete denervation is present, the nerve becomes inexcitable by the end of the first week. Recovery may be incomplete, and contractures can lead to displacement of the angle of the mouth toward the paralyzed side. Misdirection of regenerating nerve fibers sometimes leads to troublesome synkinesia; for instance, the eye winks when the patient smiles.

Diagnosis. Unilateral facial paralysis is seen in poliomyelitis, encephalitis, acute infective polyneuritis, and many forms of meningitis, both acute and chronic, but in such cases, the general setting will indicate its origin. In herpetic infection of the geniculate ganglion there is a herpetiform rash in the auditory meatus, on the pinna, and on the anterior wall of the fauces; there is often considerable pain deep in the ear, and facial paralysis follows. Facial paralysis, either unilateral or bilateral, can occur with or without swelling of the parotid gland in uveoparotid polyneuritis, a manifestation of sarcoidosis. Chronic otitis media with or without cholesteatosis is an occasional cause of facial palsy associated with deafness. Fracture of the petrous temporal bone is an obvious explanation for facial paralysis occurring at the time of an injury, but it may also occur a week or 10 days after the injury; this delayed type recovers well.

Facial paralysis of slow onset does not enter into the differential diagnosis of Bell's palsy, which is usually complete in a matter of a day or two, but it is useful to summarize some of the causes of a slowly progressive palsy. The bilateral weakness found in heredofamilial facioscapulohumeral dystrophy, myotonic dystrophy, and myasthenia gravis is unlikely to cause confusion. Lesions of the petrous temporal bone — chronic otitis media with cholesteatosis, cholesteatoma, and tumor of the glomus jugulare — can cause facial palsy and deafness. Neurinoma of the eighth nerve gives rise to deafness, vertigo, and facial weakness, followed by loss of the corneal reflex, cerebellar ataxia, and evidence of raised intracranial pressure. Leprosy is an important cause of facial palsy in Africa and the Orient. Tumor of the pons itself is a rare cause of facial paralysis and is usually associated with an abducens palsy on the same side, together with nystagmus, vertigo, and long tract signs. Bilateral facial paralysis is a late development in the bulbar palsy of amyotrophic lateral sclerosis.

Treatment. It has been claimed that the daily administration of ACTH from the first day of paralysis is valuable. In facial paralysis due to geniculate herpes, large doses of prednisone are very effective provided treatment is started within the first four days (p. 303). If the weakened muscles around the mouth are being pulled to the unaffected side, causing disfigurement, the deformity can be prevented by applying an oral splint to a tooth, with a hook projecting around the angle of the mouth on the paralyzed side. The same purpose is served, though less efficiently, by an external splint anchored over the ear. The facial muscles should receive daily massage and galvanism, but the latter must be stopped if signs of contracture appear. Facial movements can be practiced in front of a mirror as soon as there is some return of movement. Decompression of the facial nerve on its bony canal has not proved useful. Hypoglossal-facial anastomosis can prove effective in selected cases of persistent paralysis.[30]

FACIAL SPASM

Clonic spasm of the facial muscles and platysma on one side is a malady of varied etiology which afflicts adults in the second half of life (Fig. 6–15). Gardner and Sava (1962) found a definite pathological process in the cerebellopontine angle in seven of 19 cases which

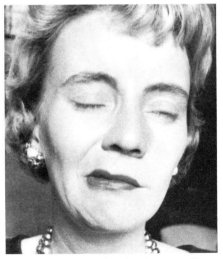

Figure 6–15. Idiopathic facial spasm. (Courtesy of Dr. A. Ornsteen.)

they explored. The spasm varies from a slight and occasional flicker around the eye or mouth to a persistent severe spasm which screws up the eye, retracts the angle of the mouth, and makes the platysma stand out prominently. It is aggravated by excitement, and ceases with sleep. It differs from psychogenic facial tic in being one-sided. In a few cases, a moderate degree of facial weakness ultimately supervenes on the affected side. The spasm can be abolished by intracranial or extracranial neurolysis of the facial nerve.[39] Recovery has also been reported following chemothalamotomy. *Tonic* facial spasm occasionally occurs in tumors of the pons. Tonic retraction of the lips on both sides occurs in the late stages of Wilson's disease.

EIGHTH CRANIAL NERVE

The eighth cranial nerve consists of two sets of fibers which are distinct as to origin, destination, and function (Fig. 6–16).

The Auditory Nerve

The auditory nerve arises from the ganglion cells of the cochlea, runs medially in the internal auditory canal beneath the facial nerve, and, after winding around the lateral border of the inferior cerebellar peduncle, ends in two nuclei in the lower part of the floor of the fourth ventricle. A fresh relay passes up in the lateral lemniscus of both sides to the medial geniculate bod-

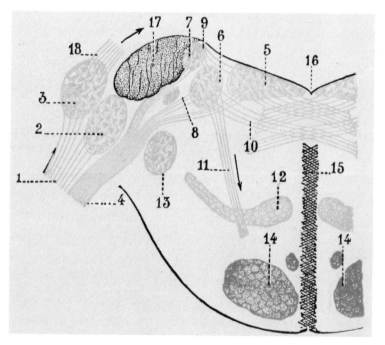

Figure 6–16. Terminal nuclei of the eighth nerve, with their upper connections (schematic). 1, Cochlear nerve, with its two nuclei; 2, accessory nucleus; 3, tuberculum acusticum; 4, vestibular nerve; 5, internal nucleus; 6, nucleus of Deiters; 7, nucleus of Bechterew; 8, inferior or descending root of acoustic; 9, ascending cerebellar fibers; 10, fibers going to raphe; 11, fibers taking an oblique course; 12, lemniscus; 13, inferior sensory root of trigeminal; 14, cerebrospinal fasciculus; 15, raphe; 16, fourth ventricle; 17, inferior peduncle; 18, origin of striae medullares. (From Goss, C. M. [ed.]: *Gray's Anatomy of the Human Body.* 27th Ed. Lea & Febiger, Philadelphia, 1959.)

ies, and from here, auditory impulses are mediated to Heschl's gyrus in the temporal lobe via the auditory radiation, which lies posterior to the internal capsule. Each temporal lobe receives afferent fibers from both sides, and this explains why unilateral lesion of the internal capsule or temporal lobe never causes deafness. Bilateral temporal lesions could—theoretically—cause total loss of hearing.

DEAFNESS

Deafness can be due to (1) disease of the middle ear—conduction deafness; (2) disease of the cochlea; (3) disease of the eighth nerve; (4) lesions of the pons. Conduction deafness is distinguished from nerve deafness by tuning fork tests: When a vibrating fork is placed in the center of the forehead the sound is heard best in the deaf ear in conduction deafness and in the good ear in nerve deafness (Weber's test). Secondly, Rinne established that in normal man as well as in patients with nerve deafness, air conduction is better than bone conduction, whereas in middle ear deafness, the reverse holds true. Absolute bone conduction, tested by holding the base of the tuning fork to the mastoid process until the patient cannot hear the sound, is reduced in nerve deafness. It is usually possible to distinguish between the nerve deafness caused by lesions of the cochlea and affections of the auditory nerve and its central pathways, because loudness recruitment[13] is present in cochlear lesions and absent or incomplete in central lesions. That is to say, in cochlear deafness, sounds which are audible may sound louder than they should. Moreover, once the hearing threshold is passed the affected ear hears as well as the other, and the intelligibility of speech does not improve with increase in loudness. In auditory nerve lesions, on the other hand, the relative deafness persists however loud the stimulus, recruitment does not usually occur, and the intelligibility of the spoken word im-

proves with loudness. Intermittent auditory stimuli are better heard than continuous tones in nerve lesions; the reverse holds in cochlear deafness. In lesions involving the *auditory nuclei in the pons*, there is severe tone perversion, recruitment may be present or absent, the pure tone threshold is normal or only slightly elevated, and the response to auditory discrimination tasks may be either normal or greatly diminished; the caloric responses are normal unless the lesion also involves the vestibular nuclei.

Cochlear deafness occurs as a result of local infection, including otitis, syphilis, senile degeneration of the cochlea, otosclerosis, mumps, typhoid, severe head injuries, thrombosis of the internal auditory artery, and abuse of salicylates, quinine, and streptomycin. It is most commonly seen in Meniere's disease (p. 115).

Auditory nerve deafness is usually due to an acoustic neurinoma and less commonly to meningitis, fracture or tumor of the petrous temporal bone, Paget's disease, and neoplastic or vascular lesions in the lateral part of the pons.

Hysterical deafness obeys no laws, but like other hysterical phenomena. it occurs against a background of neurosis, is unassociated with organic disease, and can usually be influenced by suggestion.

TINNITUS

The phrase "noises in the head" as used by patients may mean tinnitus, an intracranial bruit, or auditory hallucinations.

Tinnitus consists of a persistent noise in the ear which is described as a hissing, singing, buzzing, or whistling. It is a common accompaniment of wax in the ears, all manner of chronic aural disease, and lesions of the auditory nerve; it can also be caused by disease of the brainstem and cerebral hemispheres. It occurs in persons working in noisy surroundings, and as a result of intoxication with quinine and salicylates. Many people are able to disregard it, but it may prove a burden to individuals suffering from fatigue and anxiety, and can become the nucleus of a hypochondriacal state in obsessional subjects. Sedation, the traditional treatment, has little effect. The patient must be encouraged to ignore what cannot be helped.

An intracranial *bruit* indicates the presence of arteriovenous fistula and follows the rhythm of the pulse. Unlike tinnitus, it can usually be heard by the observer. Occasionally it occurs in severe Paget's disease of the skull, owing to the presence of wide diploic vessels, which serve as arteriovenous shunts. A bruit may be observed in normal children up to the age of about seven years; it is accentuated by arterial hypertension.

Auditory hallucinations occur in two forms. Voices may be heard, saying things which may or may not have meaning for the individual concerned; this is commonly a symptom of nonorganic psychosis, but also occurs in acute intoxications and temporal lobe lesions. An extremely brief hallucination of this type may precede a seizure. The second variety of auditory hallucinations consists of undifferentiated noises, such as whistling, bells, and buzzing, which occur now and again in patients with a lesion anywhere from the cochlea to the temporal lobe.

The Vestibular Nerve

The vestibular fibers of the eighth nerve arise in the ganglion of Scarpa, lying in the internal auditory canal, and convey information from the semicircular canals, the utricle, and the saccule. The afferent fibers pass medially with the cochlear division of the nerve, and after passing through the cerebellar pontine angle, enter the brainstem at the inferior border of the pons. Most of them terminate in the medial vestibular nucleus, the lateral nucleus (of Deiter), and the superior nucleus (of Bechterew), which are situated in the floor of the lateral recess of the fourth ventricle. A

few pass to the descending vestibular tract, which extends downward into the medulla as far as the sensory decussation. Some fibers also enter the inferior cerebellar peduncle and reach the cerebellar cortex. The vestibulospinal tract arises from the lateral vestibular nucleus. Another relay enters the medial longitudinal bundle, so establishing an important connection between the labyrinth and the nuclei of the third, fourth, and sixth cranial nerves. The temporal lobe appears to be concerned with the appreciation of vertigo as a sensation, because when seizures commence with an aura of vertigo, the lesion is usually found in this part of the brain.

In some brainstem lesions, caloric stimulation of the labyrinth produces nystagmus, pallor, and vomiting, without any subjective sensation of rotation, indicating that the afferent pathways to the thalamus and cortex have been interrupted. A similar situation is occasionally seen in patients who have attacks of pallor, sweating, staggering, and nystagmus, without any sense of vertigo. This occurs from time to time in patients with vertebral-basilar arterial insufficiency and in brainstem tumors.

Disturbances of vestibular function give rise to vertigo, incoordination of the ipsilateral limbs, past-pointing, and nystagmus. Diseases involving the internal ear or the eighth nerve commonly produce both auditory and vestibular symptoms, but since the auditory and vestibular paths separate once the nerves enter the brainstem, impairment of hearing is rarely associated with vertigo in lesions of the brain and brainstem.

VERTIGO

Vertigo may be defined as a sense of rotation or movement, either of self or surroundings, in any plane. It may amount to little more than a feeling that the ground is moving slightly, or it may take the form of a catastrophic and frightening sense of spinning. When very slight, it causes a sense of dysequilibrium without a sensation of movement, similar to what is experienced at the beginning of a caloric test of labyrinthine function, before a sense of rotation is felt. Vertigo of all degrees and origins is *usually* aggravated by movements of the head in space, and is accompanied (when severe) by anxiety, difficulty in thinking, pallor, fall of blood pressure, sweating, and nausea or vomiting. Past-pointing occurs to the side of the lesion, and the gait may be so unsteady as to prevent standing or walking. In acute cases, the patient may be hurled to the ground.

The words "dizzy" and "giddy" are applied by patients to all manner of episodes, including petit mal, syncope, and mental confusion, and care must be exercised to establish the precise features of such complaints. For instance, the "dizziness" experienced on looking down from a height is not true vertigo, but a sense of visual disorientation, compounded by fear. Similarly, the momentary visual confusion occasionally complained of by patients with diplopia or gross refractive errors when the gaze is moved from one object to another is not vertigo.

Etiology. The causes of vertigo are listed according to disease of the labyrinth, vascular disease, and neurological disorders.

The Ear

Meniere's disease
Inflammatory disease
Positional vertigo
  ("positional nystagmus")
Cholesteatosis
Eustachian tube occlusion
Obstruction of external auditory
  meatus (?)
Thrombosis of internal auditory artery
Hemorrhage into the labyrinth
Head injury

The Eighth Nerve

Vestibular neuronitis
Tumor of cerebellopontine recess

The Brainstem

Thrombosis, hemorrhage, embolism
Vertebral-basilar insufficiency
Head injury
Tumors, primary or metastatic
Multiple sclerosis
Syringobulbia
Encephalitis
Aura of migraine

The Cerebellum

Occlusion of cerebellar arteries
Cerebellar hemorrhage
Abscess

The Cerebrum

Lesions of the temporal lobe
Raised intracranial pressure
Aura of epileptic seizure

Systemic Conditions

Hepatic disease with jaundice
Hypotension
Hypertension (?)
Anemia
Carotid sinus syndrome
Cough syndrome
Drugs: Salicylates, quinine, streptomycin, Dilantin, etc.

Differential Diagnosis. There is no problem when vertigo is one of many signs pointing to gross disease of the brain or ear, but diagnosis can be difficult when it occurs as the presenting symptom.

MENIERE'S DISEASE.[14, 22] This disease, caused by edema of the labyrinth, is the most important of the aural causes of vertigo. It is usually a disease of the second half of life, but can occur under the age of 20. It is characterized by intermittent attacks of vertigo, often combined with persistent tinnitus and increasing deafness of cochlear type. Each attack may last minutes or hours. Nausea, vomiting, pallor, and sweating are present in severe attacks, and occasionally there is a fall of blood pressure sufficient to cause syncope or a convulsion. Sometimes there is difficulty in thinking during attacks. The patient prefers to remain absolutely still, with the eyes closed, and finds it impossible to walk or stand. Nystagmus is present and past-pointing will be found on the affected side. There may be a mild unilateral headache. Cochlear deafness may precede the onset of vertigo or may come on after a series of attacks, and tinnitus is usually present. There are often long intervals of freedom between bouts. As time goes on, the deafness increases and may become complete.

Symptoms differing little from the above can occur for many months as the presenting feature of a neurinoma of the eighth nerve (p. 440). Vestibular neuronitis, described later in this chapter, usually occurs in younger persons, and is not accompanied by tinnitus or deafness. In positional vertigo,[8] younger persons are affected, there is no deafness or tinnitus, and vertigo is induced only when the head is in a certan position, which is specific for each patient. Nystagmus occurring *between* attacks of vertigo excludes a diagnosis of Meniere's disease and suggests a central lesion.

Treatment. The acute attacks require sedation, and drugs such as Antivert can be used on a continuing basis in an attempt to halt them. Because hydrops of the labyrinth has been found in postmortem material, regimens directed to dehydration and restriction of salt intake are recommended, but it is doubtful whether the results justify the effort. It is similarly difficult to estimate the effect of treatment such as histamine desensitization and the use of vitamin B_{12}. In severe cases, surgical treatment can be offered; if there is no useful hearing in the ear, total destruction of the internal ear is in order. Existing hearing can be spared, however, by cutting the vestibular branch of the eighth nerve intracranially[11] or by subjecting the surgically exposed labyrinth to ultrasound. Definitive treatment of this sort is desirable in the patient who is incapacitated by recurring attacks, especially if, as sometimes happens, the liability to vertigo has induced a severe degree of anxiety and depression. Indeed, psychoneurotic features may grow so prominent as to lead the unwary into supposing that the entire condition is psychological in origin.

VESTIBULAR NEURONITIS.[6, 14] This is characterized by intermittent and sometimes persistent attacks of labyrinthine vertigo, usually in the third or fourth decade, in persons who exhibit neither deafness nor tinnitus but who show gross depression of the responses to caloric stimulation. It is attributed to a disorder of the vestibular nerve or its connections. A few patients have subsequently developed multiple sclerosis, but generally the condition is benign and can be expected to pass off after a few weeks. Sometimes the patient continues to experience transient vertigo, induced by sudden movements of the head, for many months. Attention to focal sepsis in the upper respiratory tract is advised; almost half of a series of 50 cases described by Dix and Hallpike gave a clear history of an infection at the time when the vertigo came on or presented significant evidence of chronic infection in the nose and throat.[14] The condition may perhaps be related to "epidemic vertigo," which occurs in epidemiological association with encephalitis.[41]

Miscellaneous Causes of Vertigo. Vertigo is more common in disease of the pons than in disorders of the cerebellum or cerebrum. An *acute vascular incident* in the posterior fossa, whether it be thrombotic, hemorrhagic, or embolic, can cause vertigo at the onset. In the case of vertebral-basilar stenosis, it is not always easy to be sure whether the vertigo is due to transient ischemia within the territory of the internal auditory artery, which supplies the labyrinth, or to ischemia of the brainstem. Thrombosis of the internal auditory artery can occur abruptly with vertigo, deafness, and loss of caloric responses in that ear. Occasionally, only the arterial branch to the semicircular canals is involved, in which event there is vertigo with loss of caloric responses but retention of hearing. *Multiple sclerosis, syringobulbia,* and *tumors of the brainstem* can cause episodic or persistent vertigo, but satellite symptoms and signs are usually present.

The "central" type of positional vertigo can occur as the first symptom of multiple sclerosis, but this is a rare event, and it is unjustifiable to make this diagnosis on the evidence of vertigo alone. *Posterior fossa encephalitis* (p. 314) gives rise to vertigo, vomiting, and violent ataxia, symptoms which may suggest a rapidly expanding lesion in the posterior fossa. "Dizzy attacks," sometimes amounting to vertigo, but more usually taking the form of lightheadedness on sudden changes of position of the head in space, are commonly associated with headaches in the *postconcussional syndrome*,[20] and similar symptoms may arise from *whiplash injuries.* The interpretation of this "dizziness" is difficult, but caloric and rotational tests sometimes reveal a disturbance of labyrinthine function.

A brief spell of vertigo may be part of the aura of a convulsive seizure in *epilepsy.* This has to be distinguished from a seizure occurring as a result of an abrupt fall of blood pressure. Vertigo is occasionally encountered as a result of *hypotension* caused by hemorrhage, cardiac disease, or carotid sinus sensitivity. Severe *anemia* leads to lightheadedness, and sometimes to vertigo, especially when the patient gets up suddenly from a chair. This can also occur as a result of vertebral-basilar insufficiency. Paroxysms of *coughing* in obese, middle-aged men can cause vertigo, syncope, or a convulsion. Charcot called this "laryngeal vertigo," and it seems likely that the cerebral symptoms are usually due to a fall in cardiac output during the coughing spell.

Vertigo is a familiar feature of idiosyncrasy to, or overdosage with, *salicylates, quinine and its derivatives,* and *streptomycin.* In children, episodes of violent vertigo with progressive bilateral nerve deafness and interstitial keratitis constitute *Cogan's syndrome;* the cause is unknown. It is not syphilitic, though deafness, tinnitus, and vertigo do occur in adolescents as a result of *congenital syphilis.* Invasion of the fourth ventricle by *cysticercosis* and tumors has been responsible for acute attacks of vertigo. Dizziness and true vertigo are common in *heatstroke* and heat exhaustion, probably as a result of hypotension. They also occur in *hypoglycemia* from any cause, and in the early stages of *infective hepatitis.*

THE NINTH OR GLOSSOPHARYNGEAL NERVE

The glossopharyngeal nerve conveys taste, common sensation, and motor fibers. The taste fibers come from the posterior third of the tongue, pass into the tractus solitarius, and end in the nucleus of this tract in the medulla, whence a fresh relay passes up to the thalamus and so to the cortical center for taste in the lower part of the sensory cortex.[3] Taste from the anterior two-thirds of the tongue reaches the pons via fibers which travel in the lingual nerve, chorda tympani, and the nervus intermedius to the tractus solitarius, whence a new relay crosses the midline and passes upward to the thalamus and cortex. Loss of taste is seldom caused by cortical lesions because each side of the tongue is bilaterally represented in the sensory cortex. Hallucinations of taste are sometimes experienced in temporal lobe seizures.

Common sensation for the posterior third of the tongue, the oral pharynx, tonsil, and the tympanic cavity is conveyed by the glossopharyngeal nerve, the fibers of which arise from the ganglion petrosum. The tympanic branch explains why pain is sometimes referred to the ear in disease of the posterior portion of the tongue, the tonsils, and the pharynx; it will be recalled that pain is also referred to the ear from the anterior part of the tongue and buccal cavity via the auriculotemporal branch of the lingual nerve. The motor fibers of the nerve,[16] derived largely from the upper part of the nucleus ambiguus, supply the stylopharyngeus and assist in the supply of the superior constrictor of the pharynx. Unilateral paralysis may lead to a "curtain" movement of the pharyngeal wall toward the sound side on phonation or gagging, but this is more obvious in lesions of the vagus nerve, which also supplies this muscle. Weakness and sensory loss unite to cause difficulty in swallowing solid food. The glossopharyngeal nerve is closely associated with the vagus and accessory nerves, both in the medulla and in its subsequent course through the jugular foramen, and they are usually involved together in lesions of the medulla and in the region of the jugular foramen.

Glossopharyngeal neuralgia is described in Chapter 8.

THE TENTH OR VAGUS NERVE

In contrast to its importance in visceral affairs, the vagus plays a minor role in neurological disease. Its motor fibers originate in the nucleus ambiguus and emerge from the skull, in company with the ninth and eleventh nerves, through the jugular foramen. They are destined for the elevators of the palate, the constrictors of the pharynx, the cricothyroid, and the larynx.[16] Complete unilateral paralysis is characterized by unilateral palatal palsy, a curtain movement of the pharyngeal wall, hoarseness, and some weakness of the voice; there is little dysphagia. The vagus can be involved in bulbar poliomyelitis, thrombosis of the posterior inferior cerebellar artery, a myotrophic lateral sclerosis, fractures through the jugular foramen, infective polyneuritis, syringobulbia, basilar aneurysm, and tumors. Unilateral affections of the pyramidal tract do not cause persistent disturbance of bulbar functions, but bilateral lesions of the corticobulbar fibers of the tract give rise to spastic bulbar palsy. Phonation, articulation, and deglutition are gravely embarrassed thereby, and the incapacity is usually more severe than seems justified by the degree of visible paralysis. It is seen in amyotrophic lateral sclerosis, bilateral hemiplegia from any cause, and in pseudobulbar palsy. Dysphagia can result from the extreme rigidity and akinesia of advanced Parkinson's disease.

The sensory fibers of the vagus have their cell stations in two ganglia situated in and below the jugular foramen. They convey sensation from the larynx, pharynx, esophagus, and the posterior part of the pinna and external auditory meatus. This last explains the cough which may be caused by an irritation of the meatus, and the reference of pain to the ear from the pharynx. The superior laryngeal branch of the vagus supplies the cricothyroid muscle, the chief tensor and adductor of the vocal cords; the abductors are supplied by the recurrent laryngeal branches of the vagus. Consequently, total unilateral laryngeal paralysis depends on paralysis of both the superior laryngeal nerve and the recurrent branch, and this requires a lesion of the nucleus ambiguus itself or of the intracranial part of the vagus nerve. The vocal cord is motionless, occupying the "cadaveric position" midway between abduction and adduction; the voice is weak and there is anesthesia of the affected side of the larynx.

Paralysis of the superior laryngeal nerve by itself paralyzes the adductors and leaves the abductors unopposed, but in unilateral cases the normal cord moves across the midline to close the gap, and the voice is often unaffected; there is unilateral anesthesia of the larynx. Paralysis of the recurrent laryngeal nerve causes no sensory loss, but paralyzes the abductors, and the vocal cord lies close to the midline. There is little change of voice, but there may be stridor during full inspiration. Paralysis of the left recurrent laryngeal nerve occurs in mediastinal tumor, retrosternal goiter, aneurysm of the arch of the aorta, and dilatation of the left auricle in mitral stenosis. Bilateral abductor paralysis, with consequent adduction of the cords, stridor, and hoarseness, is a dangerous condition which occurs as a result of disease of the medulla or surgical operation on the thyroid gland. Stridor also occurs from laryngospasm in infantile "croup," and, rarely, in tetany.

THE ELEVENTH OR SPINAL ACCESSORY NERVE

The accessory nerve is entirely motor, and is formed by the union of a cranial root derived from the lower end of the nucleus ambiguus, and a spinal root from a column of gray matter in the upper five segments of the cervical cord. The spinal fibers ascend between the ligamentum denticulatum and the posterior cervical roots, enter the skull through the foramen magnum, and emerge again through the jugular foramen after joining the cranial root. In the neck they anastomose with fibers from the third and fourth spinal roots. The fibers derived from the cranial component are distributed chiefly via the pharyngeal and recurrent laryngeal branches of the vagus. The spinal root supplies the trapezius and sternomastoid muscles.

Unilateral pyramidal lesions, as in hemiplegia, weaken but do not paralyze the sternomastoid and trapezius. The spinal root may be involved by poliomyelitis, amyotrophic lateral sclerosis, spinal tumors, and syringomyelia. Within in the posterior fossa, the nerve trunk is seldom involved alone, but is commonly damaged along with the vagus and hypoglossal nerves (the syndrome of the jugular foramen). After emerging from the foramen, the nerve trunk and its branches can be involved by lymphadenopathies, penetrating injuries, and surgical operations.

When the sternomastoid muscle is paralyzed, it no longer stands out as a firm band when the head is rotated toward the opposite shoulder against resistance, or when the head is flexed against resistance. Paralysis of the trapezius makes it difficult to raise the arm above the horizontal; the scapula lies further from the midline than normal, and the shoulder sags; this can give rise to a thoracic outlet syndrome on the affected side.

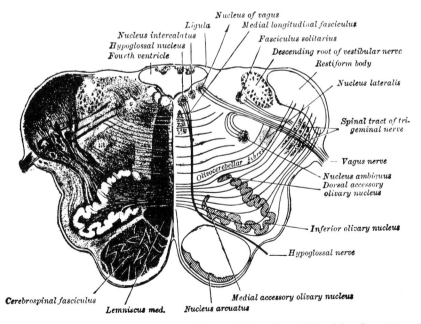

Figure 6–17. Transverse section of medulla oblongata below the middle of the olive. (From Goss, C. M. [ed.]: *Gray's Anatomy of the Human Body.* 27th Ed. Lea & Febiger, Philadelphia, 1959.)

THE TWELFTH OR HYPOGLOSSAL NERVE

The hypoglossal nerve is the motor nerve of the tongue. It originates in the hypoglossal nucleus, which lies near the midline, ventromedial to the nucleus ambiguus. The nerve fibers pass forward through the medulla and emerge in 10 or more bundles between the inferior olive and the pyramid. The nerve leaves the skull through the hypoglossal canal, after which it is joined by filaments from the first and second cervical roots. It supplies the intrinsic and extrinsic muscles of the tongue and the depressors of the hyoid bone.

Immediately after an abrupt hemiplegia from a vascular accident in the internal capsule, the protruded tongue deviates to the side of the paralysis, but this speedily passes off, and in hemiplegias of slow onset, it usually protrudes in the midline. In bilateral pyramidal lesions, the tongue becomes spastic, and this may interfere with articulation, as in pseudobulbar palsy and amyotrophic lateral sclerosis. Inability to protrude the tongue on command, without paralysis, is a form of apraxia which is sometimes seen in extensive lesions of the dominant hemisphere, and which is usually associated with motor aphasia.

A lower motor neuron lesion of the tongue gives rise to weakness and wasting; if the lesion is a progressive process affecting the hypoglossal nuclei, visible fasciculation may be seen when the mouth is open and the tongue is allowed to lie in the floor of the mouth. Protrusion is either weak or impossible. One or both nuclei may be affected by poliomyelitis, acute infective polyneuropathy, syringobulbia, and amyotrophic lateral sclerosis. Thrombosis of branches of the vertebral artery and tumors in this area commonly cause unilateral palsy. As the nerve crosses the subarachnoid space, it can be involved by meningitis, carcinomatosis of the meninges, vertebral artery aneurysm, and fractures of the base. Atrophy of one side of the tongue can occur as part of facial hemiatrophy (p. 108).

POLYNEURITIS CRANIALIS

The term *polyneuritis cranialis* should be reserved for a rare syndrome characterized by the rapid development of multiple cranial nerve palsies, slight fever, and lymphocytes in the spinal fluid, with subsequent recovery in a matter of weeks. It is doubtful whether this represents a true disease entity or not, and the greatest vigilance must be exercised to exclude other conditions which can give rise to rapidly developing paralysis of several cranial nerves, e.g., meningovascular syphilis, Gradenigo's syndrome associated with otitis media, poliomyelitis, acute febrile polyneuritis, and infiltration of the meninges and base of the skull by carcinomatosis, cholesteatoma, lymphoepithelioma, tumors of the nasopharynx, and glomus jugulare tumors.

REFERENCES

1. Altrocchi, P. H., and Menkes, J. H.: Congenital oculomotor apraxia. *Brain* 83:579, 1960.
2. Behrman, S., Carroll, J. D., Janota, I., and Matthews, W. B.: Progressive supranuclear palsy—clinico-pathological study of 4 cases. *Brain* 92:663, 1969.
3. Bornstein, W. S.: Cortical representation of taste in man and monkey. *Yale J. Biol. Med.* 13:133, 1940.
4. Brodal, A.: The hippocampus and the sense of smell. *Brain* 70:179, 1947.
5. Bruetsch, W. L.: Unilateral syphilitic primary atrophy of the optic nerves; anatomic study of two cases. *Arch. Ophth.* 39:80, 1948.
6. Carmichael, E. A., Dix, M. R., and Hallpike, C. S.: Pathology, symptomatology and diagnosis of organic affection of the eighth nerve system. *Brit. Med. Bull.* 12:146, 1956.
7. Carroll, F. D.: Symposium. Diseases of the optic nerve. *Trans. Amer. Acad. Ophth. Otol.* 60:7, 1956.
8. Cawthorne, T.: Positional nystagmus. *Ann. Otol. Rhinol. Laryngol.* 63:481, 1954.
9. Chavasse, F. B.: The ocular palsies. Some clinical sequels of ocular palsy. *Trans. Ophth. Soc. U.K.* 58:483, 1938.
10. Cogan, D. G.: *Neurology of the Ocular Muscles.* 2nd Ed. Charles C Thomas, Springfield, Ill., 1956.
11. Dandy, W. E.: Treatment of Meniere's disease by section of only the vestibular portion of the acoustic nerve. *Bull. Johns Hopkins Hosp.* 53:52, 1933.
12. DiFiore, J. A.: Diabetic oculomotor neuropathy. *Amer. J. Ophth.* 50:808, 1960.

13. Dix, M. R.: Loudness recruitment. *Brit. Med. Bull.* 12:162, 1956.

14. Dix, M. R., and Hallpike, C. S.: The pathology, symptomatology and diagnosis of certain common disorders of the vestibular system. *Proc. Roy. Soc. Med.* 45:341, 1952.

15. Dreyfus, P. M., Hakim, S., and Adams, R. D.: Diabetic ophthalmoplegia; report on a case, with post mortem study and comments on the vascular supply of the human oculomotor nerves. *Arch. Neurol. Psychiat.* 77:337, 1957.

16. Elliott, F. A.: Paralysis of the pharynx. *J. Laryng. Otol.* 70:331, 1956.

17. Falconer, M. A., and Wilson, J. L.: Visual field changes following anterior temporal lobectomy, their significance in relation to "Meyer's loop" of the optic radiation. *Brain* 81:1, 1958.

18. Fitzgerald, G., and Hallpike, C. S.: Studies in human vestibular function. II. Observations on the directional preponderance of caloric nystagmus resulting from cerebral lesions. *Brain* 65:115, 1942.

19. Friedman, A. P., Harter, D. A., and Merritt, H. H.: Ophthalmoplegic migraine. *Arch. Neurol.* 7/4:320, 1960.

20. Gordon, N.: Post-traumatic vertigo with special reference to positional nystagmus. *Lancet* 1:1216, 1954.

21. Hallpike, C. S., Some types of ocular nystagmus and their neurological mechanisms. *Proc. Roy. Soc. Med.* 60:1043, 1967.

22. Hallpike, C. S., and Cairns, H.: Observations on the pathology of Meniere's syndrome. *Proc. Roy. Soc. Med.* 31:1317, 1937.

23. Harden, A., and Pampiglioni, G.: Neurophysiological approach to disorders of vision. *Lancet* 1:805, 1970.

24. Harriman, D. G. E., and Garland, H.: The pathology of Adie's syndrome. *Brain* 91:401, 1968.

25. Hedges, T. R.: The tonic pupil. *Arch. Ophthal.* 80:31, 1968.

26. Henkin, R. I., and Powell, G. F.: Increased sensitivity of taste and smell in cystic fibrosis. *Science* 138:1107, 1962.

27. Hughes, B.: *Visual Fields.* Blackwell Scientific Publications, Oxford, 1954.

28. Hughes, B.: Chronic benign trigeminal paresis. *Proc. Roy. Soc. Med.* 138:1107, 1962.

29. Jellinek, E. H.: The orbital pseudotumor syndrome and its differentiation from endocrine exophthalmos. *Brain* 92:35, 1969.

30. Kessler, L. A., Moldaver, J., and Pool, J. L.: Hypoglossal and facial anastomoses in treatment of facial paralysis. *Neurology* 9:118, 1959.

31. King, A. B., and Walsh, F. B.: Trauma to the head with particular reference to ocular signs. *Amer. J. Ophth.* 32:191, 1949.

32. Kornhuber, H. H.: Physiologie und Klinik das zentralvestibulären Systems. *Hals–Nasen–Ohren Heilkunde.* Edited by Berendes, J., Link, R., and Zöllner, F. Georg Thieme Verlag K. G., Stuttgart, 1966.

33. Lakke, J. P.: Superior orbital fissure syndrome. *Arch. Neurol.* 7/4:289, 1962.

34. Leibowitz, U.: Epidemic incidence of Bell's palsy. *Brain* 92:109, 1969.

35. McNally, W. J., and Stuart, E. A.: Physiology of the Labyrinth: A Manual Prepared for the Use of Graduates in Medicine. American Academy of Ophthalmology and Otolaryngology, Rochester, Minn., 1967.

36. Marino, R., and Rasmussen, T.: Visual field changes after temporal lobectomy in man. *Neurology* 18:825, 1968.

37. Merritt, H. H., and Moore, M.: The Argyll Robertson pupil. *Arch. Neurol. Psychiat.* 30:357, 1933.

38. Moore, J. E.: The syphilitic optic atrophies. *Medicine* (Baltimore) 11:263, 1932.

39. Nosik, W. A., and Weil, A. A.: Selective partial neurectomy in hemifacial spasm and electrophysiologic selection of patients. *J. Neurosurg.* 13:596, 1956.

40. Paton, L., and Holmes, G.: The pathology of papilloedema: A histological study of sixty cases. *Brain* 33:389, 1910.

41. Pederson, E.: Epidemic vertigo. *Brain* 82:566, 1959.

42. Raynor, R. B.: Papilloedema associated with tumors of the spinal cord. *Neurology* 19:700, 1909.

43. Schwartz, H. G., and Weddell, G.: Observations on the pathways transmitting the sensation of taste. *Brain* 61:99, 1938.

44. Spillane, J. D., and Wells, C. E. C.: Isolated trigeminal neuropathy. *Brain* 82:391, 1959.

45. Teuber, H. L., Battersby, W. S., and Bender, M. B.: *Visual Field Defects after Pentrating Missile Wounds of the Brain.* Harvard University Press, Cambridge, 1960.

46. Tolosa, E.: Periarteritic lesions of the carotid siphon with the clinical features of a carotid infraclinoid aneurysm. *J. Neurol. Neurosurg. Psychiat.* 17:300, 1954.

47. Traquair, H. M.: *An Introduction to Clinical Perimetry.* 5th Ed. Henry Kimpton, London, 1946.

48. Traverner, D.: Bell's palsy. A clinical and electromyopathic study. *Brain* 78:209, 1955.

49. Turner, J. W. A.: Indirect injuries of the optic nerve. *Brain* 66:140, 1943.

50. Van Buren, J. M., and Baldwin, M.: The architecture of the optic radiation in the temporal lobe of man. *Brain* 81:15, 1958.

51. Walsh, F. B., and Hoyt, W. F.: *Clinical Neuroophthalmology.* The Williams & Wilkins Co., Baltimore, 1969.

52. Walsh, F. B.: Syphilis of the optic nerve. *Trans. Amer. Acad. Ophth. Otol.* 60:39, 1956.

53. Wartenberg, R.: Progressive facial hemiatrophy. *Arch. Neurol. Psychiat.* 54:75, 1945.

54. Warwick, R.: The so-called nucleus of convergence. *Brain* 81:92, 1958.

55. White, R. H.: Aetiology and neurological complications of retinal vasculitis. *Brain* 84:262, 1961.

CHAPTER SEVEN

The Epilepsies, Narcolepsy, Cataplexy, and Syncope

Epilepsy, the "sacred disease" of ancient times, was long thought to be caused by supernatural forces; the name itself, meaning "to lay hold of" or "to seize upon" carries with it a whiff of demonology, and even to this day the general public is apt to regard the malady as something which sets the epileptic apart from others. This unfortunate legacy from a less sophisticated era has unhappy social, professional, and psychological consequences for seizure-prone individuals.

Definition and Classification. Epileptic seizures are characterized by a recurrent, abrupt, brief disorder of cerebral function. Although unconsciousness and convulsions are often present, neither is essential for the diagnosis of an epileptic attack.

From the electrophysiological point of view, there are two great classes of seizures: those accompanied by a paroxysmal bilateral, symmetrically synchronous generalized EEG discharge, originating from a deep midline pacemaker, and those associated with a discharge which can be recorded from a restricted area of the scalp and which may or may not spread to the rest of the brain. The first group corresponds to "idiopathic" grand mal and petit mal, and the second to a heterogeneous collection of seizures which are referred to as focal, local, or partial epilepsy, and which usually result from a structural though not necessarily a progressive lesion at or near the site of the focal discharge.[20] Convulsions clinically resembling grand mal often result from the generalization of a discharge which started focally, and since symptoms accompanying the focal discharge may be inconspicuous, the distinction between so-called idiopathic and symptomatic seizures often depends on electroencephalography.

The following classification is primarily clinical, but it correlates approximately with electrophysiological data.

A. GENERALIZED EPILEPSIES

1. Generalized convulsions
   a. Generalized from the start (grand mal)
   b. Generalized, but with a focal onset
2. Petit mal
   a. Simple "absence"
   b. Myoclonic petit mal

B. LOCAL, PARTIAL, OR FOCAL EPILEPSIES

1. Jacksonian motor seizures
2. Jacksonian sensory seizures
3. Akinetic seizures (including "drop attacks")

4. Temporal lobe epilepsy
5. Autonomic seizures (visceral epilepsy)
6. Atypical
    a. Tonic attacks
    b. Hypsarhythmia

Incidence. Epileptic seizures occur in all races, and the sexes are equally affected. Estimates based on the examination of recruits for the armed services of the United States indicate that about five persons in 1000 are affected; a similar incidence rate is found in Europe and Britain.

Age of Onset. The incidence is highest in the first four years of life, drops in mid-adult life, and rises again after the age of 60. The first-born is more often affected than subsequent children; possibly their greater liability to birth injury contributes to this. As a general rule, the later the onset of seizures after the age of 25, the greater the likelihood of structural disease, but neither clinical examinations nor laboratory procedures disclose such disease in many individuals who develop attacks for the first time in adult life. It should be remembered, however, that although negative results may be obtained, subsequent investigation sometimes discloses the source of seizures formerly regarded as idiopathic; a slowly growing tumor, such as a meningioma or an oligodendroglioma, or a vascular malformation may be found. Therefore, periodic reexamination is desirable in all cases of late-onset epilepsy.

Etiology. Some people convulse more easily than others: At one end of the scale are the "idiopathic" epileptics who suffer from seizures without overt clinical evidence of neurological or systemic disease, and at the other end are those patients who escape seizures even in the presence of traumatic scars, tumors, birth injuries, etc. Midway between the two lie those who are free of seizures until the advent of a brain lesion or systemic intoxication. Again, some people convulse following a sudden withdrawal of barbiturates or alcohol, and others do not, and it is easier to induce convulsions by Metrazol in some patients than in others. Even in individuals who have what appears to be a built-in proclivity to convulsions, the liability to attacks varies from day to day and from year to year.

Liability to seizures is affected to some extent by heredity, especially in epileptic children with the centrencephalic EEG patterns. Metrakos and Metrakos concluded from their studies that the centrencephalic EEG pattern is an expression of an autosomal dominant gene with the unusual characteristic of very low penetrance at birth, rising to nearly complete penetrance between the ages of 4 and 16 to 17, and declining gradually to almost no penetrance after the age of 40. Lennox[36] found that if one pair of identical twins has epilepsy, the other is likely to be epileptic too, whereas this does not apply to nonidentical twins. Figures derived from various sources suggest that a child born of one epileptic parent will have about 29 in 30 chances of being normal, and if no seizures have occurred before the age of 40, the chances of continued freedom are about 39 in 40. If two epileptics marry, or if one has epilepsy and the other, although free of seizures, has a significantly abnormal EEG, the likelihood of their having epileptic or otherwise abnormal children is increased. Genetic factors are certainly most prominent in the epilepsies that arise in childhood, and the risk of epilepsy among the relatives of an epileptic child diminishes with decreasing degrees of relationship to the affected individual.

The diseases and intoxications that can cause seizures embrace virtually any condition which can affect the ganglion cells of the cerebral hemispheres, either structurally or via metabolic pathways. They occur in congenital, traumatic, infective, degenerative, and neoplastic diseases, and in inborn and acquired metabolic disorders. They also result from many conditions that arise outside the brain, such as hypoglycemia, anoxia, uremia, hepatic failure, and eclampsia.

The site of disease has an important bearing on whether seizures will occur or not. The sensory-motor cortex and temporal lobe (notably the hippocampal gyrus) have a lower seizure threshold than the frontal and parieto-occipital lobes. Furthermore, affections limited to the white matter, such as multiple sclerosis and other demyelinating diseases, do not ordinarily give rise to seizures, and when they do so, the attacks are probably the result of lesions immediately adjacent to gray matter.

Cerebrovascular disease requires special mention because it is so often invoked to explain seizures arising during the second half of life. Although degenerative vascular disease is present to a greater or lesser degree in most people over the age of 55, it is not a common cause of epilepsy. When attacks occur, they usually result from a cortical infarct, and in most cases it will have given rise to transient neurological or mental symptoms at the time of its occurrence. Seizures with a late onset should never be attributed to cerebrovascular disease until every effort has been made to rule out other possibilities, both intracranial and systemic. The most important of these other possibilities are primary and metastatic cerebral tumors.

One of the many unsolved problems of epilepsy is the etiology of the focal or diffuse glial scars which have been found on the inferomedial aspect of the temporal lobe in many patients with temporal lobe epilepsy or generalized seizures. In some cases, such "incisural" sclerosis (sometimes called "Ammon's horn sclerosis") may have occurred as the result of birth injury, whether from excessive molding of the head or from anoxia. It should be noted, however, that damage to this region does not always cause seizures.

There is evidence to suggest that violent and prolonged convulsions in infancy, from whatever cause, can give rise to brain damage as the result of anoxia. Thus, an epileptic infant who suddenly has a large number of convulsions in quick succession may emerge from them with evidence of damage to the brain and a persistent tendency to epilepsy thereafter.

Infantile convulsions have a varied etiology. The immature brain is particularly prone to seizure activity in the face of both cerebral and extracerebral disease. Seizures are common in the presence of congenital malformations, birth trauma, hypocalcemia, hypoglycemia, pyridoxine deficiency, generalized infections (pyelitis, pneumonia, gastroenteritis, etc.), and many other disorders. In general, febrile convulsions in otherwise normal infants have a better prognosis as regards the persistence of epilepsy in later life than seizures in children with congenital defects or acquired brain damage.[39] A genetic factor seems to play a part in the causation of febrile convulsions, for Lennox found that in a group of 272 individuals who had had such convulsions in infancy, the incidence of epilepsy among the relatives was twice as great as its incidence in individuals with a history of nonfebrile convulsions.[35]

Precipitating Factors. Apart from the underlying conditions, whether inherited or acquired, that give rise to seizures, there must be factors which determine why any particular attack comes on at a particular moment in time. A hint is supplied by three observations. First, seizures can be precipitated by biochemical changes, such as hypoglycemia, anoxia, hypocalcemia, hyperventilation, water intoxication, and sudden withdrawal of barbiturates or alcohol; again, sleep deprivation is another seizure-inducer in epileptics,[5] and it too presumably acts through biochemical mechanisms. It is therefore permissible to infer that chemical factors can promote conditions favorable for the occurrence of an attack. Second, emotional stress can undoubtedly precipitate seizures through some as yet unexplained psychophysiological mechanism. Third, in some persons, attacks can be triggered by a sensory stimulus which is specific for the individual; in fact, some epileptics can induce attacks at will, and actually do so for secondary gain.[1, 58] Visual stimuli which occasionally precipitate attacks include reading,[15] watching television,[21] flickering lights (for instance, alternating shadow and sunlight when driving along a road bordered by spaced trees), and sunlight reflected off water. Acoustic precipitants include a sudden loud noise, music, and the sound of bells. An even rarer type of excitant is vigorous labyrinthine stimulation;[4] this has to be distinguished from seizures arising from diseases of the temporal lobe and characterized by an aura of vertigo ("tornado epilepsy"[43]). The paroxysms of glossopharyngeal neuralgia can be followed by a convulsion;[19] in some of these, the seizure is the result of cardiac inhibition, but this has not been so in all the cases reported. Rubbing the skin at a particular site may trigger an epileptic attack, and Penfield and Jasper[44] have described a case in which pressing on the gum at a particular spot could cause a seizure in a patient with an EEG focus at the lower end of the contralateral postcentral gyrus. A light blow to the head or shoulder can precipitate akinetic or myoclonic seizures[11] ("tap seizures"). Voluntary movement can act as a precipitant. Voluntary deviation of the eyes to one side can induce a seizure. A rare but striking form of seizure induced by physical effort[18, 34, 38] (running, doing push-ups, or climbing a rope) is sometimes referred to as *paroxysmal choreoathetosis*. In one case, a boy of 16 found that after doing 10 push-ups or running 100 yards, he would suddenly experience choreoathetotic and dystonic movements of the extremities, trunk, and face, which lasted only about 15 seconds, and which were followed by complete recovery. Consciousness was retained during the attack. The patient found that if he was able to get through an initial period of exercise without having an attack, he could go on indefinitely. The attacks ceased after he started taking Dilantin on a regular basis. A psychological stimulus can be effective; thus, an attack may be brought on by a particular line of thought or by a special type of intellectual exercise such as mental arithmetic or reading.[30] Conversely, a seizure can sometimes be aborted by mental concentration.

It is sometimes possible for the patient to abort a jacksonian seizure by tightening a ligature around the wrist on the affected side as soon as the attack commences,[31] or by grabbing the forearm with his other hand, but it is not entirely certain whether this inhibitory effect is a result of the sensory stimulus of the ligature, or results from the fact that the patient has to concentrate on what he is doing.

In 1850, Hall dubbed sensory-induced seizures "reflex epilepsy" and although the term is unacceptable to the physiologist of today,[20] it does convey the idea of an attack triggered by an afferent stimulus. Animal experiments confirm that under special circumstances, sensory volleys can induce convulsive activity; for instance, if cortical inhibition is decreased by the topical application of strychnine to the sensory-motor cortex, focal or even generalized seizures can be precipitated by stimulating the skin on the opposite side of the body in the area corresponding to the site at which strychnine was applied to the cortex.

In direct contrast to the evocation of epilepsy by sensory stimuli is the frequent occurrence of grand mal seizures and EEG discharges during sleep.[13] Moreover, epileptic attacks are more likely to occur when the patient is daydreaming than when his attention and interest are closely engaged.[32]

To date, there is no single unifying explanation as to how these diverse factors determine that a seizure will occur.

Pathology. Seizures occur in a wide variety of diseases and intoxications, both cerebral and extracranial. There is no uniform pathology, any more than there is a uniform pathology for epigastric pain or headache, but study of epileptogenic cerebral cortex derived from human epileptics has disclosed focal abnormalities in the metabolism of glutamic acid, potassium, and acetylcholine which are present between seizures. The metabolic changes occurring during and immediately after a seizure are more complex, some of them being the result of the increased energy requirements of neuronal hyperactivity.[2]

Pathophysiology of Seizures. Jackson (1870) attributed seizures to an "occasional, sudden, excessive, rapid, and local discharge of gray matter," a concept which receives abundant support from electrophysiological studies by methods which were not available to him. The cells concerned may be in the cerebral cortex or in the central gray matter. Microelectrode recordings from single cells situated in epileptogenic cortical foci in man and experimental animals have disclosed autonomous, paroxysmal, high frequency discharges during interictal periods.[57] The basic cause of the discharge is an instability of the cell membrane, which leads to disorders of polarization when the neuron is subjected to alterations in its chemical environment or to excitation by nerve impulses from a distance.[47, 57] The discharge so initiated can spread widely in the same hemisphere and to the opposite hemisphere through the corpus callosum and other commissures (Fig. 7–1).

In idiopathic grand mal and petit mal the electroencephalogram during seizures usually discloses a symmetrical and synchronous discharge that seems to come from a common pacemaker situated in the midline.[20, 44] Originating from this centrencephalic focus, the discharge spreads upwards to cause a hypersynchrony of the cortical rhythm, which is seen in the EEG, and downwards via pyramidal and reticulospinal pathways to produce tonic and clonic movements in the limbs. Cutting the pyramidal tracts does not stop the tonic-clonic movements of generalized seizures derived from deep sources[56] and only decreases them when they arrive from a cortical focus. An efferent discharge via the reticulospinal tracts may explain the presence of seizure movements in a paralyzed limb.

The efferent discharge is not limited to the motor system. Although commonly obscured by the drama of a convulsion, signs of autonomic discharges are not wanting. There may be changes in the size of the pupils, sweating, erection of the nipples, piloerection, and ejection of urine and feces; the blood pressure rises, and there are alterations in cardiac rhythm and vasomotor activity (for in-

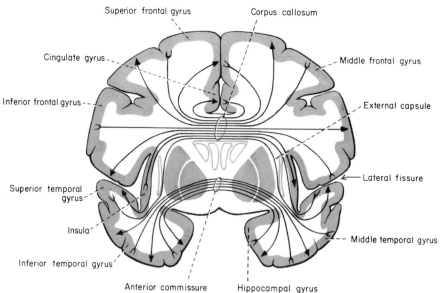

Figure 7–1. Possible anatomic pathways for the development of "mirror foci" in the opposite hemisphere. Coronal section of the brain at the level of the anterior commissure illustrating intercortical connections through the corpus callosum and the anterior commissure. (From Crosby, E. C., Humphrey, T., and Lauer, E. W.: *Correlative Anatomy of the Nervous System.* Macmillan Co., New York, 1962.)

stance, flushing of the face). In exceptional cases, which will be referred to later, these autonomic disturbances in varying combination constitute the main objective features of the seizure.[7, 10]

When a cortical epileptogenic focus has been established for some time, it can give rise to a secondary or "mirror" focus in the contralateral hemisphere (Fig. 7–1), and when this happens, seizures may persist even after the primary site of disease has been removed. Furthermore, the seizure focus, as determined by corticoencephalography, may not necessarily coincide with the lesion responsible for it, and removal of the responsible lesion rather than of the site of the discharging EEG focus may lead to the disappearance of electrical abnormalities situated at a distance from it.[17]

In a generalized convulsion, tonic spasm precedes clonic movements, and this has given rise to the idea that the persistent discharge responsible for tonic spasm leads to neuronal exhaustion, with consequent periodic interruptions of the tonic spasm and a change from tonic to clonic movements. The difficulty about this is that in some cases, clonic movements occur from the beginning. A second explanation for the rhythmical nature of clonic movements is the development of inhibition of the bulbar reticulospinal pathway during the latter stage of a seizure.[20] This is based on the concept of an inhibitory system, which is activated by the seizure and at first inhibits the bulbar discharge responsible for tonic contraction, but which leaves the cortical (clonic) component unaffected.

The disturbance of consciousness which occurs in some seizures seems to be a measure of the generalization of the epileptic discharge. For instance, consciousness is often undisturbed in focal motor or sensory jacksonian attacks, but it is lost in generalized seizures. In temporal lobe attacks (psychomotor seizures), there is often a disturbance of awareness, but the patient does not always appear unconscious in the usual sense of the word, and he may go through a complicated set of activities of which he has no subsequent recollection.

Clinical Features

PETIT MAL. This term is reserved for attacks of "absence" associated with symmetrical 3 per second spike and slow wave activity. Usually seen in children, this condition consists of a momentary break in the stream of thought and activity. Unconsciousness is so brief that it is barely noticed. The color of the face undergoes no change, and the whole episode is over in a second or two. There may be one or two attacks per month or several hundred per day; in the latter event, thinking is seriously interfered with and education may be disrupted. Sometimes the child merely stares ahead with a blank expression. In other children, the lids may twitch or droop, and myoclonic twitches may occur in the arms. When attacks last more than 5 or 10 seconds, there may be chewing movements or smacking of the lips, and the child may stumble. Drop attacks, however, are rarely the result of petit mal.

A typical absence attack may merge into a phase of petit mal automatism, which may last several minutes during which the patient may carry out simple acts and walk about in a daze.

Rarely, petit mal status occurs and may continue for hours, or even for two or three days, during which the child exhibits clouding of consciousness, slow responses, and obvious difficulty in thinking.[6] During such attacks, the EEG shows continuous spike and wave abnormalities of the petit mal type. Without the help of the EEG, it is impossible to distinguish these attacks from the somewhat similar clinical condition in which the abnormality of the EEG arises in the temporal lobe or elsewhere in the brain.[24]

Attacks are easily precipitated by hyperventilation and can also be occasioned by emotional stress and by fatigue.

True petit mal may clear up after puberty, but in many cases, it gives place to less frequent, more dramatic generalized seizures;[16] absence attacks and generalized convulsions are often seen in the same child. A significant number of individuals with petit mal have a low I.Q., according to Charlton and Yahr.

GRAND MAL. This term has come to be applied to generalized seizures in which the tonic and clonic spasms are symmetrical in their onset and in which the attacks are accompanied by diffuse, symmetrical, synchronous discharges which apparently originate in a deep midline center. Thus defined, both grand mal and petit mal have a centrencephalic origin.[20, 44] The convulsion of grand mal may differ in no way from a generalized seizure caused by a focal cortical discharge except in its EEG characteristics.

Generalized convulsions, whether idiopathic or symptomatic, are frequently preceded by an aura which seldom lasts more than a second or two, and which may occupy only a split second. The commonest aura is a curious and indescribable sensation which starts in the epigastrium and passes up into the throat and head. The sensation is usually outside the patient's normal experience, and seldom resembles symptoms from gastrointestinal disease. Electrical stimulation of the centrum medianum of the thalamus in both epileptics and nonepileptics gives rise to similar sensations.[54] The aura may be a sudden sense of a "rushing in the head." Sometimes it is of such a nature as to suggest the presence of a discharging focus in a particular area of the cortex, as for instance an abnormal sensation of movement in the face or in a limb, when the sensory-motor cortex is involved. In temporal lobe epilepsy, the aura may take many forms: an irrelevant idea or emotion, a dreamy state, a sudden experience of an unpleasant smell, a noise (a whistle, a hiss, words, music); ambient sounds may appear to quicken, or slow down, or fade away into a sudden silence. Visual sensations take the form of flashes of light or formed hallucinations, or a feeling that objects looked at are disappearing into the distance or coming nearer. The convulsive attack may be heralded by a sudden burst of laughter or by a coordinated movement such as running or turning around rapidly, or the patient may violently scratch himself, or his head and

eyes may turn to one side. It should be emphasized that the aura is not merely a warning, but an integral part of the seizure, and that in some cases it occurs without the subsequent development of a convulsion.

The aura merges into the initial tonic phase of the convulsion. No better description of grand mal has been given than that by Gowers.[25]

At the onset of the severe fit, the spasm is tonic in character—a rigid, violent muscular contraction, fixing the limbs in some strange position. There is usually deviation of the eyes and of the head toward one side, and this may amount to rotation involving the whole body and may actually cause the patient to turn around, even two or three times. The features are distorted; the color of the face, unchanged at first, rapidly becomes pale and then flushed and ultimately livid as a fixation of the chest by the spasms stops the movements of respiration. The eyes are open or closed; the conjunctiva is insensitive; the pupils dilate widely as cyanosis comes on. As the spasm continues, it commonly changes in its relative intensity in different parts, causing slight alterations in the position of the limbs. When the cyanosis has become intense, the fixed tetanic contractions of the muscles can be felt to be vibratory and the vibrations gradually increase until there are slight visible remissions. As these become deeper, the muscular contractions become more shock-like in character and the state of clonic spasm is reached in which the limbs, head, face, and trunk are jerked with violence, and through similar spasms of the muscles of the tongue and jaws, the former is often bitten. The shocks of spasm effect slight movements of the thorax so that air is expelled and saliva is frothed out between the lips. The air that enters the lungs is at first insufficient to lessen the lividity and the patient may seem to be at the point of death, but as the remissions become deeper, more air enters the chest and the lividity gradually lessens. In becoming less frequent, the contractions do not become less strong, and the last jerk is often as violent as those which have preceded it. At last, the spasm is at an end and the patient lies senseless and prostrate, sleeps heavily for a time, and then can be roused. Urine frequently, and feces occasionally, are passed during the fit.

Gowers continues elsewhere:

The posture of the limbs varies. Commonly

the arms are slightly abducted at the shoulder, the elbow and wrist are flexed, and the fingers are flexed at the metacarpal phalangeal joints and extended at the others, the thumb being adducted into the palm, or pressed against the fingers. The position is thus nearly that seen in tetany. The legs may be extended, but often there is slight flexion at the hip and knee joints. Sometimes initial extension of the legs gives place to strong flexion in the later stages of the fit. Usually the limbs of the two sides do not perfectly correspond in position, but the difference is slight. In other cases, the arms are extended and in some the fingers are flexed at all joints, the fists being clenched. In others again, instead of a combination of flexion and extension, flexion predominates throughout. The head is bent forward, the arms and legs are strongly flexed so that the fists are in contact with the chest and the knees with the abdomen. At the commencement of such flexor fits, the patient often falls forward. In rarer cases, the arms are raised above the head at the onset of the attack and may be kept in that position throughout, or put straight forward. The neck in these fits is often bent backward; the legs may be extended or one or both may be flexed. The violence of the tonic spasm is often very great; the shoulder may be dislocated by it, and when this accident has once happened, it is very apt to recur.

In addition to the motor aspects of a seizure, evidence of an autonomic nervous discharge is seen in excessive salivation, sweating, piloerection, erection of the nipples, secretion of mucus from the vagina, and voiding of urine and feces.

As the attack passes off the patient gradually passes from coma into sleep and from sleep into wakefulness, and has no memory of the events which have just occurred. Postictal headache is common, and sometimes a headache in the morning, a sore tongue, and evidence of incontinence are the sole indications that the patient has had a seizure during sleep. Severe generalized seizures are followed by aching in the muscles of the neck, limbs, and back.

Rarely, a generalized seizure is followed by a phase of automatism. The patient may get up, wander about in a confused state, and become violent; if restrained, he may injure bystanders. Or, he may walk about in a mechanical sort of way before coming to his senses. Such postictal automatism must be distinguished from (1) the organically determined psychotic states that sometimes occur for days or weeks following a series of violent convulsions and which presumably result from brain damage from anoxia, and (2) ictal automatism, in which coordinated but purposeless activities constitute the entire seizure; this is one form of temporal lobe epilepsy. Exceptionally, postictal automatism may be prolonged over several days, but it is difficult in such instances to distinguish between true automatism and a hysterical fugue or malingering; the distinction is particularly difficult when the seizure has been so slight as to pass unnoticed. The subject is further discussed below under *"Diagnosis."*

FOCAL SEIZURES (THE PARTIAL EPILEPSIES). The most important types of partial seizure are jacksonian attacks and temporal lobe epilepsy. It has already been pointed out that focal seizures may spread to produce a generalized convulsion and unconsciousness.

JACKSONIAN ATTACKS.[31] This term refers properly to unilateral seizures caused by a discharging focus in the contralateral motor cortex, and characterized by clonic movements that start in one group of muscles and spread systematically to adjacent groups, reflecting the march of the seizure activity through the motor cortex. Thus, an attack beginning on one side of the mouth spreads in turn to the muscles around the eye, the tongue, the platysma, the arm, and the leg. If it starts in the upper limb, the clonic movement usually appears first in the thumb and index finger, and then spreads progressively to the arm and face, then down the body to the leg, reaching the foot last. If it begins in the foot, it goes up the leg and down the arm. Sometimes the attack will begin with deviation of the head and eyes to the opposite side (contraversive seizure); this usually means that the discharging focus is situated immediately anterior to the motor cortex.

Following a jacksonian attack, there may be weakness or paralysis of the affected limbs (Todd's paralysis). After severe or repeated attacks, the paralysis may result from local neuronal exhaustion, but this cannot explain either the transient palsy which sometimes succeeds a very slight clonic attack or the unilateral weakness which occasionally follows a jacksonian sensory attack. An alternative explanation is that in these cases the epileptic discharge activates an inhibitory mechanism, a theory which has also been invoked to explain akinetic attacks in which weakness or paralysis is the sole feature of the seizure.

FOCAL SENSORY SEIZURES. These are less common than jacksonian motor attacks. Tingling, pins and needles, or a sensation of motion commences in the hand, face, or foot, and spreads to the rest of the affected side of the body. It may pass off without a motor component, or it may give place to either a unilateral motor seizure or a generalized convulsion with loss of consciousness. Sometimes the aura of migraine takes the form of a slowly spreading tingling sensation in one side of the body, but it can be distinguished from a sensory seizure by the fact that it lasts much longer— 15 minutes or more—and is usually succeeded by the nausea and violent headache of migraine. On some occasions, the headache does not occur, in which event it is only the extreme slowness of the "march" which serves to distinguish the two conditions.

AKINETIC SEIZURES. These are uncommon. There is a simple, abrupt loss of tone which can lead to sudden, unexpected falls, without unconsciousness. Abrupt unilateral paralysis has been described as an epileptic phenomenon, but care must be exercised not to confuse it with an abrupt transient hemiparesis resulting from carotid insufficiency; in such cases, the weakness commonly lasts much longer than in epileptic attacks.

TEMPORAL LOBE SEIZURES. Seizures associated with disease of the temporal lobe constitute one of the most important and interesting forms of epilepsy.[2, 12, 17, 23] They are common in institutionalized epileptics because the attacks often take the form of episodic, explosive disorders of behavior, which render hospital care essential. Temporal lobe seizures are variously referred to as psychomotor, psychoparetic, or psychic equivalents. They are more common in adults than in children, and although an individual attack may be exceedingly brief, some of them last several minutes—longer than the usual epileptic seizure. A psychomotor seizure consists of a series of coordinated acts which are out of place, bizarre, and serve no useful purpose. To quote four examples: A man rose from the table, micturated into the fireplace, and sat down again, without knowing what he had done. Another patient got up from a table in a restaurant and climbed into a window display of cakes and pastries. A girl experienced a sudden sense of fear which was so intense that she made attempts—often violent— to escape from her surroundings. A middle-aged woman, uttering obscenities, started to disrobe in the street.

In "cursive" epilepsy, the patient starts running about and may or may not then have a generalized seizure. Sudden brief spells of laughing may constitute the entire attack (gelastic epilepsy[28]). The fact that epileptics can suffer from transient involuntary aberrations of conduct does not mean that the occasional misdeeds of these individuals are necessarily epileptic in origin, and the greatest care has to be exercised in assessing the evidence whenever epilepsy is offered in extenuation of offenses. Criminal activity is no more common in epileptics than in nonepileptics, according to Lennox and others. Behavior problems in children are sometimes associated with a discharging temporal lobe focus and improvement may follow the use of antiseizure medication. The same is true of petit mal.[6]

Sometimes temporal lobe attacks take the form of a brief mental or emotional experience such as a feeling of misery, anger, unreality, or—rarely—happiness.

Impotence is not uncommon in patients with temporal lobe seizures.

FOCAL SEIZURES INVOLVING THE SPECIAL SENSES. These are uncommon and usually result from a lesion of the temporal lobe. *Uncinate attacks* arise from a discharging focus in the region of the uncinate gyrus, which is situated anterolateral to the pituitary fossa and is therefore apt to be involved by pituitary tumors and other lesions in the middle fossa. The attack consists of a transient hallucination of smell, usually unpleasant, which is accompanied by a peculiar dreamy state and may be associated with smacking of the lips, swallowing movements, and champing of the jaws. Sometimes there is a marked sense of déjà vu. Spread of the paroxysmal discharge from the uncinate region to the rest of the brain may cause a generalized convulsion. *Visual seizures* are rare, although a visual aura preceding a generalized convulsion is not uncommon; it may take the form of dimness of vision, hemianopia, blindness, crude flashes of light, complex visual hallucinations, or the sudden eruption into consciousness of a vivid visual memory relating to some past event in the patient's life. Whether or not a visual experience gives place to a generalized convulsion, it usually indicates an origin in the temporal lobe. Vivid Lilliputian hallucinations are sometimes associated with uncinate attacks; the patient sees highly colored diminutive figures—human or animal—during the dreamy state which is part of the seizure. *Auditory attacks* are uncommon and usually consist of noises, such as a hissing, booming, or ringing, or there may be a sudden sense that all outside sounds have ceased or that the tempo of ambient noises has suddenly accelerated or slowed down. Formed auditory hallucinations, such as a voice speaking, may occur in disease of the temporal lobe, but the hearing of voices more often results from a psychosis than from structural disease of the brain. Vertigo of abrupt onset and brief duration may be the aura of a generalized seizure arising in the temporal lobe.[43] It is distinguished from aural vertigo by the brevity of the attack and by the absence of other aural symptoms. Occasionally, aural vertigo causes either syncope or an evoked epileptic convul-

sion.[4] A generalized convulsion can be triggered by the pain of glossopharyngeal neuralgia; in some of these cases, the seizure is the result of a fall of blood pressure from vagal inhibition,[19] but in others the blood pressure is maintained and the attack falls within the category of evoked seizures.

AUTONOMIC SEIZURES. This rare type of attack has also been called "diencephalic autonomic epilepsy." Epileptic attacks in which the manifestations are largely confined to the vegetative nervous system are rare and usually result from a tumor or other lesion of the thalamus or hypothalamus. Varying combinations of the following symptoms occur, with or without disturbances of consciousness: dilatation or constriction of the pupils, flushing of the face and neck, sudden profuse sweating (sometimes unilateral),[7] piloerection and goose pimples,[10] bradycardia or tachycardia, alterations in respiratory rhythm, hiccup, yawning, sudden fever or a sense of chill, abdominal sensations sometimes amounting to pain, or a desire to defecate. The attack may or may not be accompanied by a sense of apprehension and may be followed by unconsciousness. In one case, a woman of 38 experienced repeated attacks of a severe sense of crushing discomfort in her chest, accompanied by a sense of fear. These attacks started nine months after she had suffered a severe head injury and were brought under control by treatment with Dilantin. Some of the symptoms of visceral seizures suggest an anxiety state, but they are distinguished from the latter by their brief and episodic character and by the normality of the patient between attacks. During the attack, the EEG reveals bilateral high voltage 4 to 6 cycles per second activity.

TONIC SEIZURES (MESENCEPHALIC SEIZURES, CEREBELLAR FITS, DECEREBRATE ATTACKS). These are attacks of extremely brief duration in which the extremities and trunk assume a rigid posture comparable to that of decerebrate rigidity. They occur in the presence of expanding lesions above the tentorium, with uncal herniation and compression of the mesencephalon. Tonic seizures also occur in expanding lesions below the tentorium, such as a cerebellar tumor. In the author's opinion, they should not be regarded as epileptic, but rather as brief episodes of decerebrate rigidity.

The generalized seizures caused by anoxia are characterized by unconsciousness and tonic rather than clonic movements.[20]

MYOCLONUS. The term *myoclonus* refers to brief, shocklike contraction involving one or more muscles. The contraction does not involve groups of muscles which normally work together synergically to produce voluntary movement, and the contractions do not appear simultaneously in agonist and antagonist. The movements are not cortical in origin but are thought to originate in the brainstem and, in special instances, in the spinal cord.

There are many causes of myoclonic movements, other than epilepsy. These are discussed in Chapter 2. In seizure-prone individuals, myoclonic jerks may occur in the course of an attack of petit mal. They also sometimes interrupt deep sleep in patients with grand mal.[52] Occasional myoclonic jerks occurring while drifting off to sleep are usually physiological. Repeated myoclonic movements occurring during the process of waking, or shortly thereafter, are not uncommon in children with centrencephalic epilepsy. Severe myoclonus, generalized seizures, and progressive dementia occur in progressive familial myoclonus epilepsy (Unverricht's disease), which is described in Chapter 11.

HYPSARHYTHMIA. As the name implies, this term applies to an electroencephalographic abnormality.[8, 41] It is found in infants and is characterized by high, sharp, irregularly occurring spikes in all leads, interspersed with many high voltage slow waves. It is associated with infantile spasms—frequent, sudden, jerking spasms of the eyes, neck, limbs, and trunk. Mental defect is usually present, and the condition is associated with a variety of diseases and metabolic defects, including phenylketonuria and hypoglycemia. It is important to recognize the condition because the spasms can be stopped by the administration of steroids or ACTH regardless of the etiology. The underlying condition must also receive appropriate treatment.

POSTEPILEPTIC AUTOMATISM. A seizure may be followed by a period of automatism in which the patient appears to be fully conscious but behaves in a bizarre way and has no subsequent memory of his actions. He may be violent, abusive, and unlike his usual self, carrying out antisocial actions that are out of keeping with his normal personality and habits. The cultured spinster may use indecent language. The devoted father wanders away from home. The disciplined soldier leaves his barracks without a pass. In all such cases, there is a change of personality for the duration of the automatism, and it is invariably a change for the worse, leading to purposeless clashes with authority and unashamed departures from conventional decency. Such attacks may last minutes or hours; in exceptional cases, they may be prolonged over several days, but it is necessary in such instances to distinguish between postepileptic automatism and a hysterical fugue or malingering. This is not difficult when a seizure has preceded the automatism, but if the attack has been so slight as to have passed unnoticed, the difficulty may be extreme. Important differentiating features are the presence of proved epilepsy in the past, the complete change of personality during the automatism, and the purposeless nature of the activity, which is often detrimental to the patient's interests. In malingering and hysterical fugues, the patient's behavior is an attempt to escape from some situation, whether psychological or physical, which he can no longer face. It is, in effect, a flight from reality, a series of purposive actions which are directly related to the patient's circumstances.

Postictal automatism also has to be distinguished from prolonged disturbances of behavior and thinking that result from continuous or almost continuous epileptic discharges, which may last up to 72 hours. The patient appears dazed and confused. The EEG may display spike and dome activity,[6] or bilateral spiking.[6, 24]

STATUS EPILEPTICUS. In this condition, there is a succession of generalized seizures without recovery of consciousness between them. The severe muscular exertion, continuing asphyxia, and difficulty in maintaining an adequate intake of fluid and food combine to produce a dangerous condition of exhaustion and acidosis which can prove fatal unless it is stopped. In infants and young children, status epilepticus can produce irreversible damage to the brain as the result of anoxia. A special form of status epilepticus is epilepsia partialis continua, which usually takes the form of almost continuous jacksonian motor seizures limited to one side of the body or to a portion of one side, e.g., the face and hand. This is usually seen as the result of an irritative lesion of the sensory-motor cortex, and when the attacks cease, Todd's paralysis is commonly present. At times, it is difficult to decide whether postseizure paralysis results from functional exhaustion of the cortex or from the presence of structural disease in that area.

In petit mal, a dozen or more attacks can occur within one hour, but consciousness is restored between attacks and the condition is in no way dangerous.

Personality Disorders in Epilepsy. The modern view is that there is no personality profile which is peculiar to epileptics. It is not surprising, however, that patients who are subject to periodic seizures should develop secondary neurotic symptoms as the result of frustration, a sense of being different, and inability to live a normal social and professional life. In some cases, seizures, mental deficiency, and behavior disorders are all results of maldevelopment or acquired disease, while in other instances, episodes of abnormal behavior are themselves epileptic in origin. The personality which was at one time thought to be typical of the epileptic is marked by egocentricity, boastfulness, religiosity, and moodiness; some of these features are due to overcompensation.

The control of seizures by medication or the surgical removal of a seizure focus is sometimes followed by striking improvement of personality, behavior, and intellectual function. Aside from the obvious psychological benefits derived from a lessening of seizures, it seems likely that, in some cases, an epileptogenic focus exercises a malign influence on cerebral function as a whole. This is well illustrated by the great improvement in mind and behavior seen following hemispherectomy in cases of seizures associated with hemiplegia of infantile origin;[45] the clinical improvement is accompanied by a parallel improvement in the electroencephalogram of the remaining hemisphere.

The Electroencephalogram in Epilepsy. Electroencephalography is a valuable tool so long as it is used in conjunction with careful clinical studies; it should not be allowed to dominate the diagnostic debate. For instance, it is sometimes necessary to diagnose epilepsy in the face of a normal record, and, conversely, an abnormal record does not necessarily mean that the patient's symptoms result from epilepsy.[62] Scalp electrodes may fail to pick up discharges originating in the undersurface of the brain, notably in the temporal lobe; this difficulty can be overcome to some extent by the use of sphenoidal and pharyngeal electrodes. Even then, the record may appear normal in some persons who undoubtedly are suffering from seizures, and in this connection it is significant that depth electrode studies show that abnormal activity can go on in deep structures without affecting the cortical patterns. A further limitation is imposed by the fact that in grand mal, seizure discharges are intermittent, so that a single record may disclose nothing amiss, despite good clinical evidence that the patient is suffering from seizures. The number of such false normals can be much reduced by the use of activating techniques, such as hyperventilation, sleep, photic stimulation, artificially induced hypoglycemia, the administration of Metrazol, and the administration of antidiuretic hormone and large amounts of water by mouth. Of these, the last two can produce severe convulsions and are seldom used. *Hyperventilation* can provoke diffuse slowing and paroxysmal discharges, or even a seizure, especially in cases of petit mal. The fact that in some patients seizures occur only at night emphasizes the importance of *sleep records.* A relaxed patient will sometimes drift into somnolence or sleep during a prolonged recording, and this can be facilitated by the administration of a short-acting barbiturate, a technique especially useful in children. As sleep approaches, spindling appears in the normal EEG, and abnormal discharges may appear in both centrencephalic and symptomatic epileptics; this can be especially useful in temporal lobe epilepsy, in which localized spikes sometimes appear during sleep, though they are absent in the waking state.

Photic stimulation by a flickering light can evoke parieto-occipital responses in normal persons, and in light-sensitive epileptics, paroxysmal discharges are also elicited; this usually happens in patients whose seizures arise subcortically. A moderate degree of hypoglycemia can be induced in fasting patients by administering 1 gm. of tolbutamide by mouth, and this can elicit nonspecific generalized slowing, and, in some cases, focal spikes in the neighborhood of a tumor or other lesion,[27] which may have given no other evidence of its presence (see Fig. 7–7); the hypoglycemia is easily corrected by giving the patient a sweetened drink at the end of the session. Insulin is more capricious than tolbutamide and can lead to undesirably severe reactions. Metrazol can elicit seizure discharges, but it can also produce violent generalized convulsions in normal persons, and is therefore not used except under special circumstances, as, for instance, in attempting to localize the source of psychomotor seizures when surgical interference is being planned. It is given in small repeated doses during electroencephalography, and the ad-ministration is stopped as soon as seizure discharges appear in the record.

ELECTROENCEPHALOGRAPHIC PATTERN. The electroencephalogram taken during seizures shows characteristic patterns. The petit mal seizure is characterized by synchronous bilateral, generalized, high voltage spike and wave discharges; this abnormality is seldom absent in the intervals between attacks, and it can be accentuated by hyperventilation. Grand mal seizures are usually preceded by bursts of fast low voltage spikes at the rate of 20 to 30 per sec., succeeded by high voltage slow waves during the attack, but the latter are often obscured by muscle artefacts. During the clonic phase, the frequency decreases, though the voltage may increase, and immediately following the seizure the tracing is flat or almost so, with little evidence of cortical activity; this flattening is thought to indicate a state of neuronal exhaustion. In idiopathic grand mal, the record then returns to normal, but when general convulsions are the result of a spreading discharge from a cortical focus, the attack may be preceded by a focal spike discharge, and this spiking is often present between attacks. In temporal lobe seizures, the electroencephalogram may disclose slow, high voltage, flat-topped waves in the delta range (2 to 4 per sec.); often, however, there is also low voltage fast activity superimposed on the slow waves. Gastaut and Fischer-Williams distinguish no less than eight types of epileptic discharge in temporal lobe epilepsy[20] and emphasize that the "classical" flat-topped waves are not common. Interictal spikes from the temporal lobe are common, especially during sleep; sometimes they are obtainable only from sphenoidal electrodes.

It follows from what has been said that a normal electroencephalogram between seizures does not exclude the diagnosis of grand mal or temporal lobe epilepsy, but it does argue against the diagnosis of petit mal. It must also be remembered that nonspecific abnormalities are found in the interseizure records of some epileptics and that similar

(Text continued on page 138.)

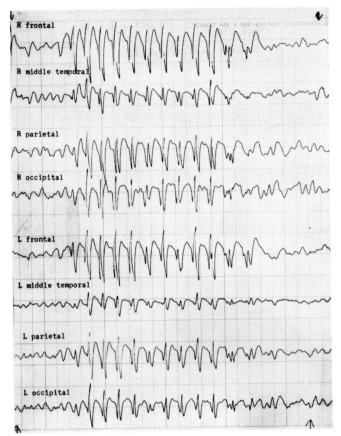

Figure 7-2. Electroencephalographic tracing in petit mal.

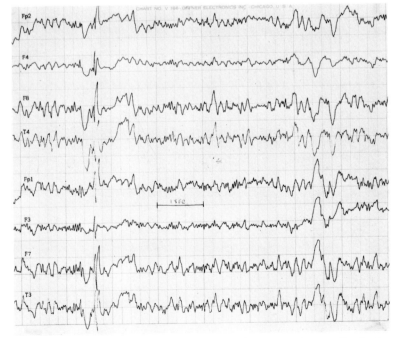

Figure 7-3. Grand mal, duration 12 years. A man of 30, with occasional generalized seizures and no evidence of cerebral disease or injury.

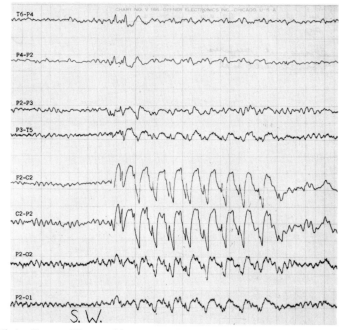

Figure 7–4. From a 17-year-old patient suffering from both grand mal and petit mal.

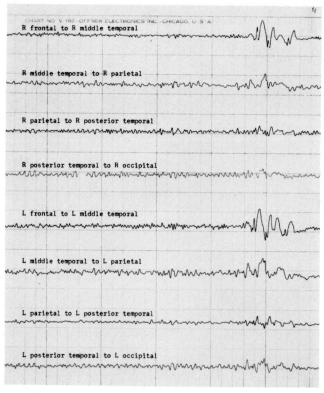

Figure 7–5. Symmetrical paroxysmal activity. The patient complained of occasional "jerks" in both arms, sometimes followed by a generalized seizure.

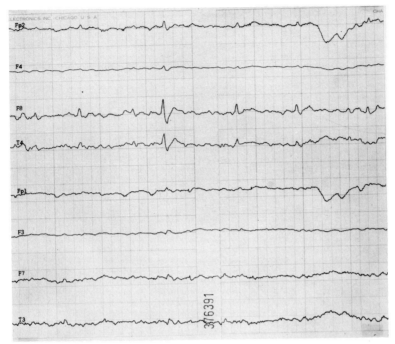

Figure 7–6.   Sharp waves from anterior and middle parts of the right temporal lobe from a patient with temporal lobe seizures.

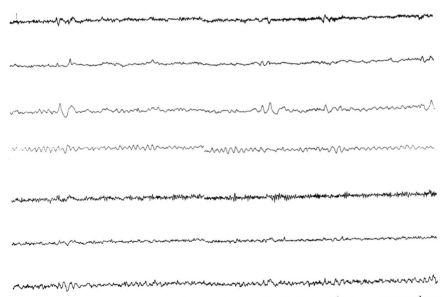

Figure 7–7.   Slow waves in right temporal region induced by Tolbutamide in an apparently normal patient. Two years later, a right-sided sphenoidal ridge meningioma was diagnosed and removed. (Courtesy of Dr. Joseph Green.)

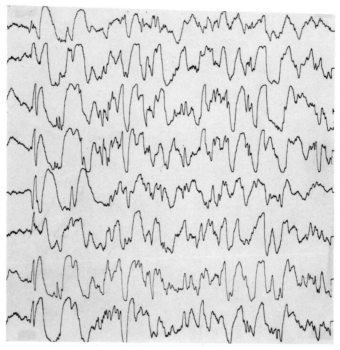

Figure 7–8. Hypsarhythmia. (Courtesy of Children's Hospital of Philadelphia.)

abnormalities occur in about 15 per cent of the normal population. Finally, the presence of a focal discharge does not necessarily mean that the responsible lesion is at that site; it may be some distance away in the same hemisphere, or even in the opposite hemisphere, but when a paroxysmal discharge occurs in relation to a focal lesion, the electroencephalogram will usually show that it started in the affected hemisphere and then spread to the opposite side.

Diagnosis. When the physician is confronted with a patient who has episodic symptoms suggestive of epilepsy, the first thing he must do is to recognize the presence of epilepsy and the second is to decide what kind of epilepsy it is and what it stems from.

The most useful means of identifying an episode as epileptic is the history, preferably reinforced by an eye-witness report. Time spent on this is time well spent, for it can give information which is unobtainable in any other way. Although epilepsy appears in many guises, it always takes the form of brief episodic disturbances of brain function (somatic, psychological, or visceral) which come on rapidly. Other episodic conditions which can mimic epilepsy are: syncope, which depends on a fall of blood pressure; aural vertigo; cerebrovascular insufficiency; hypoglycemia; narcolepsy; the aura of migraine; hysteria; and malingering.

SYNCOPE. This is discussed on page 144.

CEREBROVASCULAR INSUFFICIENCY. This is caused by stenosis of the internal carotid or basilar vertebral systems or by small emboli, and it sometimes causes episodes of neurological dysfunction or mental confusion. They include transient loss of vision in one eye, brief hemianopia, aphasia, dysarthria, hemiparesis or hemiparesthesias, attacks of sudden falling without warning, brief vertigo, attacks of confusion or amnesia, and so on. The episodes usually occur in the second half of life, consciousness is not necessarily disturbed, and they usually last longer than an epileptic episode. Sudden attacks of vertigo or staggering, or of weakness of one side of the body, may be caused, in cases of vascular insufficiency, by turning the head to one side, thereby compressing either a stenosed carotid or a narrow vertebral artery, and only by patient inquiry is it possible to trace the episodes to this particular movement.

HYPOGLYCEMIA. A fall of blood glucose, whether due to an excessive dose of insulin, endogenous hyperinsulinism, or functional hypoglycemia, may cause either unconsciousness or a convulsion, but the symptoms come on more slowly than is the case in an epileptic attack. This is further discussed in Chapter 21.

NARCOLEPSY. Narcolepsy is distinguished by the resemblance of the attacks to ordinary sleep in their onset and character, and by the fact that they last longer than an epileptic seizure. Cataplexy, often associated with narcolepsy, is characterized by sudden attacks of weakness in the limbs, induced by emotion.

MIGRAINE. If the aura of migraine is not followed by headache or vomiting, it may suggest a focal seizure, but it usually lasts longer (20 to 30 minutes), and there is no loss of consciousness during the attack.

HYSTERIA. Hysterical attacks can mimic epilepsy, and the bizarre manifestations of temporal lobe epilepsy are sometimes mistaken for hysterical conversion. In a convulsion of hysterical origin, the pupils, tendon reflexes, and plantar responses remain normal, and it is usually possible to terminate the attack by throwing water in the patient's face or by applying some other vigorous and surprising stimulus. For obvious reasons, the attack usually takes place in front of an audience. It is not followed by headaches, sleep, or muscle pain, and the electroencephalogram usually fails to show any evidence of epilepsy (unless the patient is an epileptic as well). Psychological studies will disclose positive symptoms of an underlying emotional disorder. The name hysteroepilepsy is used if both epilepsy and hysterical convulsions are present in the same case.

MALINGERING. This is seldom encountered, although individuals who have access to medical textbooks or who have witnessed a true epileptic attack can give a good rendering of the genuine article and have been known to do so when faced with military service or with some other situation from which they wish to escape.

Laboratory Aids. Petit mal is easily identified because of the characteristic electroencephalographic patterns, which occur both during and between seizures. It is less easy to be certain about grand mal, because the interseizure record is sometimes normal or almost so, but when generalized convulsions result from a focal lesion, such as a scar from a head injury or a small tumor, a focal discharge will often persist in the electroencephalogram between attacks. As was pointed out above, activating techniques increase the number of positive results in such cases. Careful history taking or the observations of witnesses will sometimes disclose that a generalized seizure had a focal onset, and this excludes the possibility of centrencephalic epilepsy. The discovery of abnormal neurological signs is even more convincing.

If there is reason to suppose that epileptic seizures are the result of local disease, every effort must be made to ascertain the cause. The spinal fluid should be examined; an increase of protein and a slight pleocytosis can be present after a succession of generalized seizures or after a head injury resulting from a seizure, but with these exceptions, significant changes in the spinal fluid indicate local intracranial disease. X-rays of the skull should be done routinely in searching for abnormal calcification, displacement of the pineal body, abnormal vascular markings, etc. When seizures occur for the first time in a patient over the age of 20, it is desirable to pursue the matter still further with arteriography, pneumoencephalography, and a brain scan. The decision as to just how far to push the investigation will depend on the circumstances in each case. It is worth noting that follow-up studies of patients developing seizures for the first time after the age of 50 show that approximately one in four cases proves to have a cerebral tumor[60]; three in four do not. In a series of patients with temporal lobe epilepsy investigated by Falconer, careful histological examination of resected temporal lobes showed focal lesions (small tumors, hamartomas, infarcts, cortical scars, etc.) in 40 of 50 patients, none of whom had objective neurological signs of disease apart from the seizures and EEG changes.

Course and Prognosis. True petit mal is usually a disease of childhood and may pass off as the brain matures, either at puberty or shortly thereafter. It may give place to generalized convulsions, or both types may be present during childhood. The febrile convulsions of infancy, occurring in otherwise normal infants, do not necessarily carry a bad prognosis.[39] However, if convulsions appear repeatedly, both with and without infections, the possibility of epilepsy later in life is considerable. Seizures occurring in brain-damaged children are likely to persist.

With regard to grand mal, it is always difficult to give a prognosis early in the patient's history. Some individuals suffer from only one or two attacks a year, and there may be complete remissions for several years at a time. Others, less fortunate, have several seizures every month, and may have to live restricted lives; but even in these cases, the frequency sometimes diminishes remarkably in later life. Traumatic epilepsy carries a variable prognosis,[46] but some idea of what is to be expected can be derived from Walker's study of 246 cases; 33 per cent of these were free of epilepsy five to 10 years after injury, and less than 50 per cent were receiving treatment.[55]

In general, epileptics have a shorter life span than the normal population. In addition to being subject to and succumbing from the same diseases as other people, they are exposed to additional risks as a result of seizures—e.g., status epilepticus, suffocation from rolling on the face during a seizure, fatal falls, road accidents, severe burns from falling into an open fire, and drowning.

Treatment. During a seizure, a resilient object should be placed between the upper and lower teeth to prevent tongue biting during the clonic stage. Removal of dentures is advisable but often impracticable. Clothing should be loosened at the neck, and the limbs should be kept out of range of hard objects against which they could be injured.

STATUS EPILEPTICUS. Status epilepticus is best treated by intravenous diazepam (Valium),[42] whether the seizures are centrencephalic in type or a result of organic disease of the brain. Provided that an airway is present to prevent lingual obstruction, the drug is remarkably safe. It avoids the respiratory and cardiovascular collapse which sometimes follows administration of intravenous hypnotics, the acute right heart failure and massive pulmonary edema which may follow intravenous injection of paraldehyde, the cardiorespiratory failure associated with the intravenous injection of local anesthetics, and both the permanent damage to the nervous system and the fatal effects on an irritable myocardium that can be produced by prolonged intravenous administration of diphenylhydantoin. The initial dose of Valium ranges from 2 to 20 mg. injected at the rate of 2 to 5 mg. per minute, repeated at 20 minute intervals if necessary. It is seldom necessary to give more than 35 mg. in a single hour. The injection should be stopped if respiratory depression results. If the seizures continue, an additional 100 mg. of the drug may be infused in 500 ml. of 5 per cent dextrose saline over 12 hours. In children, diazepam is given by slow intravenous injection in a dose of 0.25 mg. per pound of body weight, up to a maximum of 10 mg., repeated thereafter if necessary. Intravenous sodium amytal and diphenylhydantoin should be avoided in children.

Whatever drug is to be used, it is important to establish an adequate airway, and oxygen should be administered. Vital signs should be recorded at 10 minute intervals; if the temperature is rising, a hypothermic blanket or alcohol sponging should be resorted to.

If diazepam is not available, 500 mg. of sodium amytal may be given intravenously at a rate not greater than 50 mg. in 30 seconds. It should be stopped at once if hypotension or respiratory depression occurs. The third alternative is diphenylhydantoin, given intravenously at the rate of 50 mg. every 30 seconds, to a total of 500 mg. If the foregoing drugs are not available, from 200 to 400 mg. of phenobarbital can be administered by slow intravenous injection, followed by an intramuscular dose of 100 to 200 mg. at 2 to 6 hour intervals, the dose not to exceed 1000 mg. Paraldehyde may be given in doses of 5 to 10 ml. intramuscularly, or 1 to 3 ml. may be given over a period of not less than 2 minutes by intravenous injection.

Should seizures and unconsciousness persist for more than 3 hours, intravenous glucose saline should be administered.

Prophylactic treatment includes attention to general health and the administration of anticonvulsant medication. The maintenance of positive health is essential in every case. This requires a compromise between fussy interference and careless neglect, the aim being to lead as normal a life as is possible under the circumstances. Exercise in the open air, an adequate amount of sleep, and appropriate recreational activities will do more for the patient than too sheltered a life hampered by vexatious restrictions which mark the epileptic as something apart. The handicap of epilepsy is apt to create a sense of frustration, which contributes to abnormal behavior and unhealthy reactions, and any step which helps to remove the barrier between the patient and his fellows is to be encouraged, provided it does not place him in a position of special danger. Social life should be interrupted as little as possible. Dietetic restrictions are not necessary. Alcohol is usually interdicted, but small quantities taken on social occasions do no harm. Large amounts of fluid, including beer, should not be allowed, because hydration can precipitate seizures. The combination of epilepsy and chronic alcoholism is formidable, but it should

be remembered that *sudden* withdrawal of alcohol can precipitate seizures.

The choice of employment is governed by the frequency of seizures and the patient's mental capacity. Things to be avoided include driving a car and working at heights or among unshielded machinery. Seizures often seem to be more frequent when the attention of the subject is not fully engaged, so occupations which allow daydreaming and periods of idleness are less desirable than work which requires concentration. If seizures are very frequent, the patient may have to work at home, or, if home conditions are unfavorable, in an epileptic colony. This becomes desirable when epilepsy is associated with mental deficiency, psychopathic behavior, or frequent lapses into postepileptic automatism, factors which can impose an impossible burden on the relatives.

Epileptics often seek, but seldom take, advice as to the wisdom of getting married and of having a family. Epilepsy by itself is no bar to marriage, provided both partners realize what they are about, but the question of having children is more difficult. Generally speaking, if one parent is normal and the other has seizures as a result of previous insult to the brain, such as a head injury, meningitis, etc., the risk of epilepsy among the offspring is very slight. In the case of centrencephalic petit mal and grand mal, the risk is greater, and it is still greater if an epileptic marries a partner who has never had seizures but who has epileptic paroxysmal discharges in his or her EEG. A complete review of the family history of both potential parents will sometimes provide so gloomy a view of recurrent abnormality—epilepsy, alcoholism, mental defect, psychoneurosis, and social maladaptation—that there is little difficulty in concluding that the chances of transmitting some defect are so great that child adoption is preferable to childbearing.

Anticonvulsant Drugs. In the majority of cases, reliance has to be placed on antiseizure medication, but sometimes the attacks can be eliminated or reduced in number by the surgical excision of a circumscribed epileptogenic lesion of the cortex. This has been carried out successfully in cases of temporal lobe epilepsy, by amputation of the anterior portion of the temporal lobe.

Spontaneous remissions lasting for months or years are common, especially in idiopathic epilepsy, and in some cases the attacks die out altogether, particularly with petit mal. The aim of medication is to reduce or eliminate the seizures. This damping-down process must be continued until the patient has been free of attacks for at least two years before risking any reduction in medication. It is essential that treatment should be continuous and without intermission, since temporary withdrawal can release epileptic activity, with a consequent increase in the number of seizures, or it may actually precipitate status epilepticus. The continuous administration of anticonvulsant drugs has no serious ill effects if the dosage is correct and if idiosyncrasy is absent; but it is a burden to the patient and for this reason many authorities feel that it is permissible to withhold medication in the case of patients whose seizures are very infrequent—one attack per year, for instance.

The aim of drug therapy is to maintain an effective serum level of each agent. It takes several days to produce such a level. It is customary to prescribe medication three times a day, but twice a day is sufficient. The midday dose, when the patient may be at work or at school, is often a source of embarrassment, and for this reason the patient may be tempted to "forget" to take it. Blood level determinations are useful in gauging the optimum dose.

PHENOBARBITAL. A suitable starting dose for either a child over the age of 10 or an adult is 50 mg. twice a day, and this may have to be raised to as much as 200 mg. twice a day. Large doses make some patients unduly somnolent, while smaller doses may not effectively control the seizures. Drowsiness is common at the start of treatment, but usually it disappears after a time. Idiosyncrasy to bar-

biturates can produce an erythematous rash and a high temperature, but the patient neither looks nor feels as ill as would be the case if the symptoms were due to an infection.

DILANTIN (DIPHENYLHYDANTOIN SODIUM). This drug is effective in the treatment of grand mal and psychomotor epilepsy. The average daily requirement for a child under six is from 60 to 100 mg.; for an adult, 300 to 400 mg. The object is to build up and maintain an effective level of the drug in the blood, and it takes about two weeks of treatment to bring this about, so in general it is unwise to increase the dose after a shorter interval. Since Dilantin has virtually no hypnotic action, the entire daily ration can be taken at one time. It can cause mild gastric irritation, so it is best taken with meals. Toxic symptoms are occasionally encountered, whether from idiosyncrasy or from too large a dose, and include rashes, urticaria, fever, and eosinophilia; swelling and bleeding of the gums; increased growth of hair on the face and limbs; lymphadenopathy; hypochromic or macrocytic anemia and leukopenia; cerebellar symptoms, including dysarthria, nystagmus, and ataxia of gait; and, rarely, an acute psychosis.

MESANTOIN (METHYL-PHENYL-ETHYL-HYDANTOIN). This is sometimes more effective than Dilantin in the treatment of grand mal and psychomotor epilepsy, but it has a slight hypnotic action and occasionally produces serious complications, notably agranulocytosis and aplastic anemia. Monthly blood counts are necessary when it is being used. The daily intake for a child is 400 mg. and for an adult, 300 mg.

MYSOLINE (PRIMIDONE). Either alone or in combination with Dilantin, Mysoline is useful for grand mal and psychomotor attacks. The daily ration is from 150 mg. to 750 mg. for a child, and 1 to 1.5 gm. for an adult. Minor toxic reactions are not unknown; they include nausea, vomiting, dizziness, and sleepiness.

TEGRETOL (CARBAMAZEPINE). This drug is related to the phenothiazines.

It can be used for the treatment of grand mal and temporal lobe seizures, the dose for adults ranging from 400 mg. to 800 mg. a day. When the drug is first started, it is common to encounter drowsiness, nausea, and ataxia, but these soon pass off. More serious complications reported include agranulocytosis, exfoliative dermatitis, oliguria, hypotension, persistent incoordination, peripheral neuropathy, and depression. Most of the toxic reactions reported have been seen when Tegretol has been used for the treatment of tic douloureux.

TRIDIONE (TRIMETHADIONE). The drug is useful for petit mal, reducing the frequency of seizures in more than 50 per cent of all cases so treated. If the patient has both petit mal and grand mal, phenobarbitone or Dilantin should be given in addition to Tridione. The daily requirement is from 20 to 50 mg./kg. daily. Toxic symptoms include rashes and photophobia. When the drug has been given for some time, more serious complications can occur—nephrosis, aplastic anemia, and leukopenia. Regular blood counts and urinalyses are therefore mandatory.

ZARONTIN (ETHYL-METHYL-SUCCINI-MIDE). This is an effective drug for the treatment of petit mal; it is less toxic than Tridione, and it has the additional advantage of being available in liquid form. An average daily ration is 750 mg. (three capsules or 15 ml. of the fluid preparation). It can cause drowsiness, gastric upset, skin rashes, and headache.

MILONTIN (METHYLPHENYL SUCCINI-MIDE). This drug is more toxic than Zarontin. The daily requirement is in the region of 750 mg. to 1.5 gm. for a child, and 1 to 2.5 gm. for an adult.

BENZEDRINE (AMPHETAMINE SULFATE) AND DEXEDRINE (DEXTROAMPHETAMINE SULFATE). Administered in doses of 5 to 20 mg. a day, these drugs can be helpful in counteracting the somnolence produced by phenobarbital. Curiously enough, nocturnal seizures are sometimes reduced by the administration of these drugs in a slow release capsule at bedtime. If the dose is suitably adjusted, insomnia does not occur. The possibil-ity of addiction must be remembered, notably in the case of adolescents and young adults.

NARCOLEPSY AND CATAPLEXY

These two conditions (which, when present in the same case, are referred to as Gelineau's syndrome) are not usually regarded as forms of epilepsy, despite their paroxysmal nature, because they are unassociated with the types of EEG abnormalities which occur with epilepsy and because they are not controlled by the drugs that are effective for ordinary seizures. Neither of these objections is absolute, and the author subscribes to the view, carefully argued by Symonds,[51] that narcolepsy and cataplexy are variants of epilepsy.

In narcolepsy[9, 61]—a rare condition which usually starts in adolescence—the patient is liable to sudden and uncontrollable spells of what looks like normal sleep, lasting for a few minutes to an hour or two. The attacks can recur several times a day, but they do not interfere with the subsequent night's sleep. Some patients experience an aura of prodigious fatigue, while others receive no warning. Attacks are particularly common during and after meals, or when the individual is sitting quietly. In one case, the attacks frequently occurred when the patient was stopped by a traffic light, only to be wakened by the hooting of outraged motorists behind him.

Occasionally, narcoleptics experience vivid visual hallucinations when falling into natural sleep (hypnagogic hallucinations) or may suffer from occasional attacks of "sleep paralysis" when going to sleep or upon awakening. The patient is completely conscious but is totally unable to speak or move for a period of a few seconds to two minutes. One patient would recover the power to move instantly if she was touched on the face or forearm by a companion.

The EEG is usually normal between attacks but during spells of somnolence the record shows rapid eye movement (REM) sleep immediately, whereas in normal persons REM is preceded by a non-rapid eye movement phase.

Narcoleptic attacks may be simulated by tumors and other lesions of the hypothalamus and upper brainstem.[9, 33] but structural disease does not give rise to the combination of narcolepsy, cataplexy, and sleep paralysis.

Cataplexy is characterized by abrupt attacks of muscular weakness that are triggered by a *sudden* emotional stimulus, such as mirth, anger, fear, or surprise. The subject is paralyzed for a few seconds. Rarely, the weakness is confined to one group of muscles; the head may fall forward, or one limb may be affected. Sudden and unexpected confrontation with old friends caused complete paralysis of the facial muscles in one patient. When the weakness is confined to the legs, an abrupt "drop attack" is the result. The presence of narcolepsy helps to differentiate such cases from drop attacks resulting from other causes — vertebral basilar insufficiency, anterior cerebral artery insufficiency, interhemispheric tumors between the medial aspects of the frontal lobes, tumors of the third ventricle, and normal pressure hydrocephalus.

TREATMENT. Narcolepsy can be suppressed to some extent by methylphenidate (Ritalin) in doses of 10 mg. or more three times per day. Dextroamphetamine sulfate is also effective, in doses starting at 5 mg. three times per day. Ephedrine in doses of 25 to 50 mg. three times per day can also be used.

Cataplexy is more difficult to treat, but some cases respond to Imipramine (Tofranyl) and to desmethylimipramine, in doses of 25 to 50 mg. three times per day.

SYNCOPE

Fainting attacks are caused by a *sudden* fall of blood pressure when the patient is standing up, or — rarely — sitting. Unconsciousness is usually preceded by premonitory symptoms, such as lightheadedness, slight blurring of vision, sweating, nausea, and a sense of weakness. The face is pale or ashen, except in primary orthostatic hypotension. In many cases, the attack can be averted at this stage if the head is put down below the knees, or if the patient lies down. Unconsciousness lasts for a few seconds to 2 minutes and recovery is rapid, without the confusion or sleepiness seen after a seizure. If the bladder is full, enuresis may occur. Occasionally, there may be a few clonic movements of the limbs, but tonic contraction of muscles does not occur, and the tongue is not bitten. Occasionally, syncope triggers a true seizure, with tonic and clonic phases.[52]

ETIOLOGY. The most common cause of fainting in the young is prolonged standing in a hot atmosphere — as in soldiers on parade and in spectators. It may also occur on suddenly assuming the erect posture (e.g., in convalescence from prolonged illness, anemia, following splanchnectomy or lumbar sympathectomy, and as a result of treatment with hypotensive agents, phenothiazines, and amine oxidase inhibitors). Uncommon causes in the same category of acute orthostatic hypotension include adrenal and pituitary insufficiency, severe polyneuropathy from any cause, tabes, and high spinal cord injuries.

A second cause of fainting is reduced venous return to the heart, as occurs in the Valsalva maneuver, sustained coughing in obese middle-aged men (tussive syncope), stretching the arms upwards with the spine extended (stretch syncope), straining to empty a full bladder in the middle of the night (micturition syncope). There is some doubt as to whether all cases of tussive syncope and micturition syncope are explained by the effect of reduced venous return to the heart, because in some cases there has been no evidence of straining or prolonged coughing.[53] Syncope following a brief period of light-headedness can be the first symptom of large internal hemorrhage, as from a bleeding ulcer.

Cardiac causes of syncope include Stokes–Adams attacks, the onset of fibrillation, slowing of heart rate and a fall of blood pressure from carotid sinus stimulation, aortic stenosis, ball valve thrombus or tumor in the left atrium, pericarditis with effusion, and a sudden fall of blood pressure from myocardial infarction.

The role played by the central nervous system in the maintenance of blood pressure and heart rate is emphasized by the syncope which occurs from an emotional shock. Structural disease of the brain and the spinal cord can also produce intermittent hypotension with syncope. It is seen, for instance, in disease involving the hypothalamus (e.g., craniopharyngioma in adults, tumors of the third ventricle) and in lesions of the upper half of the spinal cord (trauma, tumors, syringomyelia).

The condition known as *primary neurogenic orthostatic hypotension* is characterized by inability to sustain the blood pressure while standing, without the development of pallor or tachycardia.[40] This can occur on its own, but it is more often found in association with other evidence of disease of the central nervous system. Shy and Drager[49] described four cases in which there was loss of sweating, impotence, loss of sphincter control, atrophy of the iris, external ocular palsy, parkinsonian rigidity and tremor, and muscle wasting and fasciculation as a result of a peripheral neuropathy. Others have described dysarthria, monotonous speech, pupillary irregularities, vertigo, extrapyramidal symptoms, and cerebellar ataxia. It is thought that the cause for the postural hypotension lies in the central rather than the peripheral nervous system. The hypotension is not accompanied by peripheral vasoconstriction, so the face does not become pale during the attack. The etiology of this disease, or of this group of diseases, is not known. Bannister and his colleagues[3] found that the administration of 9 α-fluorohydrocortisone is the most effective way of achieving improvement and suggested that it operates in part by producing an increase in blood volume.

Vasovagal Attacks. Gowers[26] introduced this term to describe attacks lasting for 10 to 30 minutes, in which the patient becomes ashen and complains of substernal discomfort and respiratory distress; these symptoms are sometimes accompanied by a sense of impending death. Consciousness is lost if the patient is unable to lie down. These rare but dramatic attacks lie on the borderline between epilepsy and syncope.

Diagnosis of Syncope. In theory, it should be easy to distinguish between syncope and an epileptic seizure, but if there has been no witness to the attack, the distinction may be difficult. The usual warning symptoms of syncope are absent in Stokes-Adams attacks. A few clonic movements may occur in syncope; conversely, in akinetic epilepsy, there are no abnormal movements. Urination may occur, or may not occur, in both. Pallor is usual in syncope but does not occur in primary neurogenic orthostatic hypotension. The difficulties are compounded by the fact that both syncope and epileptic seizures may occur in the same individual.

Individuals prone to syncope in response to emotion (e.g., the sight of blood) were investigated by Williams,[59] who found nonspecific EEG abnormalities in 31 per cent (as against 16 per cent of normal subjects) and episodes of fast activity in 19 per cent (as opposed to 4 per cent of normal individuals).

REFERENCES

1. Andermann, K., et al.: Self-induced epilepsy. *Arch. Neurol.* 6:49, 1962.
2. Baldwin, M., and Bailey, P. (ed.): *Temporal Lobe Epilepsy.* Charles C Thomas, Springfield, Ill., 1958.
3. Bannister, R., Ardill, L., and Fentem, P.: Treatment of idiopathic orthostatic hypotension. *Arch. Neurol.* 19:163, 1968.
4. Behrman, S., and Wyke, B. D.: Vestibulogenic seizures. *Brain* 81:529, 1958.
5. Bennett, D. R.: Sleep deprivation and major motor convulsions. *Neurology* 13:953, 1963.
6. Bornstein, M., Coddon, D., and Song, S.: Prolonged alterations in behavior associated with continuous electroencephalographic (spike-and-dome) abnormality. *Neurology* 6:444, 1956.
7. Botez, M. I., Stoica, E., and Crighel, E.: Lo-

calized sweating as the single clinical manifestation in a case of epilepsy. *Psychiat. Neurol. Neurochir.* 64:100, 1961.

8. Bower, B. R., and Jeavons, P. M.: Infantile spasms and hypsarrhythmia. *Lancet* 1:605, 1959.

9. Bowling, G., and Richards, N. G.: Diagnosis and treatment of the narcolepsy syndrome. Analysis of 75 case records. *Cleveland Clin. Quart.* 28:38, 1961.

10. Brody, I. A., Odom, G. L., and Kunkle, E. C.: Pilomotor seizures. *Neurology* 10:993, 1960.

11. Calderon-Gonzales, R., Hopkins, I., and McLean, W. T.: TAP seizures. *J.A.M.A.* 198:521, 1966.

12. Cavanagh, J. B., Falconer, M. A., and Meyer, A.: Some pathogenic problems of temporal lobe epilepsy. *Temporal Lobe Epilepsy.* Edited by Baldwin, M., and Bowling, P., Charles C Thomas, Springfield, Ill., 1958, pp. 140–149.

13. Caveness, W. F., Parsonage, M. J., and Edmond, M. M.: Convulsive seizures coincident with sleep. *Trans. Amer. Neurol. Assn.* 75:155, 1950.

14. Cobb, S., and Lennox, W. G.: *Epilepsy.* The Williams and Wilkins Co., Baltimore, 1928.

15. Critchley, M.: Reading epilepsy. *Epilepsia* 3:402, 1962.

16. Currier, R. D., Kooi, K. A., and Saidman, L. J.: Prognosis of "pure" petit mal: A follow-up study. *Neurology* 13:959, 1963.

17. Falconer, M. A., Driver, M. V., and Serafetinides, E. A.: Temporal lobe epilepsy due to distant lesions. Two cases relieved by operation. *Brain* 85:521, 1962.

18. Falconer, M. A., Driver, M. V., and Serafetinides, E. A.: Seizures induced by movement: Report of a case relieved by operation. *J. Neurol. Neurosurg. Psychiat.* 26:300, 1963.

19. Garretson, H. D., and Elvidge, A. R.: Glossopharyngeal neuralgia with asystole and seizures. *Arch. Neurol.* 8:26, 1963.

20. Gastaut, H., and Fischer–Williams, M.: The physiopathology of epileptic seizure. *Handbook of Physiology.* Edited by Field, J., American Physiological Society, Washington, D.C., 1959, Vol. 1, Section 1, Chap. 14, p. 329.

21. Gastaut, H., Regis, H., and Bostem, F.: Attacks provoked by television, and their mechanism. *Epilepsia* 3:436, 1962.

22. Gibbs, F. A., and Gibbs, E. L.: Atlas of electroencephalopathy. *Epilepsy.* 2nd Ed. Addison–Wesley Publishing Co., Cambridge, Mass., 1952, Vol. 2.

23. Gibbs, F. A., Rich, C. L., and Gibbs, E. L.: Psychomotor variant type of seizure discharge. *Neurology* 13:991, 1963.

24. Goldensohn, E. S., and Gold, A. P.: Prolonged behavioral disturbances as ictal phenomena. *Neurology* 10:1, 1960.

25. Gowers, W. R.: *Diseases of the Nervous System.* 2nd Ed. J. & A. Churchill, London, 1893.

26. Gowers, W. R.: *Epilepsy and Other Chronic Convulsive Diseases.* 2nd Ed. London, 1901.

Reissued by Old Hickory Bookshop, Brinklow, Md., 1964.

27. Green, J.: The activation of electroencephalographic abnormalities by tolbutamide-induced hypoglycemia. *Neurology* 13:192, 1963.

28. Gumpert, D., Hansotia, P., and Upton, A.: Gelastic epilepsy. *J. Neurol. Neurosurg. Psychiat.* 33:473, 1970.

29. Holowach, J., Renda, Y. A., and Wapner, I.: Psychomotor seizures in childhood. *J. Pediat.* 59:339, 1961.

30. Ingvar, D. H., and Nyman, G. E.: Epilepsia arithmetices: A new psychologic trigger mechanism in a case of epilepsy. *Neurology* 12:282, 1962.

31. Jackson, J. Hughlings: Selected Writings, Vol. 1. *On Epilepsy and Epileptiform Convulsions.* Edited by Taylor, J., Hodder and Stoughton, Ltd., London, 1931.

32. Jung, R., and Freiburg, I. B.: Blocking of petit mal attacks by sensory arousal and inhibition of attacks by a change in attention during the epileptic aura. *Epilepsia* 3:435, 1962.

33. Kamman, G. R.: Narcolepsy following epidemic encephalitis. *J.A.M.A.* 93:29, 1929.

34. Kato, M., and Araki, S.: Paroxysmal kinesigenic choreoathetosis. Report of a case relieved by carbamazepine. *Arch. Neurol.* 20:508, 1969.

35. Lennox, W. G.: The genetics of epilepsy. *Amer. J. Psychiat.* 103:457, 1947.

36. Lennox, W. G.: Sixty-six twin pairs affected by seizures. *Res. Pub. Assn. Res. Nerv. Ment. Dis.* 26:11, 1947.

37. Levin, M.: Cataplexy. *Brain* 55:397, 1932.

38. Lishman, W. A., Symonds, C. P., Whitty, C. W. M., and Willison, R. G.: Seizures induced by movement. *Brain* 85:93, 1962.

39. Livingston, S., Bridge, E. M., and Kajdi, L.: Febrile convulsions: Clinical study with special reference to heredity and prognosis. *J. Pediat.* 31:509, 1947.

40. Martin, J. B., Travis, R. H., and Vanden Noort, S.: Centrally mediated orthostatic hypotension. *Arch. Neurol.* 19:163, 1968.

41. Millichap, J. G., Bickford, R. G., Klass, D. W., and Backus, R. E.: Infantile spasm, hypsarrhythmia and mental retardation. A study of etiologic factors in 61 patients. *Epilepsia* 3:188, 1962.

42. Nicol, C. F., Tutton, J. C., and Smith, B.: Parenteral diazepam in status epilepticus. *Neurology* 19:332, 1969.

43. Nielsen, J. M.: Tornado epilepsy simulating Meniere's syndrome. Report of 4 cases. *Neurology* 9:794, 1959.

44. Penfield, W., and Jasper, H. H.: *Epilepsy and the Functional Anatomy of the Brain.* Little, Brown and Co., Boston, 1954.

45. Ransohoff, J., and Carter, S.: Hemispherectomy in treatment of convulsive seizures associated with infantile hemiplegia. *Res. Pub. Assn. Res. Nerv. Ment. Dis.* 34:176, 1954.

46. Russell, W. R., and Davies-Jones, G. A. B.:

Epilepsy following the brain wounds of World War II. *The Late Effects of Head Injury.* Edited by Walker, A. E., and Caveness, W. E. Charles C Thomas, Springfield, Ill., 1969, Chapter 20.

47. Schmidt, R. P., and Wilder, B. J.: *Epilepsy.* Contemporary Neurology Series. Edited by Plum, F., and McDowell, F. H., F. A. Davis Co., Philadelphia, 1968.

48. Sherwin, I., Geschwind, N., Abramowicz, A.: Language-induced epilepsy. *Trans. Amer. Neurol. Assn.*, 1965, p. 183.

49. Shy, G. M., and Drager, G. A.: The neurological syndrome associated with orthostatic hypotension: A clinical pathological study. *Arch. Neurol.* 2:511, 1960.

50. Slater, E., and Beard, A. W.: The schizophrenia-like psychoses of epilepsy. *Brit. J. Psychiat.* 109:95, 1963.

51. Symonds, C. P.: Cataplexy and other related forms of seizure. *Canadian Med. J.* 70:621, 1954.

52. Symonds, C. P.: Discussion on faints and fits. *Proc. Royal Soc. Med.* 43:507, 1950.

53. Symonds, C. P.: Excitation and inhibition in epilepsy. *Brain* 82:133, 1959.

54. Van Buren, J. M.: The abdominal aura. A study of abdominal sensation occurring in epilepsy and produced by depth stimulation. *Electroenceph. Clin. Neurophysiol.* 15:1, 1963.

55. Walker, A. E.: Prognosis in post-traumatic epilepsy. A ten year follow-up of craniocerebral injuries in World War II. *J.A.M.A.* 164:1636, 1957.

56. Walker, A. E., and Richter, H. A.: Cerebral peduncle in propagation of convulsions. *Arch. Neurol.* 8:581, 1963.

57. Ward, A. A., and Schmidt, R. P.: Some properties of single epileptic neurons. *Arch. Neurol.* 5:308, 1961.

58. Whitty, C. W. M.: Photic and self-induced epilepsy. *Lancet* 1:1207, 1960.

59. Williams, D.: Discussion on faints and fits. *Proc. Royal Soc. Med.* 43:510, 1950.

60. Woodcock, S., and Cosgrove, J. V. P.: Epilepsy after the age of fifty: A five year follow-up study. *Neurology* 14:34, 1964.

61. Yoss, R. E., and Daly, D. C.: Narcolepsy in children. *Pediatrics*, 25:1025, 1960.

62. Zivin, L., and Marsan, C. A.: Incidence and prognostic significance of "epileptiform" activity in the EEG of non-epileptic patients. *Brain* 91:751, 1968.

CHAPTER EIGHT

Pain in the Head, Face, and Limbs

The resolution of the many difficulties which beset the evaluation of pain in the head, face, and limbs depends more upon clinical methods than upon laboratory procedures. In most cases, the facts derived from the history and from observation provide a recognizable diagnostic pattern, but in a substantial minority the clinical picture is atypical and the interpretation of symptoms requires an understanding of what is known about the anatomy, physiology, and psychophysiology of pain. These are outlined in Chapter 1.

HEADACHE

Mechanisms. Conventional usage confines the term *headache* to discomfort in the forehead and scalp area, excluding the face below the eyebrows. The area so defined is supplied by the great occipital nerves, derived from the second cervical roots, and by the first divisions of the trigeminal nerves. The second and third divisions of the trigeminal nerve send thin tongues of sensory supply upward across the temple toward the vertex, thus explaining why pain from the jaws is sometimes referred to the temple. The brain itself, the pia arachnoid, the ependyma, and the choroid

plexuses are insensitive, but pain can be evoked from the dural sinuses, parts of the basal dura, the dural arteries, the vessels at the base, and from the trigeminal, glossopharyngeal, and vagus nerves. Displacement of these structures by an expanding intracranial mass will cause pain if the displacement occurs rapidly, but will not necessarily do so if the process is a slow one.

It is probable that the headache which occurs with subnormal intracranial pressure is also due to displacement of pain-sensitive structures since it is induced by the individual's assuming an upright position and is relieved by his lying flat. It occurs following lumbar puncture and occasionally after closed head injuries. Traction on pain-sensitive structures is responsible for "cough headache"—stabbing pain in the head induced by coughing or straining especially when the patient is upright. It can be present for a long time as the only symptom of organic intracranial disease, usually in the posterior fossa, but may also occur as a benign syndrome which starts after some generalized infective illness, lasts a few months, and then disappears. Cough headache [38] can also arise without antecedent illness in overworked middle-aged subjects, and in patients with polycythemia.

The second intracranial mechanism for the production of pain is the presence of *abnormal chemical substances* in the spinal fluid, as for instance in meningitis, in the meningism of acute lobar pneumonia and other infections, and in subarachnoid hemorrhage.

The third category of headache is due to *affections of the arteries in the scalp*, and the fourth is disease of the skull itself. The fifth group consists of patients in whom *pain is referred to the cranium from elsewhere*—eyes, teeth, accessory nasal sinuses, the upper two cervical vertebrae and nerve roots, and the muscles of the neck. Occasionally pain is referred to the head via the vagus from sources in the thorax and upper abdomen, but this seldom causes confusion because the headache is a minor element in the total clinical picture. Finally there remains a heterogeneous group of headaches for which no satisfactory explanation is forthcoming; it includes those which follow head injuries and meningitis, those which sometimes occur in severe arterial hypertension and carotid stenosis, and those caused by emotional tension.

Diagnosis. We are not here concerned with headaches which are incidental to some obvious malady, such as a cerebral tumor, or the onset of lobar pneumonia, or meningitis, but with the problem of the patient afflicted by persistent or recurrent headache without obvious cause. Though it is difficult to identify the cause in some of these cases, the majority can be traced to their source, not by laboratory procedures but by taking an accurate history and applying clinical methods of examination. Information is required as to the total duration of the symptoms; the nature, situation, and severity of the pain; whether it is continuous, intermittent, or episodic; how long it lasts, and at what time of day it comes on; what relieves and what aggravates it; whether it is accompanied by other symptoms, neurological or otherwise; the general health and past history of the patient; his social and domestic circumstances, with particular reference to sources of anxiety; his work and the conditions under which it is carried out. Such a catechism, reinforced by a systematic examination of the whole body, will usually supply the diagnosis or at least direct attention to the system which requires further investigation. It is necessary to remember that the majority of the chronic headaches encountered in sophisticated communities are not due to organic disease, and it is to this group that attention should be directed first.

Headaches Unassociated with Structural Disease

Of these, the vascular headaches, typified by *migraine*, are common and are described below. *Tension headaches* are also very common. They are described as a persistent dull ache, situated over the top of the head or in the frontal or occipital region, and are variously likened to a tight band around the head, a sense of weight, or a feeling of pressure on the head. They are aggravated by mental effort, stuffy atmospheres, and emotional stresses, and the subject often feels better in the open air. They are usually combined with a sense of mental and physical fatigue, and are caused by prolonged overwork and emotional strain. When they occur in histrionic subjects, the description of the headache tends to be perverted or exaggerated; the pain may be said to resemble that of a nail being driven into the head, or of the skull opening and shutting. Unhappily, such subjects are also prone to exaggerate headaches due to organic disease, thereby alienating sympathy and throwing doubt on the validity of their complaints.

Rare causes of headache are allergy to specific foods, hypoglycemia, oversmoking, and working or sleeping in badly ventilated rooms. Occasional headaches, occurring only on waking, may be due to an epileptic seizure during sleep. The term "psychogenic headache" lacks precision. Psychological factors produce tension headaches and play a significant part in migraine, but the term is more often used for the vague, changeable, and indefinable head pains which are common in early schizophrenia, and for "agonizing" headaches which patients with conversion hysteria describe with such composure.

Headaches Associated with Organic Disease

The headaches caused by space occupying lesions are discussed on page 427. They are usually increased by recumbency, stooping, or straining. Headaches due to temporarily lowered intracranial pressure, as for instance after a lumbar puncture, may also be aggravated by stooping and straining, but they are relieved by lying flat. Of the expanding lesions, chronic subdural hematoma often produces a very severe headache, but this is not always the case and the pain is often unaffected by posture. Pituitary tumors usually cause a bitemporal headache which is unrelated to posture at first because at this stage it is due to expansion of the sella turcica. Later, when the tumor erupts into the cranial cavity proper, the pain is usually aggravated by recumbency.

HEAD INJURIES. A common cause of headache is head injury. The pain varies in time and location from case to case and in a single patient at different times, and is sometimes associated with tenderness at the site of the original injury. Meningeal adhesions may play a part in its production, and occasionally relief or improvement follows pneumoencephalography. A somewhat similar type of headache may occur following recovery from *meningitis* and *subarachnoid hemorrhage.* Severe throbbing pain, which is often worse at night, occasionally occurs in *secondary syphilis, gummatous meningitis,* and *syphilitic osteitis of the skull.* Other *diseases of the skull* which can produce pain in the head are osteomyelitis, tumors, and Paget's disease. *Acromegaly* occasionally causes intractable stabbing pains in the face, skull, and long bones. *Hyperostosis*

frontalis interna, common in middle-aged women, is often credited with the capacity to cause headache, but since it is usually painless, pain should not be attributed to this cause until every other possibility has been excluded.

INFECTIONS. Infections of the *accessory nasal sinuses* are a fairly common cause of headache and face-ache. Infections of these sinuses are very common and it is prudent to remember that even though the evidence of sinusitis is clear, the headache about which the patient complains is not necessarily due to the infection.

Although the pain of impacted wisdom teeth and of apical disease of the molars is usually felt locally, it can be referred to the ear, the vertex, or the temple, and in rare cases is found in the temple alone as a continuous unilateral "headache." It can be aggravated by getting the patient to bite firmly on a wooden object placed between the teeth. The reference to the temple is explained by the fact that pain from deep structures such as the teeth is referred to other deep structures innervated by the same root or segment—in this case to the temporalis muscle.

SPONDYLOSIS. *Spondylosis* of the upper cervical spine is an important source of headaches in advancing years. The pain is usually occipital and—like other osteoarthritic pains—is often at its worst in the early morning after a night's rest. The neck tends to creak on movement, the neck muscles are tender, and if the second occipital root is involved, paresthesias may be experienced in the distribution of the great occipital nerve in the posterior half of the scalp. This condition is often attributed to fibrositis, a concept which would be more acceptable if fibrositis were proved to be a pathological entity. In some cases, the pain of cervical spondylosis is referred to the forehead or temple because the sensory roots of C1 and C2 establish connection with the spinal root of the first division of the trigeminal nerve.

OTHER CAUSES. *Basilar impression* (p. 197) is an occasional cause of persistent occipital pain; the deformity is recognized on lateral x-ray pictures of the skull.

Ocular headaches are usually felt in the eye or forehead. When due to disease of the eye or of the anterior part of the optic nerve (e.g., glaucoma, iritis, retrobulbar neuritis), the pain is situated in the eye itself and there are appropriate local signs of the disease. When due to errors of refraction or to muscle imbalance, there is a bilateral frontal ache which is induced by using the eyes and is therefore most obtrusive toward the end of the working day. It may, however, be experienced during weekends only in persons whose hobbies involve more eye strain than their normal work. However, the presence of a refractive error or muscle imbalance does not necessarily prove that a headache of which the patient complains is due to these abnormalities.

Headache is sometimes due to *arterial hypertension*, which can give rise to two types of discomfort—a throbbing pain induced by fatigue or excitement, and a dull headache, often occipital, which is present on waking and passes off in an hour or two. The latter often has the features of headache due to raised intracranial pressure, and is especially apt to occur in malignant hypertension with cerebral edema. Some individuals with persistent headache toward the end of the day are found to have abnormally low blood pressure, but it is difficult to assign the pain to the hypotension in view of the rarity of headache in Addison's disease or after coronary thrombosis.

Temporal arteritis, better called cranial arteritis, is a rare but important cause of severe headache, either unilateral or bilateral. It is recognized in the acute phase by the presence of tenderness and induration along the temporal arteries (p. 384). *Polycythemia vera,* with or without hypertension, can cause headaches which are usually described as throbbing, or as a fullness of the head, and which can be improved by reducing the red cell count to a normal level by appropriate treatment.

Migraine

Definition. Migraine is a form of vascular headache which consists essentially of episodic headaches of brief duration, separated by intervals of complete freedom and associated in some cases with transient neurological and gastrointestinal symptoms.[28, 31, 33, 35, 42, 45]

Incidence. Migraine is uncommon below the age of 10 years, and usually occurs for the first time during adolescence, with a maximum incidence in the third and fourth decades. It tends to become less severe as life advances, but it may occur for the first time during the menopause in women, and in men in the fifth or sixth decade. It is more frequent in females than in males and is largely an affliction of sophisticated communities. It tends to occur in persons with obsessive-compulsive trends, many of whom show hypersensitivity to stimuli such as odors and changes of temperature.[44] Although allergy rarely *causes* migraine, there is a high incidence of allergy in the family and personal history of migraine sufferers. There is also a somewhat higher incidence of epilepsy in the family history of patients with migraine than among the general population.

Etiology. Wolff[45] and his associates have shown that the ocular and other neurological disturbances which sometimes usher in or accompany the headache are caused by vasoconstriction of intracranial vessels; these symptoms can be cut short by the inhalation of amyl nitrite or carbon dioxide. The headache is caused by dilatation of arteries in the dura, pericranium, and scalp, and the tenderness of the scalp which may persist after a severe headache seems to be due to the presence of an extravasate containing plasma, a few red cells, and a polypeptide which sensitizes pain endings in the scalp. A similar polypeptide has been found in the spinal fluid following the headache. Before the attack, there is retention of sodium and water, and diuresis often occurs as the headache wears off.[4] Yet, despite all this information, there is still no precise evidence as to how these vascular and biochemical responses are evoked.

Symptoms

PREMONITORY FEATURES. Premonitory feelings of well-being or of listlessness and depression may occur. The former sensation may lead to an increase of social and domestic activities, thus providing optimum conditions for a severe attack the next day. The episode often commences early in the day, the patient being aware of the headache on waking. It cannot be too strongly emphasized that the premonitory neurological symptoms of "classical" migraine are often absent. The most common of these symptoms is an ill-defined blurring of vision in one or both eyes, but there may be an expanding arc of brilliant colors, zig-zag lines of colored lights, a central scotoma, tunnel vision, homonymous hemianopia, or even complete blindness.[14] Less common symptoms are transient diplopia, visual disorientation, transient partial aphasia, dysarthria, slowness of thought, dyslexia, complete anosmia, deafness, vertigo, unsteadiness of gait, or paresthesias which spread slowly up one arm into the face and lips, extending into the lower limb in exceptional cases. The spread of the paresthesias is slow, occupying from 10 to 30 minutes, in contrast to the spread of a jacksonian sensory attack, which is usually complete within two minutes. Monoparesis or hemiparesis may occur alone or may accompany the paresthesias; migrainous hemiplegia has been seen in several members of a family. These symptoms are often absent; on the other hand, they can occur alone, *without an accompanying headache*, in which event they are readily mistaken for evidence of focal disease in the brain. Severe migraine is often accompanied by confusion and slowing of thought.

Although most of the premonitory features of migraine can be explained on the basis of a disturbance in the distri-

bution of the internal carotid artery, in some cases the symptoms suggest a disturbance in the territory of the basilar artery and its branches. Thus, the patient will sometimes complain of bilateral loss of vision, dysarthria, vertigo, ataxia of gait, and paresthesias or weakness of the legs. Often only one of these symptoms is present. Thus, a woman aged 36 gave a 20 year history of intermittent episodes of unsteadiness of gait lasting from one to six hours, occurring about twice a month, and only occasionally accompanied by throbbing headaches, nausea, and scintillating scotomas; sometimes the headache and nausea occurred alone without unsteadiness of gait or visual disturbances, and this type of attack always started on waking in the morning, lasted all day, and was relieved by sleep. The frequency of her attacks was much diminished by the prophylactic administration of methysergide (Sansert).

Loss of consciousness, whether syncopal, epileptic, or ill-defined, sometimes occurs during the attack. It occurred in 23 per cent of Hockaday and Whitty's cases,[17] but this figure may have been influenced by the selection of cases. In the author's experience, an attack of unconsciousness during an attack of migraine is distinctly uncommon.

THE HEADACHE. This may be unilateral or bilateral, frontal or occipital, and it may spread down into the upper part of the neck. It varies in severity from discomfort to intense pain, and when severe it tends to have a throbbing quality aggravated by recumbency or by effort. It may be associated with photophobia. It usually lasts for several hours and in severe cases may extend over a day or two, but it commonly ends after a sleep. The onset is usually fairly rapid; occasionally it starts with an abruptness which may simulate a subarachnoid hemorrhage. Migrainous subjects can suffer from tension headaches as well.

Nausea is usually present at some stage of the attack, and may proceed to vomiting and prostration. Abdominal pain occasionally occurs early in the attack and if severe it may be mistaken for an abdominal emergency. Conversely, abdominal symptoms arising in a migrainous subject may be falsely attributed to migraine.

Water retention is common before and during migraine[4]; oliguria sometimes accompanies the attack, and diuresis heralds recovery. Migrainous subjects respond normally to a water load, but excrete excess sodium and chlorides during the diuresis.

The objective signs are variable. In severe cases the patient looks ill, the face may be pale or unusually pink, and there may be congestion of the conjunctiva and of the nasal mucous membrane; epistaxis may occur.

Focal disturbances are seen on the electroencephalogram during the premonitory neurological disturbances, and nonspecific abnormalities are found in about 60 per cent of all patients between attacks. An analysis of clinical and EEG features in 560 cases of migraine by Hockaday and Whitty[17] revealed an abnormality in 61 per cent, the rate being lower (56 per cent) in classical migraine with visual aura and in cases without aura, and higher (72 per cent) in cases with a lateralized nonvisual aura. Abnormal records are found in 50 per cent of cases of basilar migraine. The incidence of *lateralized or localized* EEG changes was 23 per cent in patients without aura, 31 per cent in patients with bilateral visual aura, and 47 per cent in patients with a lateralized nonvisual aura.

Course and Prognosis. Patients developing migraine early in life may lose their symptoms at puberty, but when it occurs for the first time in adolescence it is liable to recur for many years, especially during periods of stress. It is not uncommon for one type of migraine to give place to another as life goes on. Generally speaking, there is a tendency for the attacks to become less severe and less frequent with advancing age, and lengthy remissions are common. Fracture of the skull may abruptly terminate a liability to migraine; in other cases head injuries aggravate it, not only by adding a postconcussional headache to the total picture but also by impairing the subject's ability to withstand mental and emotional stresses. Migraine arising for the first time at the menopause does not *as a rule* last longer than a year or two.

In rare instances, permanent visual impairment can follow an attack[14]; it takes the form of a uniocular scotoma or a homonymous field defect. The latter can occur in the absence of arteriographic evidence of either aneurysm or arteriovenous malformation. In general, however, permanent neurological residua following what appears to have been an isolated attack of migraine suggest the presence of a vascular anomaly, especially if the headache has been consistently limited to one side of the head. Cerebral vascular accidents have been reported from time to time in the course of an attack of migraine, but they are rare.[7] They include intracerebral hemorrhage, cerebral infarction, subdural hematoma, and dissecting aneurysms of the internal carotid or middle cerebral artery.

Treatment

AVOIDANCE OF STRESS. There is no panacea for migraine. The most important single factor in prophylaxis is the avoidance of overwork and the adjustment of domestic or professional sources of emotional strain. In extreme cases of social or domestic maladjustment, psychiatric help may be needed, but the obsessional background which is so often present renders these patients resistant to psychotherapy. When overwork is responsible for increased frequency of attacks, a prolonged vacation is desirable, followed by restriction of working hours, adequate exercise in the open air, and sufficient sleep.

Overreaction to stress may be reduced by medication, and much help may be had from the continuing administration of 30 mg. of phenobarbital twice a day between attacks. Modern tranquilizing drugs seem to be equally effective in this respect.

The facts that migraine often starts at puberty, is sometimes related to menstrual periods, and is occasionally suppressed during pregnancy have prompted efforts to use various hormone preparations prophylactically. A wide variety of substances has been used, including progesterone and methyltestosterone. Recently, Lundberg[27] and others have reported favorable results without undue side effects with flumedroxone. This compound is given in doses of 10 mg. twice a day. In Lundberg's series of 239 patients, 77 reported complete freedom from attacks during the period of treatment and 137 claimed improvement. Menstrual disturbances occurred in 25.7 per cent of the women treated.

Improvement has been reported from daily injections of thiamine chloride (100 mg.), and cases have been recorded in which the administration of 1000 μg. of vitamin B_{12} three times per week has reduced the frequency and severity of attacks. The author has seen dramatic improvement in one case following this treatment, when everything else had failed. The psychosomatic aspect of migraine encourages the belief that almost any treatment administered with enthusiasm, sympathy, and confidence can lead to symptomatic improvement, and overcritical attitudes to "unscientific" therapy are out of place if the patient is demonstrably benefited.

MEDICATION. For the actual attack, bed rest in a quiet room is the best way of cutting it short. Codeine or combinations of codeine with phenacetin and aspirin may be of assistance, if taken early, but gastric absorption is usually delayed once an attack has started. Ergotamine and dihydroergotamine have a specific action in reducing vasodilation. A suitable preparation is Cafergot, which combines caffeine and ergotamine tartrate, but the efficacy of this medication depends on the ability of the stomach to absorb it. Consequently, better results are obtained when it is administered as a suppository, and it must be emphasized that early treatment is better than late. Dihydroergotamine tartrate can be given by intramuscular injection in doses of 0.5 to 1.5 mg., and this dose can be repeated within two hours if necessary. Ergotamine preparations which can be held under the tongue and absorbed are also available. Peripheral arterial spasm with loss of the pulses and even gangrene has occurred from too frequent use of ergotamine preparations by mouth, by rectum, or by injection, and it is therefore desirable that the administration of these drugs should not be left entirely in the hands of the patient.[46] The prophylactic administration of methysergide (Sansert) in doses of 2 mg. three times a day is often effective, but since the prolonged use of this drug can give rise to retroperitoneal fibrosis, it should never be used for more than three months.

If fluid retention is a marked feature of the attacks, restriction of the daily intake of salt is sometimes successful in cases which have proved resistant to all other forms of treatment.

OPHTHALMOPLEGIC MIGRAINE

Transient diplopia may occur at the onset or during an otherwise typical attack of migraine. It seldom lasts more than half an hour. The term ophthalmoplegic migraine, however, refers to an entirely different situation in which one or more attacks of unilateral severe pain behind the eye or in the forehead are accompanied by persistent diplopia, which lasts for days or weeks.[19] The third, fourth, and sixth nerves may be affected, alone or in combination, and in extreme cases there is complete fixity of the eyeball, with ptosis and enlargement of the pupil. The corneal reflex may be diminished, and in some cases there is slight sensory loss involving the first and second divisions of the trigeminal nerve, the third division escaping involvement.

Attacks occur at intervals of months or years. Carotid angiography usually fails to show either an aneurysm or a tumor in the great majority of these cases, though an intracavernous carotid aneurysm is occasionally encountered. A tumor in the region of the pituitary fossa can present in this way, but is an unacceptable explanation for recurrent attacks with intervals of freedom. On the other hand, periostitis of the superior orbital fissure, with or without ethmoiditis, can produce one or more attacks of this type, but in these cases there is proptosis on the affected side and the second division of the trigeminal nerve is unaffected. Aneurysm, tumor, and periostitis do not account for anything more than a very small fraction of the cases observed.

Tolosa [40] has described a chronic inflammatory lesion of the cavernous sinus characterized by proliferation of fibroblasts and infiltration of the septa and walls of the sinus with lymphocytes and plasma cells. The granulomatous process in this case had engulfed the abducens nerve, the carotid plexus, and the first division of the trigeminal. This process may be the explanation of some of the cases of ophthalmoplegic migraine in which there are spontaneous remissions and in which carotid angiography and exploration fail to reveal any other cause.

CLUSTER HEADACHES

Histamine Headaches, Horton's Syndrome, Nasociliary Migraine)

This common condition is characterized by attacks of severe pain in and around one eye, associated with reddening of the eye, unilateral lacrimation, and either stuffiness or running of the nostril on the affected side. The pain often awakens the patient from sleep in the middle of the night and may last one to two hours. The attacks occur at intervals of a few hours or days, and after this has gone on for one to three months, the condition passes off for months or even years, but it is apt to recur. In extreme cases there may be edema of the upper lid, with pseudoptosis. Exceptionally, the pain is felt in the cheek and lower jaw, with little or no spread to the region of the eye, but the periodicity of the attacks and the severe boring quality of the pain distinguish the condition from other types of facial pain.

Diagnosis. Unilateral lacrimation and reddening of the eye sometimes occur in association with pain in the face due to other conditions — for instance, cerebellopontine angle tumors. Repeated paroxysms of headache, perspiration, palpitation, pallor and hypertension can be caused by a pheochromocytoma; the attacks commonly last less than an hour and are particularly prone to occur during sleep in the early hours of the morning, but unlike the cluster headache, the pain is bilateral, the blood pressure is greatly elevated, and there is no lacrimation or stuffiness of the nose. Paroxysmal hypertension and episodic generalized headache can be the presenting symptoms of a cerebellar tumor.

Treatment. Horton [18] recommended histamine desensitization, but this is a tedious and often unrewarding process. The administration of dihydroergotamine by intramuscular injection is often effective. It is given in doses of 1 mg. intramuscularly, and since the attacks come on abruptly and without warning, it is prudent to use the drug prophylactically by giving an injection every evening for 10 days and then lengthening the intervals between injections until it is certain that the "cluster" has come to an end. The same drug can be used at the onset of an individual attack. Alternatively, oral preparations of ergot can be given by mouth or by suppository before going to bed. If the ergot preparations prove ineffective or are contraindicated, propranolol hydrochloride should be tried. This is a beta-adrenergic receptor blocking agent which at present is still under trial; however, the author has been impressed by its effectiveness in doses of at least 40 mg. three times a day. Its use is contraindicated in the presence of bronchial asthma and congestive heart failure.

As is to be expected, complete relief from the attacks can be obtained by cutting the sensory root of the trigeminal nerve, but this should be resorted to only when all other methods have failed, and when the attacks are very severe. Sectioning of the greater and lesser petrosal nerves has given variable results. [42]

As with migraine, fatigue and psychological stress often play a part in the production of this condition, and these factors should receive attention.

Migrainous Neuralgia

Migrainous neuralgia occurs alone or in association with migraine.[3] The pain is usually supraorbital or in the temple, lasts for hours or days at a time, and is not accompanied by the neurological or gastric symptoms of migraine. In an attack, the pain can be relieved by an injection of procaine into the supraorbital nerve, but cutting the nerve does not necessarily prevent further attacks. Similarly, intracranial section of the first division of the trigeminal nerve is not always curative, and should be avoided.

Conditions which have to be considered in the differential diagnosis include frontal sinusitis, ethmoiditis, and high cervical spondylosis. In two cases, the condition appeared to have been caused by penetrating wounds in the suboccipital region, and in one of these, removal of a metal fragment deeply imbedded in the nuchal muscles cured the frontal neuralgia (Fig. 8–1).

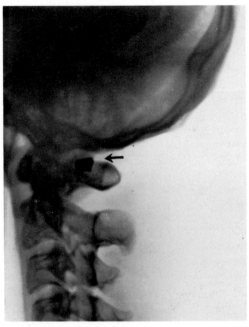

Figure 8–1. Removal of this bomb splinter cured a unilateral frontal headache, present since the time of injury.

Tic Douloureux (Paroxysmal Trigeminal Neuralgia, Fothergill's Disease)

Definition. Tic douloureux is a variety of facial neuralgia characterized by bouts of paroxysmal pain in one or more divisions of the trigeminal distribution and unassociated with either sensory loss or demonstrable pathology.

Etiology and Incidence. Tic douloureux occurs at any age after puberty, but four-fifths of all patients are between 40 and 70 years old. It is commoner in women than in men. The cause is unknown, though Harris[16] was impressed by the frequency with which infection of the teeth and sinuses was present at the inception of the disease. The term tic douloureux excludes trigeminal pain caused by gross disease of the sinuses, eyes, jaws, teeth, skull, and intracranial structures.

Demyelination and fibrotic changes have been described in the gasserian ganglion, but they are too inconstant to be considered relevant. The facts that an intravenous injection of Dilantin can interrupt an episode of trigeminal neuralgia, and that the oral administration of Tegretol can suppress the symptoms over long periods of time, have suggested that the tic is due to a paroxysmal discharge arising in the descending nucleus of the trigeminal nerve.

Clinical Features. The pain usually involves the second or third divisions of the nerve, or both, and it may spread to all three, but it is seldom confined to the first division. It is usually unilateral, but bilateral pain occurred in 17 per cent of Harris's cases and in 6 per cent of Peet and Schneider's cases.[32] Pain occurs in recurrent bouts which last days, weeks, or months, with intervals of complete freedom. During each bout the pain is intermittent, but as time goes on it tends to become persistent and more severe, with fewer and shorter intermissions.

The pain is variously described as knife-like, red-hot needles under the skin, or painful electrical shocks. The face may suddenly screw up with pain — hence the term tic. Pain occurs with or without provocation, but can often be induced by lightly touching trigger areas within the territory of the affected division. It may also be caused by talking or eating, or even by a cold draft, and it is characteristic of the condition that the pain is more easily evoked by light stimuli than by strong ones. Unilateral lacrimation and suffusion of the eye can occur, and salivation is not unknown. The pain is sometimes aggravated by stooping, coughing, or sneezing, but this is more likely to occur in the presence of an intracranial tumor or aneurysm.

There may be graying of the hair and coating of the tongue on the affected side. There is no objective sensory loss or other signs of neurological disease, and the spinal fluid is normal in all respects. Any increase of cells or protein, or any deviation from the normal electrophoretic pattern, should be regarded as evidence that the pain is symptomatic of intracranial disease.

Diagnosis. Tic douloureux is identified by the quality of the pain, its distribution, the presence of superficial trigger points, and the absence of neurological signs of structural disease. However, precisely similar pain, unaccompanied by sensory loss or other objective neurological findings, occasionally occurs during the *early* development of tumors and aneurysms, persistence of the embryonal trigeminal artery, multiple sclerosis, glioma of the pons, and syringobulbia. Frontal and maxillary sinusitis occasionally cause a stabbing pain, with tic-like periodicity, and the same is true of neoplasms of the maxilla and nasopharynx and disease of the temporomandibular joint, but generally speaking, the pain caused by these conditions differs significantly from that of tic douloureux, and there are usually accessory symptoms and signs which make the diagnosis clear. Postherpetic neuralgia and other continuous boring pains in the face are so different from the recurrent shooting pains of tic douloureux that they do not cause confusion.

Prognosis. Individual bouts of pain last days, weeks, or months, and complete intermissions lasting several months are not uncommon. The condition tends to worsen with advancing years, and is apt to undermine both health and morale. If the second and third divisions are involved, the patient ultimately becomes afraid to eat, and this can cause a severe degree of inanition.

Treatment. The treatment of tic douloureux has been revolutionized by the introduction of carbamazepine (Tegretol) which suppresses the pain though it does not cure the "disease." The oral administration of 200 mg. three times a day, one hour before meals, is effective in the majority of cases. Sometimes a single dose, taken in the morning, will protect the patient from pain throughout the day; in resistant cases, it may be necessary to give as many as 10 tablets during the day, but these high dosages should be reached gradually. Side effects in the form of nausea, dizziness, skin rashes, and marked depression of neutrophil leukocytes occasionally contraindicate the use of the drug. Dilantin can then be tried in place of Tegretol, in doses of 100 mg. three times a day, but this compound is less effective. Inhalation of Trilene affords relief during violent spasms. From 50 to 100 mg. of Demerol (pethidine), taken one-half hour before meals, may enable the patient to eat with relative comfort, but this and other habit-forming drugs should be avoided in view of the chronic nature of the ailment.

Surgical measures [42] are necessary if Tegretol produces too many side effects, or if—as sometimes happens—the patient acquires a tolerance to it. Two procedures are available: injection of alcohol into the roots or ganglion, and sectioning of the sensory root. Avulsion of the peripheral branches is seldom effective for long. The same applies to peripheral alcohol injections. When the injection of the ganglion is correctly carried out, there is complete sensory loss in the related area of skin, and in most cases there is loss of corneal sensation. The injection is sometimes followed by trophic disturbances, of which the most important are neuroparalytic keratitis, corneal ulceration, and infection of the anesthetized eye. This risk is reduced by wearing a specially constructed eye shield to protect the eye from pressure and dust, coupled with the instillation of castor oil three times a day, for the first three or four weeks. After this period, the danger of ocular damage is very much less. Tarsorrhaphy should be carried out at the first sign of conjunctival congestion.

Mandibular and gasserian injection is sometimes followed by transient loss of taste on the affected side of the tongue.

In a certain number of cases, the tic is cured but is replaced in six weeks to three months by a burning sensation, or other unpleasant paresthesias, in the affected area of the face. This discomfort cannot be relieved by further injection or by root section and it is desirable that the patient should be warned of this possibility when the question of surgical treatment is discussed.

Root section is indicated when injection fails, when there is any reason to suspect the presence of disease in the cerebellopontine angle, or when the patient lives far from surgical facilities. It is possible to do a fractional section of the nerve in accordance with the situation of the pain, but since pain can appear at a later date in the other divisions, this refinement is of doubtful value. There are obvious advantages in sparing the first division and therefore retaining the corneal reflex in patients who have no pain in that division.

Glossopharyngeal Neuralgia

Definition. Glossopharyngeal neuralgia is a rare form of neuralgia limited to the distribution of the glossopharyngeal nerve but similar to tic douloureux in the quality of the pain.[16, 23]

Etiology. The cause of glossopharyngeal neuralgia is unknown. It is very much less common than trigeminal neuralgia. The onset is usually in the fourth or fifth decade, and men are more frequently affected than women.

Clinical Features. The pain is felt in

the region of the tonsil, the pharynx, the back of the tongue and jaw, and deeply in the ear; it may be limited to one of these places. It is described as pricking, stabbing, or shooting, and occurs in intermittent spasms lasting seconds and recurring over many hours at a time. The pain can be induced by swallowing or talking or by touching the tonsil; this "triggering" is reminiscent of what occurs in tic douloureux, and it can be abolished temporarily by procainization of the tonsil and pharyngeal area. Thomson[39] and others have described the association of glossopharyngeal neuralgia and convulsions, the latter being "triggered" by the former and both being relieved by section of the ninth nerve and lower two filaments of the tenth cranial nerve. Syncope from cardiac arrest has also been reported.[23]

Glossopharyngeal neuralgia can be mimicked by carcinoma of the fauces; the condition will usually be obvious on inspection. Very rarely, a tumor of the cerebellopontine angle or a glomus tumor may present with similar pain, and the same applies to persistence of the embryonal hypoglossal artery.

Treatment. The oral administration of 200 mg. of Tegretol three times a day, or larger doses, can suppress the pain, as in tic douloureux. If this fails, or if the patient is intolerant of the drug, it is necessary to cut the intracranial section of the glossopharyngeal sensory root. In some cases, it is also desirable to divide the intermediate nerve of Wrisberg and the upper filaments of the vagus.[42]

Atypical Facial Neuralgias

A perplexing problem is often provided by a patient suffering from pain in the face and jaws which cannot be traced to any organic lesion, which lacks the characteristic features of trigeminal or glossopharyngeal neuralgia, and which cannot be classified as migrainous.[3]

TEMPOROMANDIBULAR   NEURALGIA[5] (COSTEN'S SYNDROME). This is a somewhat ill-defined syndrome occasionally found in individuals who, as a result of loss of teeth or of wearing shallow dentures, develop a derangement of the temporomandibular joint by habitually overclosing the jaws in speaking and chewing. The syndrome can also follow forcible opening of the mouth for the insertion of a gag during oral operations.

The pain varies from dull discomfort to sudden spasms of such intensity that the patient can neither eat nor talk. It is induced by moving the jaws, and is felt in one or more of the following sites: the temple, cheek, lower jaw, over the affected joint, deeply in the ear, and behind the ear in the region of the mastoid. The stabbing pain in these regions is sometimes accompanied by a dull ache at the side of the face and by a burning sensation at the side of the tongue. The symptoms are strictly unilateral and the lancinating quality of the pain, together with its "triggering" by talking and chewing, may suggest tic douloureux. However, the pain usually extends beyond the trigeminal territory, is not accompanied by tactile trigger spots, and does not usually occur unless the jaw is moved.

In some of the patients described by Costen, there were complaints of slight deafness and tinnitus on the affected side, and vertigo was also reported. Hankey,[15] reviewing 100 cases, found that these additional symptoms were conspicuous by their absence, and he noted that pain might sometimes radiate to the top of the head and down into the neck behind the angle of the jaw. In 34 per cent of his cases, the temporomandibular joint appeared to be normal on x-ray, 8 per cent showed pathological changes, and 58 per cent showed abnormal condylar movements. Ninety-seven per cent showed some form of malocclusion, and the majority of these were helped by prosthetic appliances designed to open the bite.

Intracapsular injections of hydrocortisone can help if arthritis is present.

CLONIC FACIAL SPASM WITH TRIGEMINAL NEURALGIA. This is a rare condition in which there are continuous clonic spasms of one side of the face associated with pain resembling that of tic douloureux. The facial spasm is unlike the involuntary screwing up of the face which occurs in tic douloureux, but it closely resembles idiopathic facial hemispasm. The pain can be cured by the methods employed for tic douloureux, but the facial spasm persists. Exploration of the cerebellopontine angle is advisable.

SLUDER'S NEURALGIA. Sluder[36] described cases of pain in the root of the nose, in and around the eye, in the upper and lower jaw, extending backward to the zygoma, ear, and mastoid, and even radiating into the neck and shoulder. The pain was described either as constant, with exacerbations, as cyclical, as in migraine, or as sharp and tic-like.

Campbell and Lloyd[3] draw attention to a group of patients in whom either constant or paroxysmal unilateral discomfort in the face spreads into the neck and to the mastoid region or the back of the head. Some have flushing of the affected side of the face during an attack, and localized sweating, lacrimation, and pupillary changes may also occur on the affected side. Ptosis and narrowing of the pupil may occur during the attack. Some of their patients also had migraine and were able to distinguish between the two forms of discomfort. The sympathetic symptoms, together with the liability of the pain to spread into the neck and occipital region, focused attention on the cervical sympathetic and on the possibility that skeletal factors might be responsible for triggering the attacks. Neuwith and others have found that traction on the head may temporarily banish both pain and the sympathetic disturbances. On a long-term basis, the use of a cervical collar is reported to be satisfactory in the majority of cases. Cervical sympathectomy may or may not bring temporary relief, but the attacks usually return in a year or so. Jaeger,[20] describing similar cases as sphenopalatine neuralgia, reported permanent relief from destruction of the petrosal nerves and the superior cervical ganglion. The administration of dihydroergotamine in doses of 0.5 to 1.0 mg. daily is reported to be effective in some cases.

PAIN IN THE UPPER LIMB

This account will be confined to conditions which cause pain in the upper limbs by direct involvement of the nervous system. The commonest of these is root pain caused by prolapsed discs and cervical spondylosis. Next in frequency is the aching discomfort and numbness associated with the several varieties of the thoracic outlet syndrome, including cervical ribs. Compression of the median nerve in the carpal tunnel and traumatic ulnar neuropathy are very common indeed, but pain is less prominent than paresthesias, and it is only in a minority of patients that discomfort is present in the forearm. Less common sources of pain in the upper limb include rare examples of central pain from lesions of the brain and spinothalamic tract, syringomyelia and tumors of the cervical cord, hypertrophic pachymeningitis, postherpetic neuralgia, primary and secondary tumors of the cervical spine, fracture dislocation involving cervical roots, and malignant infiltration of the brachial plexus. Neuralgic amyotrophy (paralytic brachial neuritis) is an occasional cause of severe but transient pain in the upper part of the limb.

Disease of the cervical cord is a rare cause of brachial pain. Extramedullary *tumors* (neurofibroma, meningioma) are more common than intramedullary growths, but pain down one or both arms can be an early symptom in both forms and may precede other symptoms and signs by many months. The pain is commonly accompanied by paresthesias, and ultimately by sensory loss, weakness, and sphincter symptoms, the march of events being characteristic of compression of the spinal cord. Suspicion of spinal compression is aroused when brachial pain is accompanied by tingling or a sense of coldness in the feet, "aching" or weakness of the legs, and

sphincter disturbances. Myelography may show the presence of a partial or complete block, usually with an increase of protein, and x-rays will sometimes reveal erosion of pedicles in advanced cases.

Syringomyelia is usually painless, but occasionally there are complaints of a burning or stabbing pain in one or both arms; moreover, when the cervical cord is much distended by the lesion there may be pain and stiffness of the neck. However, by the time syringomyelia causes pain in the arm and stiffness of the neck, the sensory loss, depression of tendon reflexes, and wasting are well established.

Hypertrophic pachymeningitis of the cervical region is an extremely rare cause of pain in the arms.

Postherpetic neuralgia occasionally follows an attack of herpes zoster involving one or more cervical root ganglia. The pain varies from slight to severe and is usually described as shooting or burning or as a deep ache of fluctuating severity. It is associated with an unpleasant sensitivity of the skin in the dermatomes affected, and rarely there is weakness or paralysis of a muscle or group of muscles. Such weakness dates from the onset of the herpes and is not progressive. The history of a rash and the presence of depigmented scars indicate the diagnosis.

PROTRUSION OF INTERVERTEBRAL DISCS

Pathology. Disc protrusions are common throughout the spinal column, excluding the spaces above and below the atlas, in which there is no true disc tissue. Protrusions producing symptoms are most common in the lower lumbar and midcervical areas, but root pain from thoracic herniations is not unknown.

An intervertebral disc consists of an elastic inner portion, the nucleus pulposus, invested by an outer fibrous ring, the annulus fibrosus (Fig. 8–2). The nucleus pulposus undergoes progressive desiccation after the thirtieth year, becoming less resilient as time goes on.[26]

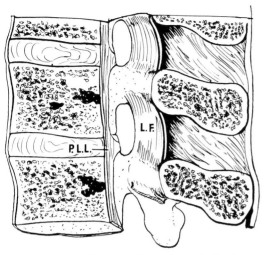

Figure 8–2. Cross section of the spinal column to show relationship of the intervertebral discs to the intervertebral foramen. LF, ligamentum flavum; PLL, posterior longitudinal ligament.

Nuclear herniation can occur through a defect in the annulus at any point of its circumference, but forward protrusions are uncommon because the anterior common ligament strengthens the disc at this point. Herniation can occur at any age, with or without trauma, and as life advances there is an additional tendency for the annulus to bulge, either in its entire circumference or in a segment of the periphery. Ultimately, calcification and even ossification can occur on the surface of these bulges, giving rise to the familiar lipping or spurring seen on x-ray photographs. Both nuclear herniations and annular protrusions can impinge on emerging roots, the spinal cord, or the cauda equina, and the adjacent vertebrae come closer together when this happens; this causes some overriding of the intervertebral articulations which eventually show osteoarthritic changes. Pressure on the roots leads to swelling and a fibrotic reaction in the dural sheaths,[13] while backward protrusions sometimes lead to the formation of dense adhesions between the posterior common ligament and the pia arachnoid. These adhesions can tether the cord, preventing it from moving upward with flexion and extension of the neck in the course of normal activity.[43]

The foramen can be narrowed by a posterolateral herniation and by flattening of the disc as a whole (Fig. 8–3). Hypertrophy of the ligamentum flavum in association with disc disease can further narrow the intervertebral foramina. Osteoarthritic spurs of the intervertebral articulations can, by themselves, narrow the foramen. In the cervical spine, osteoarthritic changes in the joints of Luschka can also play a part. These lie between the upper and lower surfaces of the bodies of the cervical vertebrae on their posterolateral aspects, directly in front of the emerging root. In advanced spondylosis the intervertebral foramen is encroached upon by these structures, and the root is displaced and becomes fibrotic.

Clinical Features of Cervical Protrusions

ONSET. The onset may be sudden or gradual, with *or without* painful stiffness of the neck.[9, 12] Pain usually extends across the back of the shoulder and down the back of the arm and forearm to the wrist, and may radiate over the scapula and into the upper part of the pectoral region; in some cases, it is felt first in the arm, or in the front of the chest, and there may be no pain in the neck whatsoever. If the eighth cervical root is involved, the pain is felt along the inner side of the arm and forearm. It is often aggravated by coughing and sneezing and by movements of the neck. The pain in the arm tends to be worse at the end of the day, when the patient has been using the limb, whereas pain in the neck is often worse on waking in the morning. Paresthesias may be present or absent. If the sixth root is involved, paresthesias are felt in the thumb and index fingers, whereas in lesions affecting the seventh root, paresthesias are usually in the index or middle fingers (Fig. 8–3). The eighth root is seldom involved, but when it is, tingling may be present in the ring and little fingers and along the ulnar border of the hand. Sometimes paresthesias precede pain. The clinical picture may be complicated by the presence of a thoracic outlet syndrome which can oc-

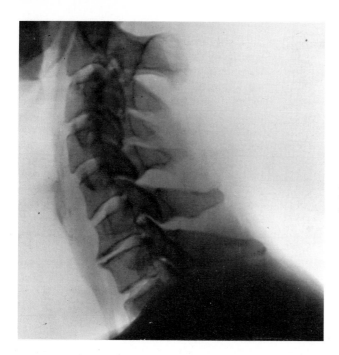

Figure 8–3. Narrowing of the interspace between C6 and C7 in a patient with severe pain in the distribution of C7.

cur if the patient holds the arm adducted and immobile in order to avoid pain.

Neck movements are usually somewhat restricted; in particular, tilting the head to the affected side may aggravate the pain in the arm. The same is true of downward pressure on the head. There is sometimes a flattening of the normal cervical lordosis. In severe cases, there is tenderness of the muscles of the shoulder, pectoral region, and arm. Pressure on trigger points in the tender muscles of the shoulder girdle may cause pain to shoot down the limb, and injections of procaine into these trigger points will sometimes relieve the patient of much of his discomfort, thereby misleading the observer into thinking that these trigger points are, in fact, the cause of the patient's complaints.[11]

Weakness or paralysis of muscles is uncommon, but pain often prevents the patient from exerting full power. Rarely, there is weakness of the triceps and the extensors of the wrists and fingers. Elderly patients with large herniations or a considerable degree of spondylosis may experience sudden paralysis of a muscle or group of muscles, e.g., wrist drop or finger drop, or weakness of the intrinsic muscles of the hand.

Sensory loss is usually limited to blunting of pinprick in the periphery of the dermatome concerned, but this is a late development. If the sixth root is involved, the biceps and supinator jerks are reduced or absent, whereas the triceps jerk is lost in lesions affecting the seventh root. In many cases, especially in the early stages, sensation and reflexes are entirely normal, and the diagnosis is made on the distribution of pain and paresthesias. On the other hand, large herniations may give rise to cord compression as well as pain in the arm,[9] and bilateral symptoms in the upper limbs is by no means rare in spondylosis.

LABORATORY TESTS. Small posterolateral herniations involving the spinal root do not interfere with the circulation of the spinal fluid, so Queckenstedt's test is negative. The constituents of the spinal fluid are often normal; a modest elevation of protein is sometimes found. If spinal compression has occurred, elevation of the protein is to be expected, and Queckenstedt's test *may* be positive. X-rays of the spine may be completely normal because a recent herniation is radiotranslucent. Because most people over 40 years have a slight narrowing of the disc spaces, with or without marginal lipping, which may be seen to extend into the intervertebral foramen in oblique views, such changes are not necessarily relevant to the patient's symptoms. Contrast myelography will usually reveal obliteration of the root sleeve or an actual filling defect at the site of the prolapse. Electromyography will sometimes show excessive irritability in the tender muscles, together with fibrillation action potentials, even in patients in whom no obvious motor impairment can be detected by clinical methods.

Prognosis. The prognosis is usually good. Pain lasts several weeks, with gradual improvement, but it may recur.

Diagnosis. Diagnosis is made on the characteristic pattern of the symptoms outlined—a linear pain extending down the limb, with or without painful stiffness of the neck, and paresthesias limited to the extreme periphery of a single dermatome. In the early stages, there is no limitation of movement, though in neglected cases a "frozen shoulder" occasionally develops, and in this event there is pain in the shoulder on rotation of the humerus and on abduction of the arm. The thoracic outlet syndrome, whether due to a cervical rib or not, usually gives rise to more diffuse paresthesias, which can be induced by placing the arm in certain postures. The pain is less severe and more diffuse, and the biceps, triceps, and supinator reflexes are commonly spared. The distinction between a spinal tumor and a cervical disc can be difficult in the early stages. A neurofibroma can give rise to intermittent attacks of pain with minimal neurological signs over a period of many months or even years, but eventually the neurological deficit associated with a tumor will appear, and the persistence of pain, together with the onward march of physical signs, will lead to the correct diagnosis. Fortunately, new growths are very much less common than disease of the intervertebral discs.

Treatment. Prompt bed rest, with a sufficiency of pillows to support the head and the affected arm in a comfortable position, is the surest way to cut short the period of incapacity. Each patient will find the position of head and arm which is most comfortable for him. Analgesics of the coal tar series are seldom adequate; codeine, Demerol, and even morphine may be needed. Radiant heat is comforting when there is much muscle spasm, but massage is contraindicated. Infiltration of "trigger" spots with procaine can give striking relief, apparently by stopping painful involuntary spasm in muscles supplied by the affected root. When severe pain has subsided, gentle passive movements of the neck and shoulder should be started, but vigorous physiotherapy is contraindicated when pain is severe. Movement of the arm is apt to aggravate the pain.

When pain persists unabated after a week in bed, continuous head traction by a halter may be tried, but this is often ineffective, or it is effective only so long as the traction is maintained. A plastic collar should be worn during convalescence. Operation is indicated when there is no sign of improvement after conservative measures have been given a trial for five or six weeks, and it should be resorted to at once if there is evidence of cord compression, rapid increase of weakness, or sensory loss in the affected arm.

CERVICAL SPONDYLOSIS

This condition can give rise to irritation of one or more cervical roots, and to compression of the cervical cord. The intervertebral discs are narrowed from above down, and there are multiple bulges around the circumference of the annulus fibrosus, which provoke the outgrowth of osteophytes from the margins of the adjacent vertebrae. The intervertebral articulations are often the seat of hypertrophic osteoarthritis, giving rise to an enlargement of the joints, which can impinge on the intervertebral foramina.

Cervical spondylosis may exist in advanced degree in patients without any symptoms, past or present, but if and when one of the protrusions occupies an intervertebral foramen, it can cause pressure on the emerging root, and this is usually accompanied by fibrous reaction in the root sheath and in the dura in its immediate vicinity. The degeneration commonly affects several discs, and for this reason the symptoms are sometimes bilateral and may point to involvement of more than one root on one or both sides.

Backward protrusion of the annulus gives rise to a transverse ridge which pushes the cord backwards. If the sagittal diameter of the spinal canal is normal or large, a good deal of cord displacement can occur without symptoms, provided that displacement occurs gradually, but if the canal is congenitally shallow, as is quite often the case, the symptoms of cord compression are likely to appear early. It is not only the height of the ridge which matters, but also the size of the canal.

Clinical Features. There is often pain and stiffness of the neck, especially in the morning after a night's rest, and when the upper cervical vertebrae are involved, as frequently happens, pain in the arm may be accompanied by early morning headaches in the occipital region. The pain in the arm is usually more diffuse than is the case in herniation of the nucleus pulposus involving a single root, and it may have a peculiar burning quality in elderly subjects. Paresthesias are often present, and their distribution may indicate that more than one root is implicated. Muscle weakness, wasting, and depression of reflexes are not common, but if present their distribution is appropriate to the root, or roots, involved. The patient often has additional symptoms referable to spondylosis in other areas of the vertebral column, and may show evidence of osteoarthritis in large joints.

The earliest symptoms of cervical cord compression by spondylosis may take the form of aching in the lower back and pain down the legs,[25] and it is important to note that there may be no pain or stiffness in the neck or pain in the arms. In such cases, the lumbar pain is not associated with rigidity (unless the lumbar discs are also involved) and the pain in the legs is more diffuse and less linear than in irritative lesions of the lumbar roots. It cannot be too strongly emphasized that at this stage there may be no neurological signs of cord compression, and that it is easy to ascribe the patient's symptoms to lumbar spondylosis, especially if a lumbar myelogram shows posterior ridging of one or more lower lumbar discs. The true state of affairs will not be disclosed unless the thoracic and cervical areas are examined by myelography. Surgical decompression of the cervical cord will usually produce immediate relief of the pain in the lower back and legs.

More often, however, displacement and compression of the cervical cord is associated with some limitation of movement in the neck, and the patient will complain of heaviness or weakness of the legs, together with burning or other paresthesias in the feet. Lhermitte's sign may be positive, but it is often negative. The lower limbs are found to be spastic and slightly weak, with exaggerated tendon reflexes and—eventually—extensor plantar responses. Posterior column sensibility is depressed, and this is followed by impairment to touch and pinprick in the feet. In time, a definite sensory level may develop, but this can be misleading since it is often several segments below the actual level of the compression. As in compression by spinal cord tumors, impairment of pain and temperature sensibility in one or both legs—suggesting an intramedullary lesion—may be the first sensory change to appear.

Severe spondylosis can displace the vertebral arteries as they lie in the cervical canal alongside the lateral borders of the discs, and plaques of atheroma may develop at these sites. It is not uncommon for these patients to exhibit vertigo on sustained forced movements of the head to one side. Indeed, the symptoms of vertebral arterial insufficiency may be so well marked as to suggest that the neurological signs are intracranial in origin.

Treatment. The treatment of cervical spondylosis is unsatisfactory since the condition is a progressive one and usually involves several discs. The natural course of the disease is intermittent, with frequent remissions, which renders it difficult to assess the value of various therapeutic procedures. In general, however, when the symptoms complained of are confined to the neck and one upper limb, gentle passive movements and various forms of heat may be used with apparent benefit. Neck traction by means of a halter relieves some patients. Wearing a plastic collar, to restrict movements of the head, can be extremely efficacious, and may lead to the relief of symptoms resulting from cord compression. The collar should be worn all day, and at night when possible.

When spinal compression has not been helped by the wearing of a collar, decompression should be attempted only after careful myelographic study to define the number and position of the offending discs. Decompression can be done by an anterior approach, which allows the removal by curettage of both the central ridge and the lateral osteophytes. Alternatively, laminectomy and bilateral facetectomy provides decompression of the dural contents, permitting the cord and its roots to move backwards.

Cervical Rib

Bony or fibrous bands arising from the transverse process of the seventh cervical vertebra and passing forward to the first rib behind the scalene tubercle are common in otherwise normal persons.[41] The brachial plexus has to cross this structure on its way to the axilla (Fig. 8-4), but in early life the shoulders are high and there is no interference with the plexus. However, if as a result of advancing age, fatigue, or injury to the trapezius, the shoulder is allowed to sag, the lower cord of the plexus is angulated

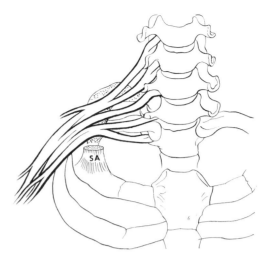

Figure 8-4. Diagram depicting the brachial plexus passing over a cervical rib (stippled). SA, stump of the scalenus anterior.

over the rib. Moreover, descent of the shoulder brings the clavicle into a more horizontal position, and both the plexus and the subclavian artery in front of it are then liable to be compressed between the rib and the clavicle in movements of retraction and abduction of the shoulder. The result of this new alignment is that the plexus is subject to friction during the course of vigorous movements of the arm and in deep breathing, and both the artery and the plexus are compressed between rib and clavicle during certain movements and in certain positions.

The intimate anatomy of the area varies greatly from case to case with a corresponding range of variability in the symptoms and signs. Any condition which induces weakness or fatigue of the muscles of the shoulder girdle can precipitate this syndrome, and the same is true of fractures of the clavicle and other injuries to the shoulder.

Symptoms and Signs. There may be motor, sensory, or vascular symptoms and signs. Pain is seldom prominent and may be absent. It is felt behind the clavicle and down the arm, usually on the inner side, and is increased by the carrying of heavy weights. It is sometimes complicated by the pain of muscle ischemia in the forearm and hands when there is compression of the subclavian artery. Paresthesias are troublesome and are usually limited to the inner border of the forearm and hand, but when subclavian compression is present, the patient's whole hand feels numb while he is doing manual work or resting with the limb in certain positions. The shoulder is depressed as compared with the unaffected side. Slight swelling of the hand and prominence of the veins are seen when the venous return is reduced at the thoracic outlet; this sometimes leads to the development of a median carpal tunnel syndrome, with paresthesias involving the thumb, index, and middle finger, and weakness and wasting involving the thenar eminence. More often weakness and wasting are confined to the muscles supplied by the inner cord of the plexus.

Paralysis of the serratus anterior, with winging of the scapula, occasionally occurs from involvement of the long thoracic nerve as it crosses a cervical rib. Raynaud's phenomenon is sometimes seen in the fingers on the affected side.

A rare but serious complication of cervical rib is the formation of an aneurysm of the subclavian artery just distal to the point where it crosses the rib or band. This can be a source of emboli to the hand. Rarely, thrombosis of the subclavian artery gives rise to severe arterial insufficiency in the upper limb. When this occurs on the right-hand side, the thrombus may extend proximally to the point of junction of the subclavian and right common carotid arteries, and detachment of a portion of the clot can give rise to cerebral embolism, or a clot may break off and pass into the vertebral-basilar system.

The symptoms fluctuate, being aggravated by use of the limb, by fatigue, and by cold weather. They may become worse during acute respiratory diseases owing to the increased rate and amplitude of thoracic movements. Improvement follows prolonged rest, especially in cases in which general fatigue and muscular flabbiness have contributed to a sagging of the shoulder.

Diagnosis. Diagnosis does not depend on the radiological demonstration of a cervical rib because such an abnormality is frequent in normal persons and, in addition, a fibrous band which may be causing the symptoms will not appear on x-ray examination. The combination of discomfort, paresthesias, muscular atrophy in the hand, slight sensory disturbances, and vascular symptoms is not found in any other condition, and difficulty arises only in early or atypical cases. Traumatic neuropathy of the ulnar nerve at the elbow leads to weakness of flexion of the little finger and wasting of the ulnar intrinsic muscles; sensory loss is minimal, and if present is confined to the little finger and the ulnar side of the ring finger and the inner border of the hand to just above the wrist. Cubitus valgus is usually present, and the ulnar nerve is tender and sometimes swollen as it lies in its groove at the elbow.

In the median carpal tunnel syndrome, both paresthesias and objective neurological findings are limited to the distribution of the median nerve below the wrist. Wasting of the small muscles of one or both hands may suggest motor neuron disease or the effects of poliomyelitis, but these possibilities are excluded by the presence of paresthesias and sensory loss. Syringomyelia involving the lower cervical segments usually causes uniform wasting of the intrinsic muscles of the hand, depression of the tendon reflexes in the arm, and dissociated sensory loss. A prolapsed disc involving the eighth cervical root is uncommon and is distinguished from the thoracic outlet syndrome by severe pain descending from the neck down the inner border of the arm and forearm, aggravation of symptoms by sustained downward pressure on the head, and absence of vascular symptoms.

Treatment. In early cases, rest to the arm and a sling to support the elbow will cause a slow recession of symptoms. Shoulder exercises to improve posture sometimes assist in recovery, but they are contraindicated by severe pain and by objective motor and sensory changes.

If vascular changes appear or wasting is present, or if pain persists despite conservative treatment, the brachial plexus should be explored to determine the anatomical situation responsible for the symptoms and, if possible, to adjust it. It may be necessary to remove the rib or a fibrous band. Dividing the tendon of the scalenus anterior allows the muscle to retract out of the way and gives the plexus and artery more room. The precise surgical measures required can be determined only by wide exposure and careful observation of the events during passive movements of the shoulder, carried out at the time of operation. The results of surgery vary; failure to relieve symptoms is not uncommon and it is therefore unwise to advocate surgery before conservative treatment has been given a thorough trial. On the other hand, the presence of symptoms of vascular insufficiency constitutes an imperative indication for the correction of subclavian stenosis or aneurysm.

Related Syndromes of the Thoracic Outlet

ABNORMAL FIRST RIB. When the first rib is malformed, it ends by joining the second rib and may resemble a cervical rib unless its origin from the first dorsal vertebra is recognized. It may give rise to the same symptoms as a cervical rib, and treatment is similar. Even a normal first rib may cause symptoms in cases of marked descent of the shoulder from any cause.

THE SCALENUS SYNDROME. The clinical picture usually attributed to the scalenus syndrome differs in degree rather than in kind from that produced by a cervical rib. Mild cases of the thoracic outlet syndrome are sometimes benefited by freeing the scalenus anterior from its attachment to the first rib. The view that the symptoms are caused by "spasm" of the scalenus anterior is untenable.

COSTOCLAVICULAR COMPRESSION. Costoclavicular compression of the brachial plexus and subclavian artery occurs in many normal persons when the arm is abducted or the shoulder is retracted or depressed. The precise position required to produce symptoms is subject to wide individual variation, but whatever it is, the radial pulse is obliterated, paresthesias are felt in all the fingers if the position is maintained for a minute or two, and a systolic bruit is heard over the clavicle. The symptoms are often induced by heavy manual work or by tasks involving use of the hand above the level of the shoulders. Treatment is as described for the thoracic outlet syndrome.

Other Affections of the Brachial Plexus

NEURALGIC AMYOTROPHY. This is an acute condition which gives rise to pain, paralysis, and minimal sensory changes (p. 176). As a rule, the pain lasts from one to 10 days.

BRONCHOGENIC CARCINOMA. Bronchogenic carcinoma of the superior pulmonary sulcus (Pancoast's tumor) sometimes spreads up to involve the upper thoracic roots, the brachial plexus, and the ribs. Severe pain is felt deep to the clavicle and may spread down the inner aspect of the arm and forearm, together with paresthesias in the same distribution. Wasting of the intrinsic muscles of the hand and Horner's syndrome may appear. Erosion of the vertebrae and the necks of the upper ribs is ultimately visible on x-ray photographs, which will also show the tumor of the lung. The pain due to these tumors is singularly resistant to treatment, and when opiates fail, it is necessary to carry out a high cervical cordotomy or thalamotomy (p. 15) in order to make the remainder of the patient's life bearable.

MALIGNANT METASTASES. Malignant metastases in the axillary and supraclavicular glands may cause severe pain down the arm; when the adenopathy is evident, diagnosis is easy, but occasionally diffuse infiltration of the plexus occurs without any palpable mass, in which event pain is slight or absent, but paresthesias, sensory impairment, and paralysis develop rapidly.

CAUSALGIA. This sometimes follows incomplete traumatic lesions of the median and ulnar nerves (Chap. 18).

THE MEDIAN CARPAL TUNNEL SYNDROME. This is a common condition caused by compression of the median nerve as it runs in its tunnel under the transverse carpal ligament. It usually occurs in middle-aged women who are engaged in vigorous manual work, especially if they are unused to such work, but it can occur at all ages and in both sexes. It can occur during pregnancy, and is common in patients with mild rheumatoid arthritis of the wrist. The syndrome has been seen in association with acromegaly and as a complication of compound palmar ganglion and of tenosinovitis at the wrist. Occasionally it occurs in association with the thoracic outlet syndrome.

The patient complains of paresthesias in the palmar aspect of the thumb and index and middle fingers and sometimes of pain in the palm; in rare cases, pain shoots up the front of the forearm. An unpleasant numbness rather than true pain is the most frequent symptom. It is aggravated by using the hands but is also prone to occur at night or early in the morning, presumably owing to the slight swelling of the upper extremity which occurs after a period of recumbency.

In moderate cases, there is slight blunting to pinprick over the median distribution in the hand. Other patients complain of weakness of the thumb, and in long-standing cases, there is pronounced weakness and atrophy of the opponens pollicis and the abductor pollicis brevis, the two radial lumbricales, and the outer head of the flexor brevis pollicis. Sometimes the first dorsal interosseous muscle is involved too. Although this situation usually takes months or even years to develop, rare cases are encountered in which almost complete paresis develops over a matter of a day or two.

Decompression of the carpal nerve is the treatment of choice in all well-established cases, and should be done as an emergency in the acute type of case described above. In patients who have mild rheumatoid arthritis, administration of 5 mg. of prednisone three times a day will often cause a remarkable remission of the neurological symptoms, and this may be sufficient to tide the patient over a period of a few months. However, it would not seem desirable to use steroids continuously over a long period for a relatively mild condition which can be effectively treated surgically. Local injections of hydrocortisone can help. When practicable, restriction of manual work suffices for the milder type of case.

ULNAR NEUROPATHY. This condition seldom causes pain, but is included here for convenience. It usually occurs as a result of recurrent minor injuries to the nerve at the elbow in persons with cubitus valgus or a shallow ulnar groove behind the medial epicondyle. There may be an ache at the elbow and along the ulnar border of the forearm, but paresthesias in the ulnar border of the hand and wasting of the interossei and hypothenar muscles are the symptoms which usually bring the patient to the doctor. There is often slight tenderness and palpable thickening of the nerve behind the elbow. Treatment is either by operative transposition of the ulnar nerve to the front of the elbow or by decompressing the nerve as it dips down beneath the twin heads of the flexor carpi ulnaris (p. 526).

Wasting of the ulnar intrinsic muscles of the hand and minimal sensory loss also occur in persons whose occupations or hobbies involve pressure on the base of the hypothenar eminence where the nerve enters the hand, e.g., professional cyclists and men engaged in using a file or a vibrating instrument such as a road drill. These distal ulnar involvements are distinguished from affections at the elbow by the presence in the latter of sensory loss over the ulnar side of the wrist and by weakness of the ulnar head of the flexor digitorum profundus.

The Shoulder-Hand Syndrome

This curious syndrome [37] is characterized by painful stiffness of the shoulder and dystrophic changes in the wrist and hand. It has been described in association with a heterogeneous collection of conditions, including myocardial infarction, pulmonary fibrosis, pulmonary tumors, cervical spondylosis, herpes zoster of the shoulder area, hemiplegia from any cause, injuries to the shoulder, electroconvulsive therapy, epileptic seizures, and injury to the hand or arm. The majority follow myocardial infarction. In some cases, no provocative agent can be found.

At first, there is painful stiffness of the shoulder, reddening and edema of the hand, and persistent burning pain. The skin of the hand is hot, dry, and tender to the slightest touch. After some months, the acute process usually subsides; the pain lessens, shoulder movements improve, and edema of the hand disappears. This may be followed by atrophy of the subcutaneous tissue and muscles, with contractures of the fingers. The skin becomes smooth, the hand is cold and blue, and the nails are thick and brittle. The fingers are stiffened in flexion and the shoulder is "frozen" in adduction; the entire upper limb wastes, and osteoporosis is seen in the long bones. These are the features of disuse. Such, at any rate, is the clinical course in neglected cases. With treatment, recovery usually occurs within a year, or in two years at most. Persistence beyond that time raises the possibility of faulty diagnosis or the deliberate prolongation of incapacity by a patient in search of secondary gain.

The underlying mechanism is not understood, but it is generally agreed that two things are necessary to initiate the condition—a painful condition in or around the shoulder, and disuse.

Treatment. Intensive physiotherapy is essential from the start. It aims at maintaining or restoring mobility to the shoulder, wrist, and fingers. In addition, Plewes and others have found it useful to expose the entire limb to heat for several hours each day by using hot air (105° F.) or hot wax. Cold dressings are used instead of heat in those patients whose symptoms are aggravated by heat. Sympathetic block and sympathectomy have not proved uniformly successful.

PAIN IN THE LOWER LIMB

The causes of pain in the lower limb fall into two groups. The first, with which we are not concerned, includes all affections of the bones, joints, ligaments, muscles, and blood vessels of the limb and pelvic girdle. The second group consists of conditions in which the pain is due to disease involving the sensory nerves and roots, the cauda equina, and the spinal cord. Since some conditions in this group do not present neurological signs early in the course of the disease, diagnosis can be difficult, but the principles set forth in Chapter 1 can help in the interpretation of the pain.

Of the diseases which directly implicate the sensory pathways, lesions of the intervertebral discs, whether in the form of prolapse or spondylosis, are by far the most common. Neoplasms involving the cauda equina, lumbar vertebrae, pelvic bones, and pelvic viscera, parasitic cysts, and tuberculous or pyogenic affections of the spine and sacrum are relatively rare. "Neuritis," which was at one time regarded as the common cause of anterior femoral and sciatic pain, has yet to be established as a pathological entity, except insofar as a local interstitial reaction may occur in peripheral nerves and plexuses in response to pressure, inflammation, or neoplastic infiltration. Meralgia paresthetica (p. 531) is a relatively common cause of uncomfortable paresthesias in the thigh, which may be accompanied on occasion by severe pain. Postherpetic neuralgia, sciatic causalgia, neuralgic amyotrophy, and spondylolisthesis are rare causes of pain in the lower limb.

Sciatica Due to Prolapse
of Intervertebral Discs

Posterolateral herniation of the fourth or fifth lumbar disc is the most common cause of acute sciatic pain. Exceptionally, a large midline herniation of the second or third lumbar disc may involve the roots of the cauda equina and give rise to sciatica on one or both sides, with or without pain in the front of the thigh. It is thought that the cause of herniation is primarily a degeneration of the disc which loses its resilience and tends to flatten out under the weight of the body above it, but the rupture is often occasioned by lifting a heavy weight, falling from a height, or by some comparatively trivial but awkwardly executed movement.

Pathological studies show that herniations can occur at any point on the circumference of the disc, although posterolateral herniations are the most common. Whatever the site, the herniation is apt to reduce the space separating the adjacent vertebrae, as is easily seen by x-ray photographs of advanced cases. It must of necessity cause subluxation of the intervertebral articulations, and this is one of the factors which cause painful spasm of the lumbar muscles. At autopsy, large herniations situated well away from the intervertebral foramen are frequently found in persons who have suffered from recurrent attacks of low back pain without leg pain. The posterior longitudinal ligament lying along the posterior surfaces of the vertebral bodies and intervertebral discs is a sensitive structure, being supplied by recurrent sensory nerves from the spinal roots. It seems likely that the back pain associated with many cases of prolapsed disc may be due in part to displacement of this ligament at the time of the herniation.

When a herniation is so placed as to impinge on the emerging root, it will cause pain of radicular distribution and will ultimately lead to swelling of the root and fibrosis of its dural sleeve. In long-standing cases, there is sometimes

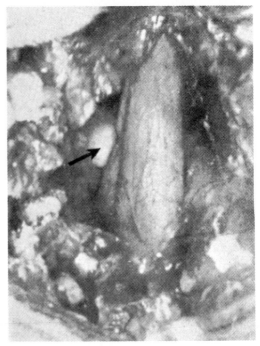

Figure 8–5. Prolapse of the fourth lumbar disc (arrow) indenting the fifth lumbar root as it leaves the dural sac.

hypertrophy of the ligamentum flavum which may itself press forward on to the root as it enters the intervertebral foramen (Fig. 8–6). Herniation of the fourth lumbar disc will involve the fifth root (Figs. 8–6, 8–7), whereas herniation of the lumbosacral disc implicates the fifth lumbar or the first sacral root, or both. Larger herniations spreading medially can involve other elements of the cauda equina as they pass downward toward the sacral foramina.

Clinical Features. Lumbar pain is usually present but may be absent. It may come on abruptly while the patient is stooping and he then has difficulty in straightening up. It is associated with painful rigidity of the lumbar spine, and may be aggravated by sneezing and coughing. It is followed immediately or after a delay of days or weeks by pain which extends across the buttock, down the back of the thigh, and down the back of the calf (first sacral), or down the lat-

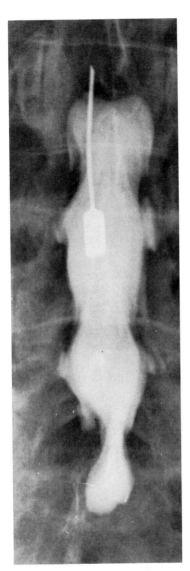

patients feel better when they are up and about. Sensations of tingling, numbness, and pins and needles are often experienced, occurring in the outer border of the foot and across the top of the toes when the fifth root is involved and on the sole of the foot when the first sacral root is implicated. Patients with long-standing pain may also complain of an ache in the groin, probably from holding the thigh slightly flexed over long periods of time. Large herniations which involve other elements of the cauda equina may cause pain in the perineum, as well as sciatica.

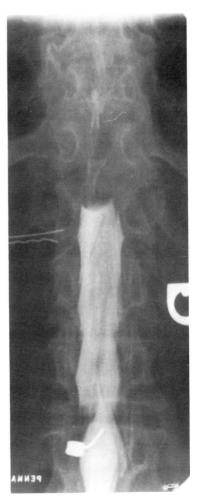

Figure 8–6. Myelogram showing bilateral medial displacement of first sacral roots by thickening of ligamentum flavum. There was no disc protrusion and the symptoms were relieved by removal of hypertrophied ligament.

eral side of the leg along the fibula (fifth lumbar). Exceptionally, it is first felt below the knee, and may be confined to a comparatively small area of the leg. The pain in the leg may be dull or lancinating. It is often aggravated by sneezing, jolting the spine, stooping, or even by rapid flexion of the neck. The pain may be relieved by lying down, but some

Figure 8–7. Myelogram showing notching of the column by herniation of the fourth lumbar disc, and obstruction at L1 caused by a meningioma.

PHYSICAL SIGNS. These vary greatly. There is usually rigidity of the lumbar spine, with obliteration of the normal lumbar lordosis, and there may be scoliosis to either side. There is often tenderness of the lumbar muscles, the buttocks, the hamstrings, and the calf, and sometimes pressure over tender points in the buttock may give rise to an exacerbation of pain down the leg, and the patient may experience considerable relief if such "trigger" areas are infiltrated with 1 per cent procaine.[10, 11] There is evidence that irritative root lesions can cause small foci of painful spasm in muscles supplied by the affected root, and procaine relieves pain by stopping this spasm. Lasègue's sign—aggravation of pain in the back and leg by raising the heel from the bed with the knee straight—is often positive, but is also present in many other painful conditions of the hindquarters. However, if the pain induced by this maneuver is further increased either by forcible flexion of the neck (which exerts upward traction on the cord) or by dorsiflexion of the foot (which pulls on the nerve and its roots), it is good evidence of a lesion in the roots, lumbosacral plexus, or sciatic nerve. These tests are almost always positive at some time or other in the history of sciatica due to irritation of a spinal root.

OBJECTIVE NEUROLOGICAL SIGNS. Such signs are usually absent in the early stages. When the herniation involves the fifth lumbar root, there may ultimately be some weakness of the dorsiflexors of the toes and foot, and occasionally foot drop may supervene. The calf muscles are flabby and may be weak when the first sacral root is involved. Fasciculation is rare. Slight wasting of the leg below the knee is common in acute cases, and the affected foot is often cold with diminished pulsation of the pulses at the ankle. It appears that vasoconstriction in response to pain occurs in these cases because there is improvement in the temperature of the foot and in the volume of the peripheral arterial pulse in pain-free intervals.[10]

SENSORY LOSS. This is usually slight or absent, amounting to no more than a blunting to pinprick and light touch over the lateral border and dorsum of the foot (L5) or on the sole of the foot and back of the ankle (S1). Widespread sensory loss suggests the presence of a very large herniation causing a lesion of the cauda equina. The Achilles reflex is reduced or lost in lesions of S1, but is unaffected when L5 alone is involved. Rarely, the patellar reflex is reduced in herniations of the fourth disc, presumably owing to an anomalous reflex pathway. Sometimes, however, herniation of the third lumbar disc will involve both the emerging third lumbar root—with loss of the patellar reflex—and the fourth and fifth roots as they pass downward toward their points of exit. Sphincter symptoms are uncommon except in large herniations involving several roots.

LABORATORY TESTS. The spinal fluid is normal in all respects in more than half of all cases; the protein content is moderately raised in the remainder. The cell count is usually normal. Manometry does not show evidence of block in the majority of cases. Plain radiographs of the lumbar spine may reveal narrowing of disc spaces, Schmorl's nodes, or lipping of the vertebral bodies; such findings indicate degeneration of the discs but do not prove that the symptoms are due to the abnormal features seen on the x-ray. Errors in localization based purely on the interpretation of physical signs are sufficiently common to render contrast myelography desirable prior to operation, although some surgeons dispense with it.

Course and Prognosis. Individual attacks last days, weeks, or months, and recurrences are frequent, often separated by an interval of many years. There is a natural tendency toward spontaneous cure which should be taken into account in assessing the value of treatment and the need for surgical intervention. Spontaneous cure appears to be due to vascularization and absorption of the herniation. Foot drop, a rare occurrence, is usually permanent, and if the ankle jerk has disappeared, it seldom returns.

Differential Diagnosis. Arthritis of

the hip causes pain in and around the joint, which is aggravated by rotation of the flexed thigh. Since the disease does not directly affect the sensory nerves, there are no paresthesias, sensation is unaffected, and the ankle jerk is preserved. Disease of the *sacroiliac joint* can cause pain in the vicinity of the joint itself and also down the back of the thigh to just below the knee, but not to the ankle. Paresthesias and objective neurological signs are absent, but Lasègue's sign is often positive. However, flexion of the neck and dorsiflexion of the foot, carried out while the leg is raised from the bed, do not aggravate the pain. Forceful rotation of the flexed thigh causes pain in the region of the joint. There are no objective neurological signs, but the patient sometimes complains of a curious feeling of instability in the leg and this may be misinterpreted as weakness. X-ray photographs seldom assist in the diagnosis of sacroiliac disease until it has been established for some weeks, or, in the case of tuberculosis, for some months. *Pelvic masses,* including the gravid uterus, can cause pain and paresthesias of sciatic distribution, but generally speaking, paresthesias are more obtrusive than pain, and foot drop is often an early symptom. During difficult labor, the lumbosacral cord can be compressed against the brim of the pelvis; in a conscious patient this causes excruciating pain down the leg, which is almost always followed immediately by foot drop and weakness of the calf muscles, though the weakness often is not appreciated until the patient first gets out of bed. Not all sciatica in a pregnant woman or associated with parturition is due to this factor, however; herniation of lumbar discs can occur late in pregnancy and during childbirth. *Pott's disease* seldom appears in the lumbar spine, but when it does so it may present with low back pain followed by sciatic radiation. Such cases may closely resemble the picture of prolapsed disc. Straight x-rays of the lumbar vertebrae do not reveal *early* tuberculous caries, and a myelogram may show a filling defect similar to that of a prolapsed disc.

There is usually a slight rise of temperature, and the sedimentation rate will be increased. *Neoplasms* of the lumbar spine, including myeloma, usually cause intense lumbar pain but comparatively little rigidity. X-rays will commonly be positive, and when the tumor is metastatic the sedimentation rate may be raised. *Tumors of the cauda equina* can cause great difficulty, and this applies particularly to a single neurofibroma which can cause intermittent sciatic pain with minimal objective neurological disturbances for months or even years. The pain-free intermissions are particularly misleading. Sciatica, usually bilateral, may occur early in the history of hemangioendothelioma of the cauda equina, but there is a rapid development of obvious neurological deficit in both lower limbs, and sphincter symptoms occur early. In countries in which the condition is endemic, *hydatid cysts* can cause lumbar pain and sciatic radiation, but the sciatica is atypical and by the time symptoms arise, there may be extensive erosion of the sacral canal or of the pedicles.

PERIDURAL AND EXTRADURAL CYSTS. Sciatica with pain in the lower back may also be caused by peridural or extradural cysts.[34] Peridural sacral cysts may be semisolid and can erode the sacrum. Extradural cysts occur in the midthoracic region and also occasionally in the sacral area; they arise from a diverticulum of arachnoid which has herniated through a dural defect; this variety usually communicates freely with the subarachnoid space. The symptoms and signs are essentially those of a prolapsed disc, but there is usually erosion of bone and expansion of the vertebral canal. Recovery follows operation.

SPINAL COMPRESSION. Intense bilateral pain in the legs can occur with spinal compression in the cervical and upper thoracic regions.[25] Generally speaking, the pain in the legs does not present the linear distribution characteristic of a root lesion; it is more diffuse, appearing in both the front and the back of the limbs. It is seen in both intramedullary and extramedullary lesions,

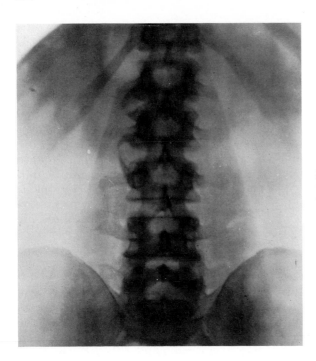

Figure 8–8. Large osteophytes outlining protrusions of disc substance between L1-L-2 and L2-L3. The patient had pain in the groin and down the leg to the knee.

including spondylosis, and may completely overshadow the symptoms and signs arising at the level of the lesion. Objective signs of spinal compression may be minimal, and it is only too easy to search for the cause of the patient's pain in the lumbar area and to ignore the higher reaches of the spinal cord. It is supposed that the pain in the legs is the result of "irritation" of the spinothalamic tracts at the site of spinal compression. It will be recalled that intense pain in the legs occurs in the presence of thrombosis of the anterior spinal artery (p. 386).

Treatment. Surgical removal of the offending disc or discs is the treatment of choice in severe, persistent cases which do not respond to conservative treatment over a period of three to six weeks. Surgery is also desirable, irrespective of the severity of the pain, if muscular weakness or sphincter symptoms develop. The sudden appearance of hesitancy of micturition or retention is an indication for immediate operation. Surgery is rather less effective for patients in whom intractable back pain is the primary problem. Spinal fusion is seldom effective, except in the presence of obvious instability of the spine.

Conservative treatment should always be tried first. Rest in bed, with adequate analgesics, is imperative, and a firm mattress or bed board is desirable. Pelvic traction, often advised, is unimpressive in its results, but it does keep restless patients in bed. Vigorous physiotherapy which includes active and passive movements of the legs is to be deplored, and deep massage of tender muscles is apt to aggravate the pain. The injection of procaine into tender spots may bring partial relief, which often outlasts the anesthetic effect of the injection. Epidural injection of 50 to 200 ml. of 1 per cent procaine in saline is usually useless, but sometimes it effects a dramatic cure, the reasons for which are not understood. Immobilization in a plaster jacket often relieves pain temporarily, but relapses are common when the plaster is taken off, and the method is unsuitable for severe cases. A well-fitting corset brings relief to mild cases, its chief virtue being that it prevents excessive flexion of the spine. Skillful manipulation of the back often gives temporary relief, and it is a curious and un-explained paradox that rapid improvement occasionally occurs when a patient, tired of medical restrictions, goes back to horseback riding, gardening, or other seemingly inappropriate occupations.

Spondylosis of the Lumbar Spine

Spondylosis of the lumbar spine is a common cause of lumbago, sciatica, and pain in the front of the thigh. Pathologically, there is degeneration of the intervertebral discs with marginal lipping, narrowing of the disc spaces, osteoarthritis of the intervertebral joints, and fibrosis of the root sheaths. Multiple protrusions are common, so the symptoms sometimes reflect involvement of more than one root.

There is often a history of recurrent lumbago, and the patient is apt to complain of stiffness and pain in the back on getting up in the morning or on rising after prolonged sitting, the symptoms improving after a little exercise. Sciatic or femoral pain is often accompanied by paresthesias, but objective sensory, motor, and reflex signs are rather less prominent than in the case of acute herniations in younger people. Furthermore, the clinical picture is sometimes confused by coincident osteoarthritis of the hip and knee.

When symptoms indicate involvement of a single root, surgery is advisable, but in the majority of cases spondylosis in *elderly* individuals is a relapsing chronic disease for which only physiotherapy and the support of a corset can be offered.

Pseudoclaudication from Compression of the Cauda Equina

Pain down one or both legs, which may mimic the pain of intermittent claudication, sometimes occurs as a result of compression of one or more roots of the cauda equina by a prolapsed disc or posterior protrusion of the annulus.[22] The patient complains of pain in the buttock, thigh, and calf on one or both sides. It is induced by exercise, or even by prolonged standing, and subsides after 20 or 30 minutes if the patient sits down or lies down. There is no clinical evidence of peripheral vascular disease and—unlike cases of true intermittent claudication—the straight leg-raising test is usually positive and there may or may not be sensory and reflex changes appropriate to root involvement. It should be noted that this condition has nothing to do with the so-called "intermittent claudication of the spinal cord" described by Déjerine in 1911, in which exercise leads to weakness and the appearance of pyramidal signs in the lower limbs. Déjerine attributed it to vascular insufficiency of the spinal cord.

There is as yet no good explanation for "pseudoclaudication" syndrome in cauda equina lesions. In 1930, Roger reported that oscillometry of the calf discloses reduced pulsation in some patients with sciatica, and in 1949, the author briefly reported that in some cases of prolapsed disc, the muscles innervated by the compromised root showed evidence of reduced arterial input.[10] This study was prompted by the case of a 42-year-old man whose sciatic pain (produced by a disc involving the fourth lumbar root) was much increased by walking, and it was found that after walking about three blocks, the pulses at the ankle on the affected side disappeared, only to return after the patient had rested for half an hour. It therefore seems possible that pseudoclaudication is due to vasoconstriction. However, most cases of pseudoclaudication from cauda equina compression have been described in middle-aged or elderly men, who are candidates for aorto-ilial insufficiency, and it is therefore desirable to carry out aortography as well as myelography in the investigation of these patients. From the practical point of view, it is necessary to emphasize that the pain of pseudoclaudication has been relieved in some cases by removing the offending disc.

Spondylolisthesis

Spondylolisthesis is often present without symptoms. In other cases, there is pain in the back, and in a minority there is unilateral or bilateral sciatica. The fifth lumbar vertebra is usually dislocated forward, and this usually happens when, as a result of a congenital anomaly, the intervertebral joints between the fifth lumbar and first sacral vertebrae run in an anteroposterior plane instead of transversely. It can also occur as a result of a fracture. Posterior displacement of the fifth lumbar vertebra on the sacrum is occasionally seen. Whether the displacement is backward or forward, herniation of disc substance often plays a part in the production of symptoms by pressing upon the fifth lumbar and first sacral roots, so that treatment involves the removal of the herniation as well as spinal fusion. The symptoms and signs may be unilateral or bilateral, and may involve the lower sacral roots in addition to the fifth lumbar and first sacral roots. Pain and paresthesias are prominent, and objective motor and sensory signs are usually to be found within the territory of the affected roots. Sphincter symptoms occur in severe cases, constituting an imperative indication for surgery. Diagnosis is made by x-ray of the lumbosacral articulation, but symptoms and signs occurring in the presence of spondylolisthesis do not necessarily result from it since the condition can be symptomless.

Anterior Femoral Pain

Pain in the front of the thighs is less common than sciatica. It can be due to disease of the hip joint, but in the majority of cases it is caused by affections of the second, third, or fourth lumbar root; pain from irritation of the fourth lumbar root frequently traverses the front of the thigh and the anteromedial aspect of the leg to the ankle. When the third lumbar root is involved by a prolapsed disc, the pain is almost always accompanied by tingling in the front of the thigh, weakness and wasting of the quadriceps, and an absent knee jerk. Lumbar pain is rather less prominent than in disc lesions at a lower level. Straight leg raising does not aggravate the pain (unless the lumbar spine is flexed thereby) because it does not cause traction on the lumbar roots. Anterior femoral pain is more commonly from spondylosis than from herniation of the nucleus pulposus. The existence of interstitial neuritis of the femoral nerve has yet to be proved.

Meralgia Paraesthetica

This condition is described on page 531.

Postherpetic Neuralgia

Herpes zoster is uncommon in the lower limb. At its onset, there is pain of radicular distribution, and the rash usually appears in three or four days. After it subsides, severe pain may persist, and paresthesias and slight sensory loss are often present. As in the case of the upper limb, anterior horn cells are occasionally involved, leading to weakness, atrophy, and loss of the appropriate tendon reflex. The history of the rash will indicate the diagnosis. As in postherpetic neuralgia elsewhere, pain may be intractable in elderly subjects, and may necessitate spinothalamic tractotomy if there is no sign of abatement within 12 months of the onset, and even then no guarantee can be given that the pain will cease (Chap. 1).

Neuralgic Amyotrophy

Neuralgic amyotrophy, common in the arm and shoulder girdle, is rare in the leg. When it occurs there is intense pain lasting for a few days, accompanied by a lower motor neuron paralysis of the muscles in which the pain has been felt;

slight sensory loss may be found in the appropriate radicular area at the onset (Chap. 20).

Neoplasms of the Cauda Equina

Symptoms. Neoplasms of the cauda equina are rare, meningiomas, small fibromas of the root sheaths, and giant tumors (p. 466) being the least uncommon. Lumbar pain is often absent in the early stages, but may occur in association with rigidity later on. Freedom from symptoms in the back may be misleading when the patient complains only of pain in the leg, especially if it is limited to the lower part of the limb, but when it is influenced by changes of posture, by movements of the spine, or by coughing and sneezing, it points to a spinal or intraspinal origin.

Pain in the leg may be unilateral or bilateral, distal or proximal. It is commonly of sciatic distribution, whatever the situation of the tumor, but it may be felt in the front of the thigh (L2–L3–L4) or in the adductors (L2–L3). It is a feature of hard, slowly growing neoplasms, and is less marked in quickly growing infiltrative masses such as the giant tumor. Paresthesias—tingling, numbness, or thermal sensations—are a common accompaniment, and may involve one or more dermatomes. Weakness and wasting are prominent; fasciculation may be seen in the affected muscles. Sensory loss is usually prominent; its distribution will depend on the roots affected, which may include the perianal area (S3–S5). Tumors situated high up in the cauda equina may interfere with all the tendon reflexes, and there may be loss of the cremasteric reflex as well; sometimes, though pain is unilateral, reflex changes are found bilaterally. Impotence arising early in the history indicates disease in the neighborhood of the conus, but it may also occur temporarily as a result of long-continued pain. Sphincter symptoms usually appear early. Remissions of pain are not uncommon, and *in an important minority pain may precede the development of neurological signs by several months.*

Diagnosis. Diagnosis depends largely on ancillary investigations. Lumbar puncture may show partial or complete block, but small tumors will be missed if too much reliance is placed on manometric findings. The protein content is usually raised, but this by itself does not mean that a tumor is present since a small increase occurs in some cases of prolapsed disc and other intraspinal conditions. A normal protein content does not exclude a small tumor. A small increase in cells may be present. X-rays sometimes show erosion of the medial aspect of one or more pedicles, but early diagnosis depends on contrast myelography. A positive reaction for syphilis in the spinal fluid may or may not be relevant, syphilitic affection of the cauda equina being extremely rare.

Treatment. Treatment is surgical. It is seldom possible to determine the operability of a case without an exploratory laminectomy, and it is wiser to undertake what may prove to be a useless operation than to refrain from doing so because of academic doubts as to the outcome.

REFERENCES

1. Blau, J. N., and Logue, V.: Intermittent claudication of the cauda equina. *Lancet* 1:1081, 1961.
2. Bull, J. W. D.: Rupture of the intervertebral discs in the cervical region. *Proc. Roy. Soc. Med.* 41:513, 1948.
3. Campbell, A. M. G., and Lloyd, J. K.: Atypical facial pain. *Lancet* 2:1034, 1954.
4. Campbell, D. A., Hay, K. M., and Tonks, E. M.: An investigation of the salt and water balance in migraine. *Brit. Med. J.* 2:1424, 1951.
5. Costen, J. B.: A syndrome of ear and sinus symptoms dependent upon disturbed function of the temporo-mandibular joint. *Ann. Otol. Rhinol. Laryngol.* 43:1, 1934.
6. Cushing, H.: The major trigeminal neuralgias and their surgical treatment based on experiences with 332 gasserian operations; varieties of facial neuralgia. *Amer. J. Med. Sci.* 160:157, 1920.
7. Daniels, L. E.: Hypertension and vascular accidents during bouts of migraine. *Postgraduate Med.* 38:381, 1965.

8. DeVilliers, J. C.: A brachiocephalic vascular syndrome associated with cervical rib. *Brit. Med. J.* 2:140, 1966.
9. Echlin, F. A.: Herniation and protrusion of intervertebral disc tissue. *Injuries of the Brain and Spinal Cord.* 4th Ed. Edited by Brock, S., Springer Publishing Co., New York, 1960, Chap. 21.
10. Elliott, F. A.: The neurological manifestations of the "rheumatic" diseases. *Proc. Roy. Soc. Med.* 42:579, 1969.
11. Elliott, F. A.: Tender muscles in sciatica; an electromyographic study. *Lancet* 1:47, 1944.
12. Elliott, F. A., and Kremer, M.: Brachial pain from herniation of cervical intervertebral disc. *Lancet* 1:4, 1945.
13. Frykholm, R.: Cervical nerve root compression resulting from disc degeneration and root sleeve fibrosis. *Acta Chir. Scand.* Suppl. 160, 1951.
14. Graveson, G. S.: Retinal arterial occlusion in migraine. *Brit. Med. J.* 2:838, 1949.
15. Hankey, F. T.: Some observations on Costen's mandibular syndrome. *Proc. Roy. Soc. Med.* 51:225, 1958.
16. Harris, W.: The facial neuralgias. An analysis of 1,433 cases of paroxysmal trigeminal neuralgia and the end results of gasserian alcohol injection. *Brain* 63:209, 1940.
17. Hockaday, J. M., and Whitty, C. W. M.: Factors determining the electroencephalogram in migraine. A study of 560 patients. *Brain* 92:769, 1969.
18. Horton, B. T.: The use of histamine in the treatment of specific types of headaches. *J.A.M.A.* 116:377, 1941.
19. Hunt, W. E., Meather, J. N., LeFever, H. E., and Zeman, W.: Painful ophthalmoplegia. *Neurology* 11:56, 1961.
20. Jaeger, R.: Sphenopalatine neuralgia? *Med. Ann. D. C.* 33:258, 1964.
21. Johnson, E. W., and Pannizzo, A. N., Management of the shoulder-hand syndrome. *J.A.M.A.* 195:108, 1966.
22. Kavanaugh, G. J., Svien, H. J., Holman, C. B., and Johnson, R. M.: "Pseudoclaudication" syndrome produced by compression of cauda equina. *J.A.M.A.* 206:2477, 1968.
23. Kjellin, K., Muller, R., and Widen, L.: Glossopharyngeal neuralgia associated with cardiac arrest and hypersecretion from the ipsilateral parotid gland. *Neurology* 9:527, 1959.
24. Knight, G.: Facetectomy in the treatment of cervical rhizalgia. *Proc. Roy. Soc. Med.* 48:595, 1955.
25. Langfitt, T. W., and Elliott, F. A.: Pain in the back and legs caused by cervical cord compression. *J.A.M.A.* 200:382, 1967.
26. Lindblom, K., and Hultqvist, G.: Absorption of protruded disc tissue. *J. Bone Joint Surg.* 32:557, 1950.
27. Lundberg, P. O.: Prophylactic treatment of migraine with flumedroxone. *Acta Neurol. Scand.* 45:309, 1969.
28. Marcussen, R. M., and Wolff, H. G.: Studies on headache. *Arch. Neurol. Psychiat.* 63:42, 1950.
29. Melzack, R., and Wall, P. D.: Pain mechanisms: A new theory. *Science* 150:971, 1965.
30. Migraine and Epilepsy (editorial). *Lancet* 2:527, 1969.
31. Pearce, J.: *Migraine.* Charles C Thomas, Springfield, Ill., 1969.
32. Peet, M. M., and Schneider, R. C.: A review of 689 cases of trigeminal neuralgia. *J. Neurosurg.* 9:367, 1952.
33. Schottstaedt, W. W., and Wolff, H. G.: Studies on headache. *Arch. Neurol. Psychiat.* 73:158, 1955.
34. Schurr, D.: Sacral extradural cysts. *J. Bone Joint Surg.* 11:60, 1955.
35. Selby, G., and Lance, J. W.: Observations on 500 cases of migraine and allied vascular headaches. *J. Neurol. Neurosurg. Psychiat.* 23:23, 1960.
36. Sluder, G.: *Headaches and Eye Disorders of Nasal Origin.* The C. V. Mosby Co., St. Louis, 1918.
37. Steinbroker, O., Spetzer, M., and Friedman, H. H.: The shoulder-hand syndrome. *Ann. Int. Med.* 29:22, 1948.
38. Symonds, C.: Cough headache. *Brain* 79:557, 1956.
39. Thomson, J. L.: Glossopharyngeal neuralgia accompanied by unconsciousness. *J. Neurosurg.* 11:511, 1954.
40. Tolosa, E.: Periarteritic lesions of the carotid siphon and the clinical features of a carotid infra-clinoidal aneurysm. *J. Neurol. Neurosurg. Psychiat.* 17:300, 1954.
41. Walsh, F. M. R., Jackson, H., and Wyburn-Mason, R.: Some pressure effects associated with cervical and with rudimentary and normal first ribs. *Brain* 67:141, 1944.
42. White, J. C., and Sweet, W. H.: *Pain and the Neurosurgeon.* Charles C Thomas, Springfield, Ill., 1969.
43. Wilkinson, M.: The morbid anatomy of cervical spondylosis and myelopathy. *Brain* 83:589, 1960.
44. Wolff, H. G.: Personality features and reactions of subjects with migraine. *Arch. Neurol. Psychiat.* 37:895, 1937.
45. Wolff, H. G.: *Headache and Other Head Pains.* Oxford University Press, New York, 1950.
46. Young, J. K., and Humphries, A. W.: Severe arteriospasm after use of ergotamine tartrate suppositories. *J.A.M.A.* 175:1141, 1961.

CHAPTER NINE

Congenital and Developmental Disorders

MENTAL RETARDATION

The measurement and classification of mental retardation presents many difficulties. An I.Q. can only indicate where an individual stands in intellectual performance compared to others in respect to the particular test used. Circumstances such as nationality, social class, and ethnic group produce variables which are difficult to allow for, and international comparisons based on I.Q. scores have little validity. Low I.Q.'s can result from both biological handicaps and psychosocial deprivation, and sometimes the two overlap. Moreover, children with overall mental retardation must be distinguished from those whose formal education is impaired by some form of minimal cerebral dysfunction[5, 32] — e.g., difficulty in learning to read or write, impairment of sight or hearing, clumsiness and difficulty in learning motor skills.

Because of these facts it is difficult to judge the incidence of mental retardation. For what the figure is worth, it is thought that about 2 per cent of the population in the United States is retarded.

ETIOLOGY. Some of the causes of mental retardation[23] are tabulated in Table 9–1. The deficiencies of this list may be illustrated by the fact that in 1967, Crome and Stern were able to tab-ulate 47 metabolic disorders, many of them involving amino acid metabolism, which may be associated with mental retardation, and a recent atlas presents pictures of 84 different conditions in which mental retardation is accompanied by a characteristic facial appearance with or without abnormalities of the skull, feet, and hands. This latter book[22] provides a useful short-cut when the physician is confronted with a retarded child with an unusual appearance.

CLINICAL FEATURES. These vary from case to case, depending upon the underlying condition and the degree of retardation. It takes an experienced observer to detect mental retardation in the first few weeks of life, but suggestive features include apathy, failure to feed, and lack of response to sounds or bright lights. Fretfulness, convulsions, and a peculiar blankness of expression are common. Suspicion that all is not well should arise if at three months the child does not lift his head while in the prone position, or does not follow an object with his eyes. Other signs are: failure to lift the head in the supine position at six months, failure to sit up at nine months, or to walk at 18 months, and failure to use words at 18 months, or to form simple sentences at three years. Mild degrees of feeble-mindedness are not

179

Table 9–1.   Mental Retardation

1. PRENATAL CAUSES

A. Developmental abnormalities, including cerebral malformations, hydrocephalus (Chap. 10), Sturge–Weber disease (Chap. 15)

B. Chromosomal anomalies: Down's syndrome, etc.

C. Genetically determined disorders:

True microcephaly	The mucopolysaccharidoses (Chap. 11)
Familial spastic paraplegia (Chap. 12)	Hyperuricemia (Chap. 11)
Hereditary mental retardation	Nephrogenic diabetic insipidus (Chap. 11)
The aminoacidurias (Chap. 11)	Tuberous sclerosis
The lipidoses (Chap. 11)	The leukodystrophies (Chap. 13)
The hypoglycemias (Chap. 11)	

D. Prenatal infections of the fetus: Syphilis, rubella, cytomegalic virus, toxoplasmosis, etc. (Chap. 14)

E. Complications of pregnancy: Eclampsia, placenta previa, hyperemesis gravidarum, severe infections

F. Other: X-radiation, radium, thalidomide

2. PERINATAL CAUSES

Anoxia	Bilirubin encephalopathy
Birth injury	Prematurity

3. POSTNATAL CAUSES

Infections (meningitis, encephalitis)	Hypothyroidism (Chap. 11)
Cerebral infarction, hemorrhage	Malnutrition
Severe head injury	Lead poisoning (Chap. 21)
Status epilepticus (Chap. 7)	

incompatible with the acquisition of speech, but poverty of vocabulary and defective enunciation are common in many such cases. Physical development is often normal in the mildest cases, but it is usually defective in the more severe degrees of mental retardation. Some types are marked by a characteristic facies.[22]

Mental Retardation and Cerebral Palsies

Mental development must always be judged with great caution in infants and children with motor disorders—e.g., athetosis—because it is often better than it seems.[8] Some degree of retardation occurs in at least 50 per cent of all patients with cerebral palsy. Others display the syndrome of short attention span, lack of concentration, restlessness and emotional instability. Some are intelligent but think very slowly and remain childish and immature in emotional life and in forming judgments.

Familial Microcephaly

This condition is inherited as an autosomal recessive trait.[29] The head is small, with receding forehead, a furrowed scalp and virtually normal dimensions of the face, nose, and ears.[3] The convolutional pattern of the brain is greatly simplified, the gyri being relatively broad, and the cerebellum disproportionately large. Mental retardation is evident from an early age. In some families, the microcephaly is associated with chorioretinopathy.

Hereditary Mental Retardation

There is a high incidence of mental retardation in families in which one or both parents are either of low intelligence or actually retarded. It is probable that this "idiopathic" group will shrink as more becomes known of the biochemical and genetic factors concerned. At the same time, it must be recognized that normal children born of such parents may suffer not only from a lack of opportunity to learn but also from poverty and consequent malnutrition[39]; protein deprivation in the first year or so of life can inhibit the maturation of the brain.

Tuberous Sclerosis
(Epiloia, Bourneville's Disease)

The term "tuberous sclerosis" refers to the neurological aspects of Bourneville's disease, in which there are abnormalities in the brain, heart, kidney, lungs, eyes, bone, and skin. This is a genetically determined disease, which falls into the group of the phakomatoses and is usually inherited as an autosomal dominant. It is characterized by the presence of congenital tumor-like malformations whose potentiality for growth does not greatly exceed that of the tissues in which they are situated.

PATHOLOGY. The lesions include rhabdomyomas of the heart, multiple "tumors" of the abdominal viscera and pleura, adenoma sebaceum of the skin, subungual fibromas, retinal phakomas,[18] and tuberous sclerosis of the central nervous system.

The brain[29] is of normal size, but some of the gyri are widened by tubers within them. The tubers may also appear as nodules on the surface of the brain and under the ependymal lining of the lateral ventricle. They are firm and vary in size from 0.5 cm. to 3 cm. in diameter. They are composed of an overgrowth of glial cells and fibers, in which are groups of large vacuolated cells of a type that is not found in the mature nervous system. Hydrocephalus can be caused by a tuber situated at the foramen of Monro or in the midbrain. Calcification is not infrequent, and areas of sclerosis are sometimes present in the skull. A diffuse infiltrative glioma sometimes arises in the course of the disease.

CLINICAL FEATURES. The three most obvious features are seizures, mental deficiency, and adenoma sebaceum of the face. Seizures usually appear within the first two years of life, mental retardation a little later on, and the skin lesions at the age of 5 or 6, or even later. However, there are many exceptions to this timetable; in particular, adenoma sebaceum may not appear until after puberty, and mental deterioration may not become evident until late childhood.

Seizures may be focal or generalized, and status epilepticus is not uncommon. In a small minority, there is also evidence of focal damage to the brain—hemiparesis, diplegia, athetosis, etc. Rapidly advancing neurological defects, however, suggest the presence of a glioma.

Mental retardation varies from slight to severe and it tends to progress. Rarely, intelligence is normal.

Adenoma sebaceum appears as a collection of small, pinkish or yellowish-pink nodules distributed in a butterfly-shaped area over the cheeks and nose. They also appear on the forehead and chin in some cases. In well developed cases, there is a fine network of capillaries over the surface of each nodule. Other skin lesions may also be encountered—café au lait spots, areas of depigmentation, pedunculated polyps, and patches of elevated, thickened and roughened areas of skin ("shagreen") in the lumbosacral region.

When retinal phakomas are present, they appear as opaque white areas, either near the disc or more peripherally in the retina.[18]

Of the visceral "tumors" which are found in this disease, few give rise to symptoms, but pleural nodules can cause spontaneous pneumothorax, and a cardiac rhabdomyoma may cause death in infancy. Many patients die in childhood and few survive beyond the twentieth year.

The cerebrospinal fluid may contain an excess of protein. Pneumoencephalography usually reveals irregularities (candle guttering) in the walls of the lateral ventricles.

TREATMENT. Seizures are treated by anticonvulsant medication. Exceptionally, it is possible to excise a seizure focus which has been localized by electroencephalography. If hydrocephalus arises, it can be treated by a ventricular-atrial shunting procedure.

Chromosomal Anomalies

Chromosomal anomalies have been found in a number of syndromes characterized by mental retardation and other abnormalities. In 1959, it was discovered that in Down's syndrome, the chromosomal content of the cells is increased by an amount equal to that of the smallest autosomes—commonly, an increase in the number of small chromosomes (Numbers 21 and 22) from two pairs to two pairs and one extra chromosome. This is known as "trisomy 21–22." Sometimes the extra chromosome becomes attached to one of the larger chromosomes, usually in group 13–15, in which event the child has a normal number of chromosomes, but the total mass is the same as in persons with trisomic Down's syndrome, from whom they are clinically indistinguishable. A large translocation chromosome, consisting of one chromosome from the 13–15 group and one from the 21–22 group, is sometimes found in the mother, who possesses only 45 chromosomes but has a normal chromosome mass. The risk for such a mother of having another child with Down's syndrome is about 30 per cent, against a 2 per cent risk for the mother of a child with trisomy Down's syndrome. Examination of the mother of a child with this condition is therefore a prerequisite for genetic counseling.

Individuals without the physical features of Down's syndrome sometimes have the trisomy 21–22 anomaly. Conversely, typical patients sometimes appear to have a normal karyotype. It is possible that some of these departures from the normal rules are the result of mosaicism, which occurs when the number of chromosomes varies in different cells in the same individual.

Trisomy for chromosomes 15–18 and 13–15 has been reported in mentally retarded individuals with visceral and somatic defects. In the "cri-du-chat" syndrome, the short arm of one of the number 5 chromosomes is absent; such children are small at birth and develop very slowly. They are microcephalic and have slanting eyes. The voice is high-pitched and resembles the cry of a kitten. In those that survive infancy, mental retardation is severe.

Anomalies of the sex chromosomes can give rise to a number of gonadal and somatic abnormalities, and mental retardation is occasionally encountered in both men and women who have more than three sex chromosomes. Behavioral scientists have been interested to note that violence and antisocial behavior are relatively common in XYY men, many of whom are much taller than their siblings.

Down's Syndrome
(Mongolism)

Down's syndrome is a clinical diagnosis based on the presence of mental retardation and a particular physical appearance. It is usually associated with triplication of the chromosome 21. Occasionally, the extra chromosome is translocated to another autosome, as has already been mentioned.

The condition is relatively common and is thought to account for about 5 per cent of severe mental retardation in persons of all ages. The chance of having a child with Down's syndrome increases with increasing age of the mother, so that after the age of 45 years, the risk is almost 2 per cent.

PATHOLOGY. The brain is small and abnormally rounded. The convolutional pattern is usually normal, but poor development of the third frontal gyrus may expose the insula. The superior temporal gyrus is very narrow in about 50 per cent of cases.[29] The cerebellum and brainstem are conspicuously small in comparison with the cerebrum. Many microscopic abnormalities have been described, but they are found in other forms of severe developmental defects of the brain.

CLINICAL FEATURES. The newborn often has feeding difficulties and is sluggish and apathetic. The appearance is characteristic. The face is round, with slanted eyes and epicanthic folds. The back of the head is flat and the head itself is small. The neck is short, the feet and hands are broad, and there is a deep "simian" transverse crease on the palms of the hands. The dermal ridges in the fingers and hands are abnormal. There is often a notable gap between the big toe and the second toe. Maldevelopment may be found in other organs of the body; Fallot's tetralogy is not infrequent. Cataracts are common in those who survive to adult life. There is marked hypotonia, which allows the child to assume improbable attitudes, but the tendon reflexes are normal.

Mental endowment usually varies between imbecility and feeble-mindedness, but occasionally a mongoloid appearance is found in otherwise normal persons, for which reason the prognosis should be guarded in infancy. The child with Down's syndrome is usually described as affable and lovable, cheerful and easy to manage, but this is by no means always the case. Presenile dementia may occur in adult patients.

Many affected children die in infancy and few survive to adult life. The chief causes of death are acute infectious diseases and congenital heart disease.

DIAGNOSIS. The diagnosis is usually obvious from the appearance of the patient. In cretinism, by contrast, the skin is dry and wrinkled, there is puffiness and swelling of the eyelids, the epiphyses unite late, the serum cholesterol is raised, and the uptake of radioiodine is reduced.

TREATMENT. There is no effective treatment for Down's syndrome. Those with a minor degree of feeble-mindedness may benefit from appropriately adjusted education,[12] but in the majority of cases, institutional care is necessary.

Other Causes of Mental Retardation

Developmental abnormalities of the brain are often incompatible with long life, and if the infant survives, varying degrees of mental deficiency are often found. The effects of infantile hydrocephalus are described in Chapter 10 and those of Sturge–Weber disease in Chapter 15.

Prenatal infection of the fetus (congenital syphilis, rubella, the cytomegalic virus, toxoplasmosis) are discussed in Chapter 14.

Diseases and intoxications occurring during pregnancy may lead to malformed offspring. They include extrauterine gestation, toxemia of pregnancy, placenta praevia, severe infections, deep x-ray or radium therapy during the first four months of pregnancy. Maternal diabetes has been incriminated in the past; it gives rise to big babies, with an increased risk of birth trauma, but this may not be the whole story. Navarrete and his colleagues[28] followed up a series of 349 women who had been delivered of a malformed infant and found that diabetes had developed later in an unusually large number of mothers—0.6 per cent in the first year, 14.8 per cent by the twelfth year, and 34.3 per cent by the twenty-fifth year. The figures were even higher when mothers who did not have clinical diabetes but who did show abnormal glucose tolerance tests were added to the score, reaching 53.1 per cent at 25 years. These findings suggest but do not prove that the early phase of the diabetic state predisposes to the bearing of a malformed infant.

The ingestion of large doses of LSD during pregnancy can give rise, in animals, to malformations of the brain and limbs. It is not yet known whether the use of this drug, either before or during pregnancy, will produce viable infants with mental retardation.

Birth injuries and anoxia during birth or shortly thereafter can cause cerebral palsy with or without mental retardation, and the risks are greater in premature than in full-term infants. It is important to emphasize that excessively quick and "easy" delivery can injure the brain by producing intracerebral lacerations and hemorrhages.

Bilirubin encephalopathy is an important cause of brain damage in the perinatal period.[7]

Malnutrition, poverty, bad education, and poor medical care are all strongly associated with mental retardation, and it is difficult to separate one cause from the other.[23] Animal experiments have shown that lack of protein during development can influence the growth of the brain, behavior, and mental performance.[39] In rats, the number of cells in the brain can be reduced by protein deprivation, both during gestation and in the postnatal period. Behavioral abnormalities have also been produced by protein deprivation in dogs and pigs. The evidence in human beings is less conclusive at the present time, but from the studies that are available, it is probable that nutritional deficiencies, especially protein deficiency in early life, can cause permanent mental retardation. If this is so, it has vast social and economic implications, both at home and abroad.

BILIRUBIN ENCEPHALOPATHY
(Kernicterus)

In 1875, Orth described yellow pigmentation of the basal ganglia, brainstem nuclei and cerebellum in fatal cases of icterus gravis neonatorum and in 1904, Schmorl named the condition "Kern Icterus." Since then, "kernicterus" has been used to designate a clinical syndrome caused by hyperbilirubinemia, whatever its cause, and characterized by mental retardation, chorioathetosis, and other features.

ETIOLOGY. Any condition of severe hyperbilirubinemia can produce kernicterus, but more than 50 per cent of all cases are caused by rhesus incompatibility, which results from the presence of a heterozygous rhesus-positive fetus in a rhesus-negative mother. This provokes the formation of maternal antibodies, which are inimical to the fetal red cells. The sensitization of the mother is a slow process so that the first-born (who starts the trouble) usually escapes ill effects, but if the succeeding child is also rhesus-positive, the antibody in the mother's serum crosses the placenta and either destroys the fetal red cells in utero, giving rise to a pale, edematous, stillborn infant at full term (hydrops fetalis) or causes a severe hemolytic jaundice shortly after birth (icterus gravis neonatorum). The first child can be affected by either of these conditions if the mother has been sensitized by a previous blood transfusion from a rhesus-positive donor.

During fetal life, bilirubin is excreted through the placenta and is dealt with by the liver of the mother, but after birth, excretion of bilirubin is dependent on the glucuronyl transferase system in the infant's liver. If the amount of bilirubin is excessive, the liver cannot conjugate and remove it with sufficient speed, and when the serum bilirubin level exceeds 18 mg. per 100 ml., there is danger of serious damage to the brain. In congenital familial nonhemolytic jaundice (the Crigler-Najjar syndrome), bilirubin accumulates because glucuronyl transferase is absent.[34]

Factors other than the quantity of bilirubin in the serum help to determine whether brain damage will occur or not. The administration of sulfonamides and salicylates displaces bilirubin from binding sites on serum proteins, thereby increasing the amount of free bilirubin and predisposing to encephalopathy. Relatively low serum bilirubin levels (12 mg. per 100 ml.) have been associated with encephalopathy in sick premature babies; conversely, relatively high bilirubin concentrations do not necessarily damage the brain in mature, healthy babies. There is some evidence that perinatal and neonatal hypoxia predisposes to the development of kernicterus in human infants, but it does not do so in the Gunn rat, a strain in which hemolytic jaundice is transmitted by a mutant recessive autosomal gene.

PATHOLOGY. Sectioning of the brain shows intense yellow pigmentation of the basal ganglia, subthalamic nucleus, mammillary bodies, inferior olive, cornu Ammonis, dentate nuclei, and (to a lesser extent) the cortex. Petechiae and hemorrhages may be present. There is a considerable outfall of cells in the basal ganglia, and those which remain show varying degrees of damage. The pigment is present in the ganglion cells and also in large phagocytes. Children who survive the acute phase show defective myelination of the white matter of the brain and spinal cord, and patchy gliosis of the basal ganglia. The liver shows central necrosis of the lobules, and the bone marrow is hyperplastic.

The localization of the pigment in certain areas of the brain, notably the basal ganglia, is not fully understood. Bilirubin staining of similar distribution has been seen in cases of septic jaundice, in experimentally produced toxic hepatitis, and in obstructive jaundice in animals. Schutta's experimental work on the Gunn rat suggests that the distribution of bilirubin staining may depend on regional differences in blood flow.

CLINICAL FEATURES. The child may appear normal at birth but is often slightly jaundiced, anemic, and edematous. The jaundice becomes intense during the first few days, and edema is apparent in the face and neck. The liver and spleen are enlarged, and the stools and urine are heavily bile stained. Signs of brain damage develop between the second and fifth day; the child becomes apathetic and sucks poorly.[17] In severely affected infants, lethargy gives place to stupor and coma, which may be interrupted by seizures and spasms of opisthotonos, with death ensuing after a few days. Less severely affected individuals show generalized rigidity, with seizures, trismus, and opisthotonos. Rigidity remains intense, and there is eye-rolling, profuse sweating, and evidence of defective temperature control. Such patients usually die in infancy. When the condition is still less severe, rigidity and choreoathetosis develop; in some cases, the movements appear in the trunk muscles, as well as in the limbs. In the mildest form, the child seems to improve for a time, showing few signs besides eye-rolling and some retraction of the head. In about the third or fourth month, hypertonia and weakness become apparent and choreoathetosis develops. Walking is delayed by a notable lack of equilibrium. Mental retardation is common and may be severe. High tone deafness is found in many cases, and there may also be impairment of ocular movements. It is generally believed that *severe mental deficiency without motor disturbances should not be attributed to bilirubin encephalopathy*, but Odell[32] and others have found a relatively high incidence of defects of cognitive functions, visual perception, fine motor coordination, and short-term memory in children who have survived neonatal jaundice and who have been treated by exchange transfusions.

COURSE AND PROGNOSIS. Early recognition and prompt treatment reduce the immediate mortality, which is otherwise in the region of 75 per cent. Untreated survivors may live for a few years, but they show a liability to infections and the poor resistance that is common to so many defective children, so that the ultimate prognosis as regards life is poor.

DIAGNOSIS. Jaundice must be differentiated from the physiological icterus of the newborn, which starts later, is less severe, and is unaccompanied by anemia, serious malaise, or enlargement of the liver. It is sometimes difficult, when dealing with a child of four or five years who has neurological symptoms, to assess the meaning of a history of neonatal jaundice in retrospect. But, if there is a positive family history, or history of neurological disability at the time of the jaundice, the jaundice is probably to blame.

TREATMENT. If a Rhesus negative mother is delivered of a Rhesus positive baby, sensitization can be prevented by the administration of antibody within 48 hours of delivery. This will prevent icterus gravis neonatorum in subsequent babies.

The treatment of icterus gravis is by exchange transfusion, which should be carried out if the serum bilirubin exceeds 18 mg. per 100 ml., and if the reserve serum albumin binding capacity falls below 50 per cent. However, these figures are approximate.

CEREBRAL PALSY

The term "cerebral palsy" is applied to a heterogeneous group of syndromes which are dominated by disorders of movement and posture.[8, 9, 14, 40] The responsible lesions are situated in the brain, the condition is permanent and nonprogressive, and the damage to the brain occurs in fetal life, during parturition, or in the neonatal period.

The reported incidence of cerebral palsy varies in different countries — about 5 per 1000 children in the United States, around 1.62 per 1000 births in the Scandinavian countries, and between 1 and 2 per 1000 of the school population in England and Wales. The disability is mild in about 50 per cent of all cases, and only about 10 per cent are severely handicapped. Some degree of mental retardation is present in 66 per cent of all cases. Seizures are common.

Not included in the above figures are the cases of *minimal cerebral dysfunction*,[5] which include the "clumsy child syndrome," the hyperactive child, and those who are slow in developing language skills.

ETIOLOGY. Prenatal causes include infection of the fetus by syphilis, toxoplasmosis, rubella, and cytomegalic inclusion body disease. Severe viral infections in the first three months of preg-

nancy (e.g., poliomyelitis) sometimes appear to be responsible, but this is unproved. Anoxic episodes, x-rays, and toxemia of pregnancy may affect the fetus. Autosomal recessive inheritance is a rare cause of nonprogressive cerebral palsy in more than one member of a family. Anoxia during parturition or arising in the perinatal period is probably the most common cause of cerebral palsy and the risk is increased by prematurity, prolonged dystocia, abnormal position of the fetus, and intracranial hemorrhage — subarachnoid, subdural, and intracerebral — which occurs in some cases, but it is difficult to know whether subsequent cerebral palsy results from the hemorrhagic complications or from coincident trauma. Subarachnoid hemorrhage can give rise to subsequent hydrocephalus.

Meningitis, encephalitis, infarction from occlusion of a major blood vessel, bleeding from an arteriovenous malformation, hydrocephalus, and hemolytic disease are important neonatal causes of cerebral palsy.

PATHOLOGY. The pathological features vary from case to case.[30, 40, 42] Four types of abnormality are found: (1) The central nervous system appears normal to the naked eye, but microscopy shows defective development of both gray matter and projection tracts, without evidence of destruction or repair. However, the absence of such evidence can be fallacious because the immature nervous system does not react to disease in the same way as does adult tissue; inflammatory reactions are not seen before the sixth month of fetal life, and brain tissue can be absorbed without leaving any evidence of scarring.[29] (2) Gross anatomical abnormalities of the brain are present. These can be due to faulty development, but this is not necessarily genetic in origin since infections of the fetus in the first trimester can lead to microcephaly, absence of the corpus callosum, and hydrocephalus. As with the first group, there may be no evidence of previous inflammation. (3) Localized or generalized atrophy of the brain, with degeneration of cells and fibers, over-growth of neuroglia, and perivascular sclerosis, may occur. When this is local-ized to one or two lobes, it is sometimes referred to as atrophic lobar sclerosis. (4) In some cases of congenital choreo-athetosis, the gray matter, the putamen, and caudate nuclei are broken up by a network of myelineated fibers; when stained by Weigert's method, the af-fected area presents a mottled appear-ance, which earned for it the name of "status marmoratus" (Vogt).

CLASSIFICATION. It is difficult to subdivide the cerebral palsies into well defined syndromes because there is con-siderable overlapping among different categories. For this reason, the descrip-tions that follow are approximate rather than exact.

CONGENITAL SPASTIC DIPLEGIA (Little's Disease)

Congenital spastic diplegia is a com-mon syndrome, which is probably caused by many disorders, including maternal illness during pregnancy, birth injury, and asphyxia. It usually affects only one member of a family.

CLINICAL FEATURES. In severe cases, the condition appears shortly after birth. Cyanosis, a feeble cry, and inability to nurse indicate that all is not well. Seiz-ures may occur. The legs are rigid, and the back may arch when the infant cries. Swallowing is defective and nutrition suffers. Early death from intercurrent infection is the usual termination.

In milder cases, the child may be re-garded as normal for the first few months and then it is noticed that he fails to hold up his head, cannot suck, and holds his legs in rigid extension and adduction when placed on his feet. Walking is de-layed by rigidity, adduction of the legs, and lack of equilibrium. The hands are sometimes stiff and clumsy, and atheto-sis may be present. The tendon reflexes may be difficult to elicit in the presence of severe spasticity. In the mildest

cases, the arms are unaffected, but the legs are stiff and clumsy, and there is a tendency to a scissors gait; bilateral equinovarus is usual. Mental retardation is common in this group.

In most cases, the incapacity results more from spasticity than from muscular weakness, and although it is usual to regard the disability as of pyramidal ori-gin, the abdominal and plantar reflexes are often normal, which suggests that the spasticity in such cases stems from damage of the reticulospinal system.

Two variants require special mention. In congenital double hemiplegia, there is spastic weakness of the arms and legs, but the former is more severe than the latter, and there is usually some degree of bulbar palsy as well. Seizures, athe-tosis, and mental retardation are usually present. In congenital bulbar palsy,[14] there is spastic weakness of the lips, tongue, and pharyngeal muscles, with consequent dysarthria and dysphagia, but the limbs are unaffected. Some cases also present supranuclear paralysis of ocular movements and difficulty in chew-ing. This condition is rare, and survival beyond the first year is uncommon.

PROGNOSIS. In mild to moderate cases, the patient may survive infancy, but his condition sometimes appears to deteriorate because the defect is brought into ever-increasing prominence with the widening range of activities expected of a growing child. The disability is sometimes aggravated by intercurrent illness. Ultimately, some degree of functional improvement may set in, until a stationary condition is reached by the sixth or seventh year.

DIAGNOSIS. Spinal paraplegia due to birth injuries is immediately obvious and is distinguished by the presence of sensory loss below the level of the lesion and a history of dystocia necessitating traction. Paraplegia occasionally results from damage to the parasagittal area of the brain as a result of excessive molding of the head, but birth injury to the head is not regarded as a common cause of congenital spastic diplegia, although it is important in the causation of infantile hemiplegia. Acute cerebral diplegia may also be caused in infancy by thrombosis of the superior sagittal sinus in a child who is normal at birth.

TREATMENT. The treatment is palliative.[12] Defective children require both care and discipline from the start. If the child is either spoiled or neglected, the most is not made of whatever mental and physical capacity is present. There is need for physiotherapy, educational exercise, and—at a later date—orthopedic treatment for the relief of contractures. Seizures are treated on the usual lines. Vigilance must be maintained to secure adequate nutrition and protection from chills and infections. When the first-born is affected, the question of further pregnancies will arise. There is always the possibility of further disasters, but the risk is a small one unless there is clear evidence of morbid inheritance. Should a second child also be defective, further additions to the family are to be avoided.

CONGENITAL ATONIC DIPLEGIA

This uncommon condition is noticed shortly after birth. The infant is abnormally still, cries little, and feeds poorly. The head lolls about in a helpless way, and the range of passive movements permitted is in excess of normal. Voluntary movements are feeble, and there is a striking sense of flabbiness when the child is held in the arms, comparable to the experience of handling an anesthetized baby. When the infant is lifted up by placing the hands in the armpits, the legs may become rigid. There is no paralysis, the tendon reflexes are normal, and the electrical responses are physiological. Voluntary movements are often ataxic. Mental deficiency and seizures are common, and kyphoscoliosis and congenital dislocation of the hips may be present. These children may improve slightly but remain disabled to some extent, and severely affected children seldom reach maturity.

Other causes of infantile hypotonia (the floppy baby syndrome)[33] are described on page 550.

SYNDROME OF CHANGING MUSCLE TONE

This is sometimes described as a "mixed form" of cerebral palsy. When undisturbed, the infant lies in the frog position and appears to be hypotonic, but the tendon reflexes are normal or increased. Mental development is severely delayed. When the infant is disturbed, for example by being handled, the limbs become spastic. The tonic neck reflex, the Moro reflex, and the sucking and grasping reflexes persist throughout childhood. Sometimes this syndrome is combined with ataxia or choreoathetosis.

CONGENITAL CEREBELLAR ATAXIA

Agenesis of the cerebellum, pons, and olives with or without defects of the cerebrum is encountered as a nonfamilial and nonhereditary condition which is manifested clinically by hypotonia, intention tremor, and nystagmus.[35] The infant is floppy and is slow in learning to hold up his head, sit up, or walk. The ataxia may appear to become more prominent in the second year, when walking is attempted. Mild mental retardation may be present.

A mild form of this condition is seen in children who are clumsy for their age. They are late in walking, and have difficulty in learning to run or hop. More sophisticated skills, such as riding a bicycle or skating, may be impossible, and the child is accident-prone.

Other causes of ataxia in infants include the Dandy-Walker syndrome, hydrocephalus, and the Marinesco-Sjögren syndrome, a genetically determined disease characterized by ataxia, retarded motor development, bilateral cataracts, short stature, and mental retardation. *Intermittent* cerebellar ataxia, coupled with a pellagra-like skin rash, is a feature of Hartnup disease (p. 218).

CONGENITAL EXTRAPYRAMIDAL SYNDROMES
(Athetosis, Chorea, and Mixed Forms)

Congenital Bilateral Athetosis. For the first few months, infants with this condition are hypotonic, and involuntary movements and abnormal postures do not develop until the fourth or fifth month. Athetoid movements invade the face, neck, arms, and legs, interfering with all voluntary movements, including speech and swallowing. There are no abnormal movements at rest, but as soon as muscles are used, movement is handicapped by athetosis and a background of fluctuating hypertonicity, which is felt as soon as the limbs are handled. In pure form, it is unassociated with the reflex disturbances of pyramidal disease, but in some cases, spasticity is present. "Mobile spasm" is an apt synonym. Occasionally, the movements are confined to the face and tongue. Deafness is sometimes present. Intelligence may be normal or defective, but in many cases it is a great deal more acute than appears at first sight, and it can be harnessed in the task of educating the child to relax and thus to control the involuntary movements. The presence of dysarthria may help to hide an underlying intelligence.

Congenital athetosis can be caused by neonatal jaundice and by severe asphyxia. Some patients, who died early, have shown the status marmoratus of Vogt.

Physical education along the lines pioneered by Phelps, starting in the third year and continuing for several years, is helpful in mild cases. Stereotaxic surgery can abolish the athetosis, but is only to be considered in the case of children with good mental endowment.[6]

Congenital Chorea. This condition is less common than athetosis and appears at about the sixth month. The movements are polymorphic and generalized. They may resemble those of Sydenham's chorea or possess a quality more akin to athetosis (choreoathetosis). There is marked hypotonia, but the reflexes are unaltered. The milestones of development are reached late. Swallowing may be interfered with. Severely affected infants die early, but those with mild impairment may survive and improve; exacerbations may occur during periods of strain and infection and after surgical operations.

HEMIPLEGIA

This is a syndrome rather than a specific disease. Very rarely, it seems to be developmental in origin, as in cerebral hemiatrophy, when the two hemispheres are unequally developed and the cortical pattern on the affected side is primitive in type. Ford has reported congenital hemiplegia in identical twins.[14] Sometimes hemiplegia arises as a result of birth trauma or asphyxia; in such cases, the hemiplegia may not be obvious before the third or fourth month, because the primitive movements of the newly born do not depend on the corticospinal path but on subcortical systems. Ford[14] studied the pathology in nine such cases; in three, there was a porencephaly which was probably the result of a vascular lesion. In three others, there was local atrophy and sclerosis of the cortex, with local thickening of the pia arachnoid. In the remaining three, there was evidence of an old subdural blood clot with atrophy of the underlying cortex.

In a third and larger group, symptoms develop acutely in infancy or the early years of childhood.[42] This is known as "acute infantile hemiplegia," and it is often the result of vascular occlusive disease, as demonstrated by arteriography. It has been supposed that, in some cases, the hemiplegia results from an unspecified "encephalitis." Abrupt hemiplegia can also occur in infants suffering from the Sturge-Weber syndrome.

ACUTE INFANTILE HEMIPLEGIA

This condition occurs in previously healthy children between the ages of six months and six years, who fall ill abruptly, with a seizure, or a series of seizures. The convulsive movements usually involve only one side of the body but may be generalized. The temperature rises steeply and stupor continues for hours or days. When consciousness returns, the child is found to be hemiplegic. The spinal fluid is normal at the outset, but there may be an increased number of leukocytes during the second week of the illness. When air studies have been performed, they have shown swelling of the affected hemisphere, followed at a much later date by enlargement of the ventricle on the affected side, associated in some cases with porencephaly.

At first, the paralyzed limbs are flaccid but they gradually become spastic. Tremor or athetosis may appear. The limbs on the affected side develop less well than normal and remain small and deformed. Seizures are apt to continue for years. If the lesion is in the dominant hemisphere, speech may be delayed. There may be a degree of retardation, though this is not always the case. Disturbances of mood and behavior are not uncommon, and may be related to the

frustration engendered by physical incapacity and frequent seizures. It is possible that subclinical seizure activity plays a role, because improvement in behavior sometimes follows when the damaged hemisphere is removed.[41]

PROGNOSIS. The mortality is low, but the outlook for complete recovery is poor.[38] Most recovery is to be expected in the legs, the arms remaining more or less useless. Seizures are treated along the usual lines. In general, hemispherectomy is indicated in patients with behavior disorders, persistent seizures, and complete hemiplegia. The indications and contraindications for this procedure are discussed by Wilson.[41]

PROGRESSIVE CEREBRAL DEGENERATION OF INFANCY
(Alpers' Disease)

First described by Alpers[1] in 1931 and sometimes called poliodystrophia cerebri progressiva, this disease occurs in early life; both familial and sporadic cases have been described. There is a loss of

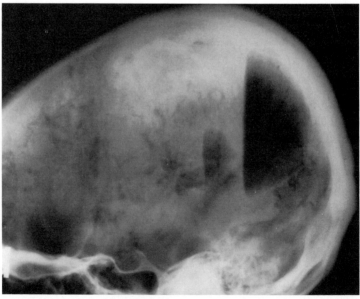

Figure 9–1. Porencephalic cyst (left parietal) communicating with trigone of left lateral ventricle in 30-year-old woman with history of birth trauma. (Courtesy of Dr. James Bull.)

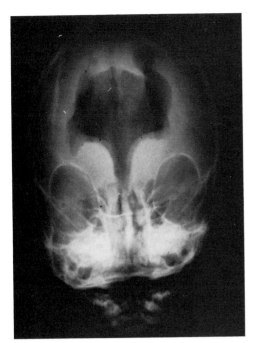

Figure 9–2. Ventriculogram showing absence of the corpus callosum. (Courtesy of Dr. Charles Kennedy.)

ganglion cells from the cerebral cortex, and sometimes the basal ganglia and cerebellum are also involved. The cortical degeneration is diffuse, and there is some proliferation of astrocytes; microglial cells laden with lipids may be seen.

The condition usually appears in a previously normal infant, and takes the form of progressive mental deterioration and failure to reach the normal milestones of physical activity. Seizures may occur, and myoclonus is common. Cortical deafness and blindness may develop, and optic atrophy has been described. Spastic weakness on one or both sides of the body, ataxia, and choreoathetosis have been reported. Mental deficiency becomes increasingly severe, and the motor disturbances progress steadily.

The disease has to be distinguished from other progressive cerebral degenerations in infants. Tay-Sachs disease may be suspected, but the retina does not show a cherry-red spot. A positive diagnosis cannot be made except by autopsy. The fact that the disease can be familial has to be brought to the attention of the

parents once the pathological diagnosis has been made.

AGENESIS OF THE CORPUS CALLOSUM

Complete or incomplete absence of the corpus callosum may exist on its own, but it is usually associated with other congenital defects of the brain. There is usually some degree of mental retardation, which is not due to the callosal lesion as such but to other defects, since the corpus callosum can be cut from end to end without causing motor disability or obvious mental symptoms (page 35).

Pneumoencephalography discloses a large third ventricle which is extended dorsally and separates the lateral ventricles (Fig. 9–2).

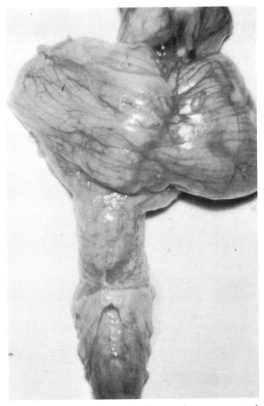

Figure 9–3. The cerebellum and upper cervical cord in a case of Arnold-Chiari malformation. (Courtesy of Department of Neuropathology, Philadelphia General Hospital.)

THE ARNOLD-CHIARI MALFORMATION

This is a rare condition. The inferior poles of the cerebellar hemispheres extend downward through the foramen magnum of either side of an elongated medulla.[13, 29] The latter is flattened, and the lower cranial nerves are stretched. The fourth ventricle extends into the canal and the outflow of the spinal fluid may be blocked, causing internal hydrocephalus.[29] The defect is almost always associated with a meningomyelocele or spina bifida occulta in the lumbosacral region. Many other associated defects of the brain and spinal cord have been found.

Symptoms usually appear in the first few months of life. There may be symptoms and signs of hydrocephalus, with or without involvement of the lower cranial nerves, and cerebellar ataxia. The clinical picture can be modified by the development of syringomyelic cavities in the upper part of the spinal cord.[25]

Treatment is by surgical decompression of the foramen magnum and upper cord.

THE KLIPPEL-FEIL SYNDROME

This rare condition is characterized by maldevelopment of the cervical vertebrae, which are reduced in number and fused together. Spina bifida or meningomyelocele may be present. The infant seems to have virtually no neck. Movements of the head are severely restricted, and the head may be inclined to one side, as in torticollis. The scapulae are elevated. Fusion of the vertebrae may extend into the upper dorsal spine, and there may be an associated dysplasia of the cervical cord, manifesting itself either as a slowly progressive spastic weakness of the arms and legs or as an inability to dissociate the movements of the hands; each movement of one upper limb is copied by the other. The latter symptom is attributed to faulty decussation of the pyramids. Neurological

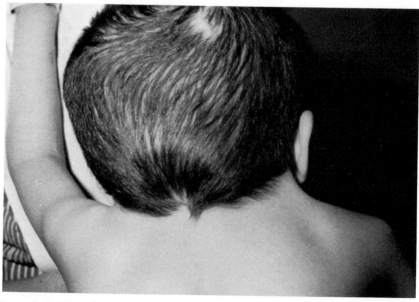

Figure 9–4. Klippel-Feil syndrome. (Courtesy of Children's Hospital of Philadelphia.)

symptoms may also result from an associated Arnold-Chiari malformation or syringomyelia.

SYRINGOMYELIA AND SYRINGOBULBIA

Syringomyelia is a syndrome of the upper spinal cord or medulla (or both), characterized by gliosis and cavitation.

ETIOLOGY. Syringomyelia has been regarded for many years as a primary disease of congenital origin, and this appeared to be supported by a high incidence of associated congenital abnormalities, which include cervical rib, kyphoscoliosis, spina bifida, platybasia, hydrocephalus, and the Arnold-Chiari malformation.[25] Another view, first advanced by Gardner,[15, 16] is that syringomyelia is caused by developmental or acquired abnormalities which obstruct the foramen of Magendie, thereby raising the pressure in the central canal of the spinal cord. In support of this view, it has been found that symptoms resulting from syringomyelia can be improved by surgical operations designed to correct the Arnold-Chiari malformation, platybasia, and other congenital lesions in the vicinity of the foramen magnum. Moreover, syringomyelia has been found in association with leptomeningeal adhesions around the roof of the fourth ventricle, and clinical improvement has followed when free flow of the spinal fluid was restored. Softening and cavitation of the cervical and thoracic spinal cord have been produced in dogs by inducing chronic adhesive arachnoiditis around the base of the brain.

PATHOLOGY.[29] In most cases, syringomyelia is found in the cervical cord, but it may extend into the upper thoracic segments. The cavity usually extends transversely across the cord, dorsal to the central canal, and often invades the ventral portions of the dorsal horns and the bases of the ventral horns. In the early stages, the cavity may be unilateral and limited to the base of one dorsal horn. Ultimately, it enlarges to involve most of the cord at that level. The cord is spread thinly around the circumference of the cavity. These anatomical variations are reflected in the physical signs, which differ widely from patient to patient.

The cavity is lined with glial scar tissue and not with ependyma. In some areas, there is more gliosis than cavitation. On inspection at operation, the cord may appear normal, but more often it appears shrunken; occasionally, it is distended.

Secondary degeneration follows in cells and tracts, notably in the spinothalamic decussation, the spinothalamic and pyramidal tracts, the dorsal columns, the anterior horn cells, and the posterior horns. In syringobulbia, the fibers relaying to the thalamus from the nuclei gracilis and cuneatus (conveying proprioception) are often involved, as are the fibers and cells of the descending trigeminal roots and the nuclei of the tenth, eleventh, and twelfth cranial nerves.

Cavitation of the spinal cord somewhat resembling syringomyelia may be found in association with trauma to the cord, spinal arachnoiditis, angiomatous malformations and spinal tumors. These cavities are sometimes spoken of as secondary syringomyelia, and they may or may not give rise to symptoms. The cavity is usually located at the base of the posterior columns or in the dorsal horns, and it does not usually communicate with the central canal of the cord. It may be small, or it may extend over several segments.

Hydromyelia, a dilatation of the central canal, is occasionally found in routine postmortems and also occurs in a large proportion of cases of meningomyelocele and the Arnold-Chiari malformation. Most of the wall is covered with ependymal cells. Hydromyelia is not thought to cause neurological symptoms.

CLINICAL FEATURES. Symptoms occasionally occur in childhood and late adult life, but the most common age of onset is between 20 and 40. The arms are usually involved first, and the first symptoms to appear are segmental in distribution. Later on, as cavitation increases, the long tracts in the white matter are involved, either by pressure or by gliosis, with consequent dysfunction below the level of the syrinx. Years may elapse between these two stages.

Because cavitation usually starts in the gray matter posterior to the central canal, often in the base of one or both posterior horns, sensory phenomena commonly precede motor disturbances. They may be unilateral or bilateral. The patient may complain of paresthesias in the hand or in the shoulder and neck, but pain is uncommon. Often the patient finds that he cannot appreciate heat, and he may burn his fingers without feeling pain. At this stage, examination will disclose marked impairment to pain and temperature, with relative preservation of touch, joint sense, and vibration. These findings may be unilateral or bilateral, and they may be limited strictly to the hand or may extend up the limb to involve the shoulder and upper part of the trunk in a jacket-like distribution. Occasionally, loss of deep pain in the affected segments is the earliest sensory sign. A curious feature of the disease is its capacity to produce sensory loss in the peripheral or proximal distribution of several adjacent segments; for instance, the loss of temperature and pain may involve the fingers and hand up to the wrist (C6, C7, and C8). As time goes on, the posterior columns and the spinothalamic tracts are implicated, producing impairment of pain and temperature below the lesion. Paresthesias and a variable degree of sensory impairment then appear in the feet and legs.

Anterior horn cell involvement is usual; it is difficult to know how this comes about in the early stages of the condition, but weakness, wasting and fasciculation in the small muscles of the hand, or (less commonly) the shoulder girdle, may appear quite early in the history. Later on, pyramidal signs appear below the level of the syrinx, but several years may pass before this happens.

The tendon reflexes related to the af-

fected segments are reduced and ultimately abolished because their intraspinal pathways are interrupted. When the pyramidal tracts are affected, the reflexes become hyperactive below the level of the lesion, the abdominal reflexes are lost, and the plantar responses become extensor.

Excess sweating may occur in the affected limb or limbs, but anhidrosis is more common. Horner's syndrome is seen in some cases of cervicothoracic syringomyelia. Sphincter symptoms are late in appearing.

Trophic effects are common in analgesic areas. Superficial burns and other injuries give rise to indolent ulceration, with subsequent scarring. Sometimes there is thickening of the subcutaneous tissue of the hand, which becomes pudgy and curiously soft (main succulente), and when this is associated with local ulceration of the fingers and sensory loss, it constitutes one type of Morvan's syndrome. Charcot's arthropathy sometimes occurs in the shoulder (Fig. 9–5) and the finger joints and wrists may also be affected.

SYRINGOBULBIA. This   can   occur

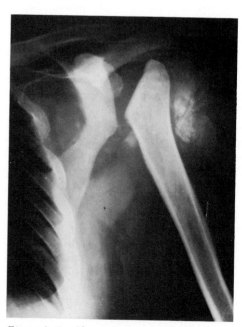

Figure 9–5. Charcot joint in a case of syringomyelia.

alone or in association with syringomyelia. There are one or more narrow slits in the medulla and lower pons; they may or may not communicate with the fourth ventricle. The symptoms include dysphagia and dysarthria from involvement of the nucleus ambiguus, with consequent unilateral weakness of the palate, pharynx, and larynx; wasting and weakness of one side of the tongue; loss of pain and temperature sensibility in the central portion of one side of the face from implication of the descending root of the trigeminal nerve; vertigo, with or without unsteadiness of gait from interference with vestibular-cerebellar connections; nystagmus; and long tract signs, which sometimes result from an associated syrinx of the cervical cord.

DIAGNOSIS. The onset in adult life, the presence of other congenital defects, the dissociated sensory loss of segmental distribution, and the vegetative and trophic disturbances are characteristic. Nevertheless, at the time the patient first seeks advice, the diagnosis can be difficult. Both extramedullary and intramedullary *tumors* can cause localized muscular atrophy and segmental sensory loss, but with tumors progression is more rapid, root pain is common, trophic disorders are infrequent because there is insufficient time for them to develop, a rise of protein in the spinal fluid usually occurs early in the disease, and myelography discloses either compression or widening of the cord. In syringomyelia, the myelogram remains normal for several years. *Cervical spondylosis* can produce wasting of muscles in the upper limb, and long tract signs, but root pain is common, gross segmental sensory impairment at the level of the lesion is unusual, and the diagnosis can be confirmed by myelography.

Cervical ribs can give rise to localized atrophy of the small muscles of the hand and sensory impairment, with or without evidence of subclavian arterial compression, and since accessory ribs are common in syringomyelia, confusion can occur. However, sensory loss in cases of cervical rib is usually limited to the ulnar side of the hand and forearm, touch is more affected than pain, the tendon reflexes in the arm are not affected, and long tract signs are absent.

Ulnar palsy gives rise to localized weakness of the interossei and the median two lumbricales, but sensory impairment is relatively slight, and touch is involved as well as pain; the nerve is usually tender behind the elbow.

Leprosy can produce sensory loss, wasting of the muscles in the upper limbs, and ulceration of the fingers, but there is thickening of the median, ulnar, and radial nerves and of the brachial plexus, and there may be patches of depigmentation on the trunk.

Syphilis can mimic syringomyelia in two ways. In hypertrophic cervical pachymeningitis (which is rare), there may be loss of sensibility, atrophy, and weakness of the upper limbs and pyramidal signs in the legs, but there will be myelographic evidence of subarachnoid block, and the serology will be positive; moreover, the progress of the disease is more rapid than is the case in syringomyelia. Secondly, gumma of the cord can give rise to the signs of an intramedullary tumor, but here again deterioration is rapid, and the serology is positive.

Amyotrophic lateral sclerosis is not readily confused with syringomyelia because it does not cause paresthesias or sensory loss.

Hematomyelia has an abrupt onset, which distinguishes it from syringomyelia; the residual signs may resemble the latter, but usually they do not progress.

TREATMENT. Surgical correction of platybasia, Arnold-Chiari malformations, and adhesive arachnoiditis around the medulla has led to clinical improvement in a number of cases. In the author's experience, radiation therapy to the affected portions of the cord has proved singularly ineffective.

CRANIOSTENOSIS

DEFINITION. Premature union of one or more cranial sutures gives rise

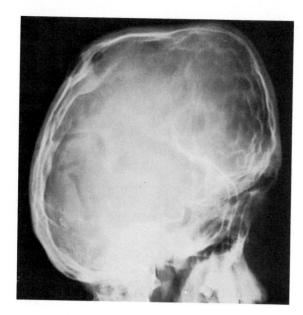

Figure 9–6.   Craniostenosis;   tower-skull.
(Courtesy of Dr. R. H. Chamberlain.)

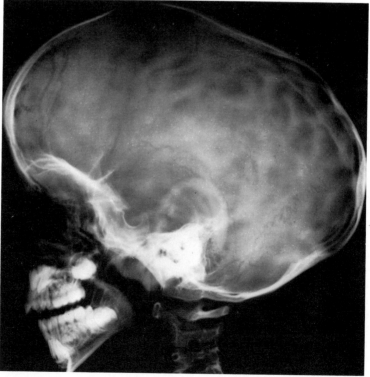

Figure 9–7.   Scaphocephaly and craniostenosis in child aged 35 months. The sagittal and coronal sutures appear fused. (Courtesy of Dr. James Bull.)

to malformation of the head and in some cases to an increase of intracranial pressure.[21]

ETIOLOGY. These conditions are sometimes familial, and may be associated with defects of development elsewhere in the body.

PATHOLOGY. At birth, the bones of the vault are still separated, but during the second six months of life, their margins begin to interlock. The posterior fontanelle closes in the second month, and the anterior fontanelle about the middle of the second year. The sutures do not normally begin to disappear until the fourth decade, and if premature synostosis occurs during infancy or childhood, the intracranial pressure is raised by the growing brain, and the skull will bulge in areas not affected by the closure of the sources. The ultimate shape of the head will then depend on which sutures are affected.

CLINICAL FEATURES

Oxycephaly. In this form, the coronal and sagittal sutures close, with the result that the skull is high, and slopes upward to a pointed vertex. The condition may be apparent in the first few weeks of life or may delay its appearance for some years. The skull is high, narrow, and pointed. The orbits are shallow, and exophthalmos is the rule. External strabismus is common. As time goes on, the headaches from increased intracranial pressure appear, and papilledema occurs. Optic atrophy with blindness is common but not invariable. Deafness, anosmia, and mental defect are common, and syndactyly is not infrequent. Radiographs reveal the typical pointed skull with synostosis of sutures, increased depth of the middle and posterior fossae, and increased digital markings in the vault. Minor degrees of oxycephaly do not interfere with normal life, but early death is to be anticipated in untreated cases.

Acrobrachycephaly. In this form, the head is high and pointed but it is wide at the base, and pressure symptoms are less common than with oxycephaly.

Scaphocephaly. This condition results from synostosis of the sagittal suture, which allows the skull to grow in length and height but not in breadth. Exophthalmos, squint, and optic atrophy occur, but in mild cases, the unusual shape of the head may be the only abnormality.

Surgical measures for the prevention of synostosis and the relief of raised intracranial pressure are sometimes successful, provided they are carried out before the age of 2 years. Exceptionally, improvement has followed operation in children up to the age of 8 years.

BASILAR IMPRESSION
(Platybasia)

The essential feature of this rare condition is upward displacement of the basilar and condylar portions of the occipital bone, with consequent reduction in size of the posterior fossa.[20, 26, 31] In severe cases, the cerebellar tonsils and the lower part of the medulla come to lie within the foramen magnum, and in consequence the lower cranial nerves are angulated and compressed en route to their point of exit from the posterior fossa. Platybasia is usually congenital in origin and is often associated with other malformations, notably stenosis of the foramen magnum, the Arnold-Chiari malformation, or fusion of two or more of the cervical vertebrae (Klippel-Feil syndrome). Familial incidence has been described.[4] Basilar impressions can also occur as a result of softening of the occipital bone in osteogenesis imperfecta, Paget's disease, rickets, and hyperparathyroidism.

CLINICAL FEATURES. The neck appears shortened and may be stiff. Neurological symptoms are absent in some cases; when present, they usually appear for the first time in early adult life, but they may start in childhood. When the condition results from Paget's disease, the onset usually occurs after the age of 50.

Compression of the cerebellum leads to nystagmus and cerebellar ataxia, with or without paralysis of the lower cranial nerves (e.g., wasting of the tongue on one or both sides). Interference with the outflow of the spinal fluid from the fourth ventricle may produce internal hydrocephalus, with symptoms and signs of raised intracranial pressure. In some cases, the odontoid process projects into the spinal canal, in which event the cerebellar ataxia is complicated by progressive spastic weakness of all four limbs, thus mimicking a tumor of the foramen magnum. A syrinx may develop in the upper part of the cord or in the medulla.

Occipital headache and pain in the upper part of the neck are common, and pain is sometimes referred to the face on one side, presumably as a result of irritation of the descending root of the trigeminal nerve.

The vertebral artery may be compressed as it passes through the foramen magnum, especially when the patient turns the head to one side, and this can give rise to transient symptoms of vertebral basilar insufficiency.

DIAGNOSIS. The effects of basilar impression may be mistaken for a tumor in the posterior fossa or at the foramen magnum. Occipito-nuchal pain and stiffness of the neck may suggest cervical spondylosis in middle-aged subjects. The diagnosis is made by x-ray.[4] A line drawn from the back of the hard palate to the posterior lip of the foramen magnum (Chamberlain's line) should lie above the atlas and axis, but in basilar impression, the odontoid process and part of the axis lie above the line.

CONGENITAL DEFECTS OF THE SPINE AND SPINAL CORD

Defective closure of the neural tube and vertebral canal in early fetal life leads to a graduated series of congenital abnormalities of the spine, spinal cord, and cauda equina.[29] The union of the vertebral arches starts in the mid-dorsal region and spreads up and down, being complete from the first cervical to the fourth sacral by the eleventh week. Defective closure of the arches is common in the lumbar and lumbosacral region, less so in the cervical region, and comparatively rare in the thoracic spine.

The simplest type is *spina bifida occulta*, which can be found at any level of the spinal column and is usually asymptomatic because the cord is not involved. Less often, it is associated with a *meningocele* (a hernia of the meninges, which appears as a rounded lump on the back), or there may be a narrow sinus leading onto the skin. The third degree of abnormality is spina bifida with a meningocele that contains either the cord or the cauda equina, depending on its site—a *meningomyelocele*. Finally, in complete *rachischisis*, neither the neural tube nor the vertebral canal closes completely, and the cord is exposed for several segments, appearing as a red ribbon lying at the bottom of a groove in the skin of the back. In *diastematomyelia*,[11] there is a cleft in the midline of the cord over a segment or two; each half is surrounded by a dural sac and is separated from its fellow by a bony septum. Spina bifida is usually present. The legs are spastic or weak. The bony septum may be seen on roentgenographic examination, and myelography discloses two separate streams of dye in the affected area.

Spina Bifida

SPINA BIFIDA OCCULTA. This lesion is very common in the lumbar region and is seldom associated with neurological symptoms. The site may be marked by a dimple, a nevus, or a deposition of fat in the overlying skin. A band of fibrous tissue may extend from the skin to the cord; this tethers the cord, and may cause symptoms as the child grows older, because the spinal column elongates faster than the spinal cord. For example, there may be complaints of pain in the back and of paresthesias in the legs induced by stooping. In other cases, there is an associated intradural lipoma or dermoid, which may produce progressive sphincter disturbances and vasomotor changes in the feet in older children and young adults. This may progress to weakness and sensory loss in the legs. In yet other cases, progressive motor, sensory, reflex, vasomotor, and trophic disturbances may occur in the legs in a previously normal child as a result of gliosis in the cord, a condition resembling but not identical to syringomyelia. Another occasional association of spina bifida occulta is a narrow sinus, lined with stratified epithelium, which extends from the skin in the midline down to the meninges. This can occur at any level, but it is usually found in the lumbosacral region. The opening on the skin is marked as a rule by a dimple or a tuft of hairy, pigmented skin. Infection of the sinus is an occasional cause of meningitis in children. Hydrocephalus is less common with isolated spina bifida occulta than it is with the more severe types of incomplete closure.

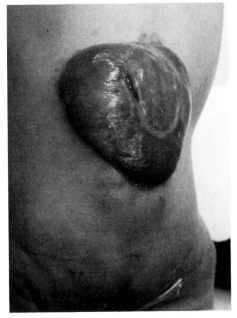

Figure 9-8. Meningomyelocele. (Courtesy of Children's Hospital of Philadelphia.)

SPINA BIFIDA WITH MENINGOCELE. This is usually found in the lower lumbar region and less often in the neck. Hydrocephalus is common, and there may be congenital deformities in other parts of the body, but the spinal cord is often spared, and any neurological disturbances are then results of the associated hydrocephalus. A meningocele may be the only abnormality present; if the walls are thin, it is a danger to life because of the liability to ulceration with consequent ascending meningitis, and it should be removed if it is certain that hydrocephalus is not present.

MENINGOMYELOCELE. This is found in the lumbar region, involving the cauda equina, and in the neck, involving the cervical cord (Fig. 9-8). It is sometimes associated with the Arnold-Chiari malformation. The sac is partly translucent, and there is often evidence of hydrocephalus. In some cases, there is no local lump to be seen. In the lumbar form, there is paralysis and atrophy of the legs, usually below the knee. Contractures are common, with consequent deformities of the feet. The tendon reflexes are depressed or absent. Sensory loss is usually present, but it is seldom severe, and it is symmetrical and radicular in distribution. Trophic disturbances—ulcers, thickening of the toenails, and coldness of the skin—are the rule when sensation is much affected. Sphincter disturbances are common. Rarely, incontinence constitutes the entire disability. When the defect is in the upper cervical region, the arms and legs are spastic, and there may be symmetrical loss of pain and temperature sensibility in the cervical dermatomes. Loss of proprioception from involvement of the posterior column can give rise to sensory ataxia. Hydrocephalus is common. When cerebellar ataxia and nystagmus are present, they result from an associated Arnold-Chiari malformation.

The course of the condition is variable; severely incapacitated patients die in infancy, but those with milder types, unassociated with hydrocephalus, may survive and lead useful lives. Occasionally the disability, present since early life, starts to progress in later childhood, and presents a picture similar to that of syringomyelia, with atrophic paralysis of the arms, spastic weakness of the legs, and dissociated sensory loss over the cervical and dorsal segments.

Treatment. Spina bifida occulta requires no treatment unless it is associated with either a skin sinus or a meningocele. A patent skin sinus is a threat to life, owing to the danger of meningitis, and should be closed. A meningocele can be very much in the way, and is liable to ulceration and rupture, with subsequent infection of the meninges. Surgical closure of the sac is sometimes (but not invariably) followed by the development of hydrocephalus or by an increase in the size of an already enlarged skull. This is likely to occur when the spinal deformity is accompanied by the Arnold-Chiari malformation, in which condition the cerebrospinal fluid reaches the spinal cord but cannot circulate over the convexity of the hemispheres; in such cases, the meningocele probably helps in the absorption of spinal fluid, and its removal is a mistake, unless something is also done to restore the free circulation of the fluid over the convexity of the brain. The ultimate prognosis depends largely upon the control of infection in the urinary tract. Culp and his colleagues [10] advise implantation of the ureters into the ileum as the most effective way of dealing with a neurogenic bladder in these cases.

CONGENITAL AFFECTIONS OF EYE AND EAR

Color blindness. Total color blindness is rare, and is usually associated with poor visual acuity, photophobia, and optic nystagmus. Red-green blindness is common; it is seldom discovered until the child starts to use crayons, and may escape notice until the patient is exposed to routine tests for color vision, such as are carried out for intending drivers, seamen, and service personnel.

Many persons with red-green blindness can recognize traffic lights because they contain elements of yellow and blue. Isolated yellow-blue blindness is very rare indeed. It is useful to remember that apparent field defects discovered during perimetry with colored objects may be the result of color blindness and not of disease of the visual pathways. Acquired color blindness occurs as a result of lesions of the retina, optic nerve, and chiasm, and the patient is aware of a deterioration of vision.

Congenital night blindness. This is a rare and often hereditary disorder in which vision is good by day and poor by night. It also occurs with retinitis pigmentosa, vitamin A deficiency, opacity of the peripheral parts of the lens, and severe papilledema. The reverse condition, in which vision is better by night than by day, usually stems from diseases affecting central vision: opacities of the center of the lens, macular lesions, and retrobulbar neuritis.

Congenital optic atrophy. This condition is rare as an isolated defect, but it is less uncommon as an association with cerebral palsy. Congenital blindness sometimes results from absence of the optic nerves. Gross defects of central vision, either unilateral or bilateral, can be caused by congenital dysplasia of the maculae and by macular coloboma. Congenital lesions of the occipital cortex are usually associated with other cerebral defects; the discs may appear normal or pale, and the light reflex is present.

Congenital word blindness and mirror writing. Difficulty in learning the symbols of written speech, despite normal intelligence and normal visual acuity, is a fairly common congenital disability, which probably depends on bilateral maldevelopment of the cortex in the region of the angular gyrus. It may occur sporadically or in several members of one family, and is sometimes hereditary. The child is usually left-handed and left-eyed, and has a natural tendency to write backwards and to reverse the letters. Mirror writing is also seen from time to time in adults suffering from right hemiplegia when attempting to write with the left hand, and with congenital diplegia and circumscribed lesions of the angular gyrus of the dominant hemisphere. Difficulty in reading and writing associated with defective calculation, constructional dyspraxia, finger agnosia, and right-left disorientation has been described by Benson and Geschwind[2] as a developmental Gerstmann syndrome in two otherwise normal adolescents.

Early recognition of word blindness is important. Failure to learn to read and write, or relative deficiency in these subjects in otherwise normal children, may result from (1) reduced visual acuity; (2) muscle imbalance in left-eyed children, who have difficulty with the left-to-right movements required in reading; (3) mental deficiency; (4) word blindness, relative or absolute, with or without mirror writing. If the nature of the difficulty is not appreciated by teacher and parents, and appropriate measures are not instituted, the child is handicapped at school and is apt to become discouraged, lazy, or aggressive. The defect can usually be overcome by individual tuition.

CONGENITAL DEFECTS OF THE THIRD, FOURTH, AND SIXTH NERVES. These include: (1) ptosis and (2) complete paralysis of the third or sixth nerve — rarely, the fourth — in which the child tilts the head to avoid diplopia; this type of torticollis differs from that which is produced by birth injury to the sternomastoid in that there is no contracture and the mobility of the neck is normal.

PUPILLARY ABNORMALITIES. These include structural abnormalities of the iris, inequality of pupils, and occasionally complete absence of the reflexes to light and convergence, a condition distinct from the tonic pupil (p. 96).

THE FACIAL NERVE. Bilateral agenesis of the seventh nuclei causes facial diplegia.[19] The face is mask-like, the skin shiny, and the eyes cannot be closed. It is often associated with agenesis of the adjacent sixth nuclei, giving rise to paralysis of the external rectus muscles. Unilateral facial paralysis in infants is usually due to birth injury.

CONGENITAL DEAFNESS. Intellectual development depends on the integrity of individual functions of the brain — vision, hearing, memory, powers of association, and so on. Absence of any one function necessarily impedes the whole to some extent. Congenital deafness isolates the child in a silent world and prevents the acquisition of speech. Consequently, intellectual development which is dependent on hearing is reduced, but mental life in other fields is less affected. It is encountered (1) as a familial condition caused by maldevelopment of the internal ear; (2) as a result of maternal rubella in the first three months of pregnancy; (3) in congenital syphilis; (4) in cretinism; (5) in kernicterus. Whatever the cause, the infant is unresponsive to noises and to the mother's voice and does not learn to speak; mental development is slow, and behavior disorders may occur. In some cases, the deafness is confined to high tones, with the result that only certain components of speech are inaudible. The child learns to use the fragments he can hear, and substitutes sounds of his own invention for the rest. The result — one form of idioglossia — is a personal language which may be intelligible to mother or nurse. Some deafmutes show a complete absence of vestibular function, but walk steadily because of a compensatory acuity of vision and proprioception; however, they are completely disoriented under water, when both proprioception and vision are at a discount, and should not be allowed to swim except under supervision. Much can be done for deaf children by speech therapy.

CONGENITAL AUDITORY APHASIA (CONGENITAL WORD DEAFNESS). In this disorder, hearing is intact, but there is inability to understand the significance of the spoken word, with consequent failure to speak properly because the child cannot appreciate and correct his own mistakes (see Chap. 3). He will either not attempt to speak at all, or will develop a personal language. This can be corrected to some extent by speech therapy, provided that intelligence and emotional stability are adequate.

REFERENCES

1. Alpers, B. J.: Progressive cerebral degeneration of infancy. *J. Nerv. Ment. Dis.* 130:442, 1960.
2. Benson, D. F., and Geschwind, N.: Developmental Gerstmann syndrome. *Neurology* 20: 293, 1969.
3. Brandon, M. W. G., Kirman, B. H., and Williams, C. E.: Microcephaly. *J. Ment. Sci.* 105:721, 1959.
4. Bull, J. W. D., Nixon, W. L. B., and Pratt, R. T. C.: Radiological criteria of familial occurrence of primary basilar impression. *Brain* 78:229, 1955.
5. Clementis, S. D.: Minimal brain dysfunction in children. *U. S. Public Health Service Publication, No. 1415,* 1966.
6. Cooper, I. S.: Relief of juvenile involuntary movement disorders by chemopallidectomy. *J.A.M.A.* 164:1297, 1957.
7. Crome, L., Kirman, B. H., and Marrs, M.: Rhesus incompatibility and mental deficiency. *Brain* 78:514, 1958.
8. Crothers, B., and Paine, R. S.: *The Natural History of Cerebral Palsy.* Harvard University Press, Cambridge, Mass., 1960.
9. Courville, C. B.: *Cerebral Palsy.* San Lucas Press, Los Angeles, 1954.
10. Culp, D. A., Bekhrab, A., and Flocks, R. H.: Urological management of the meningomyelocele patient. *J.A.M.A.* 213:753, 1970.
11. Dale, A. J. D.: Diastomyelia. *Arch. Neurol.* 20:309, 1969.
12. Deaver, G. G.: *Rehabilitation of the Handicapped Child.* Monograph IX. Institute of Physical Medicine and Rehabilitation, New York University-Bellevue Medical Center, New York, 1955.
13. DeBarros, M. C., Farias, W., Atide, L., and Lins, S.: Basilar impression and the Arnold-Chiari malformation. *J. Neurol. Neurosurg. Psychiat.* 31:596, 1968.
14. Ford, F. R.: *Diseases of the Nervous System in Infancy, Childhood, and Adolescence.* 4th Ed. Charles C Thomas, Springfield, Ill., 1960.
15. Gardner, W. J.: Hydrodynamic mechanism of syringomyelia: Its relationship to myelocele. *J. Neurol. Neurosurg. Psychiat.* 28:247, 1965.
16. Gardner, W. J., Abdullah, A. F., and McCormack, L. J.: The varying expressions of embryonal atresia of the 4th ventricle in adults. *J. Neurosurg.* 14:591, 1957.
17. Gerrard, J.: Kernicterus. *Brain* 75:526, 1952.
18. Hall, G. S.: Ocular manifestations of tuberose sclerosis. *Quart. J. Med.* 15:209, 1946.
19. Henderson, J. L.: The congenital facial diplegia syndrome: Clinical features, pathology, and etiology. *Brain* 62:381, 1939.
20. Hurwitz, L. T., and McSwiney, R. R.: Basilar impression of the skull. *Brain* 73:405, 1950.
21. Ingraham, F. D., Alexander, E., and Matson, D. D.: Clinical studies in craniostenosis: Analysis of 50 cases and description of method of surgical treatment. *Surgery* 24:518, 1948.
22. Gellis, S. S., Feingold, M., and Rutman, J. Y.: *Atlas of Mental Retardation Syndromes.* U. S. Department of Health, Education, and Welfare, U. S. Government Printing Office, Washington, D.C., 1968.
23. Kirman, B. H.: Clinical Aspects of Retardation. In *Mental Retardation. An Annual Review.* Edited by Wortis, J., Grune and Stratton, New York, 1970.
24. Laurence, K. M.: The natural history of hydrocephalus. *Lancet* 2:1152, 1958.
25. Lichtenstein, B. W.: Cervical syringomyelia and syringomyelia-like states associated with Arnold-Chiari malformation and platybasia. *Arch. Neurol. Psychiat.* 48:879, 1943.
26. List, C. F.: Neurologic syndromes accompanying developmental anomalies of the occipital bone, atlas and axis. *Arch. Neurol. Psychiat.* 44:577, 1941.
27. Matson, D. D.: Intracranial hemorrhage in infancy and childhood. *Res. Pub. Assn. Res. Nerv. Ment. Dis.* 34:59, 1959.
28. Navarrete, V. M., Rojas, C. E., Alger, C. R., and Pamiagua, H. E.: Subsequent diabetes in mothers delivered of a malformed infant. *Lancet* 2:993, 1970.
29. Norman, R. M.: Malformation of the nervous system, birth injury, and diseases of early life. *Neuropathology.* Edward Arnold, Publisher, London, 1958, Chap. 5.
30. Norman, R. M., Sandifer, P. H., Evans, E. S., and Tizard, J. P. M.: Discussion on infantile cerebral palsies. *Proc. Roy. Soc. Med.* 46:627, 1953.
31. O'Connell, J. E. A., and Turner, J. W. A.: Basilar impression of the skull, *Brain* 73:405, 1950.
32. Odell, G. B., Storey, G. N. B., and Rosenberg, L. A.: Studies in Kernicterus. III. The saturation of serum proteins with bilirubin during neonatal life and its relationship to brain damage at five years. *J. Pediatrics* 76:12, 1970.
33. Rabe, E. F.: Hypotonic infant. *J. Ped.* 64:422, 1964.
34. Rosenthal, I. M., Zimmerman, H. J., and Hardy, N.: Congenital nonhemolytic jaundice with disease of the central nervous system. *Pediatrics* 18:378, 1956.
35. Rubenstein, H. S., and Freeman, W.: Cerebellar agenesis. *J. Nerv. Ment. Dis.* 92:489, 1940.
36. Russell, D. S.: Observations on the pathology of hydrocephalus. Medical Research Council Special Report, Series 265, H. M. Stationery Office, London, 1949.

37. Sjögren, T.: Hereditary congenital spinocerebellar ataxia accompanied by congenital cataract and oligophrenia. *Confin. Neurol.* (Basel) 10:293, 1950.

38. Solomon, G. E., Hilal, S. K., Gold, A. P., and Carter, S.: Natural history of acute hemiplegia of childhood. *Brain* 93:107, 1970.

39. Stein, Z. A., and Kassab, H.: Nutrition. *Mental Retardation: An Annual Review.* Edited by Wortis, J., Grune and Stratton, New York, 1970.

40. Towbin, A.: *The Pathology of Cerebral Palsy.* Charles C Thomas, Springfield, Ill., 1960.

41. Wilson, P. J. E.: Cerebral hemispherectomy for infantile hemiplegia. *Brain* 93:147, 1970.

42. Wolf, A., and Cowen, D.: The cerebral atrophies and encephalomalacias of infancy and childhood. *Res. Pub. Assn. Res. Nerv. Ment. Dis.* 34:199, 1954.

CHAPTER TEN

Hydrocephalus

Terminology

The term "hydrocephalus" is customarily used to mean dilatation of the ventricles occurring as a result of obstruction to the flow of the cerebrospinal fluid. In the past, it was sometimes applied to the general rise of intracranial pressure which can result from thrombosis of the dural venous sinuses, as in "otitic" hydrocephalus.

An obstructive internal hydrocephalus is one in which the cerebrospinal fluid is pent up within the ventricular system by an obstruction in the third ventricle, sylvian aqueduct, or fourth ventricle. When this occurs before the skull sutures have joined, the head enlarges; in older patients, the head does not enlarge and the hydrocephalus is spoken of as "occult." Internal hydrocephalus can also result from compression of the third ventricle or brainstem by tumors in the subarachnoid space, or by a pressure cone. There is evidence that it can also be caused by compression of the third ventricle by an elongated and dilated basilar artery.[3]

The term "communicating hydrocephalus" is applied to the enlargement of the ventricles and sylvian aqueduct which occurs when the fluid can get out of the fourth ventricle, but cannot reach the sites from which it is absorbed because of leptomeningeal adhesions in the basal cisterns.[10]

The Dynamics of Hydrocephalus.[2,4,7,13,19] Despite much investigation, arguments continue as to the formation, flow, and absorption of the cerebrospinal fluid, as is made clear in Davison's monograph (1967).[4] While it is generally agreed that the choroid plexuses secrete cerebrospinal fluid, there is evidence that these are not the only source. Studies in man and animals disclose that in hydrocephalus, at any rate, only about 60 per cent of the fluid is provided by the choroid plexuses, the remainder coming from the ventricular walls, the convexity of the brain, and the spinal subarachnoid space. This is consistent with the fact that there are considerable differences in the protein and ion content of fluid recovered from the ventricles, the basal cisterns and the lumbar subarachnoid space. Moreover, fluid continues to collect in the ventricles, albeit in reduced amount, after complete surgical removal of the choroid plexus.

The present view of the flow pattern of the cerebrospinal fluid is that when it leaves the fourth ventricle, it passes through the complex system of basal cisterns and ultimately reaches the convexity of the cerebral hemispheres. It is absorbed by the arachnoidal granulations and villi which project into all the dural venous sinuses. In addition, structures similar to arachnoid villi penetrate some of the dural venous sinuses around the emerging spinal nerve roots,[5, 21] and it is supposed that this provides a second pathway for the absorption of cerebrospinal fluid.

The normal direction of flow can be changed under certain circumstances. Thus, in the presence of communicating hydrocephalus, radioactive tracers injected into the lumbar sac appear in the ventricles within three hours, which is too rapid to be explained by simple diffusion. In these cases, there must be two-way traffic, with a net flow outwards from the ventricles into the subarachnoid space.

As mentioned above, some of the intraventricular cerebrospinal fluid comes from the ependyma. In addition, the ependyma can absorb fluid and in the presence of internal hydrocephalus this absorption is increased.[2, 12] It has been suggested that this enhanced absorption may be due, in part at least, to the ruptures which occur in the ependyma when it is stretched by the enlargement of the ventricles.[12, 19] The ependyma can also absorb proteins and smaller molecules. This circumstance has been exploited by Feldberg[6] and others in studying the behavioral responses of animals to the intraventricular injection of naturally occurring compounds and synthetic drugs. Depending on the substance used, the procedure can give rise not only to autonomic and motor disturbances but also to a wide spectrum of behavioral symptoms, including agitation, sham rage, hostility, apprehension, apathy, stupor, catatonia, and hallucinations. At the time of writing, no attention has been paid to the possibility that the mental symptoms and disturbance of behavior which are so often encountered in paraventricular tumors and internal hydrocephalus may be due, in part at least, to the absorption by the ependyma of polypeptides and other breakdown products which seep into the ventricles. Substances which are usually excluded from the cerebrospinal fluid by the blood–cerebrospinal fluid barrier may also pass into the ventricular fluid under these circumstances.

The enlargement of the ventricles seen in hydrocephalus is usually attributed to the elevated intraventricular pressure, and it has been suggested that the process is aggravated by the dilatation of the choroid plexuses which occurs

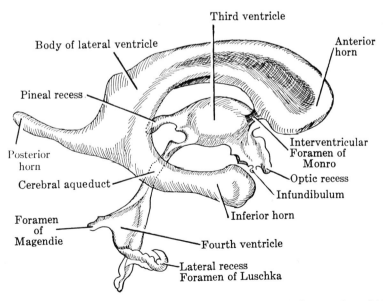

Figure 10–1. Drawing of a cast of the ventricular cavities. (From Wechsler, I.: *Clinical Neurology.* 9th Ed. W. B. Saunders Co., Philadelphia, 1963; after Retzius.)

with each arterial pulse beat. When there is free egress for cerebrospinal fluid from the ventricles, a drop of iodized oil placed in the sylvian aqueduct can be seen to move to and fro with each pulse, and it is possible that if the fluid cannot be ejected because of an obstruction, the pulsating pressure on the ventricular walls may contribute to their dilatation.

An important departure from conventional thinking on the relationship between ventricular pressure and enlargement of the ventricles was introduced by Adams and his associates,[1] who called attention to the fact that, in communicating hydrocephalus, the ventricles may continue to enlarge although the cerebrospinal fluid pressure is within normal limits. They point out that this is in accordance with Pascal's law for enclosed fluids, which states that the force on the walls of a container is equal to the product of the pressure of the fluid and the area of the wall. The larger the area, the smaller the pressure required to distend the container. Applied to the ventricular system, it means that a pressure of, for instance, 120 mm. Hg, may be well tolerated in ventricles of normal size but will prove excessive in enlarged ventricles. This law also explains why the lateral ventricles, which are large, usually expand to a greater degree than the smaller third and fourth ventricles, and why the frontal horns expand more than the smaller temporal horns. *The theory leaves unresolved the question of what caused the initial dilatation of the ventricular system*, but the validity of the concept is supported by the fact that in normal pressure hydrocephalus the symptoms often recede rapidly following shunting procedures, as was first reported by Foltz and Ward in 1956.[6a]

The cerebral circulation is reduced in both high-pressure and normal-pressure hydrocephalus,[7, 8] and is improved by atrioventricular shunting.[9] It is supposed that clinical improvement following this procedure is due, in part at least, to the increased blood flow.

Etiology of Hydrocephalus. For practical purposes, hydrocephalus is always the result of obstruction to the cerebrospinal fluid pathways, either within the brain or around the basal cisterns. An exception is the raised intracranial pressure which occurs as a result of thrombosis[20] or neoplastic infiltration[14] of the dural venous sinuses, but it is questionable whether the term hydrocephalus should apply to these conditions. It has been suspected that overproduction of cerebrospinal fluid by the choroid plexuses may contribute to hydrocephalus, but this is unproved.

The causes of obstructive internal hydrocephalus include developmental abnormalities involving the sylvian aqueduct and the fourth ventricle[22]; these are described later in this chapter. Meningitis can produce either internal or communicating hydrocephalus, and this can happen in the acute phase of the illness, immediately after the acute stage (as in posterior basic meningitis of children, and tuberculous meningitis) or after an interval. It can occur in bacterial meningitis, meningovascular syphilis, fungal meningitis, subarachnoid hemorrhage,[11] chemical meningitis, and carcinomatous "meningitis." It is not known whether viral infections can cause a delayed-onset hydrocephalus from leptomeningeal adhesions around the basal cisterns. Horrax and others have speculated whether influenza-like illnesses could be responsible for sporadic cases of posterior fossa arachnoiditis,[10] in which there is no previous history of meningitis, head injury, subarachnoid hemorrhage or other disease. Intrauterine infection, including toxoplasmosis and cytomegalic inclusion disease, can be responsible for infantile hydrocephalus.

Tumors in or adjacent to the ventricles and sylvian aqueduct are an important source of internal hydrocephalus at all ages from infancy on. Tumors can also produce internal hydrocephalus by compressing the brain from outside; this is particularly likely to occur with tumors arising in the region of the pituitary, the cerebellopontine angle, and the foramen magnum. Inflammatory granulomata arising either within the brain substance or in the subarachnoid space can mimic neoplasms in this respect.

Subarachnoid hemorrhage from an aneurysm[11] and from head injury will occasionally give rise to a communicating hydrocephalus shortly after the main event,[6a] but progressive disability immediately following subarachnoid hemorrhage may also be due to continued bleeding or to slowly spreading arterial spasm. Occasionally, a communicating hydrocephalus arises weeks, months, or even years after a subarachnoid hemorrhage, and at operation leptomeningeal adhesions containing hemosiderin are found around the base. Rarely, a large unruptured aneurysm, strategically situated, produces internal hydrocephalus. A recent report suggests that chronic adult hydrocephalus can be caused by displacement of the floor of the third ventricle by an elongated basilar artery;[3] the author has seen a similar case, whose symptoms were largely relieved by a shunt.

Leptomeningeal adhesions around the basal cisterns, commonly spoken of as chronic arachnoiditis, can give rise to a communicating hydrocephalus with the symptoms and signs of raised intracranial pressure, and it is also thought to be one cause of normal-pressure hydrocephalus with dementia.

The role of hydrocephalus in infections and tumors is discussed under appropriate headings elsewhere in this book. The following account is limited to two syndromes—hydrocephalus in early life, and normal-pressure hydrocephalus with dementia in adults.

Congenital Hydrocephalus

Enlargement of the head by progressive accumulation of cerebrospinal fluid in the ventricles can be caused by congenital malformations or by acquired disease. The congenital type may arise before birth, producing dystocia, or it may be noticed within days, weeks, or months of birth. It is usually sporadic, but familial incidence is not unknown.

Etiology. Developmental anomalies are usually to blame and are commonly to be found in the sylvian aqueduct, which may be narrowed or broken up into a number of small and inadequate

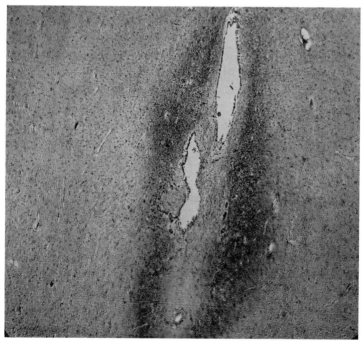

Figure 10–2. Forking of the aqueduct in a patient with congenital hydrocephalus. (Courtesy of Department of Neuropathology, Philadelphia General Hospital.)

channels, described by Russell as "forking" of the aqueduct (Fig. 10–2). In other cases, it may be occluded by a transverse septum. A less common cause is the Arnold-Chiari malformation in which the foramen magnum and upper cervical canal are occupied by extensions of the medulla and cerebellum, with the result that the cerebrospinal fluid can gain egress to the spinal subarachnoid space but not to the basal cisterns or to the convexity of the hemispheres. Any form of developmental hydrocephalus may be accompanied by other malformations, notably spina bifida with or without a meningocele or meningomyelocele, encephalocele, syringomyelia, hydromyelia, microgyria, macrogyria, absence of the corpus callosum, fusion of the hemispheres, absence of the cerebellar vermis, porencephaly, etc. In the Dandy-Walker syndrome, the escape of spinal fluid from the fourth ventricle is prevented by a membrane; there is maldevelopment of the flocculus and vermis, and the fourth ventricle is ballooned to such an extent that the posterior fossa is enlarged.

Hydrocephalus in infants may also be due to acquired disease. We are not here concerned with hydrocephalus occurring during the course of basal meningitis, dural sinus thrombosis, or intracranial tumor, but with its appearance as the main pathological event. The child may have appeared normal at birth, though this need not apply to hydrocephalus resulting from in utero infection by cytomegalic inclusion disease or toxoplasmosis. In other cases, the aqueduct is narrowed and distorted by an overgrowth of subependymal neuroglia and this process may spread to the ventricular ependyma. The outcome is a slowly progressive internal hydrocephalus of the lateral and third ventricles.

Meningeal adhesions can prevent the cerebrospinal fluid from reaching the arachnoid villi, thereby causing a communicating hydrocephalus. Adhesions from subarachnoid hemorrhage due to birth injury are thought to be responsible for some cases. The role of infection, so clear in hydrocephalus occurring during or after outspoken meningitis, is less easy to assess, but it is possible that mild attacks of meningitis and meningoencephalitis can cause leptomeningeal ad-

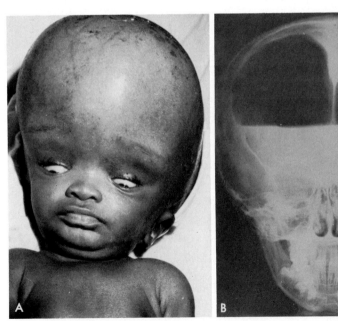

Figure 10–3. Congenital internal hydrocephalus. *A,* Outward appearance. *B,* Ventriculogram. (Courtesy of Children's Hospital of Philadelphia.)

hesions around the base in the absence of a clear-cut clinical history of post-natal infection.

Gross Pathology. One effect of hydrocephalus is to expand the skull. The bones are thin and the convolutional impressions are distinct. The clinoid processes are eroded. If the obstruction is in the roof of the fourth ventricle, the posterior fossa is enlarged. The ventricular system is dilated above the block and the overlying cortical mantle is thinned. The brain often continues to grow while the ventricles are enlarging, and the weight of the brain tissue mass may be greater in some of these children than it is in normal children of the same age [19] (Fig. 10–3).

Clinical Features. Enlargement of the head may be identified during pregnancy, at birth, or within the first few weeks of life.

Symptoms vary; in the mildest form, the head is large, but there are no other symptoms apart from occasional headache. In a well marked case, the head is obviously much too large for the body, and the face by contrast appears small and triangular. The eyes are thrust downwards in their sockets. The hair is thin, the scalp veins are prominent and the sutures are separated. The skull may be felt to pulsate.

The most common neurological symptom is undeveloped legs with spasticity. If a meningomyelocele is also present, the lower limbs are paralyzed, wasted, and cyanosed. In hydrocephalus produced by the Arnold-Chiari malformation, there may be both spasticity and ataxia of the legs.

Papilledema is rare, but strabismus and optic atrophy are common in untreated cases. Convulsions are not uncommon.

Mental retardation is common, but the child's intelligence is sometimes better than might be expected in the presence of such a gross lesion.

Course and Prognosis. In severe cases, death occurs at birth or in early infancy. A few patients appear to achieve a precarious balance between the production and absorption of cerebrospinal fluid; the head ceases to enlarge and they live for many years but are liable to a recurrence of symptoms at any time. Sometimes, in severe cases, ventricular rupture occurs, usually through the lamina terminalis of the third ventricle, and this provides a spontaneous shunt.

Diagnosis. If the head is enlarged at birth or if enlargement becomes apparent after birth, and if it is associated with spinal or other malformation, the condition is easily recognized. The site of the obstruction can be determined by ventriculography and by injecting a dye into the lateral ventricle and looking for it in the urine and the lumbar spinal fluid. It should appear in the spinal fluid in from 2 to 3 minutes and in the urine in 10 to 12 minutes. If the dye is not recovered from the spinal fluid or if its arrival is much delayed, a block in the ventricular system at or about the fourth ventricle is indicated, whereas if it appears in the spinal fluid "on time" and if its excretion in the urine is greatly delayed, the block lies outside the ventricular system.

The head may appear too large for the body in premature infants and in older infants who are suffering from severe malnutrition. True progressive enlargement may occur as a result of a neoplasm within the ventricular system but this can usually be identified by ventriculography.

Treatment. Hydrocephalus is treated by a variety of shunting procedures. The choice of method is controversial,[18,19] and it is sometimes difficult to know whether improvement following the provision of a shunt results from spontaneous arrest of the disease or from the shunt. However, there is a sufficient number of examples of rapid improvement following shunting to justify the procedure in many cases.

Occult Hydrocephalus with Dementia (Normal-Pressure Hydrocephalus in Adults)

In 1956, Foltz and Ward[6a] described patients with hydrocephalus but without increased cerebrospinal fluid pressure who improved after a shunt procedure, and in 1965, Hakim and Adams delineated a syndrome characterized by the insidious development of presenile dementia followed by mild ataxia of gait caused by communicating hydrocephalus in the presence of normal cerebral spinal fluid pressure.[1]

Etiology. In a few cases, there is a history of a subarachnoid hemorrhage,[6a] spinal anesthesia, meningitis, or head injury, but in the majority of cases there is no explanation for the leptomeningeal adhesions around the basal cisterns, which are assumed to be the usual cause of communicating hydrocephalus of this type.[1] It will be remembered that patients with verified arachnoiditis around the optic chiasm and spinal cord are often unable to recall any previous illness which might have been responsible for the condition.

Clinical Features. The condition usually affects people over the age of 50. The onset is insidious, with impairment of memory. At first, the memory loss is more inconvenient than serious, but as time goes on, it eventually interferes with daily life. Names and faces are forgotten, things are mislaid, errors are made in business, and it becomes clear both to the patient and to his friends that the failure of memory is more than can be accounted for by advancing age. Judgment, interest, and attention suffer, and the patient becomes quieter and more pliable. As a rule the social graces are retained and mood swings are uncommon. Eventually, there is a global dementia.

Headaches are rare, and the cranial nerves are not affected. There is no papilledema. There are no motor or sensory symptoms in the upper limbs, but gait gradually becomes slightly unsteady and

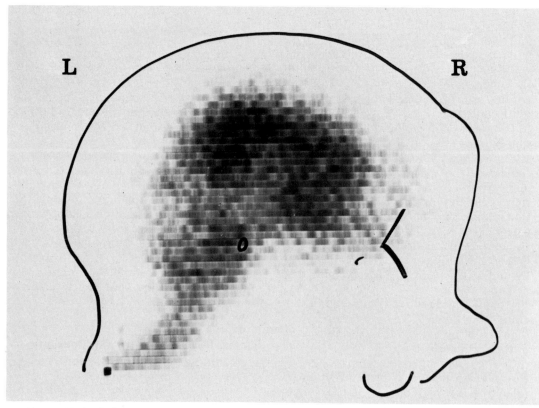

Figure 10–4. Radioisotope cisternogram of a patient with normal-pressure hydrocephalus. At 24 hours, radioactivity was confined to the ventricles.

eventually pyramidal signs may appear in the lower limbs. In some cases, however, the initial difficulty appears to be an ataxia of gait.

Both the mental and the motor symptoms fluctuate, and from time to time relatives may report that the patient seems to be improving a little, but the overall progress is downhill.

Laboratory Aids. The contents and pressure of the spinal fluid are within normal limits. Pneumoencephalography shows a communicating internal hydrocephalus, but very little air collects over the hemispheres or in the sulci. If serum albumin tagged with radioactive iodine is injected by spinal tap, it collects in the ventricular system (Fig. 10–4). It may stay there for as long as 48 hours before it starts to appear over the cerebral hemispheres. The electroencephalogram may be entirely normal, but in some cases it discloses diffuse theta and delta waves.

Differential Diagnosis. Although many conditions can cause progressive dementia in the second half of life, few of them give rise to this picture of a quietly dementing process in a patient who looks and feels well and who displays no disturbance of the pupils, cranial nerves, long tracts, or reflexes. The most important conditions to exclude are the presenile dementias of Alzheimer and of Pick. This does not depend on subtle differences in the characteristics of the dementia but on the demonstration by pneumoencephalography of enlarged ventricles and cortical atrophy. Syphilitic general paresis is excluded by examination of the spinal fluid and blood. Hypothyroidism can give rise to slowing of mind, apathy, and cerebellar ataxia without much in the way of loss of hair, increase in weight or signs of reduced metabolism. Severe involutional depression can cause enough slowing of thought to suggest an organic dementia, but the resemblance is superficial.

Slowly growing deep midline supratentorial tumors occasionally present as a gradually increasing organic dementia over a period of months before giving rise to long tract signs or evidence of raised intracranial pressure, but headache is often present and since these tumors are usually paraventricular in situation, the protein of the spinal fluid is often elevated. A tumor of the third ventricle can cause dementia without headache or papilledema and without the intermittent symptoms characteristic of a colloid cyst.[17] Non-neoplastic aqueductal stenosis may become symptomatic for the first time in adult life.[22] When a patient with presenile dementia displays arterial hypertension or is suffering from diabetes, it is only too easy to ascribe the dementia to cerebrovascular disease, but while it is true that an organic dementia can develop following repeated strokes, it is imprudent to attribute mental dilapidation to arteriosclerosis in the absence of a clear history of one or more cerebrovascular incidents. Jakob-Creutzfeldt disease can start with the features of a progressive dementia before there is any evidence of pyramidal or extrapyramidal disease, but the symptoms are relatively rapid in evolution, and motor symptoms soon appear.

Treatment. Relief of the hydrocephalus by shunting procedures produces rapid and marked improvement in the mental symptoms. However, this treatment has not been in practice long enough for the long-term prognosis to be known.

REFERENCES

1. Adams, R. D., Fisher, C. M., Hakim, S., Ojemann, R. G., and Sweet, W. H.: Symptomatic occult hydrocephalus with "normal" cerebrospinal-fluid pressure. A treatable syndrome. *New Eng. J. Med.* 273:117, 1965.
2. Bering, E. A., and Sato, O.: Hydrocephalus: Changes in formation and absorption of C.S.F. within the cerebral ventricles. *J. Neurosurg.* 20:1050, 1963.
3. Breig, A., Ekbom, K., Greitz, T., and Kugelberg, E.: Hydrocephalus due to elongated basilar artery. *Lancet* 1:879, 1967.
4. Davison, H.: *Physiology of the Cerebrospinal Fluid.* Little, Brown, and Co., Boston, 1967.
5. Elman, R.: Spinal arachnoid granulation with especial reference to the cerebrospinal fluid. *Bull. Johns Hopkins Hosp.* 34:99, 1923.
5a. Everette, James A., Deland, F. H., Hodges, F. J., and Wagner, H. M.: Normal pressure

hydrocephalus. Role of cisternography in diagnosis. *J.A.M.A.* 213:1615, 1970.

6. Feldberg, W.: *A Pharmacological Approach to the Brain from its Inner and Outer Surfaces.* Williams and Wilkins Co., Baltimore, 1963.

6a. Foltz, E. L., and Ward, A. A.: Communicating hydrocephalus from subarachnoid bleeding. *J. Neurosurg.* 13:546, 1956.

7. Greitz, T.: Cerebral blood flow in occult hydrocephalus studied with angiography and the 133 Xenan clearance method. *Acta Radiol.* 8:376, 1969.

8. Greitz, T.: Effect of brain distension on cerebral circulation. *Lancet* 2:863, 1969.

9. Greitz, T., Grepe, A. O. L., Kalmer, S. F., and Lopez, J.: Pre- and postoperative evaluation of cerebral blood flow in low-pressure hydrocephalus. *J. Neurosurg.* 31:644, 1969.

10. Horrax, J.: Generalized cisternal arachnoiditis simulating cerebellar tumor: Its surgical treatment and results. *Arch. Surg.* 9:95, 1929.

11. Kibler, R. F., Couch, R. S. C., and Crompton, M. R.: Hydrocephalus in the adult following spontaneous arachnoid hemorrhage. *Brain* 89:45, 1961.

12. Milhorat, T. H., Clark, R. G., Hammock, M. K., and McGrath, P. P.: Structural, ultrastructural, and permeability changes in the ependyma and surrounding brain favoring equilibration in progressive hydrocephalus. *Arch. Neurol.* 22:397, 1970.

13. Millen, J. W., and Wollam, D. H. M.: *The Anatomy of the Cerebrospinal Fluid.* New York, Oxford University Press, 1962.

14. Mones, R. J.: Increased intracranial pressure due to metastatic disease of venous sinuses. A report of 6 cases. *Neurology* 15:1000, 1965.

15. Oldstone, M. B. A.: Endocrinological aspects of benign intracranial hypertension. *Arch. Neurol.* 15:362, 1966.

16. Ray, B. S., and Dunbar, H. S.: Thrombosis of the dural sinuses as a cause of "pseudotumor cerebri," *Ann. Surg.* 134:376, 1951.

17. Riddoch, G.: Progressive dementia without headache or changes in the optic discs, due to tumors of the third ventricle. *Brain* 59:225, 1936.

18. Scarf, J. E.: Evaluation of treatment of hydrocephalus. *Arch. Neurol.* 14:382, 1966.

19. Shulman, K. (ed.): *Workshop in Hydrocephalus.* Philadelphia, University of Pennsylvania Printing Office, 1965.

20. Symonds, C. P.: Hydrocephalic and focal cerebral symptoms in relation to thrombophlebitis of the dural sinuses and central veins. *Brain* 60:531, 1937.

21. Welch, K., and Pollay, M.: The spinal arachnoid villi of the monkey. *Anat. Rec.* 145:1, 1963.

22. Wilkinson, H. A., Lemay, M., and Drew, J.: Adult aqueductal stenosis. *Arch. Neurol.* 15:643, 1966.

CHAPTER ELEVEN

Metabolic Disorders of the Central Nervous System

This chapter deals with some of the metabolic diseases which affect the *central* nervous system. Metabolic disorders affecting muscle are dealt with in Chapter 19 and those affecting the peripheral nervous system are described in Chapter 20. Metachromatic leukodystrophy is discussed with the demyelinating diseases in Chapter 13.

THE NEURONAL STORAGE DISEASES

In this genetically determined group of diseases, enzymatic defects lead to an excessive accumulation of normal or abnormal substances in nerve cells. Disorders of lipid metabolism are found in Tay-Sachs disease, Gaucher's disease, Niemann-Pick disease, and Hallervorden-Spatz disease.[15] Disorders of carbohydrate metabolism include Hurler's disease and related syndromes,[26] Pompe's disease, and Unverricht-Lafora myoclonic epilepsy.

In Wilson's disease, which is not usually classified as a neuronal storage disease, copper accumulates in the cells of the basal ganglia, liver, Descemet's membrane, and the renal tubules.

The Amaurotic Family Idiocies (Tay-Sachs Disease, Cerebromacular Degeneration)

In 1881, Tay described the characteristic retinal appearances found in the infantile form of this group, and in 1887 Sachs described the clinical and neuropathological features of the disease. As time went on, congenital, late infantile (Bielschowsky), juvenile (Batten), and adult (Kufs) forms were defined. It now seems likely that these variants are not determined by age alone but also by differences in the nature and distribution of the lipids.[6, 38] The most satisfactory method of coming to a diagnosis in atypical cases is brain biopsy, which permits a study of the tissue both by electron microscopy and by histochemistry. In the account which follows, the term "Tay-Sachs disease" refers to the infantile form of the disease.

Definition. This disease usually occurs in Jewish families and is inherited as an autosomal recessive trait. It is characterized pathologically by an accumulation of a ganglioside in the central nervous system, and clinically by a cherry-red spot at the macula, visual impairment, paralysis, and dementia.

Pathology. The brain is usually large, with wide convolutions. Microscopically,

213

the cells of the neurons are enlarged and rounded, and their cytoplasm has a reticular appearance. The neurons in the brain and spinal cord are distended with ganglioside, and there is diffuse demyelination in the central nervous system, the spinal cord, and the peripheral nerves. Lipid accumulates in the ganglion cells of the retina, which appears grayish in color, but since there are no ganglion cells at the fovea, this area appears as a red spot. There is demyelination of the optic nerves. The intracytoplasmic lipid material appears on electron microscopy as membranous bodies with a lamellar pattern similar to myelin. In the later stages, the deep white matter is converted into a mass of large proliferating astrocytes and microglial cells. The Purkinje cells of the cerebellum contain ganglioside and degenerate in the same way as do those of the cortex.

Clinical Features. The infant develops normally until between the third and sixth month, when it becomes noticeable that something is wrong. The child ceases to take an interest in his surroundings, no longer raises his head from the pillow, and has difficulty in turning over. The infant's cry is unusually high pitched, and there is a marked startle response to noise, characterized by flexion or extension of the legs and extension of the arms. At this stage, the muscles are hypotonic, but the reflexes are exaggerated. Nystagmus may be present. The cherry-red spot, which appears early, is also seen occasionally in Niemann-Pick disease. It is present in 90 per cent of children with Tay-Sachs disease but is apt to fade in the later stages.

During the second half of the infant's first year, he shows an evident failure of motor development, marked hypotonia, and a notable lack of interest in surrounding events. Familiar objects are no longer recognized. During the second year of life, the deterioration continues, feeding becomes a problem, and cortical blindness sets in; the pupils still react to light. The muscles are weak and fasciculation may appear because of degeneration of anterior horn cells. At this stage, tonic neck reflexes may be elicited, and the extensor plantar response of infancy persists. Seizures, including gelastic seizures, are sometimes prominent. By the end of the second year, the child is almost completely vegetative. Most children die of aspiration pneumonia between the second and third year.

When seizures develop, the electroencephalogram shows paroxysmal slow waves and single or multiple spike discharges. In the terminal stages, seizures are apt to decrease and the EEG shows a decrease of voltage and fewer spikes.

There is evidence that serum fructose-1-phosphate aldolase is lacking in patients with Tay-Sachs disease, in the mothers, and in most of the fathers.[15]

There is no treatment.

Other Types of Cerebroretinal Degeneration

Juvenile Cerebroretinal Degeneration (Spielmeyer-Vogt Disease, Batten's Disease). This condition has no special ethnic predilection and usually starts between the ages of five and seven years. The material stored within the neurons differs from that in Tay-Sachs disease. The earliest symptom is impairment of vision, and this may precede all other signs by more than a year. A cherry-red spot seldom appears; in its place, there is a fine, black, granular pigment, which starts at the macula and spreads to involve the whole of the retina—a form of retinitis pigmentosa. In a few cases, blindness has not developed. There is progressive dementia, liability to seizures, and an increasing spastic weakness. There may also be cerebellar ataxia with nystagmus, and parkinsonian rigidity has been described. Ultimately, there is dementia, paralysis, and rigidity, and death occurs before the age of 20.

Kufs's Disease. This has been described as an adult variety of Tay-Sachs disease, but it is probably a different disease or group of diseases. Pathologically, there is ballooning of neurons, with predilection for the striatum, hypothalamus, the cerebellar cortex, and the anterior horn cells. There is no increase in gang-liosides, but many neurons are filled with other lipid materials. In one group, in-tellect and vision are unaffected, the principal manifestation being progressive cerebellar ataxia, with or without pro-gressive atrophy of muscles with fascicu-lation. Other cases occur in adults with a family history of infantile or juvenile lipidosis, and these display mental deterioration and visual failure, together with cerebellar ataxia and myoclonic jerks. The analysis of material obtained from brain biopsy may eventually shed light on this group of rare conditions.

Niemann-Pick Disease

This is a disease of infancy which usu-ally leads to death in the first three years of life.[11,15] About 50 per cent of the pa-tients so far recorded have been Jewish. It somewhat resembles amaurotic famil-ial idiocy in its clinical characteristics— including the cherry-red spot—but the intracellular deposits consist of sphingo-myelin and cholesterol. There is a marked deficiency of sphingomyelin lipase. Four subgroups have been described, based on ethnic and clinical factors, but at present, this subdivision lacks biochem-ical support.

In the infantile form, the microscopic changes found in the brain are indis-tinguishable from those of Tay-Sachs dis-ease. The infant appears normal for sev-eral months, after which it is noticed that the liver and spleen are enlarging. The child becomes weaker and hypotonic and has difficulty in swallowing. A cherry-red spot may appear at the macula. In con-trast to Tay-Sachs disease, the startle reflex is not found. Many of the affected infants appear to be deaf. Seizures are not common. Death from respiratory in-fections is common.

In the juvenile form, the liver and spleen are enlarged, but the patient may survive for many years with or without evidence of central nervous system involvement.

In a third group, the disease comes on in late childhood, and the course is slower. There is no change in the blood lipids and there is no involvement of the lung. Eventually, cerebellar ataxia de-velops.

No effective treatment is known. Splenectomy has been carried out in some cases to avoid the complication of splenomegaly.

Gaucher's Disease

This disorder appears in three forms, infantile, juvenile, and adult; in the first of these, the central nervous system is involved.[15] There is an accumulation of cerebroside in many organs of the body, especially the liver and spleen. It also affects the lymph nodes, bone marrow, and the neurons. It is transmitted as a recessive trait. Usually, the child de-velops normally up to about six months and then shows progressive regression of motor and mental development. The eyes do not fix, the muscles become hyper-tonic, the head is retracted, and there is exaggeration of the tendon reflexes. The spleen enlarges. Eventually, bulbar symptoms supervene, with stridor and difficulty in swallowing, followed by decerebrate rigidity and death within the first year.

The brain does not show the lipid de-posits in neurons that are seen in Tay-Sachs disease, but there is a diffuse neuronal degeneration, and occasionally perivascular collections of Gaucher cells may be found. The serum acid phos-phatase is elevated and the diagnosis is confirmed by the presence of "Gaucher" cells in the bone marrow.

In a few cases, the onset has been in the first few years of life and progress has been slower. Intraneuronal deposits of PAS-positive material have been seen, and the ganglioside patterns and the levels of glucose cerebroside are normal.

Neurological symptoms do not develop in the adult type of Gaucher disease.

Pigmented Degeneration of Globus Pallidus and Substantia Nigra (Hallervorden-Spatz Disease)

In 1922, Hallervorden and Spatz described the syndrome which bears their names. It affected several members of one family and similar cases, both familial and sporadic, have been recorded since then. There is some doubt as to whether this is a specific disease or a syndrome. It usually comes on in childhood and is marked by progressive generalized rigidity and increasing dementia. The rigidity usually starts in the legs, spreading later into the upper limbs, face, and bulbar musculature. In some of the affected families, there has been athetosis, parkinsonian tremor, or dystonia. Some patients have developed retinitis pigmentosa. Eventually, there is mental deterioration in most cases, and death usually occurs before the thirtieth year. Pathologically, there is a brownish discoloration of the globus pallidus, and an increase of pigment occurs in the substantia nigra. Microscopic examination shows an increase of iron-containing pigment in the ganglion cells, glia, and small blood vessels. There is a moderate loss of ganglion cells, with mild reactive gliosis. Cellular loss is also seen in the cortex and in the Purkinje layer of the cerebellum. Zeman and Scarpelli found ganglioside and sphingomyelin deposits in neurons.[43]

Bassen-Kornzweig Syndrome

This is a very rare disease which is probably inherited as a recessive trait. It is the only one of the hereditary ataxias in which a specific biochemical disorder has been established—absence of beta lipoproteins and decrease of the total lipid content of the serum.

It starts as a steatorrhea in infancy or childhood, with malabsorption of triglycerides. This feature tends to improve later on, but it is followed by the appearance of retinitis pigmentosa (leading ultimately to blindness) and a neurological disability which resembles Friedreich's ataxia. There is demyelination of the posterolateral columns and peripheral nerves.[36] There is also clinical evidence of peripheral sensory neuropathy, and a cardiac myopathy. When the erythrocytes are examined in a wet smear, they appear crenated (acanthosis) and there is a reticulocytosis.

Hand-Schüller-Christian Syndrome (Xanthomatosis, Histiocytosis-X)

This rare disorder usually occurs in children and is characterized by xanthomatous deposits in the membranous bone of the skull, the orbit, and the tuber cinereum and pituitary.

The lesions consist of histiocytic granulomas in which the histiocytes are stuffed with cholesterol. The plasma cholesterol is usually normal, and the increased cholesterol content of the cells may be a secondary development because early lesions are indistinguishable from those of eosinophilic granuloma. The lesions appear in the skull, long bones, skin, viscera, lymph glands, gums, and the walls of the larger blood vessels. Plaques of demyelination, which contain foam cells, have been found in a few cases.

Clinical Features. Diabetes insipidus may arise before radiological evidence of bony changes in the skull is observable; these changes take the form of large defects in the membranous bones. Exophthalmus may be unilateral, bilateral, or absent. When the pituitary gland is involved, mental and physical growth are retarded and adiposogenital dystrophy can occur. Chronic otitis media is very common. Infiltration of the lungs gives rise to a mottled shadow resembling miliary tuberculosis. Pathological fractures may occur.

Treatment. Diabetes insipidus responds to the intramuscular administration of pitressin tannate in oil. The lesions themselves respond to x-ray therapy, but new foci are apt to appear elsewhere. The use of corticosteroids has been recommended.

THE AMINOACIDURIAS

Inherited disorders of amino acid metabolism can give rise to irreversible mental retardation.[12, 16, 27, 34] More than 30 types have been described, and others are likely to be discovered. The metabolic defects are identified by amino acid chromatography of the blood and urine.

Phenylketonuria (PKU). This condition results from an inborn error of metabolism characterized by inability to convert phenylalanine to tyrosine, owing to the absence of phenylalanine hydroxylase.[27] There is therefore a high concentration of phenylalanine in the blood. The condition is transmitted by a single recessive gene. Screening tests show that PKU occurs about once in every 20,000 births.

The gray matter of the brain is normal, but in severe cases there is diffuse demyelination. The white matter is spongy in appearance and shows loss of myelin, plus a reactive gliosis.

The infant, who is usually blond or redheaded, is listless and a poor feeder and by six months, there is evidence of retardation. The motor and sensory systems are unaffected, apart from a mild ataxia in some cases. Seizures may occur, and rigidity is occasionally encountered, but the plantar responses remain flexor. Eczema is often present. The I.Q. is below 60 in most cases.

The increased level of serum phenylalanine can be demonstrated by chemical analysis or by chromatography. The infants must be at least 4 days old and have received milk for at least 24 hours, or the level of phenylalanine will remain low, even in affected infants. A serum phenylalanine titer above 15 mg. per 100 ml., with a serum tyrosine level of less than 5 mg. per 100 ml. and urinary phenylalanine levels greater than 100 mcg. per 100 ml., confirms the diagnosis.[16] When the condition is established, as in older children, the electroencephalogram shows slowing of the background activity; spikes are seen in those who have developed seizures.

It is prudent to screen all infants during the first few days of life. If phenylketonuria is present, the infant is fed a formula with a low phenylalanine content, and the serum phenylalanine levels are measured at frequent intervals so as to be sure that they do not exceed about 8 mg. per 100 ml. Early treatment is required to prevent mental retardation, since once the latter is established, it is irreversible.

An increased level of serum phenylalanine without PKU is sometimes seen in prematurely born infants, but in such cases, the tyrosine level is also raised. This situation can be corrected by the administration of Vitamin C.

Maple Syrup Urine Disease. In maple syrup urine disease, the metabolism of leucine, isoleucine, and valine is disturbed, and the excess amino acids in the urine give it an odor resembling maple syrup.[35] Symptoms usually start in the first few weeks of life, and the infant develops convulsions, vomiting, metabolic acidosis, and—in some cases—hypoglycemia. Death usually occurs within a few months.

Tyrosinosis. In tyrosinosis, mental retardation is associated with hepatic and renal impairment, vitamin D resistant rickets, and hypokalemia.[17]

Methylmalonic Aciduria. In this condition, methylmalonic acid is excreted in the urine in amounts up to 5 gm. per day. The patients present a severe metabolic ketoacidosis and have both mental and physical retardation. The aminoaciduria can be reduced by the daily parenteral administration of 1000 mcg. of Vitamin B_{12} (i.e., a pharmacological dose);[31] a coenzyme derived from Vitamin B_{12}, among others, is needed for the metabolism of this amino acid.

Homocystinuria. Homocystinuria results from lack of cystathionine synthetase.[1] The hair is sparse, and pes cavus and genu valgum are usually present. Ectopia lentis is common. Mental retardation, however, is not always present.

The coagulability of the blood is increased, and this can give rise to thromboembolism and cortical thrombophlebitis with consequent seizures and focal neurological signs. The metabolic defect can be corrected by the administration of very large doses of pyridoxine, which acts as a coenzyme in the decarboxylation, transamination, and deamination of many amino acids.

Lowe's Syndrome. This is a recessive sex-linked disease which affects boys only. There is muscular hypotonia, mental retardation, cataracts and congenital glaucoma, metabolic acidosis, and rickets. Many amino acids are found in the urine, and a hyperchloremic acidosis is caused by defective ammonia formation in the kidneys.

Hartnup's Disease. This rare condition, named after the family in which it was first recognized, is inherited through a recessive gene and is characterized by renal aminoaciduria and excessive excretion of indole compounds.[2] It is thought that the transport of tryptophan across the cells of the jejunum and proximal renal tubules is defective.[28] The striking features of the disease are a pellagra-like rash following exposure to sunlight, intermittent attacks of cerebellar ataxia, and an organic confusional state. Despite the cerebellar signs, muscle tone is increased and the tendon reflexes are brisk. The condition tends to improve as the child grows older, but in some cases, mental retardation is permanent. The diagnosis is confirmed by the urinary findings. The administration of nicotinamide is said to exert a favorable influence on the skin lesions and on the neurological signs.

HYPERURICEMIA

This disturbance of uric acid metabolism, sometimes called juvenile gout or the Lesch-Nyhan syndrome, is inherited as a sex-linked recessive trait, and occurs only in boys.[5, 33] It results from a deficiency of inosinate pyrophosphate phosphoribosyl transferase. Areas of perivascular demyelination are found in the cerebrum and cerebellum. There is thickening of the walls of blood vessels, some of which are occluded. These children are retarded in early infancy, and by the end of the first year, choreoathetosis and spasticity appear. A curious feature of the disorder is a tendency to self-mutilation; the patients bite their fingers and lips and so produce sores which are slow to heal. Uric acid stones often form, and urinary tract infection is difficult to control. The serum uric acid level is elevated. Measures to reduce the level of the uric acid in the blood do not bring about any significant improvement in the neurological signs. It remains to be seen whether early recognition and treatment of the hyperuricemia will prevent damage to the brain.

DISORDERS OF CARBOHYDRATE METABOLISM

Hypoglycemia. Repeated, prolonged attacks of hypoglycemia can give rise to mental retardation.[21] This can occur as the result of (1) hyperinsulinism, (2) adrenal insufficiency, (3) pituitary insufficiency, (4) hepatic disease, (5) the aminoacidurias, notably maple syrup urine disease, (6) glycogen storage diseases—von Gierke's disease, Pompe's disease, Forbes' disease (Cori type 3), Cori type 6 glycogen storage disease, and deficiency of glycogen synthetase, (7) inability to metabolize galactose, leucine, and fructose, (8) "idiopathic" infantile hypoglycemia—a heterogeneous group the causes of which have still to be determined, and (9) the malabsorption syndrome.

Galactosemia. This is an inborn error of metabolism transmitted as an autosomal recessive trait and characterized by the absence of an enzyme which is essential for the conversion of galactose to glucose in the liver.[7, 9, 20] High blood levels of galactose stimulate insulin production and thereby produce episodes of hypoglycemia. The infant appears normal at birth, but after a few days of milk feeding, it starts to suffer from vomiting, diarrhea and lethargy. The liver enlarges and jaundice appears, followed by ascites. Cataracts develop in some cases, and if milk feeding is continued, mental retardation will result. Seizures may occur. The blood glucose is reduced and the galactose level is increased. The presence of galactose in the urine can be demonstrated by paper chromatography. The disease is treated by instituting a galactose-free diet, which may have to be continued for several years; in later life, milk is usually tolerated.

Intolerance to fructose is inherited as an autosomal recessive trait. Symptoms are first encountered in infancy, when the child has been placed on cow's milk. There is vomiting, diarrhea, and failure to thrive, and the liver enlarges. Episodes of hypoglycemia give rise to seizures and coma. The fructose tolerance test produces a fall in blood glucose and inorganic phosphorus levels. The condition is treated by strict restriction of fructose in the diet.

MUCOPOLYSACCHARIDOSES

Abnormal storage of acid mucopolysaccharides has been described in a number of conditions, of which the best known is Hurler's syndrome (gargoylism).[19, 24, 26] Mental retardation also occurs in the San Filippo and Morquio-Ullrich types of mucopolysaccharidosis.[16]

Hurler's Syndrome. This condition is inherited as an autosomal recessive trait. There is a widespread deposition of mucopolysaccharides in the neurons of the brain, spinal cord, and peripheral ganglia, in the Küpffer cells of the liver and spleen, in the intima of large and medium sized arteries, and in the myocardium. There is a deficiency of a specific beta-galactosidase enzyme.

The condition is easily recognized in the second or third year. The patient is a dwarf with a relatively large head. The nose is flat and the nostrils flare widely. The lips are thick, the eyes wide-set, the hair coarse and abundant, and the neck short. The limbs too are short and the range of movement is limited. The joints are large and irregular, the long bones are undeveloped and irregularly thickened, and the phalanges are cone-shaped. There is often kyphosis, owing to wedging of thoracic or lumbar vertebrae. The spleen and liver are enlarged. The cornea is rendered opaque by a deposit in the posterior layers. There may be progressive mental deterioration, increasing difficulty in walking because of weakness and spasticity, and seizures. The disease is steadily progressive, death occurring before the tenth year, usually from a respiratory infection or cardiac failure.

Hunter's syndrome[24] is transmitted as a sex-linked recessive trait. It resembles Hurler's syndrome, but the cornea is not affected, the heart seldom so, and the patients tend to survive longer.[16]

In all types of mucopolysaccharidosis there is increased urinary excretion of acid mucopolysaccharides. No effective therapy is available.

NEPHROGENIC DIABETES INSIPIDUS

This is a genetically determined disturbance of water and salt metabolism which results from lack of response of the kidney tubules to the antidiuretic hormone.[41] It is presumed to be transmitted as a sex-linked recessive trait, since male infants mainly are affected.

Symptoms appear in early infancy. Dehydration leads to a high fever, restlessness, vomiting, and constipation. The infant grows slowly and is both mentally and physically retarded. These cases are distinguished from those in which diabetes insipidus is caused by lack of antidiuretic hormone by the failure to respond to pitressin. The condition is treated by a low protein diet (1 to 2 gm. of protein/kg. of body weight per day) and the provision of an abundant fluid intake. Chlorothiazide in doses of 50 mg./kg. of body weight per day decreases the volume of urine and increases osmolarity.[16] If dehydration is severe when the child is first seen, 2.5 per cent dextrose in water is given intravenously. Death can occur as a result of acute dehydration, and in those that survive, the brain damage is permanent.

UNVERRICHT-LAFORA DISEASE
(Myoclonic Epilepsy)

This rare heredofamilial disorder is characterized by the onset in childhood of seizures, myoclonic movements, mental deterioration, and a variety of neurological signs. It is inherited as an autosomal recessive trait and is the result of an inborn error of metabolism, which leads to the accumulation of intracellular and extracellular PAS-positive bodies that are probably derived from glycogen.[18]

Pathology. The inclusions are found throughout the nervous system but are particularly common in the red nucleus, substantia nigra, thalamus, and dentate nucleus. They are also present in the myocardium and liver. In some clinically similar cases, Lafora bodies have been absent. There is widespread loss of nerve cells, with consequent gliosis.

Clinical Features. The disease starts in childhood. The first symptom may be petit mal, generalized convulsions, or myoclonic movements. The myoclonus consists of either violent or minor shock-like contractions of individual muscles or muscle groups that are most marked in the proximal portions of the limbs and in the trunk. They may also occur in the face, larynx, pharynx, and diaphragm. They interfere with voluntary movements. As time goes on, the patient may also develop intention tremor and cerebellar ataxia or generalized extrapyramidal rigidity. Mental deterioration may come on early or late, and in some cases, it ends in complete dementia. The disease is slowly progressive and except in mild and abortive cases, the patient usually dies within 20 years of the onset.

Laboratory Aids. The diagnosis can be established by liver or brain biopsy;

muscle biopsy is less reliable. Electro-encephalography shows severe diffuse dysrhythmia, with generalized 3 per sec. wave and high voltage spike complexes, some of which are related to the myoclonic jerks. Both the electroencephalographic abnormalities and the myoclonic shocks can sometimes be precipitated by stroboscopic photic stimulation.

Diagnosis. There is no difficulty in recognizing the fully developed syndrome when a family history of the disease is available, but in the early stages, the problem is less simple. It is a serious diagnosis to make in view of the bad prognosis. Occasional mild myoclonic jerks are quite common in epileptic patients, especially in those with petit mal. In subacute sclerosing encephalitis, there is mental deterioration and myoclonus, but the disease is nonfamilial, convulsions are rare, involuntary movements are more rhythmical and slower than those of myoclonus epilepsy, and survival for over one year is rare.

Treatment. Both the seizures and the myoclonus may be controlled to some extent by anticonvulsive agents.

HEPATOLENTICULAR DEGENERATION
(Wilson's Disease)

Wilson's disease is characterized by extrapyramidal symptoms, cirrhosis of the liver, and a ring of greenish pigmentation in Descemet's membrane near the junction of the cornea with the sclera.[42] It results from an inborn error of metabolism, transmitted as an autosomal recessive trait. There is a high incidence of consanguinity in affected families. There are marked differences in the relative severity of damage to the brain and liver in different families, and in some members, severe liver cirrhosis occurs in the absence of any neurological disorder.

Pathology. Degeneration is found in the putamen, the caudate nucleus, the dentate nucleus, the cerebellum, and the cerebral cortex. In rapidly advancing cases, there is actual cavitation of the putamen and pallidus, whereas in the more common, slowly progressive type, there is loss of neurons and diffuse gliosis in these areas. Large protoplasmic astrocytes (Alzheimer's giant cells) are found scattered through the affected areas of the brain. There is portal cirrhosis of the liver, which is enlarged at first but soon shrinks; acute interstitial hepatitis has been recorded. The spleen is enlarged because of portal congestion. There is a deposition of copper granules in Descemet's membrane.

Copper is absorbed from the intestinal tract in excessive amounts, but it is not converted to ceruloplasmin at an appropriate rate and unbound copper is therefore deposited in the liver cells, brain, renal tubules, and elsewhere.[39] The deposits of copper in the renal tubules lead to an aminoaciduria in some cases. There may also be excessive excretion of uric acid, phosphate, and bicarbonate because of the renal damage.

Clinical Features. The disease is uncommon. It occurs in both sexes and is usually diagnosed between the ages of 10 and 25 years; but it can occur in early childhood or as late as the fifth decade. The disease comes on insidiously and usually runs a slow course over a period of several years, but exceptionally, death occurs a few weeks or months after the onset of symptoms. In general, the earlier the onset, the more rapid the progress. In children and young adolescents, choreoathetotic movements appear in the face and hands, or there may be a coarse, flapping tremor when the limbs are partly relaxed. These movements are increased by voluntary movement. Gait may be disturbed by involuntary movements in the lower limbs. Writhing, dystonic movements may appear in the face, neck, and trunk.

Parkinsonian rigidity may occur early or late and is associated with poverty of movement, a masklike face, and dysarthria. As Wilson pointed out, there may be excessive retraction of the lips when smiling.

The hepatic element is often silent, but in some cases there is a history of recurrent dyspepsia or jaundice and occasionally ascites and splenomegaly appear late in the disease. In less than 10 per cent of cases, evidence of liver disease precedes the onset of neurological signs.

If the patient lives long enough—and this applies to most cases—the Kayser-Fleischer ring appears in the cornea. It starts as a brownish-red or greenish crescent of pigmentation in the limbus and eventually extends to form a complete ring. Slit-lamp examination of the cornea will often reveal the ring when direct observation fails to do so.

Some degree of mental dilapidation is usually present, and involuntary laughing and crying is common. The retraction of the lips referred to above is particularly evident during these episodes.

In the terminal stages, tonic "fits" may occur, in which the neck and back arch, the limbs are extended, the lips are drawn back, and there may be difficulty in breathing and swallowing; consciousness is retained. The tendon reflexes are normal or exaggerated, and the plantar responses are usually flexor but may be extensor. Sensation and sphincter control are unaffected.

Laboratory Aids. The spinal fluid is normal. Serum copper is reduced below the normal level of 86 to 112 mcg. per 100 ml., but there is an elevation of "free" serum copper levels. Ceruloplasmin is much reduced below the normal level (27 to 38 mg. per 100 ml.), and urinary copper exceeds the normal level (0 to 26 mcg. in 24 hours). There is often a considerable excretion of amino acids. The concentration of copper in the liver is increased, as can be determined by liver biopsy.

Diagnosis. The concurrence of liver damage, extrapyramidal symptoms, and corneal pigmentation is pathognomonic of Wilson's disease, but difficulty may be experienced if corneal pigmentation and hepatic involvement are not obvious, because progressive extrapyramidal symptoms, coupled with pathological laughter, dysarthria and dementia, can occur on a familial basis in other very rare diseases which come on in childhood—e.g., progressive pallidal degeneration and Hallervorden-Spatz disease.

All siblings of an affected member of the family should be examined for clinical and biochemical evidence of the disease,[37] so that appropriate treatment may be carried out before the disorder becomes symptomatic.

Prognosis. The disease may be acute, subacute, or chronic, but it is always fatal unless treated. In the days before treatment was available, more than 50 per cent of patients died in from 1 to 6 years; exceptionally, untreated cases have survived for more than 20 years.

Treatment. The object of treatment is to decrease absorption of copper from the intestinal tract and to increase its excretion in the urine. By appropriate dietetic restriction, it is possible to reduce copper intake to about 1 mg. per day; furthermore, the administration of 40 mg. of potassium sulfide with each meal will restrict the absorption of copper. With regard to chelating agents, penicillamine has replaced BAL because it is easier to administer and has fewer side effects.[30, 40] It is given in doses of 1 to 4 gm. per day in divided doses on an empty stomach. There is slight risk of optic neuritis, which can be reduced by administering Vitamin B_6. Other side effects can be controlled by corticosteroids. If penicillamine is given early enough, neurological disability regresses and the patient remains symptom-free as long as maintenance treatment is continued.

CRETINISM

Cretinism is a state of hypothyroidism beginning in fetal life (as opposed to myxedema supervening in a previously normal individual).[4] It occurs in an endemic form in iodine-deficient areas, and sporadically in other zones. The endemic cretin usually has a goiter, which is absent in the sporadic type. Histological examination of the brain reveals degeneration of cortical cells.

The cretin can usually be recognized at birth or shortly thereafter, and the signs become increasingly obvious as time goes by. The infant is apathetic and somnolent, the skin thick and dry, the lips full, the tongue large and protruding, the hands and feet are cold, and the pulse is slow. The hair is sparse and coarse. Closure of the fontanelles is delayed, and the bones fail to grow in length; the epiphyses unite late. The abdomen is obese and pendulous, and layers of fat appear over the clavicles, in the axillae, and between the scapulae. Hernia is common. The hands are square and the fingers spatulous. Mental retardation usually becomes obvious by the end of the first year. Cerebral diplegia is sometimes present in cretins and is said to be more frequent among children of women suffering from hypothyroidism than in others.

Treatment. Treatment is by the administration of thyroid extract by mouth, starting with 15 mg. per day and increasing the dose as needed. If treatment is started in the first six months, mental and physical development proceed fairly satisfactorily, but if treatment is delayed, the child remains below the mental and physical standards of his fellows.

CEREBELLAR ATAXIA IN MYXEDEMA

Cerebellar ataxia is sometimes seen in adults with untreated hypothyroidism[22, 29] —in primary myxedema; Hashimoto's thyroiditis, following overtreatment for thyrotoxicosis, myxedema secondary to chromophobe adenoma of the pituitary, and Sheehan's syndrome. The author has seen a case in which the disorder seems to have been precipitated by the prolonged use of Lithium for manic depressive psychosis.

Ataxia is usually confined to instability of gait, but there may also be nystagmus, dysarthria, and intention tremor. In some cases, ataxia is associated with a mild sensory polyneuropathy. There is often generalized muscular weakness, and the muscles relax slowly when the tendon reflexes are elicited. Deafness is not uncommon. Mental slowing can be sufficient to cause a suspicion of dementia, even when the systemic signs of hypothyroidism are not marked. The protein of the spinal fluid commonly is increased.

The explanation for the ataxia is uncertain. Round bodies containing glycogen, designated "neural myxedema bodies," have been found in the cerebellum of a patient with longstanding myxedema and ataxia,[29] but the influence of reduced cardiac output, retarded cerebral blood flow, and reduced oxygen and glucose consumption may play a role. Thyroid replacement therapy usually leads to a complete recovery.

WALDENSTRÖM'S MACROGLOBULINEMIA

This is a rare disease of late adult life which affects both sexes.[3, 13, 25] It is characterized by general malaise, shortness of breath, a hemorrhagic diathesis, and neurological lesions of vascular origin. There is lymphocytic infiltration, and enlargement, of the lymph glands, liver, and spleen. It is thought that the lymphocytes are the source of the macroglobulins. Blood viscosity is greatly increased by the presence of 5 gm. per 100 ml. (or more) of globulins with a molecular weight between 400,000 and 1,000,000. The erythrocyte life span is shortened.

The onset is usually insidious, with malaise, loss of weight, pallor, and anemia. There may be bleeding from the nose or the gastrointestinal tract. Visual impairment can result from retinal hemorrhages or from retinal venous thrombosis. Enlargement of the liver and spleen has been present in about 50 per cent of cases published thus far.

The neurological spectrum includes: seizures, cerebral hemorrhages with appropriate localizing signs, multifocal infarctions both above and below the tentorium, an acute organic psychosis, intraspinal hemorrhages with consequent paraplegia, and a predominantly sensory type of peripheral neuropathy.[13] Examination of the conjunctival vessels by biomicroscopy discloses massive sludging and capillary stasis. There is often an associated anemia and thrombocytopenia, and the sedimentation rate is high.

The diagnosis can be established only by ultracentrifugation or immunoelectrophoresis of the serum. Macroglobulinemia can also occur in multiple myelomas, in lymphatic leukemia, and in lymphosarcoma. The molecular weight of the gamma globulin in myeloma is in the region of 160,000 but it can be as high as 1,000,000 in some lymphomas.

Treatment. The oral administration of 4 to 8 mg. of chlorambucil daily can produce a remission of the symptoms. Plasmaphoresis can be used to tide the patient over the critical period, as when sight is threatened or acute neurological symptoms have arisen.

REFERENCES

1. Ainsworth, D. C., and Dent, C. E.: Homocystinuria. *Brit. Med. Bull.* 25:42, 1967.
2. Baron, D. M., Dent, C. E., and Jepson, J. B.: Hereditary pellagra-like skin rash with temporary cerebellar ataxia. *Lancet* 2:421, 1956.
3. Bayrd, E. D., Hagerdorn, A. B., and McGuckim, W. F.: Macroglobulinemia: Its recognition and treatment. *J.A.M.A.* 193:724, 1968.
4. Benda, C. E.: *Mongolism and Cretinism.* Grune and Stratton, Inc., New York, 1949.
5. Berman, P. H., Balis, M. E., and Dancis, J.: Congenital hyperuricemia. *Arch. Neurol.* 20:44, 1969.
6. Bori, P. F., Hooghwinkel, G. J. M., and Edgar, G. W. F.: Brain ganglioside pattern in three forms of amaurotic idiocy and in gargoylism. *J. Neurochem.* 13:1249, 1966.
7. Brandt, M. J., and Tolstrup, M.: Problems in the diagnosis of hereditary galactosemia. *Acta Pediat. Scand.* 56:85, 1967.
8. Chou, S. M., and Thompson, H. G.: Electron microscopy of storage cytosomes in Kufs's disease. *Arch. Neurol.* 23:489, 1970.
9. Cornblath, M., and Schwartz, R.: *Disorders of Carbohydrate Metabolism in Infancy.* W. B. Saunders Co., Philadelphia, 1966.
10. Cremer, G. M., Goldstein, N. P., and Paris, J.: Myxedema and ataxia. *Neurology* 19:37, 1969.
11. Crocker, A. C., and Farber, S.: Niemann-Pick disease: A review of 18 patients. *Medicine* 37:1, 1958.
12. Crome, L. C., and Stern, J.: *Pathology of Mental Retardation.* Little, Brown and Co., Boston, 1967.

13. Dayan, A. D., and Lewis, P. O.: Demyelinating neuropathy in macroglobulinemia. *Neurology* 16:1141, 1966.
14. Field, R. A.: Glycogen deposition diseases. *The Metabolic Basis of Inherited Diseases*, Edited by Stanbury, J. B., Wyngaarden, J. B., and Frederickson, D. S., McGraw-Hill Book Co., Inc., New York, 1960.
15. Freeman, J. M., and McKhann, G. M.: Degenerative diseases of the nervous system in childhood. *Advances Pediat.*, 16:121, 1969.
16. Gamstorp, I.: *Pediatric Neurology*. Appleton-Century-Crofts, New York, 1970.
17. Gemtz, J., Linblad, B., and Lindstedt, S.: Dietary treatment in tyrosinemia. *Amer. J. Dis. Child.* 113:31, 1967.
18. Harriman, D. G., Millar, J. H., and Stevenson, A. C.: Progressive familial myoclonic epilepsy in three families; its clinical features and pathological basis. *Brain* 78:325, 1958.
19. Henderson, J. L.: Gargoylism. *Arch. Dis. Child.* 15:201, 1940.
20. Holzel, A., Komrower, G. M., and Schwartz, V.: Galactosemia. *Amer. J. Med.* 22:703, 1957.
21. Ingram, T. T. S., Stark, G. D., and Blackburn, I.: Ataxia and other neurological disorders of severe hypoglycemia in childhood. *Brain* 90:851, 1967.
22. Jellinek, E. H., and Kelly, R. E.: Cerebellar syndrome in myxedema. *Lancet* 2:225, 1960.
23. Jervis, G. A.: Juvenile amaurotic idiocy. *Amer. J. Dis. Child.* 97:663, 1959.
24. LeRoy, J. G., and Crocker, A. S.: Clinical definition of the Hurler-Hunter phenotypes. *Amer. J. Dis. Child.* 112:518, 1966.
25. Logothetes, J., Silverstein, P., and Coe, J.: Neurologic aspects of Waldenström's macroglobulinemia. *Arch. Neurol.* 3:564, 1960.
26. McKussick, V. A., et al.: The genetic mucopolysaccharidoses. *Medicine* 44:445, 1965.
27. Menkes, J. H.: The pathogenesis of mental retardation in phenylketonuria and other inborn errors of amino acid metabolism. *Pediatrics* 39:297, 1967.
28. Milne, M. D., Crawford, M. A., Girao, C. B., and Loughridge, L. W.: The metabolic disorder in Hartnup disease. *Q. J. Med.* 29:407, 1960.
29. Price, T. R., and Netsky, M. D.: Myxedema and ataxia; cerebellar alterations, and "neural myxedema bodies." *Neurology* 16:957, 1966.
30. Richmond, J., Rosenoer, V. M., Tompsett, S. L., Draper, I., and Simpson, J. A.: Hepatolenticular degeneration (Wilson's disease) treated by penicillamine. *Brain* 87:619, 1964.
31. Rosenberg, L. E.: Inherited aminoacidopathies, demonstrating vitamin dependency. *New Eng. J. Med.* 281:145, 1969.
32. Rosenthal, L. M., Zimmerman, H. J., and Hardy, M.: Congenital non-hemolytic jaundice with disease of the central nervous system. *Pediatrics* 18:378, 1956.
33. Sass, J. K., Itabashi, H. H., and Dexter, R. A.: Juvenile gout and brain involvement. *Arch. Neurol.* 13:639, 1965.
34. Scriver, C. R.: Inborn errors of amino acid metabolism. *Brit. Med. Bull.* 25:35, 1969.
35. Snyderman, S. E.: The therapy of maple syrup urine disease. *Amer. J. Dis. Child.* 113:68, 1967.
36. Sorbrevilla, L. A., Goodman, M., and Kane, C. A.: Demyelinating cerebral nervous system disease, macular atrophy, and acanthocytosis (Bassen-Kornzweig syndrome). *Amer. J. Med.* 37:821, 1964.
37. Sternlieb, I., and Scheinberg, I. H.: Diagnosis of Wilson's disease in asymptomatic patients. *J.A.M.A.* 183:747, 1963.
38. Svennerholm, L.: The gangliosides. *J. Lipid Res.* 5:145, 1964.
39. Walshe, J. M.: The physiology of copper in man and its relation to Wilson's disease. *Brain* 90:149, 1967.
40. Walshe, J. M.: Treatment of Wilson's disease with penicillamine. *Lancet* 1:188, 1960.
41. Williams, R. H., and Henry, C.: Nephrogenic diabetes insipidus transmitted by females and appearing during infancy in males. *Ann. Int. Med.* 27:84, 1947.
42. Wilson, S. A. K.: Progressive lenticular degeneration: A familial nervous disease associated with cirrhosis of the liver. *Brain* 34:295, 1911-1912.
43. Zeman, W., and Scarpelli, D. G.: *J. Neuropath.* 17:622, 1958.

CHAPTER TWELVE

Degenerative Diseases of the Central Nervous System

THE SENILE AND PRESENILE DEMENTIAS

This group includes the presenile dementias of Alzheimer and Pick and senile dementia. It does not include the dementia which results from repeated vascular accidents, deep midline tumors,[24] and other diseases of the brain in which dilapidation of the intellect is a secondary or incidental feature.

Senile Dementia

This condition is usually thought of as coming on after the age of 70. The patient looks far older than his actual age; there is loss of hair, atrophy of the skin and muscles, loss of weight, tremor, poor posture, and eventually an uncertain shuffling gait.

Pathologically, there is general atrophy of the brain, widening of the sulci, loss of gray matter, and slight glial overgrowth.[41] Scattered throughout the brain are minute argyrophil senile plaques with an amorphous core, surrounded by interlacing glial fibrils. Measurement of regional blood flow discloses an overall reduction, but the reduction is greatest in the gray matter.[50]

Clinically, the patient shows a progressive narrowing of interests, slowing of mental processes, difficulty in assimilating new ideas, and increasing failure of memory.[55] In the so-called simple dementia, which is the most common form, there is a slow but steady intellectual loss, without significant affective changes; there may be episodes of confusion. In other cases, there are not only failure of memory and lack of attention, leading to disorientation of time and place, with consequent disorders of behavior, but there also may be profound depression or agitation, hypochondriacal ideas, persecutory or expansive delusions, and auditory hallucinations. The patient may be excessively restless. Dirty habits, hoarding of rubbish, and spitefulness make difficulties for those looking after such patients.

The course of senile dementia is progressively downhill into mindlessness. The process may be accelerated by head injuries, general infections, and vascular accidents, or by emotional factors such as bereavement or removal to unfamiliar surroundings.

The differential diagnosis presents difficulties. Alzheimer's disease and Pick's disease can occur in the senium, but the distinction is of academic interest since nothing can be done for either. Arteriosclerotic dementia[2, 55] should be diagnosed only when there is a

225

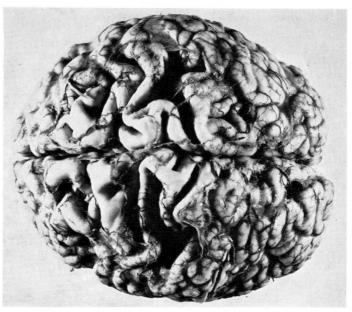

Figure 12–1.   Cortical atrophy. (Courtesy of Ayer Laboratory, Pennsylvania Hospital.)

history of one or more strokes. Of practical importance is the fact that a chronic subdural hematoma may arise in the course of senile dementia, aggravating the symptoms. Occasionally a cerebral tumor (including, surprisingly, a craniopharyngioma) can masquerade as a senile dementia,[52] but the chance of successful surgical intervention in such cases is small because of the patient's age. Dementia caused by low-pressure communicating hydrocephalus (p. 209) occurs at a somewhat earlier age and is not accompanied by the external appearances of senility.

There is no treatment for senile dementia apart from the provision of adequate nutrition and the general supervision of the patient. Nocturnal restlessness is very troublesome in some cases; on the whole, it is better controlled by the use of chloral, bromide, or alcohol than by barbiturates or tranquilizers.

Alzheimer's Disease
(Presenile Dementia)

Alzheimer first described the clinical and pathological features of the disease in 1907. As judged by the autopsy material at mental institutions, it accounts for between 2 and 7 per cent of the organic psychoses in the second half of life, but the prevalence rate is probably higher than this figure would suggest because a certain number of patients die of intercurrent disease before their condition justifies admission to a mental hospital.

Etiology.   The cause of the disease is unknown. Familial incidence has been reported, but the majority of cases occur sporadically. It is slightly more common in women than in men.

Pathology.   The brain is shrunken, the gyri small, and the ventricles enlarged.[41] The atrophy is generalized, unlike the situation in Pick's disease, in which it is limited to one or more lobes. Histologically, there is diffuse degeneration and disappearance of ganglion cells in the cortex, with a moderate increase of glial cells. A special characteristic is the prominence of Alzheimer's neurofibrillary degeneration, which is found in the cells of the cortex, Ammon's horn, and elsewhere; it is also found, albeit to a very much more limited extent, in senile dementia and in a wide spectrum of other neurological disorders. Argyrophil senile plaques are almost always present in Alzheimer's disease. The blood vessels commonly exhibit some degree of arteriosclerotic degeneration. Regional blood flow is reduced in both gray and white matter.[50]

Clinical Features. The symptoms usually appear for the first time in the 50's, but can occur earlier or later.[27] Because the disease often arises in menopausal women, many accounts refer to prodromata such as hot flashes, dizzy attacks, and headaches, but these symptoms should probably be regarded as coincidental. The earliest symptoms of the disease are the result of impaired memory and attention. The patient becomes forgetful, and this results in a falling off of efficiency in household tasks or in business. Objects are mislaid and names forgotten; familiar faces and surroundings may no longer be recognized. On shopping expeditions, the patient cannot remember what to buy, or how much, and makes mistakes in her accounts. The capacity to comprehend complex situations and ideas declines as the result of faulty powers of association and memory. This may be aggravated by defective memory for the meaning of words. Judgment is impaired because it depends partly on the correct perception of the current situation and on the ability to compare it with memories of like situations in the past, a process dependent upon memory and powers of association. Attention suffers, with consequent distractibility; the patient skips from one unfinished task to another and from one conversational topic to another. Restlessness is often conspicuous, possibly as the result of distractibility. On the other hand, perseveration is sometimes encountered.

The patient may be depressed at first, particularly if he retains enough insight to recognize that his powers are failing. When insight has failed, mood may be either elevated or flat.

Eventually specific disturbances appear in relation to the functions of speech and language. There is difficulty in recalling names and words, in the ability to understand complex sentences, and in reading. Because of the dyslexia, the patient often stops reading, but may deny that he has any difficulty and say that he finds newspapers and books dull (an explanation which is correct in patients with narrowing interests). In time, marked motor and sensory aphasia develops, accompanied in most cases by some degree of dysgraphia. There is difficulty in comprehending the meaning of pictures, and visual agnosia may extend to faces, utensils, and garments, with consequent disorders of behavior.

Apraxia and senseless repetitive activities are not uncommon, but with this exception, motor capacity remains good for a long time. However, the face ultimately becomes expressionless, movements are slow, and the gait is shortstepped and shuffling. Cranial nerves and sensation are unaffected. In the final stage, the patient is reduced to a vegetative life, with a total loss of comprehension and speech. Movements are purposeless, and primitive responses, such as the grasp reflex and the sucking reflex, appear. Eventually there is double incontinence.

The disease usually terminates in about four years, but it may run its course more rapidly; exceptionally, it has been known to last over 10 years.

Laboratory Aids. The spinal fluid is normal. Electroencephalography usually discloses diffuse bilateral slowing late in the disease, but it is nonspecific in character. Once the condition is well established, pneumoencephalography shows enlargement of the ventricles and collections of air in widened sulci (Fig. 12–2). Such pooling of air is more generalized than in Pick's disease.

Diagnosis. Diagnosis can be difficult in the early stages when the signs of mental deterioration are slight. In some, the family or business associates are the first to notice decreasing efficiency and unusual behavior. Such aberrations are often falsely attributed to stresses and emotional conflicts. In others, the patient appreciates his own deficiencies and develops symptoms of anxiety, but at this stage, tests of memory, attention, association, vocabulary, and calculation

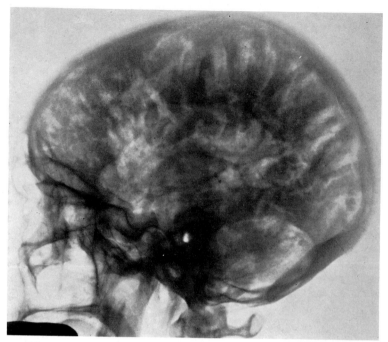

Figure 12–2. Alzheimer's disease. Pneumonencephalogram showing accumulation of air in the cortical sulci, and slight enlargement of the lateral ventricle. (Courtesy of Dr. Brodie Hughes.)

will usually disclose a profile of defect which is more or less specific for organic disease. However, it is seldom easy to convince the patient of the need for such procedures at this early stage, since insight is often lacking.

Once the presence of progressive dementia is established, an attempt has to be made to determine its cause. Senile dementia occurs in older groups and is slower in its course, and the patient almost always looks far older than his age. In Pick's disease, cortical atrophy is apt to produce aphasia or symptoms of frontal lobe involvement at an early stage, and generally speaking, memory is better preserved than in the more global Alzheimer's disease. Pneumoencephalography may disclose localized atrophy in the anterior half of the temporal lobes, or in the frontal region, but this is an unreliable method of distinguishing Pick's disease from Alzheimer's disease. There is no certain means of distinguishing between the two except by autopsy. In neurosyphilis (general

paresis), the course is usually far more rapid than in the presenile dementias, there are positive neurological signs to be found, and changes in the spinal fluid and a positive serology provide definitive evidence.

A cerebral tumor may cause mental deterioration before the appearance of headaches, papilledema, or focal motor or sensory dysfunction. The rapid evolution of most cerebral tumors usually clarifies the situation before long, but slowly growing neoplasms, notably meningiomas and occasionally a craniopharyngioma or glioma, can cause serious mental disorders for a considerable time before giving rise to localizing signs. In one series studied, the incidence of autopsy-proved brain tumors in mental institutions was twice that in general hospitals.[52] It follows from this that every case of presenile dementia should be thoroughly investigated by air studies and angiography, and it is desirable to emphasize that complete visualization of the third ventricle, using an opaque medium if necessary, is essential in these cases. Tumors of the frontal lobe and of deep midline structures are the most likely to cause mental symptoms without neurological signs.[24]

The slow development of dementia may be due to "normal pressure" communicating hydrocephalus (p. 209) in which the ventricular system is dilated but cortical atrophy is absent. It is important to establish this diagnosis, since the mental deterioration can often be halted or reversed by shunting procedures.

Metastatic carcinomatosis of the meninges can give rise to a predominantly mental symptomatology, without headaches or neck stiffness, but the rapid evolution of the disease and changes in the spinal fluid distinguish these cases from the more slowly evolving disturbances of the presenile dementias.

In more than 50 per cent of all cases of arteriosclerotic dementia, the onset is sudden because of a cerebrovascular accident, and the course of the disease is punctuated by partial remissions and abrupt or rapid exacerbations. Such abrupt incidents are uncommon in Alzheimer's disease or Pick's disease, though rapid deterioration can occur as a result of infections, operations, or intoxications. Seizures are more common in arteriosclerotic dementia than in the other presenile dementias, and focal neurological symptoms are often present. Arteriography is seldom helpful, because even though stenosis of major arteries in the neck or within the head may be disclosed, it does not follow that the patient's mental symptoms result from vascular insufficiency. There is, as yet, no method of assessing small vessel disease in the brain or of identifying reduced transcapillary diffusion which would interfere with the nutrition of the ganglion cells. The diagnosis of arteriosclerotic dementia is helped, but only to a limited extent, by the presence of hypertension and evidence of renal, peripheral, cardiac, or retinal vascular disease.

Occasionally, a chronic subdural hematoma causes mental deterioration in elderly subjects over a period of weeks or even months, and it is not necessarily associated with headache or evidence of raised intracranial pressure. The symptoms fluctuate from day to day or even from hour to hour, but the speed of deterioration is greater than is usual in the presenile dementias, and spontaneous recovery can occur. The routine use of arteriography in the investigation of organic dementia will insure against this mistake.

There are other rare forms of organic dementia whose nosological status is uncertain. Subacute spongiform encephalopathy,[49] a rare disease characterized pathologically by diffuse destruction of both ganglion cells and astrocytes of the cortex, may cause an organic dementia. It often starts with focal neurological symptoms, such as aphasia, paralysis of one or more limbs, cortical blindness, seizures, or myoclonus, but the first symptom may be mental deterioration. The disease runs a rapid course, death usually occurring in a matter of weeks or months, so that even in the cases which start with mental symptoms, the early development of focal neurological symptoms and signs enables them to be distinguished from the presenile dementias.

It is usually stated that chronic alcoholic degeneration can be distinguished from other forms of presenile dementia but in the author's experience, it can be extremely difficult to assess the parts played by alcoholism, the psychopathy which may have led to the alcoholism, coincident arteriosclerosis, senescence, and nutritional deficiencies. If the condition fails to progress, or if the patient actually improves following withdrawal of alcohol and the provision of an adequate diet and supplemental thiamine and vitamin B_{12}, the part played by alcohol comes into focus.

Treatment. There is no method of treating Alzheimer's disease. It runs its course in anything from two to 10 years. In the cases which progress slowly, it is often possible to keep the patient at home for a considerable portion of that time, but removal to an institution should

not be too long delayed, because looking after these patients can impose a
great burden on relatives.

Pick's Disease

Pick's disease is a more uncommon
type of presenile dementia than Alzheimer's disease, and like the latter, it
usually appears in the fifth or sixth decade, but it can occur in the senium.

Pathology. Atrophy starts either in
the frontal cortex or in the temporal
lobe; ultimately it affects both and may
spread back to the parietal lobe, but it
is not as generalized as in Alzheimer's
disease.[41] If the temporal lobe is involved, atrophy starts anteriorly and
spreads to involve the whole of the middle and inferior gyri and the anterior
third of the superior gyrus, the posterior
portion escaping. There is diffuse loss
of ganglion cells within the affected parts
of the brain, and this is most marked in
the outer three layers of the cortex. There
is corresponding shrinkage of the subcortical white matter, a circumstance
which led early workers to refer to the
condition as lobar sclerosis. Atrophy of
the caudate nucleus is also seen in some
cases. Many of the ganglion cells are
swollen, and contain argyrophilic inclusions (Pick cells). Gliosis is more
marked than in either Alzheimer's disease or senile dementia. Both senile
plaques and neurofibrillary changes are
present, but not to the same extent as in
Alzheimer's disease; some coincident
arteriosclerosis may be present.

Clinical Features. Though most
cases are sporadic, the disease sometimes affects more than one member of
a family. The symptoms[27] are those of a
slowly developing organic dementia,
but the mode of onset varies according
to whether atrophy begins in the frontal
lobe, in the temporal lobe, or in both
simultaneously. The onset is insidious.
Frontal involvement leads to inattention
and loss of interest, with consequent deterioration of domestic, professional,
and social activities. The patient be-

comes careless in dress and habits and
oblivious of social niceties, and may
display sexual aberrations. In this disorder, intellectual capacity—memory
in particular—may be quite well preserved, but lack of attention, initiative,
and interest leads to impairment of performance in learning. Abstract thought
is also impaired, partly because of faulty
powers of association. Generally speaking, there is inertia, apathy, and loss of
affect, but occasionally the patient is
euphoric and hyperactive. When the disease starts in the temporal lobe, some
degree of aphasia is an early feature;
the patient cannot recall names, objects,
or persons, and has difficulty in understanding complicated sentences. This
may go on to a severe degree of motor
and sensory aphasia. Occasionally dyslexia and dysgraphia occur early. At
first, the patient tends to keep quiet
because of his difficulties in speech, but
later on there may be perseveration of
speech, echolalia, and palilalia. If the
disease also involves the parietal lobe
of the dominant hemisphere, some degree of motor apraxia may develop. The
symptoms of frontal, temporal, and parietal disease may be mixed in any proportion, and the total result is dementia
with a prominent disorder of speech
function.

As the patient deteriorates, other
neurological symptoms sometimes develop. Seizures, extrapyramidal rigidity
and involuntary movements, and disturbances of gait may be seen, but true
pyramidal signs are rare. Ultimately
the picture is one of total mental dilapidation, purposeless movements, grasping and sucking reflexes, and a steady
descent into a vegetative state.

Laboratory Aids. The spinal fluid is
usually normal, but increases in the total
protein level and lymphocyte count
occasionally are reported. As in Alzheimer's disease, pneumoencephalography discloses pooling of air in the
sulci of the frontal and temporal lobes
and dilatation of the ventricular system,
which is most marked in the anterior
horns of the lateral ventricles.

Diagnosis. In the early stages of the

disease, Pick's disease must be differentiated from other causes of dementia of middle or advanced life. Such differentiation is discussed with Alzheimer's disease. In the cases which display an early disorder of speech, it is possible to distinguish them from Alzheimer's disease, but in most instances, the distinction is impossible without autopsy.

The average duration of the disease is between two and seven years. There is no treatment.

Paralysis Agitans
(Parkinson's Disease)

Parkinson's disease is a slowly progressive disease of late adult life, characterized pathologically by degeneration within the nuclear masses of the extrapyramidal system, and clinically by tremor, akinesia, and rigidity. Similar symptoms, occurring as a result of encephalitis lethargica, cerebral arteriosclerosis, and other diseases, are known as *parkinsonism*.

Etiology. The cause is unknown. Though it is not commonly regarded as a familial or hereditary disease, more than one case may appear in a family. It afflicts both sexes, usually occurs over the age of 50, and recognizes no racial barriers. It is the second most common neurological ailment in the United States and is exceeded only by cardiovascular disease and arthritis as a cause of chronic incapacity.

Pathology. There are no macroscopic changes in the brain apart from those resulting from coincident arteriosclerosis and senile changes in aging patients. Microscopically, the most important lesions are found in the substantia nigra. The most severe lesions are in the zona compacta, where groups of pigmented cells disappear. Lewy bodies are present, notably in the substantia nigra and locus coeruleus. Similar lesions are found in other melanin-bearing nerve cells in the brainstem. Less constantly, degenerative changes are found in the globus pallidus, the substantia innominata, and the hypothalamic nuclei. There is some degree of neuronal loss in the cortex, but the corticospinal tracts are unaffected. The essential lesion is in the substantia nigra.

Clinical Features. The onset is insidious. Rigidity and akinesia may precede tremor, and it is in this group that early diagnosis is difficult. Akinesia imparts a peculiar stillness to the appearance of the patient, who fidgets less, is sparing of gesture, does not swing the arm in walking, and has a fixed, unblinking stare. Movements become more deliberate, and one movement does not flow automatically into another; there is a slight delay between the act of taking spectacles out of a case and putting them on. The patient, having got up out of a chair, may stand still for a second or two before commencing to walk, and in more advanced cases the first few steps may be short and awkwardly performed. Despite the akinesia, very rapid movements are possible if the patient is caught off guard; some patients will actually catch a ball thrown at them, provided the action is unpremeditated.

The second major component of the syndrome is rigidity. This affects both extensors and flexors. It persists throughout the entire range of passive movement, and is usually cogwheel in character. When it appears first in the legs, it produces a feeling of heaviness; if the upper limb is affected, the patient notices difficulty in carrying out fine movements, and his writing suffers; the pen is pressed too hard on the paper, and the letters are small and irregularly formed. This may be mistaken for writer's cramp. As the disease advances, rigidity invades the face, lips, tongue, neck, and trunk, imposing an attitude of generalized flexion, with the chin sunk on the chest, the arms adducted and flexed at the elbows, and slight flexion of the knees. The neck is stiff, and the gait loses its spring and becomes shuffling and short-stepped. In some cases, this attitude of flexion throws the center of gravity too far forward, and the patient has to take rapid steps to keep himself from falling on his face (festination);

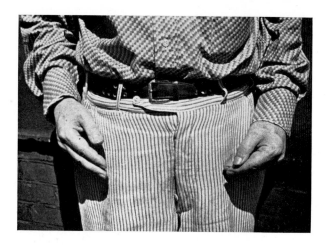

Figure 12–3. The hands in parkinsonism. (Courtesy of Dr. A. Ornsteen.)

a slight push from behind will propel him across the room before he is able to stop. Rigidity of the muscles of mastication may interfere with eating to such an extent that malnutrition results. Rigidity of the lips and tongue produces dysarthria; in addition, there is early loss of the modulations of speech, and the voice becomes monotonous. It is also weak; this weakness, together with the spastic dysarthria and a tendency to run one word into another, may render the patient all but unintelligible. Rigidity and akinesia prevent swallowing of saliva, which therefore drools from the mouth. In contrast to the rigidity of the face and the loss of expression, the eyes remain singularly alive, and ocular movements are unaffected.

Tremor usually appears after rigidity and akinesia; occasionally it is the first symptom, and rarely, it is absent throughout. It is a coarse, rhythmic, to-and-fro oscillation, which usually appears first in the hand as the typical "pill-rolling" movement of the fingers. It may also involve the lower jaw, head, and lower limb. It is a tremor of postural fixation, occurring when the limb is held in any given posture. Typically, as the hand rests on the arm of a chair or knee, rhythmic three-to-four per second movements develop, but when the patient is asked to move the arm, the tremor disappears, only to reappear when some other fixed posture is maintained. However, intention tremor is sometimes pres-

ent as well. Tremor disappears entirely during sleep, and is aggravated by anxiety and excitement. In severe cases, it persists throughout voluntary movements and greatly interferes with function.

Muscular power is unaffected at first, but in the later stages it is diminished, partly because movement is impeded by rigidity. Disuse may contribute to the weakness. Atrophy does not occur except as a part of the generalized wasting of the body, which takes place late in the disease. Neither somatic sensation nor the special senses are affected; diminution of vibration sense in the legs, often found in aging persons, is not the result of the disease. Deep and superficial reflexes are unaffected, although it may be difficult to elicit the tendon reflexes when rigidity is severe. Sphincter disturbances are rare, but frequency of micturition, especially at night, may be a troublesome symptom.

Intellectual deterioration may occur in the late stages as a result of coincident cerebral arteriosclerosis, but it is not a part of the disease per se. Emotional changes, on the other hand, are extremely common and are properly viewed as a reaction to frustration, dependence on others, and an appreciation of the hopelessness of the situation. When rigidity is extreme, there is often a compelling desire for frequent changes of position, which can be brought about only by a nurse or companion. The very inability to move seems to engender an excessive desire to do so. It is not surprising that many of these patients are demanding and depressed.

Laboratory Aids. The spinal fluid is normal. Nonspecific generalized abnormalities are recorded in the electroencephalogram in about 33 per cent of patients.

Prognosis. The disease progresses relentlessly over two or three decades. Within five years, 25 per cent of patients are severely disabled by the disease and by the tenth year this has increased to 66 per cent. By the fourteenth year, more than 80 per cent have either died or are severely disabled.[31] The shortened life expectancy is indicated by a mortality rate three times that of the general population of the same sex, age, and race. Major causes of death are bronchopneumonia and urinary infections but, as is to be expected in this age group, malignancy, vascular disease, and accidents occur with a frequency equal to that in the general population. Stereotaxic operations for the relief of symptoms have not substantially increased life expectancy, and the long-term effect of treatment with L-dopa remains to be seen.

Diagnosis. The onset is so insidious that the change may not be noticed by physicians or relatives who are in constant touch with the patient, although the diagnosis may be obvious to a new acquaintance. There is no difficulty when the characteristic tremor is the presenting symptom, but akinesia and rigidity are often the first to appear, and the stillness of the body, the fixed expression, and the deliberateness of movement will indicate the presence of an extrapyramidal disease. It is then necessary to distinguish the disease (paralysis agitans) from other causes of parkinsonism.

Encephalitis lethargica (von Economo's disease) was common between 1918 and 1925. It was followed in some cases by symptoms of parkinsonism after five to 20 years. It may be indistinguishable from Parkinson's disease, but in some cases the patient also ex-

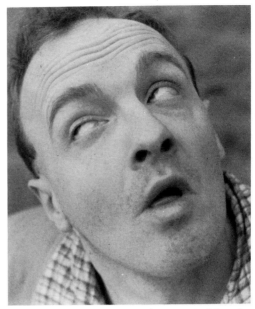

Figure 12–4. Oculogyric crisis caused by phenothiazine intoxication. (Courtesy of Dr. Douglas Goldman.)

hibits tics and torsion spasms, disorders of respiratory rhythm, oculogyric crises, seborrhea of the face, and sialorrhea. It is generally thought that encephalitis lethargica is virtually nonexistent today, but since 1940, the author has seen four cases of parkinsonism developing in middle age after an attack of encephalitis of unidentified type.

A common cause of mild parkinsonian rigidity today is the use of tranquilizer drugs, notably the phenothiazines. Some patients also develop oculogyric crises (Fig. 12–4) and spasmodic involuntary movements (e.g., retraction of the head and protrusion of the tongue). The symptoms usually disappear rapidly when the drug is withdrawn.

Arteriosclerotic parkinsonism is sometimes seen in old age. The onset may be insidious, but the course is often punctuated by major or minor vascular accidents, and the clinical picture is sometimes complicated by the presence of symptoms not seen in paralysis agitans— pyramidal weakness, dementia, pseudobulbar palsy, hemianopia, paresis of conjugate movement of the eyes, and other indications of focal disease.

A cerebral tumor arising deeply within the hemispheres may produce unilateral parkinsonian features in the early course of its development, but it very rarely produces a masklike face (which appears to require bilateral disease) or the characteristic tremor or cogwheel rigidity; nevertheless, it has to be considered when extrapyramidal symptoms develop in the arm or leg over a short period of time.

Senile tremor usually appears first in the head, and is often limited to it; when it spreads to the limbs, it is increased by volitional movements. Rigidity is absent. Familial tremor is usually seen in one or both hands; it is increased by voluntary movement and is unassociated with rigidity, and there is a family history of the condition. As in other familial conditions, the phenomenon of anticipation may be seen, i.e., the tremor appears at an earlier age in successive generations.

Severe head injuries may give rise to tremor and extrapyramidal rigidity as an immediate sequel, but the tendency is toward recovery, and there is no justification for attributing paralysis agitans to injuries received many years before. Acute carbon monoxide poisoning can give rise to progressive parkinsonism, usually accompanied by some degree of dementia. Chronic manganese poisoning occurring as a result of occupational exposure over a prolonged period can also give rise to parkinsonism, which may be complicated by pyramidal symptoms of cerebral origin or by subacute myelopathy with clinical evidence of damage to the spinal cord. Extrapyramidal syndromes occurring in children and adolescents do not enter into the differential diagnosis of paralysis agitans, which is a disease of late adult life.

Treatment. There is no way of arresting the disease, and treatment must be directed toward alleviating symptoms. At the time of writing, the most promising method is by the oral administration of L-dopa.[5, 15, 45, 51]

Of the chemical substances thought to be concerned with neural transmission within the central nervous system, dopamine is present in largest amount in the striatum, putamen, and substantia nigra. In patients with parkinsonism, the concentration is much reduced in these areas.[51] Dopamine given by mouth does not reach the central nervous system, but L-dopa does so. Cotzias took advantage of this fact to administer gradually increasing small doses of L-dopa to patients with paralysis agitans and postencephalitic parkinsonism, and since this first successful trial, an increasing body of evidence has accumulated to show that this is, to date, the best method of controlling the symptoms. L-Dopa has a somewhat greater effect on akinesia and rigidity than on tremor. The effective dose ranges from 3 to 8 gm. daily; the optimum dose must be determined for each patient. Though L-dopa is well tolerated by parkinsonian patients, there are a significant number of side effects. When therapy starts, nausea and vomiting are common, and cardiac arrhythmia and hypotension may be encountered. Following long-term administration, the most frequent side reactions are choreiform or athetotic movements, especially of the face.[5, 44] Psychiatric side effects include restlessness, aggression, hallucinations, mania, and impairment of memory.[33]

In some patients, the combined administration of L-dopa with an anticholinergic agent produces better results than either drug alone.

Amantadine hydrochloride has been found useful in some cases. This is an antiviral agent which may protect against influenza A-2 and which by chance was found to reduce the rigidity and tremor and akinesia of parkinsonism. As in the case of L-dopa, amantadine seems to help akinesia and rigidity more than tremor. In a series of cases of Parkinson's disease studied by Schwab and his colleagues, amantadine caused improvement in 66 per cent; 29 per cent showed no improvement, 2 per cent became worse, and in 3 per cent the effects were uncertain. Side effects include insomnia, "nervousness," loss of appetite, and dizziness. Understandably, both L-dopa and amantadine are less effective in severely handicapped patients than in those with less serious disability.

If neither L-dopa nor amantadine can be given, a modest degree of relief from tremor and rigidity can be achieved by the administration of belladonna alkaloids or synthetic compounds with a belladonna-like action.[25] Trihexyphenidyl (Artane) is given orally, starting with 2 mg. a day and increasing by 2 mg. per day until a total of 20 to 30 mg. is being given in divided doses. Dryness of the mouth, nausea, blurring of vision, and—occasionally—confusion and hallucinations indicate that the limit of tolerance has been reached. Cycrimine hydrochloride (Pagitane), biperiden, and procyclidine hydrochloride (Kemadrin) are analogues of trihexyphenidyl and are equally useful. If side effects are induced by any one member of this series, they are usually induced by all of them.

Antihistamines are sometimes helpful, especially when rigidity is a major problem, and they can be given in conjunction with the above group of drugs. Dextroamphetamine is sometimes used, especially for oculogyric crises in the postencephalitic variety of parkinsonism. Imipramine (Tofranil) has a use as a mood elevator, and meprobamate can be used for mild sedation. Small doses of phenobarbitone (30 to 60 mg.) can also be used to induce mental relaxation. Sedatives are useful because anxiety and embarrassment tend to augment both rigidity and tremor.

Muscle relaxants have no place in the treatment of parkinsonism. Salivation can be reduced by the use of propantheline bromide or belladonna.

Stereotaxic surgery can reduce the tremor of Parkinson's disease. Tremor—and to a lesser extent, rigidity—can be reduced by lesions in the medial aspect of the globus pallidus, the ventrolateral nucleus of the thalamus, the substantia nigra, and midbrain tegmentum. A unilateral surgical lesion ameliorates symptoms on the opposite side of the body. There are no hard and fast criteria for the selection of cases at the present time, but, generally speaking, the best indication for surgery is the presence of marked and predominantly unilateral parkinsonism in relatively young subjects who show no gross evidence of arteriosclerosis and who are normotensive. Gross bilateral disease, severe akinesia, marked dysarthria and dysphagia, and evidence that the disease is rapidly advancing are contraindications. Although the mortality rate of this operation is less than 2 per cent, the risk of hemiplegia while attempting to place a surgical lesion so near the internal capsule is ever present and, in general, operation should not be carried out unless tremor and rigidity constitute a substantial handicap to the patient, and unless L-dopa has proved ineffective.

General supportive measures are important.[25] The patient should be encouraged to take as much physical exercise as his condition permits, within the limits imposed by fatigue. Gentle massage and passive stretching of the affected limbs are comforting at all times, and when rigidity is severe, frequent changes of posture afford the patient much relief. When eating becomes a burden, concentrated foods and supplemental vitamins are required to maintain nutrition. Infections of the prostate, bladder, and upper urinary tract are not uncommon and may be a source of nocturnal restlessness.

Juvenile Paralysis Agitans of Hunt (Pallidal Atrophy)

Juvenile paralysis agitans is a very rare disease.[53] It is usually familial, but sporadic cases have been reported. However, in the absence of postmorten evidence, it is difficult to be sure that sporadic cases are not examples of Wilson's disease. The pathological changes found in the few cases that have come to autopsy include degeneration of the large cells in the basal ganglia, accompanied by gliosis; the liver is normal.[32, 60] The symptoms usually start before the age of

15 and consist of typical parkinsonian tremor and rigidity, which progress very slowly over many years, but which can ultimately lead to considerable incapacity.[64] Retinitis pigmentosa has been present in some cases.

Dystonia Musculorum Deformans

Torsion dystonia is a rare disease characterized by slow, powerful twisting and writhing movements of the body, with a predilection for the muscles of the trunk and limb girdles.[20, 23, 35] It is inherited as an autosomal recessive mutant trait in Jews and as an autosomal dominant in non-Jewish people. Somewhat similar movements, the symptomatic dystonias, have been reported from time to time in a number of diseases involving the basal ganglia[23, 30]—for example, encephalitis lethargica and Wilson's disease—and also in phenothiazine intoxication.

Pathology. After close scrutiny of the pathological evidence, Zeeman has concluded that the inherited variety of torsion dystonia is not associated with "tangible pathological abnormalities detectable by light microscopy."[23] On the other hand, Davison and Goodhart[20] reported the results of postmortem examination of four patients; they describe widespread degenerative changes affecting the caudate nuclei and putamen, with a lesser degree of involvement of the dentate nuclei, thalamus, substantia nigra, and cerebral cortex. It seems likely that the dystonia in these cases may have been symptomatic of some other disease.

Clinical Features. The onset of the disease is gradual, with symptoms appearing for the first time in late childhood or early adolescence. Exceptionally, it starts in infancy or early adult life. The first symptom may be persistent hypertonicity of the calf muscles, producing plantar flexion and inversion of the foot. The feet are inverted and their plantar surfaces are concave. When the

trouble spreads to the legs, bizarre abnormalities of gait appear and walking is disturbed not only by spasm in the legs but also by contraction of the lumbar muscles which increases the lumbar lordosis and may rotate the pelvis. There may also be a tendency to flex the thighs, which means that the patient has to bend forward in putting the foot to the ground. The movements spread upward to involve the shoulder girdles and the face, interfering with the use of the upper limbs and with speech.

In other cases, the dystonia first involves the face and neck muscles, or it may start in the muscles of the trunk, with consequent opisthotonos or a torsional movement.

When the patient is in quiet surroundings, the spasms are much reduced, but any excitement or anxiety greatly increases them, producing dysarthria, facial grimacing, torticollis, torsion of the trunk, and forceful extension and rotation or flexion of the limbs. Attempts to use the limbs bring on spasms, and, although there is no real paralysis, the patient has the greatest difficulty in performing any movement. Sensation and reflexes remain normal.

Many of these children are intellectually gifted and show great courage in facing their handicap, but ultimately some deterioration may occur. In general, the disease is progressive, but there may be periods in which it remains stationary for a long time, and temporary remissions have been reported.

Diagnosis. Similar symptoms can occur as a result of epidemic encephalitis, Wilson's disease, the juvenile form of amaurotic familial idiocy, Hallervorden-Spatz disease, etc. In the early stages, hysteria has to be considered, especially when the first symptom is spasmodic torticollis. Since all involuntary movements resulting from organic disease are aggravated by emotional factors, any observed relationship between the movements and situations with a high emotional content do not prove that the condition is hysterical. On the other hand, involuntary movements of hysterical origin are easily influenced by suggestion, and there is usually positive evidence of a disturbed emotional background.

Treatment. L-Dopa has proved disappointing, but a combination of L-dopa and haloperidol may be more effective. The most promising form of treatment is by chemo- or cryothalamotomy, as judged by Cooper's experience with 164 cases.[14, 23]

Huntington's Chorea
(Chronic Progressive Chorea)

Huntington's chorea usually starts in adult life, and is characterized pathologically by degeneration of the cerebral cortex and basal ganglia, and clinically by mental deterioration and choreiform movements. Rigidity appears in some cases.[10, 13, 41, 43]

Incidence. The disease is rare, but has been described in all races. It was introduced into America by two brothers and their families who emigrated to Long Island in 1630, and it has been estimated that between 1632 and 1932, approximately 1000 cases could be traced to these two families. The disease is transmitted by a dominant gene,[53] the sexes are affected equally, and the disease may be transmitted by either sex. In some families, only one or two members are affected, while in others, almost all the offspring develop the disease. Occasionally it skips a generation.

Pathology. The brain is small, with cortical atrophy and dilatation of the lateral ventricles.[41] There is atrophy of the corpus striatum, mainly in the putamen and to a lesser extent in the caudate nucleus; degeneration is also found in the thalamus and brainstem. In the atrophic areas, the number of small nerve cells is decreased, the large ganglion cells being spared; sometimes the cellular outfall in the caudate nucleus is so great as to cause status spongiosis. There is reactive gliosis. The blood vessels in the affected area show secondary degenerative changes, and in actively progressive cases, fat-filled histiocytes may be seen in the perivascular spaces. The cerebral cortex shows a general reduction in neuronal population, especially in layers 3, 5, and 6, with inconspicuous changes in the cells that survive.

Clinical Features. The age of onset may be at any time from infancy to old age, but in the majority, symptoms start between the ages of 30 and 50. Motor disturbances usually precede signs of mental deterioration, but in some cases, the reverse is true. At first, there are complaints of clumsiness and restlessness. There may be slight intermittent shrugging of the shoulders, twitching of the fingers, or grimacing. As time goes on, the choreiform movements become more severe, affecting the face, trunk, and limbs, and these come to interfere with voluntary movements of the hands and with walking. The movements are abrupt and pleomorphic. In addition to facial grimacing, there are irregular flexion and extension of the hands, difficulty in sitting or standing because of involuntary movements which throw the patient off balance, causing sudden falls, and dysarthria Choreiform movements are increased by emotion and are reduced when the patient is sitting quietly by himself. They disappear during sleep.

Muscle tone is usually normal, but a few cases have been described in which parkinsonian rigidity was the outstanding feature, chorea being either minimal or absent. It is usually seen in children and young adults,[10, 13] but rigidity may also supervene at a late stage of the disease. The rigidity is thought to be due to damage to the globus pallidus.

Mental deterioration may precede the involuntary movements, but commonly it appears some years after chorea has developed. There is failure of memory and difficulty in concentration, leading to a considerable loss of mental efficiency, of which the patient is at first aware. Disorders of mood are prominent: irritability, anxiety, profound apathy, and attacks of violence may occur. Eventually, there is progressive dementia with loss of insight. Seizures are uncommon.

The disease is slowly progressive, choreiform movements becoming more severe and mental deterioration increasing. The average duration of life between the onset and death is about 15 years. It has been noticed that there is a considerable incidence of suicide in the affected members of the family; this may be the result of impulsive behavior or because the patient with insight who has observed the deterioration of other members of his family is unable to face life any longer.

Laboratory Aids. The spinal fluid is normal. In the established disease, the EEG shows theta and beta waves, but may eventually become flat. Sometimes EEG abnormalities are present before clinical signs appear. Pneumoencephalography discloses enlargement of the lateral ventricles—the result of degeneration of the caudate nucleus.

Diagnosis. Sydenham's chorea occurs in children and is not a progressive disease. It may be accompanied by delirium, but this is an acute affair, quite unlike the slowly progressive dementia of Huntington's chorea. Senile chorea occurs in the fifth or sixth decade and is not familial; choreic movements are prominent, but are unaccompanied by mental deterioration.

Treatment. There is no treatment for the disease. Choreiform movements can be reduced to some extent by the administration of haloperidol or trifluperidol. The presence of the disease in the family should be regarded as an absolute contraindication to the production of children by any member of the afflicted families, whether the would-be parent is normal or not.

HEREDOFAMILIAL ATAXIAS

In 1898, Whyte remarked that even in Friedreich's disease, which is the best defined clinicopathological type of heredofamilial ataxia, each family has its own special traits. Moreover, even in a single sibship, there may be a wide variation in the symptoms and signs.[9] Pratt[53] pre-

sents a bewildering array of more than 20 different clinicopathological types of heredofamilial ataxia. Wide variation also occurs in the method of transmission, which compounds the difficulties encountered in genetic counseling. Moreover, there are no guidelines for forming a basis of such counseling for a given family until a sufficient number of siblings have been affected to establish the pattern for that particular family. Since there is no method of treating any of these conditions at the present time, and since it is usually impossible to foretell how many siblings or how many generations will be affected, the logical advice to affected families is to avoid having children, and unaffected relatives should avoid the potential perils of consanguineous marriages.

Friedreich's Ataxia

This is the most common type of hereditary ataxia. It is usually transmitted as a recessive trait and is characterized pathologically by degeneration of the posterolateral columns of the spinal cord, occasionally with involvement of the cerebellum.

Pathology. The characteristic pathological features are degeneration of axons and myelin sheaths in the posterior columns, spinocerebellar tracts, and lateral corticospinal tracts.[4, 29] In advanced cases, there may be degeneration of the dorsal roots and peripheral nerves and loss of cells in Clarke's column. The cerebellum usually appears normal, but some cases display atrophy of the Purkinje cells and dentate nuclei.

Clinical Features. Friedreich's ataxia occurs in all races and in both sexes. Symptoms usually appear for the first time between the ages of 5 and 14 but may be delayed until adult life. There is an insidious onset of clumsiness of gait; in some cases, the parents report that the child has never been agile and was late in learning to walk. Within a year or two, ataxia appears in the upper limbs, and eventually a cerebellar dys-

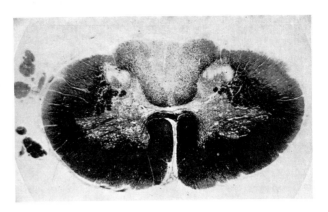

Figure 12-5. Friedreich's ataxia illustrating posterior and lateral column degeneration. (From Wechsler, I.: *Clinical Neurology.* 9th Ed.)

arthria develops. Nystagmus is usually present. The ataxia results partly from the loss of the spinocerebellar tracts and partly from loss of position sense.

The ataxia is complicated by weakness and occasionally this progresses to almost complete paralysis of the legs. Atrophy of muscles is common late in the disease, but in some cases it appears early and is out of proportion to the rest of the symptoms (Levy-Roussy syndrome). Vibration sense is impaired early, followed by defective joint sensibility in the feet and later in the hands. Advanced cases occasionally show peripheral impairment of cutaneous sensibility.

The reflexes in the legs are usually absent; rarely, they are preserved throughout the course of the disease. Reflexes in the arms are usually retained for a longer period, but ultimately they, too, are depressed and may disappear. The plantar responses are extensor; the abdominal and cremasteric reflexes are usually preserved.

Nystagmus is common; it may be horizontal, vertical, or rotary and sometimes is of the fixation type, oscillation appearing before the eyes are brought to rest on an object. Optic atrophy may occur. Oculomotor paralysis, deafness, and labyrinthine disturbances have been reported from time to time but are uncommon. Mental faculties are usually retained, but in a few cases progressive deterioration has occurred. Seizures are somewhat more common in persons suffering from this disease than in the general population.

Skeletal abnormalities are usually present. Pes cavus may be present before the other features of the disease appear, and equinovarus deformities are common. Kyphoscoliosis develops late.

The heart is sometimes enlarged, and there may be cardiac murmurs and an abnormal electrocardiogram. Progressive myocardial degeneration may occur.[59] Siblings sometimes exhibit only myocardial disease and club feet.

Autonomic disturbances have been reported—paroxysmal tachycardia, disturbances of respiratory rhythm, paroxysms of vomiting, periodic hyperthermia, glycosuria, sexual impotence, and impairment of sphincter control. Diabetes mellitus is relatively common in Friedreich's ataxia.

The cerebrospinal fluid is usually normal.

Course and Prognosis. The clinical course of the disease is variable, but in the majority of cases, incapacity is complete by the age of 20 or 25. Death usually occurs as a result of intercurrent infection or cardiac disease. Occasionally, the disease appears to stop advancing for as much as five or 10 years at a time. The life expectancy is normal in abortive forms of the disease.

Treatment. There is no means of influencing the disease. Educational exercises for the correction of ataxia may help temporarily and orthopedic operations are sometimes indicated for correction of gross deformities of the feet, when it is considered that such deformities are playing a significant role in the difficulty with walking. Immediately following such operations, the gait is usually worse for a time.

Hereditary Cerebellar Ataxia With Spasticity (Olivopontocerebellar Atrophy with Spinal Cord Involvement)

This group of disorders, which were defined by Sanger-Brown and by Marie at the end of the nineteenth century,[53] differ from Friedreich's ataxia in that the symptoms come on in the second or third decade or even later. The tendon reflexes are exaggerated, and optic atrophy is not uncommon. In most of the families studied, inheritance has been by a dominant trait.

Pathology. There is degeneration of the cerebellum, cerebellar peduncles, and olivary nuclei, and of the corticospinal and spinocerebellar tracts.[29] The posterior columns are not conspicuously involved. In some cases, there is atrophy of the optic nerves and degeneration of other cranial nerves.

Clinical Features. The onset occurs in adult life, with progressive ataxia of gait and a later appearance of incoordination of the hands. There may be dysarthria, and impairment of vision from optic atrophy or oculomotor palsy. The tendon reflexes are hyperactive, and the plantar responses are extensor. Deformities of the feet and spine are not as common as in Friedreich's ataxia.

Behr, and later van Bogaert, described a heredofamilial disease in *children* characterized by ataxia of the limbs, spasticity of the legs, and optic atrophy.[53] The visual loss, which may antedate the ataxia and spasticity, can take the form of (1) bilateral scotomas which gradually expand to involve the rest of the field, (2) more rapid loss of vision, resulting in blindness in a short time, or (3) a slowly progressive, concentric constriction of the fields of vision.

Progressive Cerebellar Degeneration (Olivopontocerebellar Atrophy, Cerebello-olivary Degeneration, Late Corticocerebellar Atrophy)

In these conditions, the spinal cord is unaffected, although there are intermediate cases in which degeneration of the posterior columns, spinocerebellar or corticospinal tracts provide a link with Friedreich's ataxia.[28, 29, 53]

The symptoms appear in adult life and take the form of a slowly progressive cerebellar ataxia of the extremities and trunk. There is nystagmus, scanning speech, intention tremor, slowness and clumsiness of voluntary movements, and ataxia of gait. In the early stages, the cerebellar incoordination which is so prominent when the patient is up and about disappears when he lies down, and, since nystagmus is often absent at this stage of the disease, the unwary observer may suspect conversion hysteria.

Mental deterioration has been reported in some of these cases.

The differential diagnosis of cerebellar ataxia in middle life is simple if there is a family history of the disorder, but in sporadic cases, it is necessary to exclude multiple sclerosis, the progressive cerebellar degenerations associated with alcoholism and visceral carcinoma, and posterior fossa tumors.

Ataxia Telangiectasia (Louis-Bar Disease)

This rare disease is characterized by progressive cerebellar ataxia and by telangiectases which are first noticed on the conjunctiva. The cases are usually confined to one sibship. Inheritance may be by a recessive trait, but this is by no means definite.[53]

Pathology. The cerebellum shows severe loss of Purkinje cells and diffuse rarefaction of the granular cell layer. The dentate nuclei are atrophic. In addition, focal demyelination has been found in the corpus callosum, the upper and middle cerebellar peduncles, the optic tracts, and the medulla.[58] Demyelinized hemosiderin-laden glial scars are found around capillaries, and there may be dilated veins in the white matter of the cerebrum.

Clinical Features. Ataxia is noticed in the first two or three years of life, and before the age of six, dilated blood vessels appear in the peripheral part of the exposed portion of the conjunctiva. Eventually, telangiectases appear on the pinnae and on the butterfly area of the face, neck, and limbs. Some degree of mental retardation is usual, and body growth may also be retarded. Speech may be impaired by cerebellar dysarthria, and there is a coarse nystagmus in all directions of gaze. As the disease develops, choreoathetosis may appear. Eventually, the ataxia of the legs makes it impossible for the child to stand or walk. The tendon reflexes are reduced, and the plantar responses are flexor. Sensation is not affected.

These children are very prone to sinusitis and pneumonia, and serum gamma globulin levels are usually low. The urine has been found to contain a polypeptide consisting mainly of proline and hydroxyproline.

Treatment. Great care must be exercised in controlling infections by antibiotics. Bronchiectasis is a danger. To date, most of these children have died from infections early in life. They also display an unusual tendency to develop leukemia, lymphosarcoma, and ovarian tumors.

Familial Spastic Paraplegia

Pure examples of familial spastic paraplegia are uncommon.[9, 53] Strümpell reported two families with dominantly inherited spastic paraplegia starting in the third decade, and at autopsy degeneration was found to be confined to the pyramidal tracts in the spinal cord and to the columns of Goll. However, other families have shown considerable variability as regards the nature of the disability. A family reported by Bickerstaff contained examples of pure spastic paraplegia, tetraplegia, hemiplegia, localized amyotrophy and retrobulbar neuropathy. In other families, the paraplegia has been complicated by ataxia. It has also been associated with mental retardation, progressive dementia, ichthyosis and mental deficiency, central retinal degeneration and mental deficiency, diffuse amyotrophy, hereditary sensory polyneuropathy, and extrapyramidal dystonia.[53] The term "familial spastic paraplegia" is properly applied only to cases with uncomplicated spastic paraplegia. The age of onset is not a criterion, since it can begin anytime from birth to the sixth decade.

Clinical Features. Males are more frequently affected than are females. The first symptom is weakness and stiffness of the legs; the patient tends to walk on the toes and gait may eventually become scissored as a result of adductor spasticity. The reflexes are brisk, clonus is present at the ankles, and extensor plantar responses are the rule. As the disease progresses, spasticity extends to the upper limbs, which become stiff and clumsy, with brisk reflexes. Spastic dysarthria has occurred in a few patients. Ultimately, the patient is unable to walk or to stand.

The course of the disease is very slow, and some patients have lived to an advanced age. So long as the arms are unaffected, the patient is able to make a living in a sedentary occupation.

Hereditary Optic Artrophy (Leber's Syndrome)

This disorder is characterized by the rapid development of bilateral central scotomas and optic atrophy in the late teens or early twenties.[7, 28, 36, 53] Occasionally, it has occurred before puberty or in middle age. There is considerable doubt as to whether it represents a disease sui generis.[53] In the first place, its mode of inheritance is unusual.[53] The disease and the carrier state are not transmitted by the male line and of the children of affected families, some 50 per cent of the males and 30 per cent of the females are affected. Second, the onset is rapid, which is unusual in hereditary diseases. Third, visual failure may be preceded—or succeeded after a considerable delay—by a variety of other neurological symptoms. Thus, in one family, an affected woman had five children, three of whom had this disease, and two of the three had symptoms and signs indistinguishable from multiple sclerosis.[39] In another series of 10 patients with Leber's optic atrophy, nine had clinical manifestations of other neurological lesions.[62] In a large pedigree described by Bruyn and Went,[12] visual failure of this type was preceded by nonprogressive athetosis and spasticity, and other patients have been described in whom the visual failure was followed after many years by spastic paraplegia. Cases such as those described by Ford,[28] in which both males and females were affected by a *slowly* progressive central scotoma, should probably be excluded from the group.

Pathology. There is destruction of the ganglion cells and nerve fibers of the retina, together with demyelination of the papillomacular and perimacular fibers in the optic nerves and optic tracts.[38]

Clinical Features. Mistiness of vision is the first complaint. It usually comes on in one eye a few days before the other and may be associated with headache and a sense of lightheadedness or dizziness. Vision deteriorates rapidly, so that visual acuity falls to 20/200 within a few weeks, or even more quickly. Visual loss takes the form of a dense central scotoma. In the most acute cases, there is swelling and reddening of the optic discs. Impairment of vision progresses for weeks or months and then stops, leaving the patient with severe depression of central vision.

Diagnosis. The diagnosis is not difficult when there is a positive family history of bilateral hereditary retrobulbar neuritis, but in the absence of such a history, the condition may be mistaken for neuromyelitis optica or multiple sclerosis.[39] Bilateral central scotomas, which occasionally occur early in the history of pernicious anemia, and which can precede the anemia, usually occur later in life, and vision deteriorates slowly. Tobacco-alcohol amblyopia, which is characterized by bilateral central scotomas, is unlikely to play a part in the visual loss of an adolescent. Compression of the optic chiasm can produce bilateral central field defects, but the scotomas are usually limited to the temporal fields, and a family history is lacking.

Treatment. There is no treatment, but when the incapacity has stabilized, the patient's life and habits must be adjusted in the knowledge that vision will not return to normal.

AMYOTROPHIC LATERAL SCLEROSIS
(Progressive Muscular Atrophy, Motor Neuron Disease)

Definition. Amyotrophic lateral sclerosis is a progressive disease of adult life characterized pathologically by degeneration of the anterior horn cells of the spinal cord, the motor nuclei of the lower cranial nerves, and the corticobulbar and corticospinal tracts. Clinically, there is paralysis of both upper and lower motor neuron types; sensation is unaffected. Aran (1850) and Duchenne (1853) described progressive muscular atrophy in which the main impact of the disease was on the lower motor neurons, and in 1869, Charcot and Joffrey gave the name "amyotrophic lateral sclerosis" to the more common cases in which atrophic paralysis is associated with signs of corticospinal tract disease. Duchenne (1860) recognized the bulbar form. The term "motor neuron disease" was introduced by Walsh to cover all varieties—spinal, bulbar, atrophic, and spastic—and this term is widely used in the British literature. "Chronic poliomyelitis," a misleading synonym, is still encountered in some European texts. In Europe the condition is often called "Charcot's disease."

Incidence. The disease is uncommon before the age of 30, and usually starts in the fifth or sixth decade. It is much more common in men than in women and has an incidence rate of approximately 1.4 per 100,000 population in the United States.[37]

Amyotrophic lateral sclerosis is common among the Chamorros on the island of Guam, among whom the incidence rate is 143 per 100,000 population. The clinical picture resembles classic motor neuron disease, but there is a pronounced familial incidence, and in some cases it is accompanied by parkinsonism and dementia.

Etiology. The cause is unknown. As early as 1881, Hammond suggested that it might be genetically determined, and this appears to be the case with the Chamorros, but it seldom occurs in more than one member of a family in other races. Only about 40 families have been reported in which many members have been affected over two or more generations; in most instances, inheritance was dominant. However, very few autopsies have been reported in this group, and since the disease has taken a very prolonged course in some of them, its relationship to "ordinary" motor neuron disease is doubtful. A protracted course is also seen in familial juvenile amyotrophic lateral sclerosis.

Trauma (including electric shock), although often invoked, is not a cause of the disease; it may direct attention to muscles which have been becoming weak; furthermore, as with other chronic neurological conditions, severe generalized trauma (such as occurs in traffic accidents, for instance) aggravates the symptoms.

The possibility that slow viruses may be involved in the pathogenesis of this disease is being investigated at the present time.

Syndromes resembling amyotrophic lateral sclerosis have been reported in the course of mercury and manganese poisoning, after gastric resection, following prolonged hypoglycemia, in uremia, and in hyperthyroidism, acromegaly, and visceral carcinoma and syphilis. It is possible that in these cases the association is coincidental.

Pathology. The outstanding features are degeneration of the corticobulbar and corticospinal tracts, mainly below the midbrain, and loss of anterior horn cells and the motor cells of the trigeminal, facial, vagal, and hypoglossal nuclei.[11, 17,]

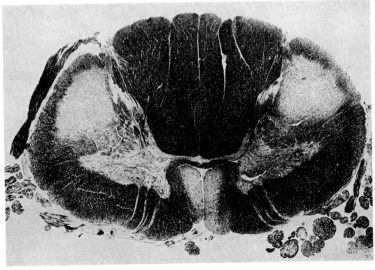

Figure 12–6. Amyotrophic lateral sclerosis. (From Wechsler, I.: *Clinical Neurology.* 9th Ed.)

[21, 42, 57] The ocular motor nuclei are not affected. Degeneration is also seen in the precentral and postcentral cortex and basal ganglia, and in the spinocerebellar, cerebellar, vestibulospinal, and reticulospinal tracts. As is to be expected from the involvement of the anterior horn cells, there is degeneration of motor fibers in the peripheral nerves, but segmental demyelination and remyelination have also been found in peripheral nerves.[21] The muscles show the typical appearance of neurogenic atrophy. In subacute and chronic cases, there is evidence of attempted regeneration, in the form of sprouting nerve fibers within the muscles.[65]

Clinical Features. Amyotrophic lateral sclerosis usually starts with muscular weakness, cramps, fasciculation, and atrophy, which appear first in the upper limbs, but which may involve any muscle or group of muscles in the body (Fig. 12–7).[46] The most common presentation of all is wasting and weakness of the intrinsic muscles of the hands; the thenar and hypothenar eminences waste, the

interosseous spaces become hollow, and atrophy of the lumbricales causes furrows to appear between the flexor tendons in the palm of the hand. Weakness and wasting then spread to involve the muscles of the forearm. In other cases, the deltoid and spinati are the first to become weak (Fig. 12–7); the triceps, latissimus dorsi, upper half of the trapezius, and the clavicular portion of the pectoralis major are often spared for a long time. Exceptionally, weakness and wasting occur first in the abdominal muscles, erector spinae, or lower limbs. Dyspnea on exertion, from weakness of the respiratory muscles, can be the presenting symptom, leading to false suspicions of cardiac disease or emphysema.[46, 47] In other cases, spastic weakness of the legs is the first thing noticed; they feel heavy and tire easily, and *cramps are often conspicuous.* It may be months before atrophy and weakness appear in the upper limbs. Occasionally, slowly progressive spastic hemiparesis ushers in the disease. Sphincter symptoms are rare, and appear late. There are no paresthesias, and objective

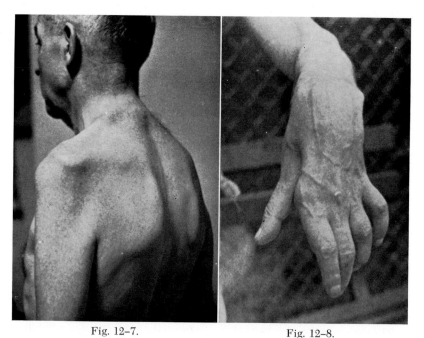

Fig. 12–7.   Fig. 12–8.

Figure 12–7.   Muscular atrophy in amyotrophic lateral sclerosis. (Courtesy of Dr. A. Ornsteen.)
Figure 12–8.   The hand in amyotrophic lateral sclerosis. (Courtesy of Dr. A. Ornsteen.)

sensory changes do not occur. An important feature of the disease is early and persistent exaggeration of the stretch reflexes, including the jaw jerk; the paradox of brisk reflexes in a limb which shows atrophy, weakness, and fasciculation is therefore highly suggestive of this disease. Extensor plantar responses appear early. As time goes on, weakness spreads to the trunk and neck, and ultimately to the face and bulbar muscles. The mind remains clear until the end.

Bulbar palsy is usually present in the later stages of amyotrophic lateral sclerosis, but sometimes it initiates the disease. The first symptom is usually the gradual appearance of slurring of articulation as a result of weakness or spasticity (or both) of the lips and tongue; paralysis of the palate may impart a nasal tone to the voice. Later on, there is weakness of the adductor muscles of the vocal cords, with the result that ultimately the glottis cannot be closed and the voice loses the normal "stops" between words, which are telescoped into each other. Weakness of the masseters interferes with mastication, and swallowing is impaired by weakness of the tongue and the muscles of the floor of the mouth; the pharyngeal constrictors sometimes escape, and the pharyngeal reflex may be abnormally brisk. Weakness of the pterygoids makes it difficult to open the mouth, or the mouth may hang open because of weakness of the masseters. Of the muscles of the face, the orbicularis oris is most severely affected. Movement of the eyes is not impaired, and the pupillary reflexes remain normal. The tongue varies in appearance; if the cells of the hypoglossal nuclei are involved, the tongue is weak and atrophied and shows conspicuous fasciculation, whereas when corticobulbar degeneration predominates, it is narrow and pointed, the jaws open with difficulty, and there is severe interference with phonation, mastication, and swallowing. In these spastic cases, pathological weeping and laughing are sometimes seen; the expression of the emotions is much exaggerated, and uncontrollable laughing and crying occur

without adequate reason. The patient is fully aware of the fact that his laughter and weeping are exaggerated. This can occur in any condition in which there is bilateral degeneration of the corticobulbar tracts.

Progressive muscular atrophy is the least common form of the disease. The atrophy may remain localized to one part of the musculature for many months or even for a year or two, or it may spread slowly or rapidly to involve the entire body. There is wasting, weakness, and fasciculation, but although the tendon reflexes may be exaggerated in the early stages, spasticity is inconspicuous and the plantar responses may remain flexor, although degeneration of the corticospinal tracts is always present. Ultimately, the tendon reflexes disappear.

Course and Prognosis[40, 47] The disease is inevitably fatal, but the duration of life from the onset of symptoms varies widely. On the average, patients live about four years, but cases commencing with bulbar palsy can prove fatal within a year, while those without early bulbar involvement and with much spasticity in the lower limbs may survive for eight or nine years. The course is apt to be very rapid in the rare, nonfamilial juvenile cases.[53] A much longer survival time is seen in the familial type in Guam and in the rare familial variety found elsewhere in the world.[26, 53]

Laboratory Aids. The spinal fluid is normal in all respects, and the electroencephalogram is not affected. Electromyography can supply early information as to the presence of denervation. When degeneration of the lower motor neuron begins, insertion of a needle electrode evokes a prolonged discharge of electrical activity in the form of large spikes of short duration. Fine fibrillation potentials are present at rest. During voluntary contraction, there is a reduction in the number of motor unit action potentials, but they are increased in both duration and amplitude; the reason for this is not known, but it has been suggested that the disease may selectively destroy small motor units, leaving the larger ones intact. It has also been thought that sprouting nerve fibers[65] may innervate adjacent denervated muscle fibers and thus contribute to the unusual features of the electromyogram. The conduction time in motor nerves is reduced, but sensory nerves are unaffected. Cumings[17] found abnormalities of pyruvate metabolism in 15 of 36 patients, aminoaciduria in six of eight, and a raised sedimentation rate in 16 of 35.

Differential Diagnosis. Widespread fasciculation of coarse type is sometimes seen in otherwise normal persons and is of no significance if the muscles in which it occurs are neither weak nor wasted. This is known as benign fasciculation.

Wasting of the small muscles of the hands, which so often is the first sign, is distinguished from similar changes caused by lesions of the ulnar and median nerves by the absence of paresthesias and sensory loss and by the fact that the atrophy is not, as a rule, confined to either the median or the ulnar distribution. Wasting of the hand owing to presence of a cervical rib is associated with tingling and numbness in the ulnar border of the hand and forearm. Cervical spondylosis is a relatively common cause of spastic weakness of the legs and lower motor neuron weakness of the upper limbs, but usually there is a history of pain in the upper or lower limbs and paresthesias in the feet and hands. Confusion will not arise if paresthesia or sensory impairment is present, because these do not occur in amyotrophic lateral sclerosis. A brisk jaw jerk and bulbar symptoms rule out cervical spondylosis as a cause of the neurological deficit in the arms and legs. When doubt remains, contrast myelography is necessary to exclude this and other causes of spinal cord compression. A cerebral tumor can be mimicked when amyotrophic lateral sclerosis starts with slowly progressive spastic hemiparesis, without atrophy or fasciculation. Cases starting with spastic weakness of the legs have to be distinguished from the progressive type of multiple sclerosis, notably in patients over the age of 40 years, but there will often be an early history of diplopia or some indication of a previous attack, and

paresthesias or depression of vibration sense in the feet will serve to exclude amyotrophic lateral sclerosis. Peroneal muscular atrophy can cause confusion when there is no family history of the disease or when it involves the small muscles of the hands first, but its extremely slow progress and early depression of tendon reflexes will suggest the correct diagnosis. Dystrophia myotonica is easily separated by the presence of myotonia, early wasting of the sternomastoids, and the family history. The muscular dystrophies usually start in childhood, are familial, progress slowly, seldom start in the hands, and are unassociated with increased tendon reflexes or other pyramidal signs. In the rare Erb's syphilitic paraplegia, spastic weakness of the legs develops very slowly over the years, accompanied by disturbances of bladder function, but without sensory loss. The serological test for syphilis will be positive in the blood and spinal fluid in untreated cases.

Treatment. There is no way of halting the disease. Massage is comforting, but strenuous physical exertion and over-energetic physiotherapy aggravate the situation. If swallowing is difficult, semisolid foods are easier to manipulate than are solids or liquids, and careful oral hygiene is needed to keep the mouth clear of food debris. Belladonna may be required to help keep the mouth reasonably dry if dribbling is a problem. Small doses of Prostigmine occasionally seem to help symptomatically, but there is no evidence that steroids, vitamin E, vitamin B_{12}, or any other form of medication has the slightest effect on the disease. In the presence of respiratory difficulties, life can be prolonged by use of a respirator. When weakness of the intercostal muscles is present, acute respiratory distress can develop rapidly in response to pulmonary infections.

FAMILIAL JUVENILE AMYOTROPHIC LATERAL SCLEROSIS

This condition is rare. It differs from the acquired disease in starting in the first or second decade of life, in its presence in several members of a family, and (usually) in having an extremely protracted course.[26] Although in many cases the symptoms remain stationary for long periods, in others the degeneration is rapid and death occurs from bulbar palsy or respiratory failure and terminal pneumonia.

The pathology differs in no respects from the ordinary nonfamilial type of the disease occurring in adults, and the clinical features are much the same, apart from the (usually) extremely slow development of the disease. The first symptom is spasticity of the legs, so it is easily mistaken for familial spastic paraplegia. As time goes on, atrophy and fasciculation appear in the muscles of the legs, and the symptoms spread to the trunk and upper limbs. Occasionally, bulbar palsy is the first symptom. Ultimately, there is the usual combination of atrophy, fasciculation, and pyramidal signs. There is no sensory loss. Mental deterioration sometimes occurs, and this suggests a link with the type of amyotrophic lateral sclerosis combined with dementia seen among the Chamorros.

REFERENCES

1. Adams, R. D., and Kubik, C. S.: Symposium on multiple sclerosis and demyelinating diseases; morbid anatomy of the demyelinating diseases. *Amer. J. Med.* 12:510, 1952.
2. Allen, E. B.: Psychiatric aspects of cerebral arteriosclerosis. *New Eng. J. Med.* 245:677, 1951.
3. Alter, M., Talbert, O. R., Allison, R. S., and Kurland, L. T.: The geographic distribution of multiple sclerosis. *J. S. Carolina Med. Ass.* 56:209, 1960.
4. Baker, A. B.: Friedreich's ataxia: A clinical and pathological study. *Amer. J. Path.* 10:113, 1934.
5. Barbeau, A.: Importance and pathogenesis of abnormal movements during L-dopa therapy of Parkinson's disease. *Neurology* 20:377, 1970.
6. Bearn, A. G.: Wilson's disease: An inborn error of metabolism. *Amer. J. Med.* 22:747, 1957.
7. Bell, J.: Hereditary optic atrophy. *Treasury of Human Inheritance*, Vol. 2. Cambridge University Press, Cambridge, 1931.
8. Bell, J.: *Treasury of Human Inheritance.* Cambridge University Press, Cambridge, 1934.
9. Bell, J., and Carmichael, E. A.: On hereditary ataxia and spastic paraplegia. *Treasury of Human Inheritance.* Cambridge University Press, Cambridge, 1939, Vol. 4, Part 3, p. 141.
10. Bittenbender, J. B., and Quadfasel, F. A.: Rigid and akinetic forms of Huntington's chorea. *Arch. Neurol.* 7:275, 1962.
11. Brownell, B., Oppenheimer, D. R., and Hughes, J. T.: The central nervous system in motor neurone disease. *J. Neurol. Neurosurg. Psychiat.* 33:338, 1970.
12. Bruyn, G. W., and Went, L. N.: A sex linked heredodegenerative neurological disorder associated with Leber's optic atrophy. Part 1. Clinical studies. *J. Neurol. Sci.* 1:59, 1964.
13. Campbell, A. M. G., Corner, B. Norman, R. M., and Urich, H.: Rigid form of Huntington's disease. *J. Neurol. Neurosurg. Psychiat.* 24:71, 1961.
14. Cooper, I. S.: Dystonia reversal by operation on the basal ganglia. *Arch. Neurol.* 7:132, 1962.
15. Cotzias, G. C., Papavasiliou, P. S., and Gellene, R. Modification of Parkinsonism—chronic treatment with L-dopa. *New Eng. J. Med.* 280:337, 1969.
16. Critchley, M.: Observation on essential (heredo-familial) tremor. *Brain* 72:113, 1949.
17. Cumings, J. N.: Discussion on motor neurone disease. *Proc. Roy. Soc. Med.* 55:1021, 1962.
18. Curzon, G., Godwin-Austen, R. B., Tomlinson, E. B., and Kantameneni, B. D.: The cerebrospinal fluid homovanillic acid concentration in patients with Parkinsonism treated with L-dopa. *J. Neurol. Neurosurg. Psychiat.* 33:1, 1970.
19. Davison, C.: Spastic pseudosclerosis (cortico-pallido-spinal degeneration). *Brain* 55:247, 1932.
20. Davison, C., and Goodhart, S. P.: Dystonia musculorum deformans. A clinicopathological study. *Arch. Neurol. Psychiat.* 29:1108, 1933; 39:939, 1938.
21. Dayan, A. D., Graveson, G. S., and Robinson, P. K.: Schwann cell damage in motor neurone disease. *Neurology* 19:242, 1969.
22. Denny-Brown, D.: *The Basal Ganglia and Their Relation to Disorders of Movement.* Oxford University Press, London, 1962.
23. Eldridge, R. (Ed.): The torsion dystonias. *Neurology* Vol. 20, Part 2, p. 154, 1970.
24. Elliott, F. A.: The corpus callosum, cingulate gyrus, septum pellucidum, septal area and fornix. *Handbook of Clinical Neurology.* Edited by Vinken, P. J., and Bruyn, G. W., North-Holland Publishing Co., Amsterdam, 1969, Vol. 2, Chapter 26.
25. England, A. C., and Schwab, R. S.: Management of Parkinson's disease. *Arch. Int. Med.* 104:439, 1959.
26. Espinosa, R. E., Okihiro, M., Mulder, D. W., and Sayre, G. P.: Hereditary amyotrophic lateral sclerosis. *Neurology* 12:1, 1962.
27. Ferraro, A.: Presenile psychosis. *American*

Handbook of Psychiatry. Edited by Arieti, S., Basic Books Inc., New York, 1959, Chap. 52.

28. Ford, F. R.: *Disease of the Nervous System in Infancy, Childhood, and Adolescence.* Charles C Thomas, Springfield, Ill., 1960.

29. Greenfield, J. G.: *Neuropathology.* Edited by Greenfield, J. G., Blackwood, W., McMenemey, W. H., Meyer, A., and Norman, R. W., Edward Arnold Publishers, Ltd., London, 1958, pp. 545–548.

30. Hertz, E.: Dystonia. *Arch. Neurol. Psychiat.* 51:305, 319, 1944; 52:20, 1944.

31. Hoehn, M. M., and Yahr, M. D.: Parkinsonism: Onset, progression, and mortality. *Neurology* 17:427, 1967.

32. Hunt, J. R.: Progressive atrophy of the globus pallidus. *Brain* 40:58, 1917.

33. Jenkins, R. B., and Groh, R. H.: Mental symptoms in Parkinsonian patients treated with L-dopa. *Lancet* 2:177, 1970.

34. Jervis, G. A.: Juvenile amaurotic idiocy. *Amer. J. Dis. Child.* 97:663, 1959.

35. Johnson, W., Schwartz, G., and Barbeau, A.: Studies on dystonia musculorum deformans. *Arch. Neurol.* 7:301, 1962.

36. Kjer, P.: Hereditary optic atrophy with dominant transmission. *Danish Med. Bull.* 3:125, 1956.

37. Kurland, L. T.: Epidemiologic investigation of amyotrophic lateral sclerosis. III. *Proc. Mayo Clin.* 32:449, 1957.

38. Kwittken, J., and Barest, H. D.: The neuropathology of hereditary optic atrophy: The first complete anatomic study. *Amer. J. Path.* 34:185, 1958.

39. Lees, F., MacDonald, A. M., and Turner, J. W. A.: Leber's disease with symptoms resembling disseminated sclerosis. *J. Neurol. Neurosurg. Psychiat.* 27:415, 1964.

40. MacKay, R. P.: Course and prognosis in amyotrophic lateral sclerosis. *Arch. Neurol.* 8:117, 1963.

41. McMenemey, W. H.: The dementias and progressive diseases of the basal ganglia. *Neuropathology.* Edited by Greenfield, J. G., Blackwood, W., McMenemey, W. H., Meyer, A., and Norman, R. W., Edward Arnold Publishers, Ltd., London, 1958, Chap. 8.

42. McMenemey, W. H.: Discussion on motor neurone disease. *Proc. Roy. Soc. Med.* 55:1021, 1962.

43. Minski, L., and Guttmann, E.: Huntington's chorea, a study of 34 families. *J. Ment. Sci.* 84:21, 1938.

44. Mones, R. J., Elizan, T. S., and Siegel, G. J.: An analysis of L-dopa induced dyskinesias in 152 cases of Parkinson's disease. *Neurology* 20:405, 1970.

45. Muenter, M. D.: Double-blind placebo-controlled study of levodopa therapy in Parkinson's disease. *Neurology* 20(Part 2):6, 1970.

46. Mulder, D. W., Miller, R. D., Lambert, E. H., Sayre, G. P., and Colon, L. T.: Symposium on amyotrophic lateral sclerosis. *Proc. Mayo Clin.* 43:427, 1957.

47. Muller, R.: Progressive motor neurone disease in adults. Clinical study with special reference to course of disease. *Acta Psychiat. Neurol. Scand.* 27:137, 1952.

48. Netsky, M. G., Spiro, D., and Zimmerman, H. M.: Hallervorden-Spatz disease and dystonia. *J. Neuropath. Exp. Neurol.* 10:125, 1951.

49. Nevin, S., McMenemey, W. H., Behrman, S., and Jones, D. P.: Subacute spongiform encephalopathy. *Brain* 83:519, 1960.

50. Obrist, W. D., Chivian, E., Cronquist, S., and Ingvar, D. H.: Regional cerebral blood flow in senile and presenile dementia. *Neurology* 20:315, 1970.

51. O'Malley, W. E.: Pharmacologic and clinical experiences with L-dopa: A symposium. *Neurology* 20(Part 2):66, 1970.

52. Patton, R. B., and Sheppard, J. A.: Intracranial tumors found at autopsy in mental patients. *Amer. J. Psychiat.* 113:319, 1956.

53. Pratt, R. T. C.: *The Genetics of Neurological Disease.* Oxford University Press, London, 1967.

54. Robertson, E. E.: Progressive bulbar paralysis, showing heredofamilial incidence and intellectual impairment. *Arch. Neurol. Psychiat.* 69:197, 1953.

55. Rothschild, D.: On clinical differentiation of senile and arteriosclerotic psychoses. *Amer. J. Psychiat.* 98:324, 1941.

56. Scott, M., and Brody, J. A.: Benign early-onset Parkinson's disease: A syndrome distinct from classic postencephalitic Parkinsonism. *Neurology* 20:400, 1970.

57. Smith, M. C.: Nerve fiber degeneration in the brain in amyotrophic lateral sclerosis. *J. Neurol. Neurosurg. Psychiat.* 23:269, 1960.

58. Terplan, K. L., and Krauss, R. T.: Histopathological brain changes in association with ataxia and telangiectasia. *Neurology* 19:446, 1969.

59. Thilenius, O. G., and Grossman, B. J.: Friedreich's ataxia with heart disease in children. *Pediatrics* 27:246, 1961.

60. van Bogaert, L.: Contribution clinique et anatomique à l'étude de la paralysie agitante juvenile primitive. *Rev. Neurol.* 2:315, 1930.

61. Walshe, J. M.: Treatment of Wilson's disease with penicillamine. *Lancet* 1:188, 1960.

62. Wilson, J.: Leber's hereditary optic atrophy—some clinical and etiological considerations. *Brain* 86:347, 1963.

63. Wilson, S. A. K.: Progressive lenticular degeneration: A familial nervous disease associated with cirrhosis of the liver. *Brain* 34:295, 1911–1912.

64. Winkelman, M. W.: Progressive pallidal degeneration. *Arch. Neurol. Psychiat.* 27:1, 1932.

65. Wohlfart, G.: Collateral regeneration from residual motor nerve fibers in amyotrophic lateral sclerosis. *Neurology* 7:124, 1957.

CHAPTER THIRTEEN

Demyelinating Diseases

This chapter deals with two groups of diseases of unknown origin in which demyelination is the oustanding pathological feature. Some of these diseases, notably multiple sclerosis, neuromyelitis, optica, and acute encephalomyelitis, display patchy destruction of normally formed myelin. Schilder's disease is included in this group, although the demyelination is diffuse. A second group, the leukodystrophies, is composed of cases in which there is a defect in the formation of myelin, which stems from genetically determined metabolic disturbances. This group includes the metachromatic leukodystrophies, Krabbe's disease, Pelizaeus-Merzbacher disease, and two very rare entities, the spongy sclerosis of Canavan[21] and hyalin body sclerosis of Alexander.

Multiple Sclerosis

Definition. Multiple sclerosis is a disease of adolescence and adult life characterized pathologically by the intermittent development of plaques of demyelination in the white matter of the spinal cord and brain, and clinically by correspondingly varied disabilities, the nature of which depends on the site of the lesions.

Distribution. The disease is especially prevalent in cold and temperate re-

gions of the Northern hemisphere and is rare in tropical and subtropical zones.[3, 27] Similarly, in the Southern hemisphere, the disease is reported with decreasing frequency as the equator is approached. Nevertheless, areas of both high and low prevalence are found which cannot be related to latitude or climate; for instance, the disease is almost unknown in Japan, which lies between 30 and 50 degrees north, but it is prevalent in the United States, much of which lies in a comparable geographic zone. Within the United States, it is much more prevalent in the North than in the South, and Kurland has shown by careful surveys that this difference is not race-linked. The disease is almost unknown in white South Africans who have never traveled abroad, but occurs in those who have left their native country; in Israel, the great majority of sufferers from multiple sclerosis are immigrants from Europe. The significance of these epidemiological facts is unknown.

Incidence. The disease is slightly more common in women than in men, and the maximum incidence is between 20 and 40. It is rare before puberty,[17] and seldom appears for the first time after 50. Siblings are affected in less than 3 per cent of all cases. Kurland estimates that the prevalence rate in the United States varies from 10 per 100,000 in the South to about 50 to 75 per 100,000 in the North;

the prevalence rate for Canada and northern Europe is similar to that of the northern part of the United States.

Etiology. The cause is unknown. Infection by a neurotropic, slow virus is a possibility which is engaging attention at the present time. The hypothesis of a spirochetal origin lacks proof. Allergy or hypersensitivity has been invoked because the initial attack occasionally follows an acute infection, the injection of serum, or vaccination, and also because patchy demyelination can be produced in experimental animals by injecting them with homologous brain extracts, fortified by a variety of adjuvants. However, the lesions so produced deviate in some particulars from those of multiple sclerosis, and the resultant disease is an acute affair rather than a remittent and chronic illness.

Bodily injury is occasionally followed, within a day or two, by the first symptoms of multiple sclerosis, or by relapse of a case in remission.[30] This does not mean that trauma causes the disease; the writer has seen cases in which the first *symptoms* of tabes dorsalis and of amyotrophic lateral sclerosis appeared within days of significant bodily injury, so that if there is any link between injury and these diseases, it is either nonspecific or coincidental.

Pathology. The essential lesion consists of a clearly defined patch of demyelination with secondary edema and round cell infiltration; it usually measures a few millimeters across, and is capable of forming larger plaques by coalescence with adjacent foci.[1, 29] The disease shows a special predilection for the white matter under the ventricular ependyma, the optic nerves, the junction between the cortex and subjacent white matter, the brainstem, and the white matter of the spinal cord. The cells of the ventral horns, though sometimes enclosed in a patch of the disease, usually remain healthy, which explains the absence of atrophic weakness of muscles from the clinical spectrum of the disease. Old and recent lesions often exist side by side. The former appear as small grayish

areas, firm to the touch and surrounded by normal tissue, while fresh patches have a pinkish appearance and often appear as a crescent on the circumference of the original lesion. This appearance led Greenfield to suggest that the new areas of demyelination might represent the extension of an infective process from the old areas.

Microscopically, the fibers traversing each plaque show demyelination, the axis cylinders often remaining viable. There is local infiltration by small round cells, and the adventitia of the blood vessels is distended by fat-laden compound granular corpuscles. Older lesions appear as a scar, with naked axis cylinders threading through a latticework of neuroglial tissue. Although the disease often affects the spinothalamic tracts and the medial and lateral lemnisci, anything more than transitory loss of pain and temperature sensation is unusual. The simultaneous presence of both old and new lesions mirrors the fluctuations and changing symptomatology of the disease from onset to termination. However, it must be emphasized that the number and dissemination of the lesions is far greater than would be anticipated from clinical examination, and that correlation between symptoms and lesions is poor.[34] Normal function may be retained despite extensive demyelination, and lesions may precede symptoms by considerable periods of time.

Symptoms and Clinical Course. Multiple sclerosis is usually recognized by its behavior rather than by any constant constellation of clinical signs. In most cases, and particularly in people under 40, the disease is characterized by remissions and exacerbations and by the presence of symptoms indicating multiple lesions within the central nervous system. After middle age, the disease tends to be more steadily progressive. The disorder may manifest itself by disturbances of mind, mood, speech, cranial nerves, motility, sensation, and sphincters. Of these, the most common are retrobulbar neuritis, ataxia, weakness of pyramidal origin, and paresthesias. For all practical purposes, it is true to say that the peripheral nerves are never involved.

MENTAL SYMPTOMS. Mild reactive depression is common and understandable. Occasionally, there is an elevation of mood with undue cheerfulness and excessive cordiality; this euphoria can be very striking. Minor degrees of intellectual deterioration are not uncommon in the later stages of the disease;[26] rarely, severe dementia occurs early and requires hospitalization. Bergin[7] has reported the case of a patient in whom catastrophic dementia occurred early in the disease, and the writer has seen two patients who had been admitted to a mental hospital because of an organic psychosis of rapid onset and who showed mild but distinctive neurological signs of multiple sclerosis.

SEIZURES. Focal or generalized seizures occasionally occur, and Drake and Macrae have estimated their incidence as about 30 times greater than in the general population.[14] This figure is a little misleading because in most cases in which seizures occur they are neither persistent nor frequent, and their contribution to the general disability produced by the disease is usually inconspicuous.

DISORDERS OF SPEECH. True aphasia, either sensory or motor, is rare. On the other hand, dysarthria is common, and can be due to ataxia of cerebellar origin, bilateral involvement of the corticobulbar tracts, or both. The patient with longstanding cerebellar dysarthria finds it convenient to break down words into their constituent syllables, pausing fractionally between syllables, and this gives rise to the characteristic "scanning" speech. In rare cases, there are repeated attacks of dysarthria and ataxia, with or without diplopia, lasting less than a minute.[4] The attack is sometimes precipitated by hyperventilation. Similar attacks of "periodic ataxia" have been described in familial cerebellar ataxia, the Guillain-Barré syndrome, and diseases of the brainstem.[13] Although no abnormalities have been discovered in the electroencephalogram in the cases

studied thus far, the brevity of these "seizures" and the fact that they can often be relieved by carbamazepine (Tegretol) suggest the presence of an intermittently discharging focus.

CRANIAL NERVE PALSIES. These are common. The sense of smell is rarely affected. On the other hand, sight is often disturbed, either by retrobulbar neuritis or by diplopia. When the *optic nerve* is involved, loss of central vision comes on rapidly, and if the lesion is close to the eyeball, there may be local pain, which is aggravated by moving the eye. If the lesion is considerable it can impede the venous return from the retina, and mild papilledema develops on the affected side—the so-called optic neuritis of multiple sclerosis. Visual loss is central, in the form of a scotoma, with sparing of the peripheral fields, but in severe cases almost total blindness of one eye may develop. The blurring of vision usually clears up in a few days or weeks, leaving pallor of the temporal half of the optic discs; the temporal situation of the pallor is determined by the fact that in most cases the condition affects the macular fibers, which pass to the temporal side of the disc. Pallor without a history of visual loss is likely to be physiological. When the disease affects both sides, it usually does so in series rather than together; simultaneous involvement usually means that the lesion is in the chiasm, but this is rare. Multiple sclerosis rarely causes complete or permanent blindness. Hemianopia due to a plaque in the optic tract or optic radiation is rare.

OCULAR MOVEMENTS. Diplopia lasting for hours or days, with or without visible strabismus, is one of the common features of the disease. Pupillary inequality, or loss of the reflex to light or convergence, is rare, and ptosis is uncommon. In advanced cases with bilateral disease of the supranuclear pathways, there may be weakness of conjugate ocular movement in one or more directions, with or without diplopia. Internuclear ophthalmoplegia (p. 91) is not uncommon, and is more often seen in this disease than in any other. Nystagmus, usually due to brainstem or cerebellar involvement, is very common. It is usually seen on lateral deviation of the eyes, and it may also occur on looking upward. It may be horizontal, vertical, or rotatory. In some cases, fine oscillations occur even when the eye is looking directly forward. Monocular nystagmus on lateral deviation is highly suggestive of multiple sclerosis.

THE TRIGEMINAL NERVE. The face is sometimes the site of unilateral tingling or subjective numbness without anything more than the most fleeting of objective sensory impairment. Of greater importance is the occasional occurrence of trigeminal neuralgia, differing in no way from idiopathic tic douloureux and amenable to the same treatment. Its frequency is rather greater than can be accounted for by coincidence, and it is important to search carefully for evidence of multiple sclerosis in all cases of trigeminal pain of this type. The motor function of the fifth nerve is not affected except as a part of the spastic bulbar palsy which sometimes occurs late in the disease.

THE FACIAL NERVE. This usually escapes; rarely, there is weakness of the lower face on one side from pyramidal involvement.

THE EIGHTH NERVE. Hearing is rarely affected, but bilateral nerve deafness can occur—and hearing can be recovered. Attacks of vertigo with or without vomiting are common and are due to a lesion of the proximal portion of the vestibular nerve or the root entry zone in the pons. In some cases, vertigo is experienced when the head is placed in certain positions; the sense of rotation develops after a second or two. Unlike the positional vertigo of labyrinthine disease (p. 101), the sense of rotation can be induced by several positions of the head, and tends to continue as long as the head is held in that position. In rare instances, there is a total loss of caloric responses on the affected side.

THE NINTH, TENTH, ELEVENTH, AND TWELFTH CRANIAL NERVES. These are seldom affected directly, but speech and swallowing are often disturbed by spasticity and weakness in the late stages of the disease. Repeated transient attacks of dysarthria and ataxia have already been mentioned.

THE MOTOR SYSTEM. Motor functions can be disturbed by spastic weakness, cerebellar ataxia, intention tremor, and sensory ataxia. The anterior horn cells and the peripheral nerves escape. A little clumsiness of the hands with a tendency to drop things for no apparent reason is often an early symptom; at this stage it may be difficult, if not impossible, to detect weakness, ataxia or sensory impairment. Another common early symptom is a sense of clumsiness, stiffness, or heaviness of one or both legs; the patient tends to stumble, and the legs feel tired by the end of the day. These symptoms may be transient and remittent, or they may gradually progress to a condition of marked incapacity. There may be improvement in one limb, with concurrent deterioration in another. The clumsiness, weakness, and slight spasticity imposed by corticospinal tract disease may be further aggravated by cerebellar ataxia, in which event there is a marked falling off of manual dexterity, and intention tremor develops. The ataxia from cerebellar or spinocerebellar lesions may be aggravated, in turn, by impairment of proprioception; in some cases, the ataxia is more sensory than cerebellar in type. The gait may be spastic, ataxic, or both. There is exaggeration of the tendon reflexes, early loss of the abdominal reflexes, and extensor plantar responses; these may be present during intermissions, when the patient believes himself to be free of incapacity. As the disease progresses, weakness and spasticity increase, and walking becomes impossible. At this stage, atrophy of disuse may appear, and the legs are held adducted and flexed at the hips and the knee. Rarely, cerebellar ataxia with intention tremor dominates the scene; the patient is unable to lift a cup to his mouth, to hold a pen, or to dress himself because of violent tremor, and walking is impossible because of incoordination of the legs or trunk.

SENSATION. Sensory symptoms are more common than sensory signs. Paresthesias, described as pins and needles, coldness, or numbness, are felt in the hands, feet, face, or trunk. Their recurrence from time to time in the past history of any patient with neurological disability provides a suggestive clue as to the identity of the disease. Paresthesias which invade the limbs when the neck is flexed indicate a lesion in the upper cervical region (Lhermitte's sign); this also occurs in tumors, cervical spondylosis, and subacute combined degeneration of the cord. Pain in the form of headache or discomfort in the trunk or limbs is not a common feature of the disease, with the important exception of trigeminal neuralgia. Loss of vibration sense in the legs is the most common objective sensory disturbance, and impairment of postural sensibility in the feet and hands is not uncommon. Only in rare cases is there any considerable loss of pain and thermal sensibility, but occasionally it is sufficiently deep and extensive to suggest a transverse lesion of the cord, or it may be confined to one limb with a distribution which suggests that the root entry zone of the spinal cord has been involved by a patch of demyelination; in such cases, the tendon reflexes are lost in that limb. With this exception, loss of the tendon reflexes does not occur as a result of uncomplicated multiple sclerosis.

OTHER SYMPTOMS. Sphincter symptoms are usually absent in early cases, or are limited to hesitancy or precipitancy of micturition, but retention and overflow incontinence may occur in the later stages. Other disturbances of the autonomic nervous system are exceptional, but attacks of vomiting for which there seems to be no other explanation sometimes occur in the course of the disease. Vomiting also occurs during attacks of vertigo, caused by a plaque in the brainstem or the proximal portion of the vestibular nerve. Horner's syndrome is occasionally seen. Impotence is common. Attacks of unexplained fever, sometimes amounting to hyperpyrexia, can occur. Such incidents are characterized by the fact that the patient feels and looks relatively well, in contrast to what would be the case if the fever were due to infection.

Laboratory Data. The spinal fluid pressure is normal. There is moderate lymphocytic pleocytosis—usually less than 30 cells—in about one-third of all cases. The protein content is raised in only about one in four cases; it seldom exceeds 70 mg. per cent. On the other hand, there is often a rise of gamma globulin, and in some of these cases, it is sufficient to give a positive colloidal gold precipitation test.[16] The presence of a first zone curve in the absence of a history of syphilis and negative serological tests for that disease is suggestive of multiple sclerosis. The electroencephalogram shows slight diffuse abnormalities in many cases, but the changes are nonspecific, and this form of investigation is unrewarding, except insofar as it may help to exclude the presence of other diseases.[24]

Course and Prognosis. Multiple sclerosis is always a potentially serious disease, but its course is so variable that in the early stages it is impossible to predict what is going to happen to any given patient.[9, 10, 28, 29] More than half of all cases pursue a remittent course, while in the remainder the disease is slowly progressive. The latter is especially likely to be true in patients over 40. The duration of the remissions varies between several months and 30 or more years. A total course of 20 or more years is not uncommon, and the patient may remain capable of productive work for a large portion of that time, a point to be remembered when asked for a prognosis by the patient or his relatives. In McAlpine's study of 241 patients, about one-third died within 10 years, one-third were disabled, and the remaining one-third were capable of normal employment and domestic life despite the presence of symptoms.[28, 29] In a few cases—and fortunately these are very rare—death can occur within two months of the onset. Infections and surgical operations are sometimes, but not invariably, followed by an exacerbation of the disease. Pregnancy is often said to have a similar effect, but it must be remembered that the artificial termination of pregnancy can be followed by the deterioration which it is designed to avoid.[33] Nevertheless, this course may have to be advised to avoid adding another baby to the burdens of an already incapacitated mother.

Death is usually due to intercurrent disease, notably respiratory infections.

Diagnosis. The disease is recognized by its clinical features. When the course is remittent and the evidence of multiple lesions is definite, the diagnosis is obvious, but difficulties arise in progressive cases without remissions, and also when the presenting symptoms can be explained by a single lesion.

Neurosyphilis may display its versatility by simulating multiple sclerosis, but it can be excluded by an examination of blood and spinal fluid; cerebrovascular syphilis can occur with a normal spinal fluid and a positive blood serology, but the risk of misdiagnosis is reduced by the circumstance that vascular syphilis commonly presents as cerebral or spinal thrombosis of abrupt onset, and by the fact that all the symptoms and signs can be attributed to a single lesion. Hemiplegia, the commonest result of cerebral thrombosis from vascular syphilis, is seldom seen on its own in multiple sclerosis. Acute transverse myelitis of syphilitic origin can closely mimic a similar situation sometimes seen in multiple sclerosis, but serological tests of blood and spinal fluid will indicate the nature of the underlying lesion.

Postinfectious and postvaccinal encephalomyelitis can usually be distinguished by the onset of symptoms following vaccination or an infectious disease, and by the subsequent freedom from relapses. Moreover, it is only in the rarest of cases that multiple sclerosis develops before puberty, whereas encephalomyelitis usually occurs in children. Schilder's disease is usually distinguished by an onset in early life, severe rapid mental deterioration, focal cerebral symptoms, and a rapidly progressive course.

Cerebellar tumor may be suggested by nystagmus, dysarthria, and ataxia of the limbs, but in multiple sclerosis headaches are absent, there are usually other signs (such as an extensor plantar response or loss of vibration sense in the feet) to indicate lesions outside the cerebellum, and the pressure of the spinal fluid is normal. Cerebral tumor may be suspected in the rare cases of multiple sclerosis which start with progressive hemiparesis or jacksonian or generalized seizures. If neither the history nor the examination of the nervous system provides evidence of lesions elsewhere, recourse must be had to angiography, brain scanning, and pneumoencephalography. Spinal compression, especially in the upper cervical region, can mimic multiple sclerosis, including the production of nystagmus; it usually gives rise to an increase in the cerebrospinal fluid protein, and complete or incomplete block on manometry, but if there is any reason for doubt, myelography is necessary. Multiple sclerosis and cervical cord compression from spondylosis—both common diseases—may be present in the same patient. Tumors of the cerebellopontine angle, which may present with features as diverse as tic douloureux, attacks of vertigo, or a sense of imbalance, are easily mistaken for multiple sclerosis in the early part of their course because the symptoms and signs of raised intracranial pressure are often absent, and the symptoms may be intermittent.

It is doubtful whether the type of retrobulbar neuritis which is seen in multiple sclerosis occurs in any other condition. The classic central scotoma with or without edema of the disc, coming on rapidly and passing off within days or weeks, leaving some degree of temporal pallor, should be regarded as evidence of multiple sclerosis until the contrary is proved. It must be emphasized, however, that in some cases of retrobulbar neuritis, other evidence of multiple sclerosis fails to develop. In one series, 49 per cent of patients remained free from other symptoms over a 20 year follow-up.[9]

Friedreich's ataxia is readily distinguished by familial incidence, ataxia, early depression of the tendon reflexes in the legs, and the characteristic deformity of the feet. Amyotrophic lateral sclerosis presenting as slowly progressive spastic paraparesis may cause difficulty in middle-aged persons until the appearance of atrophy and fasciculation makes the diagnosis clear.

Subacute combined degeneration of the cord, with spasticity, paresthesias, and loss of vibratile sensibility in the feet, can simulate multiple sclerosis, but there is evidence of polyneuropathy and there is a positive response to vitamin B_{12} therapy. Myasthenia gravis can cause difficulty when diplopia is the presenting symptom, but it is distinguished by the characteristic relationship to fatigue and a positive Tensilon test.

Psychoneurosis is often suspected at first because there are often no objective neurological signs to substantiate the patient's complaint of paresthesias, transient disturbance of vision, dizziness, etc. The fact that the patient is emotionally disturbed does not necessarily prove that all his symptoms are psychogenic, and the fact that he is or has been under stress may be irrelevant. A vague past history of "nervous breakdown" in patients with multiple sclerosis often turns out to have been an attack of the disease, the organic nature of which was not recognized at the time.

Treatment. There is no known means of combating multiple sclerosis, nor of inducing a remission. There is, therefore, no justification for subjecting the patient to expensive, elaborate, and fanciful therapeutic rituals. If a placebo is necessary, it should at least be innocuous. There is no evidence that steroids are effective for chronic cases, but there may be some merit in giving 40 units of ACTH by intramuscular injection daily for 10 or 14 days during acute exacerbations of the disease.[31] Thalamotomy can bring about an abatement of severe action tremor, and this operation is justifiable when such tremor is the main incapacitating feature of the disease. When severe spasticity of the legs interferes with their use, or makes nursing care difficult by reason of adduction or flexion contractures, the interruption of conduction in the lumbar roots by intrathecal injections of phenol can be useful, but great care has to be exercised to avoid inducing severe sensory loss and bladder symptoms. Current forms of medication for the relief of spasticity are almost always totally ineffective, but patients sometimes express confidence in Valium.

Adequate nutrition, prompt treatment of intercurrent infections, and avoidance of overfatigue are indicated. Massage and exercises, if not too vigorously prosecuted, are comforting to severely incapacitated individuals. Above all, every effort should be made to maintain the patient's morale and to keep him at work. Generally speaking, the lay public has an exaggerated idea of the terrors of this disease because it hears about the disasters but not about the many persons who pursue a useful working life for many years.

Neuromyelitis Optica (Devic's Disease)

Definition. Neuromyelitis optica is a rare disease which occurs in children as well as in adults. It is characterized by massive demyelination of the optic nerves and spinal cord, occurring either together or in series.[22, 38]

Etiology. The condition is variously regarded as a type of multiple sclerosis or as a form of acute disseminated encephalomyelitis. Those who survive the acute attack do not, as a rule, develop subsequent evidence of demyelination in other parts of the nervous system.

Pathology. There is severe demyelination of both optic nerves (or of the chiasm) and of the spinal cord. In the latter, it may be confined to a few segments, usually in the cervical region, but in severe cases it extends throughout the greater part of the cord, and cavitation may occur. There may be a few small areas of demyelination in the subcortical white matter as well. Perivascular infiltration with lymphocytes occurs.

Clinical Features. Sometimes the illness begins with a sore throat or febrile disturbance, but in other cases there is no such antecedent. The ocular symptoms may precede, accompany, or succeed the spinal symptoms, but there are seldom more than a few days or weeks between these events. The eyes become painful, and this symptom is followed by the rapid development of bilateral large central scotomas, which sometimes expand rapidly to produce complete blindness, but which usually leave a small amount of peripheral vision. If the disease is situated in the optic nerve close to the eye, there is vascular engorgement and edema of the discs. Even if the visual loss is severe, it can improve to an astonishing degree within days or weeks, leaving in its wake some degree of optic atrophy, with or without a mild degree of visual impairment; in some cases, however, a severe degree of visual defect persists.

The cord symptoms are often ushered in with pain in the back and limbs, followed by the rapid development of a complete or incomplete transverse lesion of the cord, with flaccid paralysis, sensory loss, and loss of sphincter control. If the cervical cord is involved, quadriplegia results. Flaccid paresis may give way to spastic paralysis; the tendon jerks become exaggerated, and the plantar responses are extensor, but in the most severe cases, when the motor pathways are completely destroyed, there is paraplegia-in-flexion. The temperature and pulse may be elevated. Occasionally the spinal cord signs are minimal.

In some cases, the spinal fluid is normal. In others, there is pleocytosis, including both polymorphonuclear cells and lymphocytes. There may be an excess of globulin. Ford has observed partial obstruction on myelography, with a later return to normal; this is presumably due to edematous swelling of the cord.

The course of the disease is variable. Some cases go downhill rapidly, but others improve to a remarkable degree as regards both eyesight and spinal symptoms. When recovery or partial recovery has occurred, the question arises whether further attacks are to be expected. If the disorder in any particular case is a manifestation of multiple sclerosis, further symptoms are likely to occur, but since in adults there is no way of distinguishing between the two, prognosis should be guarded. In children below the age of 10 years, however, multiple sclerosis rarely if ever develops at a later date.

Diagnosis. There is no difficulty in making a diagnosis of bilateral retrobulbar neuritis; large bilateral scotomas, with or without papilledema, form a distinctive picture. There is more difficulty in coming to a conclusion when transverse myelitis precedes retrobulbar neuritis. It is necessary to exclude the possibility of syphilitic transverse myelitis, acute hematomyelia, and acute epidural abscess. Myelography may reveal a subarachnoid block in all these conditions, and exploratory laminectomy may be justified to rule out disease which might be amenable to surgery, such as epidural abscess.

Treatment. There is no specific treatment. Either ACTH or steroids should be given in the acute stage to reduce the local inflammatory response. The patient should receive the meticulous medical and nursing care appropriate to any case of acute paraplegia, with special attention to the prevention of pressure sores and urinary infection.

Schilder's Disease
(Encephalitis Periaxialis Diffusa)

Schilder's disease is a rare disorder in which there is massive demyelination of the white matter of the cerebral hemispheres, causing progressive dementia, seizures, loss of vision, and motor and sensory disturbances. It is usually sporadic, but familial incidence has been seen.

Pathology. The lesions are most conspicuous in the white matter of the cerebral hemispheres. The demyelination may be localized to one or more lobes, or may be diffuse and bilateral.[35, 37] The nerve cells and U fibers of the cortex are usually spared, but the white matter of the cerebellum is involved, and in some cases patchy demyelination occurs in the brainstem and spinal cord. The optic nerves and chiasm are often affected. Because of the destruction of the corticospinal tracts in the brain, there is secondary degeneration of these tracts in the spinal cord. Microscopic examination reveals extensive demyelination with destruction of axis cylinders and varying degrees of astrocytic proliferation. In the worst cases, the destruction may be so extensive that cavities form within the white matter. Baló and others have described cases in which there are concentric rings of demyelination with relatively preserved white matter within them.

Clinical Features. About half of all cases start before the age of 14; in children, males are more affected than females. Symptoms and signs depend upon the distribution of the lesions and on the rapidity with which the disease progresses. In children the onset may be with convulsions, or with headache, vomiting, vertigo, and papilledema, or with focal neurological deficits, including hemianopia, cortical blindness, hemiplegia with or without hemihypalgesia, cerebellar or extrapyramidal features, pseudobulbar palsy with dysarthria and dysphagia, or cranial nerve palsies. In acute cases (which can simulate a cerebral tumor), the entire course of the disease may last not more than a few weeks, but it is more usual to see progressive degeneration with death within three years of the onset. In the last stages, there is complete dementia, with quadriplegia or decerebrate rigidity. On the other hand, mental symptoms may be the first to appear.

In adults, it is unusual to encounter convulsive seizures or the clinical signs of increased intracranial pressure. Aphasia, apraxia, extrapyramidal symptoms, cerebellar syndromes, and bilateral pyramidal signs are more likely to be seen.

In acute cases, the spinal fluid is under increased pressure, and there may be some increase of protein and moderate lymphocytic pleocytosis. In the more chronic cases, the fluid is normal apart from an increase in gamma globulin.

Course and Prognosis. In the acute cases, death can occur within two weeks, but in the majority of cases the duration is from one to three years. Exceptionally, the disease becomes chronic, the patient living for as long as 20 years.

The diagnosis can be very difficult. It is suggested by a progressive march of neurological symptoms, whose distribution suggests disease in both hemispheres. The intermissions which characterize multiple sclerosis do not occur, and cortical blindness, seizures, and progressive mental dilapidation are very uncommon in multiple sclerosis. In the rare cases which present with symptoms and signs of raised intracranial pressure, a brain scan and angiography are necessary to exclude the presence of a tumor.

There is no treatment for the disease.

Metachromatic Leukodystrophy

This is the least uncommon of all the inborn errors of myelin metabolism.[5, 6, 8, 20] It occurs in young children as a rule, though it may appear in adult life. It is usually sporadic in incidence, but more than one member of a family can be affected.

Pathology. The brain feels firm, but on sectioning it may appear normal to the naked eye. There is diffuse demyelination, which includes the subcortical U fibers; the degeneration is most marked in the fiber systems which mature last, notably the corticospinal tracts. There is considerable loss of the nuclei of the interfascicular oligodendroglia, and throughout the affected area there are small granular masses of lipid material which stain with polychromatic basic blue dyes. This peculiarity of staining, plus the degeneration of the oligodendroglia, distinguishes the disease from other forms of diffuse sclerosis. Metachromatic material is also seen in the epithelium of the renal tubules, the liver, and peripheral nerves. The basic pathological process is the accumulation of sulfatide, probably due to a genetically determined lack of the enzyme aryl-sulfatase A.

Clinical Features. Metachromatic leukodystrophy presents in a variety of clinical forms, of which the commonest is the late infantile form.[20] The child develops normally until about 12 to 14 months, at which time some difficulty with gait appears. By two years, the child not only has difficulty in walking but also displays defective manual dexterity. Muscular weakness may be aggravated by ataxia or by spasticity, and in some cases hypotonia is marked. Involvement of the peripheral nerves can lead to the loss of the Achilles reflexes, with hyper-reflexia elsewhere. There may be nystagmus or dysarthria. These symptoms are followed by mental deterioration, convulsions, and loss of vision. Eventually, the patient is totally paralyzed and death occurs within a year or two of the onset.

In some cases, the disease appears at the age of 6 to 8 years, usually presenting with ataxia, with or without mental impairment.

Another variant of the disease, presenting with dementia, has been reported in adults, and in these cases the accumulation of sulfatides in gray matter has been more striking than the pronounced accumulation in white matter in the late infantile form.

Laboratory Aids. The lowered content of aryl-sulfatase in the urine serves as a simple screening test for the disease, and diagnosis is confirmed by the demonstration of metachromatic material in nerve fibers, e.g., the sural nerve, or in specimens obtained by rectal biopsy. The protein content of the cerebrospinal fluid is usually elevated.

Pelizaeus-Merzbacher Disease

This is a slowly progressive heredo-familial disease of the central nervous system which usually appears in the first few months of life.[37] Exceptionally, the onset of symptoms is delayed until adult life. It occurs in families over several generations and usually affects males.

Pathology. There is diffuse and more or less symmetrical demyelination in the cerebral white matter, brainstem, and cerebellum; the spinal cord is less affected. The gray matter and axis cylinders are relatively well preserved. There is intense gliosis within the area of demyelination — so intense that some authorities have suggested that it might be responsible for the degeneration of the myelin sheaths. A curious feature of the disease is the preservation of myelin sheaths adjacent to some of the small blood vessels.

Clinical Features. The first signs to appear are nystagmus, tremor or rolling of the head, and paucity of movement. There is delay in the development of the ability to sit erect, stand, and walk. Demyelination of the corticospinal tracts within the brain is responsible for the appearance of progressive spastic weakness of the limbs, which is frequently compounded by cerebellar degeneration in the form of intention tremor and (in older children) dysarthria. Involvement of the extrapyramidal system yields cogwheel rigidity of the limbs, parkinsonian facies, tremor, or choreo-athetotic movements. Mental deterioration often becomes apparent at about the sixth year. Sensation is preserved.

Although the course is usually progressive, there may be prolonged periods of temporary arrest, or even partial remission. Survival into middle age is not infrequent.

There is no treatment for the disease.

Diffuse Cerebral Sclerosis of Krabbe and Scholz

Krabbe's sclerosis[25, 37] is a very rare familial disease characterized pathologically by rapidly progressing diffuse demyelination of the brain, accompanied by the appearance of large, multinucleated cells (globoid cells) around the small vessels of the white matter. These cells contain PAS-positive material and are pathognomonic of the disease. Segmental demyelination also occurs in the peripheral nerves.

The infant appears healthy at birth, but symptoms appear by the fourth or fifth month. The child becomes irritable and somewhat rigid. This is followed by tonic seizures, generalized convulsions, cortical blindness and deafness, pseudobulbar palsy, quadriplegia, and progressive dementia. Death occurs in from one to two years after onset.

Scholz has described a related familial disorder. In his cases, the onset was not until about the eighth year, and although its pathological basis was demyelination of the white matter, the early symptoms — sensory aphasia and cortical blindness — were more consistent with a cortical pathology. Within months, the limbs become spastic and weak, pseudobulbar palsy develops, and choreiform and athetotic movements may occur. Ultimately, the child becomes blind, deaf, demented, and completely paralyzed, and death usually occurs within a year of the onset.

In some cases, the cerebrospinal fluid protein is elevated, with increase in albumin, a low gamma globulin, and a normal colloidal gold reaction.

Acute Postvaccinal and Postinfectious Encephalomyelitis

This condition is an acute disorder characterized pathologically by diffuse perivascular demyelination and clinically by symptoms of meningeal irritation and focal damage to the brain and spinal cord. It can occur during or after infection by measles, rubella, mumps, chickenpox, and influenza, and also after vaccination against smallpox and rabies.[18, 32] Sometimes what appears to be the same disease occurs without any known infective or other antecedent, and this is spoken of as spontaneous acute disseminated encephalomyelitis.[36]

Etiology. There is no evidence that the disease is due to viral invasion of the nervous system, but because the postvaccinal form has occurred in almost epidemic form in Holland and England, it has been suggested that vaccination may aggravate a latent neurotropic virus. Another view is that the disease represents an allergic or hyperergic response to unidentified agents. This is based on the fact that somewhat similar pathological changes can be produced in experimental animals by the injection of brain extracts fortified with various adjuvants, but the relevance of this "experimental allergic encephalomyelitis" to the human disease has yet to be proved.[40]

Pathology. There is edema and congestion of the brain and spinal cord, with marked perivascular lymphocytic cuffing. Lymphocytes and plasma cells are also found some distance from the vessels. There is a striking degree of perivascular demyelination which is especially conspicuous around the small veins. The lesions are usually scattered throughout the white matter of the cerebrum, cerebellum, brainstem, and spinal cord, but sometimes they are concentrated in one particular area. A few lesions may also be found in the gray matter.

Incidence. It is difficult to generalize about the incidence of acute encephalomyelitis following vaccination because it differs greatly in different parts of the world and at different times. There were 45 cases and four deaths following vaccination of five million people in New York in 1947, but much higher figures have been reported from time to time from other countries. It rarely occurs below the age of one year or after age 30, and is commoner following revaccination than after primary vaccination.

Clinical Features. In most cases, the symptoms develop 10 to 12 days after an exanthem or vaccination, but the latent period may be shorter or longer. The onset is sudden, with headache, malaise, fever, and vomiting; in some cases, drowsiness is conspicuous from the start, and convulsions may occur in children. Signs of meningeal irritation develop rapidly, and they are soon accompanied by evidence of multiple focal lesions of the brain, spinal cord, or both. These may include ocular palsies, trismus, flaccid paralysis of one or more limbs, retention of urine, and sensory loss. Lesions of the spinal cord may simulate acute transection of the cord or an incomplete Brown-Séquard syndrome, and in some cases the clinical features suggest a transverse myelitis alone, without cerebral involvement. Peripheral neuropathy has occasionally occurred as the sole feature of the disease.

The spinal fluid may be normal, or there may be an excess of lymphocytes and protein. The electroencephalogram shows diffuse slow activity which may persist for some weeks after clinical recovery has taken place.

The mortality has varied greatly from time to time, but the figure usually given is from 10 to 25 per cent. Death is due to medullary paralysis coming on within a few days of the onset. Residual defects in survivors are rare, but occasionally motor incapacity in the form of hemi- or monoparesis persists, or there may be a blunting of intellectual acuity. In children, there may be a change of character, and in severe cases at all ages, the disease is followed by a period of intense mental and physical fatigability.

Diagnosis. Not all neurological symptoms occurring during or after infectious fevers are due to encephalitis. Whooping cough may be accompanied by cerebral hemorrhage, and cerebral abscess may occur in the course of scarlet fever, chickenpox, or smallpox. Cerebral embolism can occur in scarlet fever. Another difficulty is that encephalomyelitis can occur following an infection which was so mild as to have passed unnoticed. If the signs of meningeal irritation are conspicuous, the condition may be mistaken for bacterial meningitis, but in this case, the reduced glucose content of the spinal fluid in the latter is helpful. Thrombosis of the dural sinuses occurring during or after prolonged infective illnesses in children may cause convulsions, unconsciousness, and hemiplegia; in such cases, the spinal fluid is bloodstained, pneumoencephalography shows the ventricles to be small, and the venous phase of an arteriogram will disclose partial or complete blocking of the affected sinus.

Treatment. There is no specific treatment for the condition, but large doses of steroids or ACTH have been recommended. For an adult, the daily dose is the equivalent of 300 mg. of cortisone; this can be reduced after a week.

Acute Hemorrhagic Leukoencephalitis (Acute Necrotizing Hemorrhagic Encephalopathy)

The disease, first described by Hurst,[23] probably represents an extremely acute variety of acute encephalomyelitis.[36] Pathologically, the swollen and edematous brain is studded with minute hemorrhages which are usually of the ball or ring type and are related to necrotic venules or thrombosed capillaries. In the early stages of the disease, there is exudation of neutrophil leukocytes, which are later replaced by mononuclear cells. Demyelination occurs around both normal and diseased vessels. The most characteristic feature is necrosis of the vessel wall and the presence of a fibrinous exudate both within the wall and spreading into the neighboring tissues. The small veins are most affected, but the arteries may be involved as well. The meninges are infiltrated by neutrophils, lymphocytes, and histiocytes.

Clinically, the disease is marked by fever, severe headache, and vomiting. There may be convulsions, and the patient rapidly sinks into unconsciousness with or without focal signs, such as hemiplegia or diplegia. There is polymorph leukocytosis in the blood, and the cerebrospinal fluid contains a large number of cells, of which the majority may be neutrophil leukocytes. Its protein content is increased, but the glucose and chlorides are normal, a point of some importance diagnostically since the condition may simulate acute bacterial meningitis. The disease is likely to be fatal in one to six days.

Differential Diagnosis. A somewhat similar clinical picture can be presented by herpes simplex encephalitis. In the latter disease, if the patient survives long enough, there will be a rise of the serum complement fixation antibody titer to herpes simplex, but it should be noted that Martin and his colleagues have reported a case in which this rise occurred but in which biopsy material established the diagnosis of acute hemorrhagic leuko-encephalitis. It is possible that in such cases the disease was not caused by the direct effect of the virus on the brain but by an immunological mechanism. Since there is some evidence that surgical decompression has therapeutic value in both conditions, the procedure affords an opportunity of obtaining tissue for examination, and this can provide the correct diagnosis.

Treatment. In addition to decompression, large doses of steroids should be given.

REFERENCES

1. Adams, R. D., and Kubik, C. S.: Symposium on multiple sclerosis and demyelinating diseases; morbid anatomy of the demyelinative diseases. *Amer. J. Med.* 12:510, 1952.
2. Alexander, W. S.: Progressive fibrinoid degeneration of fibrillary astrocytes with mental retardation in a hydrocephalic infant. *Brain* 27:373, 1949.
3. Alton, A., and Allison, R. S.: Geographic distribution of multiple sclerosis. *World Neurol.* 1:55, 1960.
4. Andermann, F.: Paroxysmal dysarthria and ataxia in multiple sclerosis. *Neurology* 9:211, 1959.
5. Austin, J. H.: Metachromatic form of diffuse cerebral sclerosis. *Neurology* 10:470, 1960.
6. Austin, J., Armstrong, D., Finch, S., Mitchell, C., Stumpf, L., and Briner, D.: Metachromatic leucodystrophy. *Arch. Neurol.* 18:225, 1968.
7. Bergin, J. D.: Rapidly progressing dementia in disseminated sclerosis. *J. Neurol. Neurosurg. Psychiat.* 20:285, 1957.
8. Black, J. W., and Cumings, J. N.: Infantile metachromatic leucodystrophy. *J. Neurol. Neurosurg. Psychiat.* 24:233, 1961.
9. Bradley, W. G., and Whitty, C. W. M.: Acute optic neuritis: Prognosis for development of multiple sclerosis. *J. Neurol. Neurosurg. Psychiat.* 31:10, 1968.
10. Cater, S., Sciarra, D., and Merritt, H. H.: The course of multiple sclerosis as determined by autopsy proven cases, *Res. Pub. Ass. Res. Nerv. Ment. Dis.* 28:471, 1950.
11. Collier, J., and Greenfield, J. G.: The encephalitis periaxialis of Schilder. *Brain* 47:489, 1924.
12. Cooper, I. S.: Neurosurgical relief of intention tremor due to cerebellar disease and multiple sclerosis. *Arch. Phys. Med.* 41:1, 1960.
13. DeCastro, W., and Campbell, J.: Periodic ataxia. *J.A.M.A.* 200:892, 1967.
14. Drake, W. E., Jr., and Macrae, D.: Epilepsy in multiple sclerosis. *Neurology* 11:810, 1961.
15. Espir, M. L. E.: Paroxysmal dysarthria and other transient neurological disturbances in disseminated sclerosis. *J. Neurol. Neurosurg. Psychiat.* 29:323, 1966.
16. Freedman, D. A., and Merritt, H. H.: The cerebrospinal fluid in multiple sclerosis. *Res. Pub. Ass. Res. Nerv. Ment. Dis.* 28:428, 1950.
17. Gall, J. C., Hayles, A. B., Siekert, R. G., and Keith, H. M.: Multiple sclerosis in children. A clinical study of 40 cases with onset in childhood. *Pediatrics* 21:703, 1958.
18. Greenberg, M.: Complications of vaccination against smallpox. *Amer. J. Dis. Child.* 76:492, 1948.
19. Hagberg, B., Sourander, P., and Svennerholm, L. Diagnosis of Krabbe's infantile leucodystrophy. *J. Neurol. Neurosurg. Psychiat.* 26:195, 1963.
20. Hagberg, B., Sourander, P., Svennerholm, L., and Voss, H.: Late infantile metachromatic leucodystrophy of the genetic type. *Acta Paediat.* 49:135, 1960.
21. Hogan, G. R., and Richardson, E. P.: Spongy degeneration of the nervous system (Canavan's disease). *Pediatrics* 35:284, 1965.
22. Holmes, G.: Discussion on diffuse myelitis associated with optic neuritis. *Brain* 50:702, 1927.
23. Hurst, E. W.: Acute hemorrhagic leucoencephalitis, a previously undefined entity. *Med. J. Austral.* 2:1, 1941.
24. Jasper, H., Bickford, R., and Magnus, O.: The electro-encephalogram in multiple sclerosis. *Res. Pub. Ass. Res. Nerve. Ment. Dis.* 28:421, 1950.
25. Krabbe, K.: A new familial infantile form of diffuse brain sclerosis. *Brain* 39:74, 1916.
26. Langworthy, O. R., Kolb, L. C., and Androp, S.: Disturbances of behavior in patients with disseminated sclerosis. *Amer. J. Psychiat.* 98:243, 1941.
27. Leibowitz, V., Shavon, D., and Alter, M.: Geographical considerations in multiple sclerosis. *Brain* 90:871, 1967.
28. McAlpine, D.: The benign form of multiple sclerosis. A study based on 241 cases. *Brain* 84:186, 1961.
29. McAlpine, D., Compston, N. D., and Lumsden, C. E.: *Multiple Sclerosis.* E. & S. Livingstone, Ltd., Edinburgh, 1955.
30. Miller, H.: Trauma and multiple sclerosis. *Lancet* 1:848, 1964.
31. Miller, H., Newell, D. J., and Ridley, A.: Mul-

tiple sclerosis: Treatment of acute exacerbations with corticotrophin (ACTH). *Lancet* 2:1130, 1961.

32. Miller, H. G., Stanton, J. B., and Gibbons, J. L.: Para-infectious encephalomyelitis and related syndromes. *Quart. J. Med.* 25:427, 1956.

33. Muller, R.: Pregnancy in disseminated sclerosis. *Acta Psychiat. Neurol. Scand.* 26:397, 1951.

34. Namerow, N. S., and Thompson, L. R.: Plaques, symptoms, and the remitting course of multiple sclerosis. *Neurology* 19:765, 1969.

35. Poser, C. M.: The differential diagnosis of diffuse sclerosis in children. *Amer. J. Dis. Child.* 100:380, 1960.

36. Russell, D. S.: The nosological unity of acute hemorrhagic leucoencephalitis and acute disseminated encephalomyelitis. *Brain* 78:369, 1955.

37. Schumacher, G. A.: The diffuse scleroses. *Clinical Neurology.* 2nd Ed. Edited by Baker, A. B., Paul B. Hoeber Div., Harper & Row, New York, 1962, Chap. 25.

38. Stansbury, F. C.: Neuromyelitis optica (Devic's disease). *Arch. Ophthal.* 42:292, 465, 1949.

39. Symposium on disseminated sclerosis. *Proc. Roy. Soc. Med.* 54:1, 1961.

40. Wolf, A., Kabat, E. A., and Bezer, A. E.: The pathology of acute disseminated encephalomyelitis produced experimentally in the Rhesus monkey and its resemblance to human demyelinating disease. *J. Neuropath. Exp. Neurol.* 6:333, 1947.

CHAPTER FOURTEEN

Infections of the Nervous System

BACTERIAL INFECTIONS

General Features of Acute Bacterial Leptomeningitis

Mode of Entry. Purulent meningitis[86] is commonly due to blood-borne infection, but it can also result from the inward spread of infection from the middle ear, mastoid, and accessory nasal sinuses, and from the direct introduction of organisms into the skull as a result of penetrating wounds or compound fractures. Fracture of the posterior wall of the frontal sinus, the cribriform plate, or the petrous bone allows bacteria to enter the subarachnoid space if the dura has been torn, and meningitis may occur either within a few days or after an interval of months or years, and it may recur. The possibility of this portal of entry must be remembered in patients with meningitis (other than the meningococcal variety) who have had a head or facial injury in the past. Organisms can also be introduced into the subarachnoid space by spinal tap, and by intrathecal injections of spinal anesthetics and contrast media; gram-negative bacteria such as *Bacillus proteus, Pseudomonas pyocyanea,* and *Escherichia coli* are usually responsible for subacute meningitis in these cases.

General Pathology of Purulent Meningitis. The leptomeninges are involved by an acute inflammatory process with pus formation. Initially, there is meningeal hyperemia followed by an infiltration with polymorphs, which appear in the spinal fluid. If the disease is unchecked, the polymorphonuclear leukocytes break up, and histiocytes, plasma cells, and fibrin appear. The blood vessels are involved by acute vasculitis, and thrombosis within small vessels can give rise to local infarctions.

The combined effect of the infection and the vascular lesions is to produce multiple areas of focal destruction over the surface of the brain and in the ventricular ependyma; the ependymitis can give rise to stenosis of the aqueduct and hydrocephalus. In the later stages of the disease, there is fibrous organization of the purulent exudate, with meningeal adhesions and diffuse glial scarring.

In children (and occasionally in adults) there can be loculation of fluid over the vertex after the acute infection has subsided. The yellowish fluid contains leukocytes and a large amount of protein, but it is sterile; it is surrounded by an ever-thickening membrane and constitutes one form of subdural hygroma.

Symptoms of Purulent Meningitis. The onset is marked by chills and severe headache. There is often vomiting and

263

photophobia. The temperature rises rapidly, and the pulse and respiration rates rise appropriately; in pneumococcal infections, respiration may be disproportionately fast even in the absence of pneumonia. In children, convulsive seizures may occur at the onset. In fulminating cases, there may be acute delirium almost from the start.

Irritation of the meninges in the posterior fossa and the upper part of the spinal cord causes reflex contractions of the posterior neck muscles; there is resistance to flexion of the neck, but the head can be moved from side to side quite easily in all but the most severe cases. In children, the head may actually be retracted. If the hip is passively flexed to a right angle and an attempt is then made to extend the knee, the hamstrings go into spasm (Kernig's sign), because the movement of the leg causes traction on the cauda equina and inflamed meninges. Flexion of the hips and knees occurs in response to attempts to flex the neck (Brudzinski's sign).

Diagnosis. Headache and evidence of meningeal irritation occur in meningism, meningitis, subarachnoid hemorrhage, and encephalitis with a meningeal reaction. In *meningism* there is headache and rigidity of the neck without change in the constituents of the cerebrospinal fluid. It occurs in children and occasionally in adults as a result of acute infective illnesses, e.g., streptococcal tonsillitis, pyelonephritis, and lobar pneumonia. The headache may be so severe as to overshadow the symptoms of the primary disease. Meningism usually passes off within 24 hours.

Subarachnoid hemorrhage usually starts more abruptly than meningitis, but sometimes the onset is gradual and the picture may be further confused by the presence of moderate pyrexia and leukocytosis due to subarachnoid bleeding at the base. The diagnosis is confirmed by spinal tap.

Many forms of *encephalitis* are accompanied by headache, mild neck stiffness, pyrexia, and an excess of lymphocytes in the spinal fluid. Similar meningeal signs are common, especially in children,

in acute poliomyelitis, acute disseminated encephalomyelitis following the specific fevers, and *cerebral abscess.* In these conditions, signs of neurological dysfunction occur almost from the start, although in the case of poliomyelitis there may be a delay of one to three days before the paralysis appears. However, in virus diseases doubts are resolved by the discovery of a lymphocytic response and normal sugar content in the cerebrospinal fluid. All bacterial infections of the meninges reduce the sugar content, and in tuberculous meningitis, the chloride level is usually subnormal at an early stage.

Confirmation of the presence of meningitis, and identification of the responsible microorganism, depends on the examination of the spinal fluid. It is important that sufficient fluid should be sent to the laboratory for a cell count, estimation of protein, glucose, and chlorides, and bacteriological examination. When the cerebrospinal fluid appears clear or merely hazy, it is desirable to examine for yeasts with methylene blue or India ink, and to culture the fluid on Sabouraud's medium for fungi and on Lowenstein's medium for tuberculosis.

Prognosis. The outlook for acute purulent leptomeningitis depends upon the nature and number of the invading organisms, their sensitivity to antibiotics, and the possibility of removing the source of infection. Untreated, the mortality of meningococcal meningitis is high, especially at the beginning of an epidemic, and pneumococcal and streptococcal meningitis is almost always fatal. The prognosis and treatment of different forms of purulent meningitis will be dealt with under the appropriate headings.

Treatment.[71, 86] Bacterial meningitis is a medical emergency, and not more than an hour should elapse between the time diagnostic measures are begun and specific treatment is started.

Attention must be given to the maintenance of a good airway, to water and electrolyte balance, and to the treatment of seizures. Dehydration can lead to renal damage if sulfonamides are used.

Adults require from 2 to 2.5 liters a day, children proportionately less. Measurement of the specific gravity of the urine provides a rough guide to whether the patient is receiving too much water or too little, and is useful when laboratory facilities are not available. Hyponatremia, hyperkalemia, and hyperglycemia must be looked for and treated. If seizures occur, sodium diphenyl hydantoin should be given intramuscularly (5 mg./kg. body weight for a child, 100 mg. for an adult); sodium phenobarbital, sodium diphenyl hydantoin, or diazepam (Valium) can be given for status epilepticus, as described on page 140.

Specific treatment must be started as soon as possible. If there is doubt as to the identity of the responsible organism, a broad spectrum antibiotic should be given at once, pending the results of bacteriological examination.

PENICILLIN G.   This antibiotic is effective against most gram-positive and a few gram-negative cocci. It is therefore one of the most useful drugs in the treatment of meningitis, but increasing numbers of persons are becoming penicillin-sensitive, and care must always be taken to establish whether or not this is the case before administering it. There is considerable variation in the dosage advised by various authorities, but an average dose for an infant is 250,000 units every three hours, and for an adult 1,000,000 units every three hours.

AMPICILLIN.   This drug is effective against both gram-negative and some gram-positive organisms. It is given by intramuscular injection or intravenous infusion in doses of 150 to 200 mg./kg. of body weight per day.

SULFONAMIDES.   These drugs are valuable. Sulfadiazine is to be preferred, and a blood level of 10 to 15 mg./100 ml. of blood is aimed at. If an effective level is to be obtained promptly, the first dose should be large and should be given intravenously in saline. For an infant, a suitable dose is 100 mg./kg. body weight in 100 to 300 ml. saline; for an adult, 5 gm. in 1000 ml. saline. These can be repeated in 12 hours. If given orally, an initial dose of 100 mg./kg. body weight is suitable for an infant, and 4 gm. for an adult, the maintenance dose being 30 mg./kg. body weight every four hours for an infant, and 1 gm. every four hours for an adult. To avoid complications from crystallization of sulfadiazine in the renal tubules, fluid intake must be well maintained, and it is desirable to keep the urine alkaline by giving 10 to 15 gm. of sodium bicarbonate every 24 hours, or 1 to 2 liters of a one-sixth molar solution of sodium lactate can be given intravenously in adults. Watch should be kept for the presence of albumin and hematuria. Occasionally sulfonamides produce drug fever, nausea, vomiting, dermatitis, leukopenia, anemia, joint pains, and peripheral neuropathy.

STREPTOMYCIN.   This is used chiefly in the treatment of influenza, proteus, pyocyaneus, and tuberculous infections. A suitable adult dose is 1 to 1.5 gm. every 12 hours intramuscularly, and for a child, 25 mg./kg. body weight every 12 hours. The intrathecal dose for an adult is 50 mg., usually given daily, in 10 ml. saline, and for a child, 25 mg. daily in 5 ml. saline. Vertigo, nystagmus, and deafness *may* occur if therapy is continued longer than three weeks; streptomycin can destroy both the cochlea and the labyrinth. Some organisms become resistant, and this should always be looked for during long-continued periods of administration.

TETRACYCLINES.   Three members of this group, tetracycline, oxytetracycline, and chlortetracycline (Aureomycin) are active against a wide range of infection including *Staphylococcus aureus*, streptococci, pneumococci, *Hemophilus influenzae*, and gram-negative bacilli such as the coli-aerogenes group. They are said to be effective in the treatment of lymphogranuloma venereum. The oral dose is 500 mg. every six hours for an adult and 15 mg./kg. body weight every six hours for a child. The tetracyclines can be given intravenously in doses of 500 mg. every 12 hours for an adult, and 15 mg./kg. body weight for a child.

CHLORAMPHENICOL.   This is a potentially dangerous drug which can cause blood dyscrasias and other complications.

The risk must be weighed against its undoubted usefulness against *H. influenzae* and the *Salmonella* group. The oral dose for an adult is 1.5 gm. initially, followed by 750 mg. every six hours; the intravenous or intramuscular dose is 1 gm. every 12 hours. For a child, the oral dose is 750 mg. initially, followed by 25 to 30 mg./kg. body weight every six hours. It should not be administered to infants.

BACITRACIN. This drug has a therapeutic spectrum somewhat similar to that of penicillin, and is also effective against some strains of gram-positive cocci which are resistant to the latter. However, bacitracin has a tendency to produce albuminuria, hematuria, and nitrogen retention. It is given intramuscularly to adults in doses of 25,000 units every six hours, and by the same route to children in doses of 200 to 400 units/kg. body weight every six hours.

ERYTHROMYCIN. Erythromycin is useful for the treatment of penicillin-resistant staphylococci and nonhemolytic streptococci, as well as against pneumococci and *H. influenzae*. The dose for an adult is 500 mg. orally every six hours, or 750 mg. intravenously every 12 hours. The dose for a child is 6 to 8 mg./kg. body weight by mouth every six hours, or 20 mg./kg. intravenously every 12 hours.

POLYMYXIN B. This compound is specific for gram-negative bacterial infections, notably *Pseudomonas aeruginosa*, and *H. influenzae*. It can be given orally to adults in doses of 100 mg. every six hours and intramuscularly in doses of 30 mg. every six hours. For children, the oral dose is 3 to 5 mg./kg. body weight every six hours and if given intramuscularly, 0.75 mg./kg. body weight every six hours.

AMPHOTERICIN B. This agent is useful against mycotic infections of the nervous system. It is given very slowly in doses of 0.25 to 1 mg./kg. body weight diluted in 1000 ml. of 5 per cent glucose solution. Giving it more rapidly may produce pyrexial reactions, and after a few days of treatment, there may be renal toxicity, as evidenced by albuminuria, hematuria, and a rising blood urea level. If administration is stopped, renal function is restored. There is as yet insufficient experience to know how long the drug has to be continued in the treatment of these very persistent infections.

Meningococcal Meningitis

Meningococcal meningitis, formerly called cerebrospinal fever or spotted fever, arises as a result of a meningococcal bacteremia. Sporadic cases can occur, but it is usually encountered in epidemics, especially in the winter and early spring, the infection being spread by carriers who harbor the organisms in the nasopharynx. Droplet infection accounts for the rapid spread of epidemics in overcrowded barracks and schools. The incidence of the disease is greatest in the first year of life, after which it declines until adolescence; there is a sharp peak between the ages of 15 and 25, after which it declines again. It is rare over the age of 50.

Pathology. There is bacteremia at the onset. The organism usually settles in the meninges and produces meningitis, but it may multiply in the bloodstream and produce a fulminating septicemia which overwhelms the patient before the signs of meningitis have time to develop. The appearance of the brain to the naked eye is that of pyogenic meningitis, and microscopy shows widespread meningoencephalitis with diffuse capillary thromboses, small hemorrhages, and degeneration of nerve cells. Severe meningococcal infection has a particular tendency to produce petechial hemorrhages in the brain and skin. In the fulminating septicemic type, massive hemorrhages are sometimes found in the adrenals.

Clinical Features. The disease starts swiftly with headache, photophobia, and signs of meningeal irritation, sometimes preceded by a sore throat and joint pains. The meningeal signs commonly appear within the first few hours, and the temperature rises sharply. Herpes febrilis is often seen on the lips, less often on the trunk. In some cases, a fine purpuric eruption develops during the first 24 hours; erythematous and maculopapular rashes are less frequent. A rash is seen in only about 30 per cent of all cases.

With spread of the disease from the meninges to the brain, clarity of mind gives place to confusion and delirium. Diplopia is common. The optic discs usually remain normal unless the meningitis lasts for more than a week, in which event a rise of intracranial pressure can give rise to papilledema. The fifth, seventh, and eighth cranial nerves may be involved. Seizures are not uncommon as an early symptom, especially in children. Paralysis of limbs is rare.[95] A characteristic short, sharp cry (the meningeal cry) is common in children. If coma supervenes, extensor plantar responses will be present.

Laboratory Findings. The spinal fluid is under increased pressure; during the first 24 hours, it may be clear or slightly hazy, becoming turbid and purulent thereafter. A count of 1000 to 2000 polymorphs is not uncommon. There is also an increase in the mononuclear cells but not to the same extent as in the polymorphs. In fulminating cases, the cell count of the fluid may be low. Both intra- and extracellular meningococci are found in gram-stained smears of the centrifuged deposit. They may not be demonstrable on a slide during the first day, but will usually be obtained if the spinal fluid is incubated for 24 hours. The protein is much increased, and glucose rapidly disappears. The chloride content is usually reduced to the region of 650 to 700 mg. per cent. In the presence of spinal subarachnoid adhesions, and when internal hydrocephalus has been caused by adhesions around the base, a dry tap may be encountered. The blood shows polymorph leukocytosis almost from the beginning, and meningococci can sometimes be cultivated from the blood in the first 24 hours.

Complications and Sequelae. Prompt, energetic treatment usually prevents complications and sequelae. Complica-

tions outside the nervous system include acute arthritis of large and medium size joints, pericarditis and myocarditis, albuminuria and hematuria, orchitis and epididymitis, and infection of the eye in the form of iritis, choroiditis, or panophthalmitis. Glycosuria can occur at the height of the disease from involvement of the hypothalamus. Deafness, vertigo, and tinnitus can occur from infection of the inner ear; defective equilibrium due to involvement of the labyrinth usually passes off after weeks or months, but deafness is apt to be severe and permanent.

A fulminating *septicemic type* of meningococcal infection can occur. The onset is abrupt, with high fever, vomiting, stupor, and coma. In infants, there may be persistent convulsions. A petechial rash develops within a few hours, and death may occur within two days if treatment is not instituted immediately. The condition should be suspected in any comatose, febrile patient who has diffuse petechiae on the skin. The organism will be obtained from the blood and in smears from the centrifuged deposit of the spinal fluid.

Meningococcal septicemia is one cause of the Waterhouse-Friderichsen syndrome, which is characterized by collapse, purpura, and hemorrhage into the adrenals. In some epidemics, it has occurred in as many as 2 per cent of all cases. There is severe prostration, coma, low blood pressure, and petechial hemorrhages which can coalesce and lead to local gangrene of the skin if the patient lives long enough. Death usually occurs within 24 hours. The syndrome can occur in the absence of hemorrhage into the adrenal glands, and it is probably due to overwhelming toxemia and septicemia.

Neurological sequelae occur in less than 7 per cent of adequately treated cases. Permanent mental impairment and change of personality, once common and distressing sequelae, are now rare. However, many patients complain for some months of intermittent headaches, fatigability, irritability, dizziness, and impairment of memory, symptoms attributable to the encephalitis which accompanies severe meningitis. The diplopia, facial palsy, aphasia, and hemiparesis which can occur during the course of the disease usually pass off completely and rapidly.

Meningeal adhesions formed during the organization of the exudate occasionally cause persistent and slowly progressive neurological symptoms. They are responsible for the special clinical features of chronic posterior basic meningitis, which usually occurs in infants between the ages of four months and three years. Obstruction to the foramina of the fourth ventricle produces an internal hydrocephalus of gradual onset, and this is accompanied by low-grade fever, vomiting, anorexia, and great irritability. The head is retracted and opisthotonos may develop. The head enlarges, and optic atrophy can occur with or without antecedent papilledema. The infant becomes severely emaciated, and the condition is fatal unless it is treated. The organism is seldom found in the spinal fluid, which shows only a moderate pleocytosis.

Opticochiasmal arachnoiditis can cause an intermittently progressive loss of vision in both eyes.[36] *Spinal arachnoiditis* can lead to constriction of the spinal cord, interfering with the blood supply over many segments.[11] It can also lead to the formation of one or more loculated cysts (meningitis serosa circumscripta). The clinical picture is one of progressive spastic weakness of the legs, with sensory impairment and sphincter disturbances which start weeks or even years after the illness. Spinal tap often gives inconclusive evidence of block, but myelography will disclose the condition. A *flaccid weakness of limb muscles* is sometimes encountered,[88] without impairment of sensation, and this is apparently due to an involvement of the anterior horn cells. This can occur at the height of the disease but can also appear later on as the result of spinal arachnoiditis.

Treatment. During epidemics in closed communities, the carrier rate can be reduced and the case incidence lowered if everyone is given 0.5 gm. of sulfadiazine twice a day for two days; this should be extended to newcomers too.

For treating the disease itself, sulfonamide drugs or penicillin G is used. Sulfadiazine is commonly used because of its high therapeutic index and low toxicity. Fluid intake must be adjusted to keep a good urinary flow, and the urine should be kept alkaline to avoid deposit of sulfadiazine crystals in the urinary tract. The initial dose is calculated on the basis of 0.05 to 0.1 gm./kg. body weight, and it should be given in the form of the sodium salt dissolved in distilled water as a 5 per cent solution. One half of the initial dose should be injected every eight hours until the patient can take it by mouth in doses of 1 to 2 gm. every four hours. This dose should be continued for about a week after symptomatic recovery has occurred. If the patient can swallow from the start, sulfadiazine can be given in doses of 3 gm. every 24 hours for infants over two months old, ranging up to 9 gm. a day for an adult. This treatment can be combined with the administration of penicillin G in doses of 1,000,000 units twice daily by intramuscular injection. Sulfadiazine and penicillin can be given together in fulminating septicemic cases. In the presence of severe purpura and a fall in blood pressure, the patient should be given cortisone, Levophed, and blood transfusion. Intraspinal injections of sulfonamides can be dangerous, and intrathecal penicillin is not necessary.

Retention of urine is not uncommon when consciousness is impaired; since the patient will not complain thereof, the state of the bladder must be watched and catheterization resorted to if necessary.

Pneumococcal Meningitis

Pneumococcal meningitis usually arises as a result of spread of infection from the ears, paranasal sinuses,[31] upper respiratory tract, or lungs. It is not uncommon following fracture of the skull. Some cases occur without any known source of primary infection. It is most common in the very old and the very young.

The pathology, clinical features, and laboratory findings are the same as in other forms of acute purulent meningitis, but smears of the sediment from the centrifuged spinal fluid show gram-positive diplococci which give a positive Neufeld reaction.

Untreated, over 90 per cent of all patients die, and even with vigorous therapy, the mortality is in the region of 30 per cent. The prognosis is poor when the disease occurs in patients already debilitated by pneumonia, lung abscess, or bacterial endocarditis.

Treatment. Penicillin is the most effective drug for pneumococcal meningitis, but many authors recommend that it be combined with one of the sulfonamides. This is a prudent procedure until the sensitivity of the organism is known; when this information is available, therapy can be altered accordingly. If penicillin is used alone, it is given in doses of 1,000,000 units every two hours by intramuscular injection for two days, followed by the intramuscular administration of 3,000,000 units twice a day for as long as necessary. If the patient is sensitive to penicillin, sulfadiazine should be given in full doses, as for meningococcal meningitis, and broad-spectrum antibiotics may have to be added.

Intrathecal penicillin is seldom needed, but if it is to be used, not more than three intraspinal injections should be given, at 12-hour intervals. Crystalline penicillin G is dissolved in 10 ml. of physiological saline solution and injected at the rate of 1 ml./minute after withdrawing a comparable amount of spinal fluid. For infants under two years, the dose should not exceed 5000 units. For children between two and 10 years, 10,000 to 15,000 units may be given, and for adolescents, 15,000 to 20,000 units is advised. For adults, the dose should not exceed 30,000 units. Larger doses can cause seizures and myelopathy, and arachnoiditis may occur as a sequel.

Erythromycin can be used. The dose for children is 100 mg./kg. body weight and for adults, 1 gm. every six hours. It can cause phlebitis unless properly dissolved and given in dilute solution. Each dose should be added to 50 to 100 ml. of saline or dextrose solution and allowed to run in as rapidly as possible.

Acute infections of the ear and sinuses usually settle down under treatment, but with chronic mastoiditis, surgery may have to be resorted to. When infection has taken place via a dural tear following a fractured skull, surgical repair of the dura should be undertaken to prevent a recurrence of the meningitis. The treatment of pneumococcal meningitis should be continued until the patient has been free of symptoms for at least a week and the cerebrospinal fluid is normal.

Streptococcal and Staphylococcal Meningitis

Streptococci account for about 7 per cent of all cases of purulent meningitis. It is usually a complication of ear or sinus infections, and in some cases there is a cerebral abscess in addition to the meningitis. Treatment is the same as for pneumococcal meningitis, together with such surgical measures as are needed to eradicate the primary focus.

Staphylococcal meningitis is usually a complication of staphylococcal infection elsewhere in the body and may follow cavernous sinus thrombosis, mastoiditis, epidural or subdural abscess, and osteomyelitis of the long bones. It is one of the most difficult forms of meningitis to treat, and the mortality rate is high. Pending sensitivity tests, the patient should be treated either with sodium methicillin or ampicillin or by erythromycin with chloramphenicol. If the organism is found to be sensitive to penicillin G, this drug should be used in a total daily dose of 12 to 24 million units in aqueous solution. Treatment should be continued for at least two weeks after the infection has subsided.

Influenzal Meningitis

At the present, influenzal meningitis is the third most common type of acute purulent meningitis in childhood in the United States, accounting for some 18 per cent of all cases. It is due to infection by gram-negative *H. influenzae* and in its primary form is usually a disease of infancy and early childhood; in adults it is uncommon, but may follow sinusitis, mild upper respiratory infections, pneumonia, or fracture of the skull. The clinical picture is that of purulent meningitis lasting from 10 to 20 days, but occasionally the course is more protracted, and in such cases, cranial nerve palsies and hydrocephalus may occur. Positive blood cultures are often obtained in the acute phase, and the organism can be obtained from the spinal fluid which shows the usual polymorphonuclear response, low sugar content, and reduction of chlorides.

The prognosis is variable. Untreated, most patients die. Inadequate treatment can lead to a protracted course and permanent defects, including paralysis of cranial nerves, seizures, mental deficiency, and hemiparesis. With energetic treatment, promptly administered, the mortality rate is under 5 per cent.

TREATMENT. Ampicillin is effective. Some authorities prefer streptomycin, starting with a single intrathecal injection of freshly prepared streptomycin in 10 ml. of saline. It has been shown that this will usually sterilize the spinal fluid within 12 hours. For infants under two years of age, the intrathecal dose is 15 to 25 mg., for young children 25 to 50 mg., and for adults 50 to 75 mg. The single intrathecal injection of streptomycin is followed by a daily intramuscular dose of 20 to 40 mg./kg. body weight for two weeks. This must be accompanied by a sulfonamide given by mouth. Chloramphenicol may be used in place of streptomycin either alone or in combination with a sulfonamide, but it should not be given to children. The adult dose is 50 mg./kg. of body weight per day. It should be given by intravenous injection at first and by intramuscular injection later on, and must be continued for two weeks. The blood should be examined every day for evidence of toxic effects on the bone marrow.

Subdural hygroma sometimes occurs in infants with influenzal meningitis. Its presence is suggested by prolonged unexplained fever, vomiting, seizures, and lack of alertness despite adequate antimicrobial therapy, as judged by the improvement in the spinal fluid. Under these circumstances, a bulging fontanelle is suggestive. Aspiration of the fluid through the fontanelle relieves the symptoms; sometimes it has to be repeated.

Meningitis Caused by Other Gram-Negative Organisms

Meningitis in infants is often due to *Escherichia coli* and other enteric organisms. In the elderly, gram-negative bacteria from the colon or genitourinary tract can cause meningitis, and in debilitated individuals, the temperature and meningeal signs may be inconspicuous, the clinical picture being dominated by a confusional state or delirium. At all ages, bacteremia due to gram-negative organism is an important cause of septic shock.

Since identification of the specific organism and determination of its sensitivity to antibiotics are rarely possible until after 48 hours, it is desirable to choose a drug with the widest antimicrobial range of action. Ampicillin is generally effective against the common gram-negative bacillary infections. The dose for infants under two weeks of age is 100 mg./kg. body weight daily, given parenterally. Adults should be given 1 gm. every three hours.

Penicillin in daily doses of 40 to 60 million units has been successful in treating meningitis due to a number of gram-negative bacilli which are insensitive to other antibiotics.

Meningitis due to *Pseudomonas* organisms may occur as a complication of spinal anesthesia, head injuries, neuro-surgical operations, or urinary tract infections. The treatment of choice is polymyxin B sulfate. It must be used both intrathecally (2 to 4 mg. per day) and intramuscularly (2.5 mg./kg. body weight daily) and since these infections are very obstinate, treatment by both routes should be continued until the spinal fluid becomes normal. Renal function should be monitored throughout the administration of this drug.

Meningitis can be caused by *Mima polymorpha*, a gram-negative pleomorphic bacillus which is easily confused with members of the Neisseria group. The meningitis has no special clinical characteristics but it is important to distinguish the bacillus from the Neisseria because it is often resistant to penicillin and sulfonamides and responds only to the tetracyclines.

Tuberculous Meningitis

Tuberculosis causes lymphocytic meningitis which runs a subacute course and is always fatal unless treated. It rarely occurs before the age of six months, is most common in childhood and early adult life, and is seldom encountered after 40.

Pathogenesis and Pathology. The bacillus is carried to the central nervous system by the blood stream, usually from a focus in mediastinal or abdominal lymph nodes, but it can be derived from any infected organ of the body. The meninges are usually infected directly from a caseous lesion in the nervous system, but any such focus must have been the result of a blood-borne dissemination of the organism. In rare instances an infant born of a mother with miliary tuberculosis is found to have miliary tuberculosis, with or without meningitis.

On naked-eye examination, the meninges at the base of the brain and around the spinal cord are thickened and cloudy, and there may be a yellow gelatinous exudate at the base of the brain. Ulti-mately, this becomes organized, with the production of dense fibrous adhesions around the base. Tiny miliary tubercles may be visible in the meninges or inside the brain. The ventricles are sometimes dilated, and their ependymal lining is granular.

On microscopic examination, the appearance is similar to that seen in other miliary tuberculous foci except for a tendency to show more neutrophilic leukocytes than in classic lesions. There is a predominance of mononuclear cells and lymphocytes, plasma cells, and epithelioid cells. Definite tubercles are present, but giant cells are uncommon. The blood vessels show adventitial inflammation and thickening of the intima. The same lesions are found in the ependyma and choroid plexuses. Eventually there is proliferation of fibroblasts and thickening of the meninges, and in patients who have survived for some time as a result of chemotherapy, one or more sizable tuberculomas may be found within the brain substance or in the meninges.[7]

Clinical Features. The onset is almost always insidious, so much so that it may be days or even weeks before meningitis is suspected. In this prodromal state there are anorexia, malaise, a modest degree of pyrexia, and lack of energy or irritability. Headache may be absent or slight. It is likely that these early symptoms are due to dissemination of infection, but it must be emphasized that clinical evidence of active disease elsewhere in the body is seldom forthcoming. With progressive invasion of the meninges, headache increases in severity, and a little rigidity is found in the neck. Temperature spikes up to 102° or more now appear, and the pulse may be rapid, though later on, with rise of intracranial pressure, it may be relatively slow in proportion to the pyrexia.

The child complains of photophobia, becomes drowsy, and lies curled up in bed, resenting examination. With rise of intracranial pressure, the headache becomes more severe, and exacerbations of pain lead to a shrill meningeal cry. In infants, the fontanelles bulge, but when the sutures are closed, the rise of intracranial pressure becomes apparent in swollen optic discs. Convulsions are not uncommon in the early days of the disease in children.

Inflammatory involvement of the third, fourth, and sixth cranial nerves leads to diplopia, and infarction due to angiopathy may lead to the sudden appearance of hemiparesis, monoparesis, aphasia, or dementia. Choroidal tubercles can often be found if the pupils are dilated. They appear as ill-defined, small, pale, yellow areas which later become white, and they ultimately become surrounded by pigmentation. In the terminal stages, the patient is in coma with retraction of the neck, incontinence, and rising pulse and respiratory rates.

Laboratory Findings. A positive tuberculin test is found in the majority of cases. X-rays of the lungs may or may not show evidence of miliary tuberculosis or a localized lesion.

The cerebrospinal fluid pressure is normal during the prodromal phase, but ultimately it increases. The fluid is clear but may have an opalescent appearance if the cell count is high. When left to stand, a fine fibrin clot forms. The cell content varies from 50 to 500 cells/cu. mm., the majority being lymphocytes. The protein is raised to an average of about 200 mg. per cent, and the sugar content falls progressively from the start of the disease. The chloride content is reduced in the majority of cases, and this is progressive; it may be normal in the prodromal period. With these findings, absence of growth when the fluid is inoculated onto ordinary culture media is highly suggestive of tuberculous meningitis; treatment should be started at once, without waiting until the diagnosis is confirmed by finding the bacillus in the spinal fluid or by guinea pig inoculation.

Diagnosis. The vagueness of the first symptoms makes it easy to miss the diagnosis in the early stages since the signs do not necessarily point to the nervous system at all. Once a diagnosis of meningitis has been made, it must be distinguished from other meningeal infections.

Acute pyogenic meningitis starts more acutely, the signs of meningeal irritation are more prominent, and the spinal fluid response is polymorphonuclear in type; the organism responsible for the disease will be found in smears and on culture.

A predominantly lymphocytic reaction in the spinal fluid is encountered in acute lymphocytic choriomeningitis and other virus infections, in syphilitic meningitis, in yeast meningitis, and in some cases of carcinomatous infiltration of the meninges. In viral meningitis, no organisms can be found in the spinal fluid, and the chloride and sugar content are normal. Acute syphilitic meningitis is rare; the sugar content of the fluid is normal and the serology is positive in both blood and fluid. Both the clinical features and the cerebrospinal fluid findings in yeast meningitis are identical with those of tuberculous meningitis, showing a fall of sugar and a predominance of lymphocytes, and the distinction is made by finding the typical budding yeast organism by the India ink technique or by culture on blood agar or Sabouraud's medium. In carcinomatosis of the meninges, the spinal fluid contains an excess of lymphocytes and polymorphs and reduced sugar. Pyrexia may or may not be present. Tumor cells can sometimes be seen. In the so-called serous meningitis associated with aural or sinus infections, both lymphocytes and polymorphs are found in the blood, but the fluid is sterile and the sugar content is normal; it can evolve into typical purulent meningitis. Cerebral abscesses and tumors abutting on the ventricular or subarachnoid surface can give rise to headache and a lymphocytic excess in the spinal fluid; obvious focal signs will usually indicate the true nature of the disease and further information can be obtained from contrast studies.

Prognosis and Course. Before the discovery of streptomycin and isoniazid, tuberculous meningitis was a fatal disease, death usually occurring within three to four weeks of the onset. With modern treatment, a cure rate in the region of 80 per cent can be expected in children under the age of 12, but the prognosis is worse in patients over 40. At any age, the chance of survival is much reduced if the patient is in coma by the time treatment is started. The presence of either miliary or localized tuberculosis elsewhere in the body does not materially affect the immediate prognosis of tuberculous meningitis. Relapses can occur months or years after the original attack, and in children recovery from meningitis may be followed a year or two later by the appearance of one or more intracranial tuberculomas, which act as space-occupying lesions.

In a few instances, recovery from the acute disease has been followed by endocrine disturbances — hypogonadism, delayed bone maturation, obesity from hyperphagia, and precocious sexual development. Radiological evidence of calcification in the region of the hypothalamus has been recorded in some of these cases.[7]

Treatment. A combination of streptomycin, para-aminosalicylic acid, and isoniazid is the treatment of choice at the time of writing. For children, isoniazid is given in doses of 20 to 30 mg./kg. body weight/day in divided amounts; an adult requires 500 to 750 mg./day. Pyridoxine should be given as protection against the polyneuropathy of isoniazid-induced pyridoxine deficiency. Streptomycin is given intramuscularly in doses of 50 mg./kg. body weight/day for a child; adults should receive 2 gm. daily, but because of the risk of damaging the cochlea and labyrinth, this should be reduced after two weeks to 1 gm. thrice weekly for an adult and proportionately less for a child. The use of intrathecal streptomycin has been largely abandoned. Para-aminosalicylic acid has the least antituberculous activity of the three agents, but is useful because it sustains isoniazid blood levels by competitive acetylation and excretion and reduces the rate at which drug resistance develops. It is given orally or intravenously at the rate of 200 mg./kg. body weight/day, which usually amounts to about 12 to 14 gm. a day for adults.

Treatment with para-aminosalicylic acid and isoniazid should continue for two years in order to prevent relapse. The prolonged use of streptomycin can damage the internal ear. Para-aminosalicylic acid can produce anorexia, nausea, and diarrhea; when this happens, the drug should be withdrawn, and when the

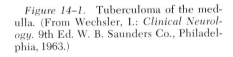

Figure 14–1. Tuberculoma of the medulla. (From Wechsler, I.: *Clinical Neurology.* 9th Ed. W. B. Saunders Co., Philadelphia, 1963.)

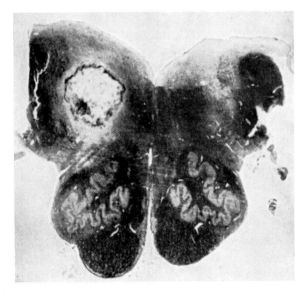

symptoms have subsided, therapy is resumed up to the level of tolerance. Administration of ACTH in doses of 20 to 50 units twice daily has been recommended to inhibit the development of inflammatory adhesions at the base of the brain, but many authorities consider this unnecessary.

Tuberculoma

Tuberculomas big enough to produce symptoms are rare in the United States and Western Europe, but are reported to constitute from 6 to 16 per cent of verified intracranial "tumors" in Portugal and some parts of South America.[7] One or more of these granulomas can grow to a considerable size within the brain, usually in the posterior fossa, during the course of tuberculous meningitis when treatment has not been fully successful (Fig. 14–1). In other cases, they present as intracranial space-occupying lesions without any evidence of meningitis; surgical removal is usually followed by infection of the meninges, but this can be successfully dealt with by appropriate medication. Occasionally, a tuberculoma will calcify and become visible radiographically.

Listeriosis

Infection with the gram-positive bacillus, *Listeria monocytogenes*, commonly spreads from contaminated animals and in consequence the disease is most common in rural communities. It develops following inhalation, ingestion, or direct contact with contaminated food or animal products. Pathologically, it is characterized by disseminated granulomata and focal necrosis or suppuration. Lesions develop in the liver, intestinal tract, skin, mucous membranes, lung, heart, spleen, lymph nodes, placenta, meninges, and brain. The fetus may be infected, and listeriosis is a well recognized cause of abortion or of babies with congenital defects. Susceptibility to the infection is increased by debilitating diseases, pregnancy, and the administration of adrenocorticosteroids.

Meningitis is the most commonly recognized form of listeriosis and it does not differ in any significant way from other forms of bacterial meningitis. The diagnosis rests on isolation of the microorganism from the spinal fluid and from the rising agglutinin titer in the serum. In culture, the organism can be confused with diphtheroid bacilli.

A second and less common form of the disease is an encephalitis which usually has its main impact on the brainstem and is characterized by malaise, nausea, vomiting, and the development of multiple brainstem lesions. Pathologically, there are multiple areas of suppurative encephalitis, pronounced perivascular cuffing lymphocytes and patchy fibrinoid necrosis of the small vessels of the brainstem.

Ampicillin is the drug of choice for listerial infections but the tetracyclines and erythromycin are also effective. Untreated listeria meningitis has a mortality rate in the region of 70 per cent.

Intracranial Abscess

Intracranial suppuration has become comparatively rare since the introduction of chemotherapy because it is now usually possible to control sources of infection, such as otitis media, mastoiditis, sinusitis, bronchiectasis, and contamination from penetrating wounds of the scalp.

Etiology. Pyogenic bacteria can gain access to the brain by direct invasion and by hematogenous spread from other organs. There are two forms of direct invasion, the more obvious of which is a penetrating wound which carries infected material into the extradural or subdural space or into the brain itself; growth of the bacteria is favored by damage to the tissues and by the presence of in-driven bone fragments, hair, skin, and foreign bodies. The second and more common method of direct invasion is spread of infection from adjacent sites of disease, notably otitis media, sinusitis, mastoiditis,[31] and osteomyelitis of the skull. The infection may march boldly inward, infecting and destroying the bone and the dura, but usually it reaches the brain by spreading along the perineural spaces of the cranial nerves or via communicating veins as a septic thrombophlebitis. Infection can also spread through the sutures.

Metastatic abscesses, single or multiple, are almost exclusively intracerebral and hematogenous, and arise from septic conditions elsewhere. The lung is the usual source, but abscesses in the brain also follow bacterial endocarditis, septicemia, and pelvic suppuration. Cerebral abscess is relatively common in the presence of congenital heart lesions with cyanosis (Fallot's tetralogy in particular) without overt evidence of systemic infection. Infected emboli, precursors of brain abscess, are also believed to reach the brain via the spinal epidural venous plexus.[13]

Pathology. Extradural collections of pus occur beneath areas of osteomyelitis, ethmoidal or frontal sinusitis, and infections of the ear and mastoid.[31] Infection from the ear may pass upward toward the temporal lobe or backward into the posterior fossa. The dura usually limits the spread of pus, but diffuse subdural collections can occur in combination with both extradural and intracerebral abscesses. A loculated abscess within the subarachnoid space is rare but is sometimes seen in the basal cisterns, in the interpeduncular space, around the internal auditory meatus, and over the cribriform plate. Intracerebral abscess usually results from intravascular or perivascular spread from infected sinuses, bone, or soft tissues of the face and neck. There may appear to be an area of intact dura between the source of the infection and the abscess, but microscopy reveals that infection has passed these barriers by spreading inward around the cranial nerves or along communicating vessels.

Cerebral abscess usually occurs in the white matter, the cortex appearing to act as a barrier to its spread; if an abscess bursts, it usually does so into the ventricles and not onto the surface of the hemisphere. It starts as suppurative encephalitis. If virulence is high or the patient's resistance is low, the infection spreads rapidly, with severe edema and rapid death. In more favorable cases, liquefaction and peripheral walling-off occur, so that ultimately there is a collection of pus within a dense glial capsule which may eventually calcify. A small abscess can be absorbed, leaving a glial scar. However, a natural cure presupposes that the patient is able to survive the acute rise of intracranial pressure which occurs at the height of the disease, and this is something that rarely happened before the days of antibiotics. In posttraumatic abscess occurring immediately after injury, the same train of events can occur; but when an abscess develops after a considerable delay, pus forms within a dense glial capsule and there may be no rise of intracranial pressure. In such cases rupture of the abscess with escape of pus into the brain, ventricles, or subarachnoid space may be the first intimation of its presence. Abscesses from local infections and from penetrating injuries are usually single and situated near the source of infection, whereas the metastatic variety is often multiple.

Bacteriology of Cerebral Abscess. Infections derived from the ears and paranasal sinuses may be due to staphylococci, pneumococci, streptococci, Vincent's bacillus, and meningococci. Coliform organisms can reach the sinuses as a result of bathing in contaminated swimming pools and can thus be responsible for cerebral abscess. Metastatic abscesses are caused by an even greater variety of organisms; in addition to those named above, the infection may be due to yeasts, the typhoid bacillus, *Entamoeba histolytica*, and many others. Streptococci, staphylococci, and pneumococci are by far the most common.

Clinical Features. The clinical features are determined by the presence of a focal expanding lesion within the cranium and the presence of a septic focus in the skull, face, or elsewhere in the body. In the majority of cases, this background of infection is clinically obvious whether it be in the ear, the accessory nasal sinuses, the cranial vault, the skin (boils and carbuncles), the heart valves, or the lung (bronchiectasis, pneumonia) or pelvis, and the patient will usually have been under treatment for some such condition at the time when the signs of intracranial spread occur. However, metastatic abscesses of the brain can be derived from a clinically inconspicuous source of infection elsewhere in the body. Consequently, the patient may *or may not* have fever, a raised sedimentation rate, polymorph leukocytosis, and local symptoms from the original infection. In acute cases, the patient looks ill.

Invasion of the brain is often ushered in by a rise of temperature and a severe headache which may be on the side of the abscess. There may be focal epileptic seizures, leaving in their wake some degree of motor or sensory impairment. If the cerebellum is involved the headache is commonly occipital, and transient vertigo and ataxia may occur. This stage of invasion may be followed by a latent period when symptoms are either absent or confined to headache, slight drowsiness, and irritability. If the condition is untreated, the headache becomes worse, appropriate focal cerebral or cerebellar signs become more conspicuous, and the signs of rising intracranial pressure appear—drowsiness, mental confusion, papilledema, and slowing of the pulse rate. If still untreated, a pressure cone will develop, often quite suddenly; this is especially likely to occur in abscess of the temporal lobe.

VARIATIONS ACCORDING TO SITE. Focal signs vary with the site of the abscess. Frontal abscesses may have little in the way of neurological signs until the process spreads back to involve the motor pathways, in which event hemiparesis involving the contralateral leg, arm, and face becomes apparent. Temporal lobe abscesses tend to produce weakness of the face and arm, but the leg is usually spared. In the case of otogenic temporal lobe abscess, there is slight weakness of the contralateral face, tongue, and arm, and depression of vision in the upper quadrants of the contralateral homonymous visual fields; this can develop into complete hemianopia. At first the field defects may not be obvious on confrontation, though some visual inattention in the contralateral half fields may be noted; perimetry gives early and conclusive evidence of damage in this area. Dysphasia is present if the dominant hemisphere is affected. When the cerebellum is involved there is nystagmus and ipsilateral ataxia. If the infection has spread from the ear, nystagmus and vertigo are more likely to be due to the aural infection than to the cerebellar lesion.

When the abscess has resulted from spread of infection from adjacent structures, some evidence of meningeal irritation is likely to be found, but in metastatic abscess meningeal signs are usually absent. Metastatic abscesses commonly occur in the distribution of the middle cerebral artery and produce severe contralateral paralysis with or without sensory loss (Fig. 14–2). When septic embolism has occurred in the posterior cerebral distribution, there is usually severe contralateral sensory loss together with homonymous hemianopia.

Intracranial *extracerebral* abscess takes a different form. Extradural collections of pus produce minimal neurological signs, and evidence of raised intracranial pressure may be absent until a late stage. On the other hand, subdural abscesses produce widespread effects, as, for instance, complete aphasia, hemiplegia, and hemianesthesia. This may occur even when intracranial pressure is normal and in the absence of any vascular complications in the subjacent cortex; the reason for the disturbance of cerebral function is not clear. Subarachnoid abscess is usually incidental to meningitis arising from infection of the overlying bone. Focal signs are minimal, and the intracranial pressure is not usually raised. An exception is the local abscess which may underlie an infected

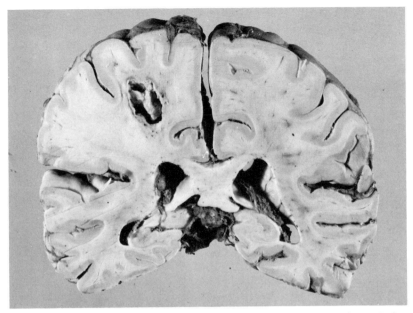

Figure 14–2. A metastatic brain abscess in the right hemisphere. (Courtesy of Ayer Laboratory, Pennsylvania Hospital, Philadelphia.)

area of radiation necrosis, for here the evidence of brain damage may be severe and widespread, probably because both the brain and the blood vessels have suffered from the radiation effects.

Laboratory Aids. There may or may not be a polymorphonuclear leukocytosis in the blood. The sedimentation rate is often but not always raised. Electroencephalography shows changes similar to those found in any rapidly expanding lesion and is not particularly helpful. X-ray of the skull may show evidence of disease in the mastoid or paranasal sinuses; lateral shift of the pineal gland is seen if the abscess is situated in the anterior compartment and is large. Of the contrast studies available, brain scanning is the most accurate and the least traumatic. Of the alternative methods, angiography is the next best. It discloses displacement of blood vessels and a vascular blush around the abscess. It is less reliable in subdural and cerebellar abscesses.

Spinal tap carries with it the risk of inducing a pressure cone either immediately, at the time of the tap, or within a few hours, as the result of continued seepage of spinal fluid through the hole made by the needle. Nevertheless there are circumstances under which it is desirable to examine the fluid, and the procedure is justified if there is nothing to suggest the presence of a pressure cone. The pressure of the spinal fluid is increased in almost all cases, and the protein content is moderately increased if the abscess is adjacent to the ventricular or subarachnoid surface. In the early stages of suppurative encephalitis, the cell count is increased, with a predominance of polymorphonuclear leukocytes, but in the case of a metastatic abscess situated deep in the substance of the brain, the cell count may be normal. With encapsulation, the number of cells in the spinal fluid drops, and lymphocytes predominate. The glucose and chloride contents are normal unless the infection has invaded the subarachnoid space and produced meningitis, in which event the glucose level is reduced.

Differential Diagnosis. In the presence of infection of the ear, nasal sinuses, or skin of the face, scalp, or neck, the signs of an expanding focal lesion of the brain usually signify an abscess, but these same conditions can give rise to infective thrombophlebitis of the lateral and sagittal sinuses, and this can cause a rise of intracranial pressure and focal signs. The pressure rises because the venous sinuses are blocked, and focal damage to the brain occurs if the infection spreads in retrograde fashion to the brain or if perivenous hemorrhage occurs. There may be obvious signs of infection—rigors and high temperature—but in some cases these features are absent. Arteriography will settle the matter, because in sinus thrombosis there is imperfect filling of the affected sinus. A rapidly growing tumor such as a glioblastoma can mimic a cerebral abscess, and it should be noted that the presence of an expanding intracranial mass in the presence of infection of the sinuses does not necessarily mean that the two are related.

It can be difficult to differentiate brain abscess from nonsuppurative encephalitis, notably that caused by *herpes simplex*, but sharply limited focal lesions are unusual in the latter, the rise of cerebrospinal pressure is seldom marked, and there is usually, but not always, lymphocytosis in the spinal fluid; brain scanning or arteriography may have to be carried out to resolve the question.

Treatment. The treatment of suppurative encephalitis and brain abscess has been revolutionized by the introduction of chemotherapy. It is usual to combine penicillin G with sulfadiazine until encapsulation occurs, which is usually within about 10 days. During this period, and especially in the early stages, sharply rising intracranial pressure may threaten life, but it can usually be controlled by aspiration of the abscess. The intravenous administration of hypertonic solutions (e.g., manitol) greatly reduces intracranial pressure for a short time, but this is followed by a rebound effect, so this type of therapy is inadmissible except to tide the patient over an hour or two pending surgical interference. Another emergency measure is subtemporal decompression for cerebral abscess, or suboccipital decompression for cerebellar abscess. Once

an abscess has been localized by contrast studies, pus can be aspirated and antibiotics instilled into the cavity, pending an attempt at total removal, capsule and all. Its size and shape can be delineated by injecting Pantopaque into it preoperatively.

If seizures develop, the patient should be given 100 mg. of Dilantin four times a day; barbiturates can be used, but they sometimes induce somnolence when given in effective doses, and this may obscure the clinical picture. It is wise to prescribe antiseizure medication on a prophylactic basis even in patients who have had no convulsions.

Extradural abscess is treated by simple drainage and the use of antibiotics and chemotherapeutic agents. *Subdural abscess* is difficult both to diagnose and to treat, requiring drainage through multiple burr holes.

Prognosis. Untreated cerebral abscess is virtually always fatal. The mortality in cases treated by antibiotics, chemotherapy, and surgery varies from 10 per cent to 45 per cent, the highest death rate being in cases associated with pulmonary infection. Survivors may develop seizures, and this is particularly likely if convulsions have occurred during the acute stage.

Acute Spinal Epidural Abscess

A rare but important condition, spinal epidural abscess is easily recognized and easy to treat, but it can lead to life-long disability or death if neglected.[4]

Pathology. The infection usually reaches the spinal epidural space via the blood stream from staphylococcal infections of the skin or elsewhere. Though usually staphylococcal in origin, any pyogenic organism can produce an epidural abscess. The primary lesion is thought to be an infective thrombosis of the epidural veins, and this can spread widely upward and downward from its point of origin, especially over the dorsal and lateral areas of the thoracic epidural space. Occasionally it starts as osteomyelitis of the spine, spreading secondarily to the epidural space, in which event the abscess lies anterior to the cord. The infection can penetrate the dural barrier to produce meningitis or localized intramedullary abscess, but this is rare.

Macroscopically, the condition varies from a series of localized pockets of pus to a more solid granulomatous collection in the case of infections of low virulence. The cord shows superficial necrosis with softening over several segments in fatal cases.

Clinical Features. There is usually an antecedent history of a boil or other local staphylococcal infection. Pain develops in the back and is aggravated by movement. It may be extremely severe, in which case it is accompanied by spasm of the paraspinal muscles. Sometimes it radiates into the lower limbs, and if the abscess is in the lower cervical spine (an uncommon event), there may be root pain down one arm. The vertebral spines in the affected area are very tender to deep pressure.

After a few days, symptoms of spinal cord compression develop. Weakness of the legs is the first symptom to appear, but this is sometimes preceded by retention of urine. Complete paraplegia can develop within 24 to 72 hours, but in some cases, paralysis develops abruptly in the course of a few minutes, presumably because of thrombosis of the spinal arteries.

Paresthesias develop in the feet and spread up the legs, and are followed by sensory impairment. The tendon reflexes in the lower limbs may be exaggerated at first, but they are soon lost, even when the lesion is in the thoracic cord. This may be the result of systemic toxemia. The plantar responses are extensor.

In acute cases, the temperature is elevated, as is the pulse. There is usually a polymorphonuclear leukocytosis.

In subacute cases, the pain in the back may go on for as long as two weeks before neurological symptoms develop,

and if pain extends down the back of one leg only, the condition may mimic sciatica due to a prolapsed lumbar disc.

Spinal tap should be performed cautiously in case pus is encountered on inserting the needle; the needle should be connected with a syringe, and suction should be applied as the epidural space is approached. If pus is not encountered, the needle is advanced in the usual way. There is usually complete, or almost complete, subarachnoid block, and the spinal fluid is yellow or cloudy. There may be a moderate pleocytosis and increased protein, but the sugar content of the fluid is normal, and cultures are usually sterile unless the infection has spread to the subarachnoid space. Myelography is essential and should not be delayed once the condition has been suspected.

Diagnosis. Acute transverse myelitis, which is more common than epidural abscess,[4] may mimic the latter. It is often preceded by a history of upper respiratory infection, and there may or may not be pain in the back and root pain. Manometric block is more common in epidural abscess than in transverse myelitis and myelography will usually disclose a complete block. However, acute swelling of the cord in acute transverse myelitis may also produce a myelographic block. X-ray evidence of vertebral osteomyelitis excludes the possibility of acute transverse myelitis, but in the early stages of an epidural abscess, the x-rays usually appear normal. The spinal fluid findings are more or less the same in the two groups, but in general there tends to be a higher white cell count in the presence of myelitis. If, after reviewing the evidence, it is not possible to distinguish between the two conditions, laminectomy should be performed to settle the matter.

Epidural metastases can produce pain in the back and cord compression, but the symptoms evolve less rapidly than in epidural abscess. Hemorrhage from a spinal angioma can give rise to abrupt, acute pain in the back, together with slowly or rapidly progressing signs of cord impairment. There is usually blood in the spinal fluid, but the author has seen two cases of acute intramedullary hemorrhage in patients with multiple cutaneous telangiectasia in whom the spinal fluid was normal.

Thrombosis of the anterior spinal artery is not preceded by local pain or by pyrexia. The onset of the cord symptoms is abrupt, and the paralysis may be accompanied by severe pain in the legs, owing to involvement of the spinothalamic tracts. The posterior columns are spared, whereas they are usually heavily implicated in posteriorly situated epidural abscesses.

Treatment. The patient should be given large doses of penicillin together with a wide-spectrum antibiotic, and the abscess should be drained. When paraplegia is complete and the onset has been sudden, the outlook for recovery is usually poor, though there have been notable exceptions to this. When neurological symptoms are slight and recent, recovery can be expected if adequate treatment is instituted at once.

Intramedullary Spinal Abscess

This rare condition[38] is usually the result of hematogenous spread from elsewhere, such as abscess of the lung, bronchiectasis, infection of the genitourinary tract, staphylococcal skin infections, or osteomyelitis. The abscess is usually in the thoracic cord and spreads longitudinally over several segments. Multifocal lesions are sometimes encountered. The cord is soft, swollen, and red. Encapsulation is rare.

The clinical features are those of rapidly oncoming weakness of the legs in a patient with evidence of generalized infection; the symptoms of infection may be obscured if antibiotics have been given. Segmental pain at the site of the abscess may be present or absent. Weakness of the legs develops over a few days. The early spastic phase gives place to total flaccidity, together with sensory loss below the level of the lesion. Spinal manometrics shows a partial or complete block. The protein level is high, and there is a modest excess of leukocytes in the fluid. Cultures may be positive or negative. Myelography confirms the presence of an intramedullary mass.

Treatment by systemic chemotherapy, and aspiration of the abscess must be carried out promptly if it is to be effective. Chloramphenicol should be combined with large doses of penicillin. Complete recovery is the exception rather than the rule.

Leprosy

Definition. Leprosy[28] is an infectious disease, peculiar to man, with an incubation period of not less than a year and a chronic course; it is caused by *Mycobacterium leprae,* which invades the skin, mucous membranes, bones, viscera, and nerves, giving rise to granulomas, destruction of tissue, and nerve palsies (Fig. 14–3). There are two main types of the disease. The first, tuberculoid leprosy, occurs in resistant subjects and is characterized by anesthetic cutaneous macules and patchy polyneuritis; such patients are seldom infectious to others and the prognosis is relatively good. The second type, lepromatous leprosy, is a more serious form; resistance is low, granulomatous ulceration is the rule, and bacilli are discharged in large numbers from the lesions. Neuritic manifestations may occur, but they are usually a late development and the condition is then known as mixed or borderline leprosy.

Etiology. The organism is an acid-fast nonmotile bacillus which cannot be cultured. It is not readily contagious, but there is no truth in the frequently repeated statement that prolonged and intimate contact is essential for the transmission of the disease. Children are more susceptible than adults. Leprosy is common in Asia, Africa, India, and the Pacific Islands, and rare in North America,

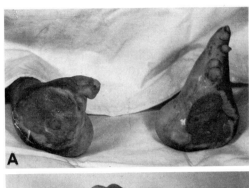

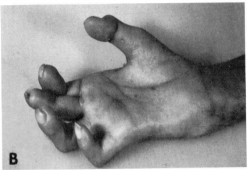

Figure 14–3. Leprosy. (Courtesy of Dr. Henry Schutta.)

Western Europe, and the British Isles. The World Health Organization has estimated that there are about 10 million cases, and that 25 per cent of patients are severely disabled. It is considered that there are over one thousand cases in the United States; 103 new cases were discovered in 1964.[24]

Pathology. The organism spreads through the lymphatics of the corium and subcutaneous tissue, producing a local inflammatory reaction and enlargement of the regional lymph glands. Superficial granulomas of the skin and of the mucous membrane of the nose, mouth, larynx, and eyes are apt to ulcerate and to become secondarily infected, with consequent loss of tissue. A few bacilli are found in the peripheral nerves, which increase in thickness and ultimately show degeneration of the axons. The organism is obtained from nasal smears and from skin granulomas; it is seldom found in the depigmented macules of nerve leprosy.

Clinical Features. The disease is often ushered in by a prolonged period of malaise, depression, and fatigue,

which may be punctuated by irregular bouts of fever with profuse sweating.[24,28] Alternating dryness and hypersecretion of the nasal mucosa, neuralgic pains in the limbs, headache, and great weariness are common features of the early phase. Then come more definite indications of what is amiss. The patient or his friends may notice depigmented patches, usually on the trunk, which have an erythematous border and a pale center. These patches show early impairment of sensation, lose their hair, and do not sweat. Occasionally, neurological symptoms precede skin changes.

The nerves most often attacked are the ulnar, common peroneal, facial, and great auricular; the radial, median, posterior tibial, and sciatic nerves are less often involved. There is superficial sensory loss, muscular paresis with atrophy, and loss of sweating in the territory of the affected nerves. Proprioception is usually well preserved, so sensory ataxia is rare. The nerve trunks are enlarged and cordlike; they are tender in the early phases, but become insensitive later. Trophic changes supervene in anesthetic areas, with ulceration and loss of tissue in the hands and feet. Contractures of paralyzed muscles add to the deformities produced by local ulceration. The neurogenic weakness of muscles is sometimes increased by a lepromatous myositis. Facial palsy, often starting as a paralysis of the orbicularis oculi, may be the first sign of leprosy. Ectropion is common. Inability to close the eye helps to produce corneal ulceration, and this risk is greatly increased if the cornea is rendered insensitive by infection of the trigeminal nerve. Paralysis of the tongue, palate, and larynx may occur. The reflexes are seldom disturbed, but a symmetrical polyneuritis is sometimes found in advanced cases.[24] Although the bacillus has been found in the brain, mental changes—other than a reactive depression—are unusual.

The clinical picture of nerve leprosy, as described above, may be complicated by lepromatous nodular lesions. These start as an outbreak of brownish-red spots, which come and go, but ultimately take the form of persistent macules which extend in area and become increasingly indurated. Unlike the maculae of nerve leprosy, the patches are raised and show a preference for the exposed parts of the body. Thickening of the lobes of the ears, nose, cheeks, and forehead coarsens the face; the scalp and the palms of the hands usually escape. Nodules appear in the mucous membranes of the mouth, nose, and eye. Ulceration and fibrosis proceed concurrently to produce great disfigurement.

Diagnosis. The organism can be obtained from the granulomas. The Wassermann reaction may be positive, but the Kahn test is negative in the absence of syphilis. The cerebrospinal fluid is normal except for an elevation of globulins.

Diagnosis is easy provided the possibility is kept in mind, but sporadic cases encountered in countries where the disease is rare are apt to be missed in the early stages. The differential diagnosis of the lepromatous lesions includes syphilis, yaws, ringworm, tinea, lupus vulgaris, fibrosum molluscum, gangosa, and naso-oral leishmaniasis. Leukoderma is distinguished from the maculae of tuberculoid leprosy by the fact that the depigmented areas sweat normally and are not anesthetic. Palsy of individual nerves or groups of nerves may suggest a wide range of possibilities, including syringomyelia, Morvan's disease, progressive muscular atrophy, cervical rib, Bell's palsy, and hypertrophic neuritis, but a careful search of the skin carried out in a good light will often disclose maculae, and there is usually some patchy thickening of the peripheral nerves.

The diagnosis is best confirmed by biopsy of a thickened cutaneous nerve or skin.

Prognosis. Without treatment, patients with lepromatous leprosy deteriorate steadily and die about 15 years from the time the disease is first recognized. On the other hand, patients with tuberculoid leprosy tend to recover, apart from residual nerve damage, within a year or two, provided the skin is not heavily involved. If skin lesions are numerous, the disease runs a more protracted course, with repeated relapses, but spontaneous remission is still possible. With chemotherapy, the disease can be arrested in virtually all patients.

Treatment. The sulfones have revolutionized the treatment of this disease. They are given either by mouth or parenterally, but the details of treatment are beyond the scope of this book. In tuberculoid cases, it may take a year or two to achieve satisfactory results, while in lepromatous cases it takes longer. If side effects prove too severe to allow continued treatment with the sulfones, amithiozone or dihydrostreptomycin can be of use, although in the opinion of some authorities they are less effective than the sulfones.

Diphtheritic Polyneuropathy

Infection by *Corynebacterium diphtheriae* may occur in the fauces, nose, larynx, conjunctiva, vulva, and prepuce, and may complicate wounds or sores on the skin. The bacillus excretes a neurotropic exotoxin which gives rise to degenerative changes in the myelin sheaths and axons of peripheral nerves and retrograde changes in the motor cells of the spinal cord and brainstem.

Clinical Features. Diphtheritic polyneuropathy is rare in communities in which inoculation against diphtheria is practiced. The commonest site of infection is the throat, which shows a diphtheritic membrane, but it must be emphasized that the faucial symptoms may be so slight as to pass unnoticed. A week or two later, there is blurring of vision due to paralysis of accommodation, and weakness of the palate may impart a nasal quality to the voice. These symptoms are followed in the course of the next two or three weeks by evidence of involvement of peripheral nerves, the longest neurons being affected first. Paresthesias and weakness start in the feet, spreading later to the upper limb. The muscles are weak, hypotonic, and tender, and incapacity for movement is further aggravated by the presence of sensory ataxia due to the effect of the toxin on the proprioceptive nerve fibers. Peripheral cutaneous loss is usually slight. The distal reflexes are lost early. In a few cases, there is paralysis of facial, pharyngeal, and external ocular muscles. Weakness of the diaphragm can give rise to shallow breathing, or even to a fatal attack of dyspnea, but death is more often due to cardiac failure.

When diphtheritic infection involves superficial wounds of the skin, it produces a chronic sore, and the skin around it becomes numb. This may be followed by weakness of accommodation and by the gradual appearance of the symptoms and signs of peripheral neuropathy. In both faucial and other forms of the disease, the protein of the spinal fluid is usually increased, but there is no pleocytosis.

Diagnosis. Diagnosis may be difficult when the initial diphtheritic infection was not detected. Acute febrile polyneuritis is often preceded by a sore throat, but there is no antecedent blurring of vision, and there is usually a delay of only three or four days between the throat infection and the onset of the polyneuropathy.

Prognosis. The mortality rate may be as high as 30 per cent following faucial diphtheria, but is low following infection of the skin.

Treatment. Treatment entails bed rest until recovery is well on the way, with daily physiotherapy. The damage has been done by the time polyneuritis occurs, so that theoretically there is no need for antitoxin, but some clinicians believe in giving 50,000 units on three consecutive days as soon as the diagnosis is made. It is a wise measure in suspected cases of cutaneous diphtheria, whether cultures taken from the sores are positive or negative.

Tetanus

Tetanus is caused by *Clostridium tetani*, a spore-bearing anaerobe. The organism is widely distributed in cultivated soil and is found in the feces of many animals, notably the horse, and in some human beings. Infection arises through contamination of wounds, scratches, and burns. Occasional sources of the disease are vaccination, infection of wounds by contaminated sutures, infection of the umbilical stump in newly born infants, and puerperal sepsis. Contamination of penetrating wounds provides optimum conditions for the growth of the organism, which is favored by anaerobic conditions and the presence of foreign bodies and necrotic tissue. The bacillus does not usually spread beyond the site of infection, but bacteremia has been recorded in a few cases. The exotoxin liberated by the organism contains several components which can be separated by electrophoresis, but only one of these gives rise to tetanic spasm.[108]

There is still controversy as to how the poison gets into the nervous system, but the balance of the experimental evidence favors hematogenous spread to the muscles and central nervous system. The toxin can pass the blood-brain barrier. It is also possible that the poison may spread up the perineural spaces.

Pathology. The occurrence of histopathological lesions in the central nervous system has been debated, and most investigators have failed to find any morphological changes in striated muscle. In patients not treated by muscle relaxants, the fine structure of the contractile elements in the sarcoplasmic reticulum is normal. However, in the muscles of the intoxicated mouse and of patients with tetanus, increased numbers of dense granules have been found in the mitochondrial matrix.[108] To date, no abnormality in the enzyme systems has been identified in experiments with highly purified neurotoxin. The localization of toxin in the sarcoplasmic reticulum and transverse tubular system of skeletal muscle—structures which are known to be involved in the contraction-relaxation cycle of muscle—suggests that the toxin may work at this site.

Clinical Features. The incubation period varies from a few hours to about a week, but it may be several weeks if the patient has received a prophylactic injection of antitoxin. The site of infection may become inflamed but often shows no change. There may or may not be premonitory malaise and a little fever for a day or two before the onset of tetanic spasm, and the patient is often irritable and restless during this period.

The first muscles to be affected are the masseters; a feeling of stiffness of the jaws is complained of, and there is some difficulty in opening the mouth (trismus). This is followed by stiffness of the neck, dysphagia, and retraction of the lips (risus sardonicus). In some cases there is elevation of the brows, or the eyes may be partly closed by spasm of the orbicularis. As the toxin spreads, the muscles of the limbs become stiff and the abdomen boardlike; the respiratory movements of the chest are reduced, and the limbs are held in extension.

Intermittent tetanic spasms are superimposed on this background of persistent stiffness. The spasms are painful; reciprocal innervation is overridden, so that extensors and flexors are pulling against each other. The spasms are precipitated by noise and by handling the patient but also occur spontaneously. Pain in the back is common. In severe cases, the contraction of spinal muscles can cause opisthotonos, and spasm of the abdominal muscles can produce emprosthotonos. Spasms of the glottis and respiratory muscles cause attacks of cyanosis which can end in sudden death.

In severe tetanus,[63] overactivity of the sympathetic nervous system is sometimes prominent. The symptoms include hypertension and tachycardia, which can be either episodic or sustained. There may be episodes of pyrexia, profuse sweating, peripheral vasoconstriction, cardiac dysrhythmias, raised cardiac output, and exaggerated circulatory responses to common stimuli.

Some cases of severe tetanus have no premonitory signs, and the illness starts rapidly with generalized tetanic spasms which continue periodically throughout the illness. The reflexes are unaffected between spasms, but for obvious reasons they cannot be elicited when the limbs are rigid.

Consciousness is not disturbed at first, the patient lying in fear of the next spasm, but in severe cases, there may be disorientation, hallucinations, and terminal loss of consciousness.

In *local tetanus* the picture is different. Occurring as a rule in patients with partial protection, tetanic stiffness is limited to the affected limb or—in cephalic tetanus—to the face and neck. If it occurs in the arm or leg, the muscles become stiff, and the limb may be as rigid as a piece of wood. The rigidity persists during sleep. Spasms are mild or do not appear at all; consequently local tetanus is usually painless. Constitutional disturbances and sweating are usually absent. This condition may be very puzzling, especially when it occurs weeks or months after a minor wound. It is usually seen in wartime as the result of penetrating wounds.

The cephalic form of local tetanus differs from other types in that local paralysis occurs, with or without tetanic spasms. There may be ptosis and paralysis of external ocular muscles, facial weakness on one side and facial spasm on the other, or paralysis of the tenth and twelfth nerves. The paralysis may take months to disappear. The term splanchnic tetanus has been applied to the bulbar palsy which sometimes follows abdominal wounds; presumably it is due to the spread of toxin from the abdomen via the splanchnic branches of the vagus to the medulla.

In severe cases there is a fall of carbon dioxide combining power, a metabolic acidosis.[63] Ketonuria and a rise of blood urea are common, and are probably due to insufficient caloric intake. There is a tendency for sodium to be retained and potassium to be excreted in excess of intake. Hyperglycemia may occur, probably as a response to stress.

Course and Prognosis. Tetanus is a grave disease. The overall mortality is in the region of 50 per cent.[63] The prognosis is bad in cases with a short incubation period, rapid generalization, spasm of the glottis and respiratory muscles, and high fever. It is worse over the age of 40 than in younger persons. The outlook is good in local tetanus and in cases without generalized spasms. Some 90 per cent of all deaths occur within the first 10 days of the illness, and it is a melancholy fact that the death rate in severe forms of the disease is not significantly lowered by the best of modern treatment.

Diagnosis. Trismus is sometimes caused by painful conditions of the teeth, jaws, and tonsillar region, and has occurred in sundry cases of encephalitis, but satellite symptoms and signs will usually serve to exclude tetanus. The convulsions of strychnine poisoning come on more rapidly, are more generalized, and are unaccompanied by rigidity between spasms. In rabies there is a history of being bitten by a rabid animal, the muscles are relaxed between spasms, there is no persistent rigidity, and spasmodic dysphagia is the most prominent symptom. In tetany, spasms are peripheral and symmetrical, affecting the hands and feet first, and the characteristic position of the hand is readily recognized; trismus is usually absent. Local tetanus in one limb can be mistaken for hysterical conversion, but the rigidity of the limb is constant, persisting during sleep and under pentothal. The electromyogram shows activity during "rest" and there is a long-lasting after-discharge.

Treatment. The wound should be widely excised. In adults, 500 to 1000 units of tetanus immune globulin (human) should be given daily, to a limit of approximately 10,000 units. If it is unavailable, horse serum antitoxin is given in doses of 100,000 to 200,000 units, precautions being taken to identify and treat hypersensitivity. Antibiotics are needed not only for their effect on the tetanus organism itself, but also against other bacteria which may be in the wound and for the prevention of pneumonia. Penicillin and tetracycline are the most effective.[45]

The patient should be kept in a quiet and darkened room. Barbiturates are suitable for the sedation of mild cases. Curare can be used to produce muscle relaxation, but the drug must be handled by experts and should not be used unless facilities are available for artificial ventilation.[45, 91] Symptoms due to sympathetic overactivity are difficult to control. Chlorpromazine is commonly used, but it has recently been found that better results are obtained by using propranolol with bethanidine.

Fluid and electrolyte balance should be controlled by appropriate treatment. The maintenance of an effective airway is essential; it is better to carry out tracheostomy too soon than too late. Untreated, asphyxia is the usual cause of death. The assistance of an anesthetist is essential in handling severe cases.

Botulism

Botulism is due to intoxication by a series of protein neurotoxins elaborated by *Clostridium botulinum*. Of the six antigenic types of the organism, four (Types A, B, E, and F) are the principal causes of the disease in man. The notion lingers on that imperfectly cooked sausage is the usual cause of the disease (the term "botulism" comes from the Latin "botulus," meaning sausage), but home-preserved foods, vegetables, fruit, fish, condiments, and meat have accounted for most outbreaks in the United States over the past 50 years.[21] Infection by Types A and B is usually associated with the ingestion of home-canned vegetables, fruit, or meat products, but Type E botulism commonly follows the ingestion of fish.

Clostridium botulinum is an anaerobic, gram-positive bacillus which produces heat-resistant spores. Toxin production can occur at temperatures as low as 38° F.; it follows that intoxication is usually the result of the ingestion of improperly cooked food.

Pathology. Selective binding of botulinus A toxin at neuromuscular junctions has been demonstrated by Zacks and Sheff.[107] No histopathological changes have been found in the central nervous system.[106, 107, 108]

Clinical Features. The possibility of botulinus intoxication should be considered in patients who develop acute cranial nerve impairment followed by descending symmetrical weakness of the limbs. The impact of the intoxication is on the motor and autonomic nervous systems; the mind and the sensory system are not involved.

The onset of symptoms can begin as soon as a few hours or as late as eight days after ingestion of contaminated food, but the usual time lapse is 18 to 36 hours. The earlier the onset, the worse the prognosis. Fever is absent early in the disease, but may develop later, with pulmonary or other complications. Gastrointestinal symptoms, notably vomiting and diarrhea, usually initiate the illness. They are soon followed by diplopia, dysarthria, and dysphagia. The pupils become dilated and do not react to light or convergence. Weakness rap-

idly spreads to the skeletal muscles, from above down. The head cannot be lifted from the pillow, respiration becomes enfeebled, and the limbs become weak. Weakness rather than paralysis is the rule; movements may be carried out once but cannot be repeated—a fatigability reminiscent of severe myasthenia gravis. Despite this weakness, the peripheral tendon reflexes are depressed rather than lost, and sensation is unaffected. Profuse sweating and tachycardia occur. The mucous membranes of the mouth and pharynx are dry.

Laboratory Aids. The cerebrospinal fluid is normal. The most effective way of confirming the diagnosis is to demonstrate toxicity of the patient's serum in mice and to prove the specificity of the toxin by neutralization tests with botulinus antitoxin. However, in view of the high mortality rate of the disease, a combination of gastrointestinal symptoms and cranial palsies is sufficiently suspicious to justify immediate treatment pending the resolution of academic doubts.

Prognosis. Between the years 1960 and 1967, 155 cases were reported in the United States, with a mortality of 21.2 per cent. If large amounts of the infected food have been ingested, death usually occurs within four to eight days from respiratory paralysis, circulatory failure, or pulmonary complications.

Diagnosis. The most obvious clue to diagnosis is when vomiting and cranial palsies come on in several people who have partaken of the same meal. Isolated cases, as in persons who live alone, are less easy to identify. The rapid onset of cranial nerve palsies may suggest thrombosis involving the brain-stem, the rare type of Guillain-Barré syndrome which starts by involving the cranial nerves, brainstem encephalitis,[18] bulbar poliomyelitis,[75] or poisoning by organic phosphorus compounds.

Treatment. The sooner antiserum is given, the better the prognosis. The patient should receive polyvalent ABE antitoxin at once, not waiting until laboratory tests determine which type is responsible. Monovalent E and bivalent AB antitoxin should be reserved for use after the specific toxin has been identified in a given outbreak. These preparations can be obtained, night or day, from the National Communicable Disease Center, Atlanta, Georgia. Commercial houses commonly stock antitoxin against Types A and B. For Type ABE, the recommended dose is 8 ml. (21,000 units) intravenously and 8 ml. intramuscularly, the latter repeated in 2 to 4 hours if symptoms persist. Since all these preparations are of equine origin, hypersensitivity reaction must be anticipated and treated. There is no time for desensitization. Type F toxin is seldom encountered in the United States, but the appropriate antiserum, developed in the State Serum Institute in Denmark, is also available from the National Communicable Disease Center, in Atlanta.

Botulism can be prevented if all concerned in the preparation of food take proper precautions. Food stored in jars or cans which has a rancid odor, or in which gas has formed, should not be eaten. The toxin is destroyed by boiling.

Whooping Cough

The neurological complications of whooping cough usually occur in infants under two years. There are two groups of cases. In the first, there are numerous perivascular petechial hemorrhages which may be combined with massive intracerebral or subarachnoid hemorrhages. The second group displays diffuse loss of neurons in the brain.

The first type is usually ushered in by convulsions, which may occur at any stage of the disease. The seizures may be general or focal and are often followed by hemiparesis, monoplegia, or diplegia. A fatal issue is common in such cases and survivors may be left with persistent brain damage.

In the second type, the onset is less abrupt and the course of the disease much slower. There is extensive degeneration of nerve cells in the cortex and elsewhere, without evidence of vascular lesions. It is likely that the damage is the result of cerebral hypoxia. There is increasing stupor, with convulsions, and generalized rigidity. Between seizures, there are muscular twitchings. There is usually a lymphocytic pleocytosis in the spinal fluid. Death may occur early or the infant may survive in a demented state for several months.

VIRAL DISEASES OF THE NERVOUS SYSTEM

Viruses commonly attack the brain and spinal cord; *Herpes zoster* is the only one which is known to affect posterior root ganglia and peripheral nerves. They are a common cause of nonsuppurative encephalitis and lymphocytic meningitis. Some are prone to occur in epidemic form, the seasonal incidence being dictated by the life cycle of arthropod vectors, such as the mosquito and the tick, while others are sporadic in their incidence. They can also be divided into those which are predominantly neurotropic, and those in which spread to the central nervous system is an inconstant and usually subsidiary event.

The list of viruses which are known to infect man is constantly increasing, but it is thought that the viruses responsible for the various types of encephalitis that occur in restricted areas of the world may have a common ancestor, the course of the disease being modified by environmental factors, such as the animal reservoir and the type of vector.

In recent years, there has been increased interest in the role of maternal virus infection in the production of fetal abnormalities. Among the infections which are known to cause neural sequelae in the human fetus are rubella, poliomyelitis, and cytomegalic inclusion disease. At the experimental level, the rat virus is able to produce specific injury to the immature Purkinje cells, with consequent ataxia, in the suckling rat and hamster.[69]

A third focus of contemporary interest

is the possibility that "slow viruses" may be responsible for certain chronic neurological diseases, such as amyotrophic lateral sclerosis and multiple sclerosis.

Slow viruses are classified according to the type of disease they cause and not according to any intrinsic property of the viruses themselves. They exhibit an incubation period of months to years and cause diseases which pursue a regular and protracted course, usually to a fatal conclusion. Most of the known slow viruses affect the nervous system. They may be divided into two groups; the first is one in which the agent has been transmitted either to an experimental animal or to a tissue culture system, and the second group comprises diseases in which there is a morphological basis for suspecting slow viruses to

be the cause, but in which no virus has been isolated.

The first group includes seven diseases (see Table 14–1). *Scrapie*,[47, 54] a disease of sheep, is characterized pathologically by diffuse degeneration of gray matter. The perineuronal gray matter becomes spongy and the astrocytes hypertrophy. Demyelination is not marked. *Mink encephalopathy* is a disease which is also marked by status spongiosus. *Kuru*,[47, 54] a human disease marked by cerebellar ataxia, has been produced in chimpanzees injected intracerebrally with brain tissue from human cases and has been passed serially to chimpanzees. Here again, the pathology is dominated by spongy degeneration of the gray matter, as in scrapie. The disease is limited to members of the Fore-speaking tribe in New Guinea, and passage from one indi-

Table 14–1. *Viral Diseases of the Nervous System*

CLASSIFICATION

1. *NEUROTROPIC VIRUSES*

Epidemic Forms	*Sporadic Forms*
Acute anterior poliomyelitis	Lymphocytic choriomeningitis
Equine encephalitis	Pseudolymphocytic choriomeningitis
Eastern Type	Herpes zoster
Western Type	Rabies
Venezuelan Type	Louping ill
Japanese B encephalitis	Rift valley fever
Russian tick-borne encephalitis	Western Nile encephalitis
St. Louis encephalitis	B-virus of monkeys
Australian X encephalitis	

2. *VISCEROTROPIC VIRUSES WHICH CAN INVADE THE NERVOUS SYSTEM*

Herpes simplex	Yellow fever
Mumps	Dengue fever
Coxsackie viruses	Psittacosis
Echo viruses	Cytomegalic inclusion disease
Infective hepatitis	Lymphopathia venereum

3. *"SLOW VIRUSES"*

Scrapie (sheep)	Kuru (man)
Mink encephalopathy	Progressive multifocal leukoencephalopathy (man)
Visna (sheep)	Subacute sclerosing panencephalitis (man)
	Jakob-Creutzfeldt disease (man)

4. *PRESUMED VIRAL INFECTIONS OF THE NERVOUS SYSTEM*

Encephalitis lethargica	Cat-scratch disease
Infectious mononucleosis	"Brainstem" encephalitis
	Encephalomyocarditis

vidual to another is thought to be brought about by cannibalism, it being the custom to eat the brain of dead members of the tribe. However, since individuals who apparently have not partaken have been known to develop the disease, there may be other routes of infection. *Visna*, a neuropathy of sheep, is characterized by meningeal and encephalitic infiltration, proliferation of cells of the reticuloendothelial system, and widespread demyelination; the gray matter is not affected. *Subacute sclerosing panencephalitis* (also known as Dawson's inclusion body encephalitis, Van Bogart's sclerosing leukoencephalitis, and the panencephalitis of Pette-Doring) is a disease of children and young people with an insidious onset and a progressive course, marked pathologically by patches of demyelination, degenerative changes in the neurons of the cortex, basal ganglia, and brainstem, and Type A inclusion bodies within the nuclei of neurons and oligodendroglia (p. 312).

Jakob-Creutzfeldt disease, also known as spastic pseudosclerosis, is characterized clinically by the insidious onset in middle life of progressive pyramidal and extrapyramidal symptoms together with organic dementia. Pathologically, there are primary changes in the gray matter, with secondary degeneration of the corticospinal tracts. It has been successfully transmitted to chimpanzees by direct brain inoculation from human patients. *Progressive multifocal leukoencephalopathy* has not yet been successfully transmitted to laboratory animals, but it is believed to be a viral disease because of the presence of intranuclear structures in the oligodendrocytes; these inclusions resemble virions of the Papova group of viruses (p. 311).[109]

Poliomyelitis

Etiology and Epidemiology. There are three strains of virus, Type I (Brunhilde), Type II (Lansing), and Type III (Leon), each of which can cause the disease.[80] Poliomyelitis is worldwide in distribution. The highest incidence used to be in communities with a high standard of hygiene, but the situation has changed for the better since the introduction of vaccines. It occurs all the year round, but sporadic, regionally limited epidemics are common in nonimmunized societies and usually start in the spring or summer. In such epidemics, the number of paralyzed persons may reach two per 1000 population; many others who are infected do not develop muscle weakness. Spread of the disease is thought to be by contact with infected persons, notably asymptomatic carriers and patients in the preparalytic stage. Even convalescents excrete large quantities of the virus in the feces, and this obviously serves as a source of infection. The virus can be spread by water and food, but it cannot survive for long outside living cells.

The usual portals of entry are thought to be the upper respiratory and gastrointestinal tracts. The disease can follow tonsillectomy, and the majority of such cases are of the bulbar type. Rarely, intrauterine infection has occurred. Poliomyelitis can be contracted during the neonatal period, but it is uncommon under the age of six months because many infants possess immunity derived from the mother. The majority of patients are below the age of 10, but the number of adult cases has been increasing in recent years. Multiple cases in a family do occur but not to the extent seen in other viral infections. The disease tends to appear in its paralytic form among the physically vigorous members of the family or community, and it has been suggested that active exercise of a limb in the preparalytic stage can determine the subsequent appearance of paralysis in that limb. There is also some evidence that the major brunt of paralysis falls on a limb which has been the site of a recent injection of serum. Paralytic poliomyelitis is about three times as common in pregnancy as it is in nonpregnant women of the same age group, and the offspring of infected mothers show an unduly high proportion of congenital defects.[22]

The virus can be obtained from the pharynx in the first few days of infection, but it may persist in the feces during the illness and for weeks or even months thereafter. It is very rarely obtained from the blood in man.

Pathology. The virus is neurotropic and has an affinity for the gray matter of the spinal cord, brainstem, and cortex (in that order), but the inflammatory response also spreads out into the white matter to some extent. The lumbar enlargement is more often affected than other parts of the nervous system. The lesions are characteristically patchy and asymmetrical, and even at the microscopic level, diseased and healthy cells are found side by side. The predilection for motor cells of the anterior horn and brainstem determines the clinical characteristics of the disease—a patchy, flaccid paresis or paralysis of lower motor neuron type. The virus also invades the large cells of the reticular formation and this may be responsible for the muscle spasm which is often seen in the early stages of the disease. The hypothalamus, subthalamic nucleus, substantia nigra, thalamus, and motor cortex are often involved as well, albeit to a varying degree.

Microscopically, the meninges show slight lymphocytic infiltration in the early stages of the disease. The anterior horn cells and their cranial homologues are diseased or destroyed; later, there is a reactive inflammatory response with marked congestion and lymphocytic infiltration, which gives place to microglial proliferation and ultimate gliosis and scarring. The inflammatory response spreads into the white matter, but there is no demyelination or primary destruction of axis cylinders. Many of the affected nerve cells recover in the course of four to six weeks.

Clinical Features

PREPARALYTIC STAGE.[80] The incubation period is not known for certain, but it is usually five to 14 days. Then comes the preparalytic stage with pyrexia, headache, malaise, gastrointestinal upset, upper respiratory symptoms, and (usu-

ally) polymorphonuclear leukocytosis. These symptoms may last for a day or two and then clear up entirely. It has been estimated that in some epidemics the percentage of infected persons who do not develop paralysis may be as high as 75 per cent. The prodromata may pass directly into the stage of meningeal irritation, but in a few cases, the initial symptoms clear up for a day or two, only to recur thereafter, producing a double-humped temperature curve. The meningeal stage may or may not be marked by headache, pains in the neck and back, aching in the limbs, prostration, drowsiness, and extreme irritability. Sometimes there is severe vomiting, suggesting bulbar involvement. The temperature may be elevated or normal. The neck is slightly stiff, and there is often a positive Kernig sign. Spinal rigidity is marked in children, who are reluctant to flex the neck or the spine because of the pain induced. The meningeal stage, during which there is lymphocytosis in the spinal fluid, lasts for two to seven days, and the patient may then recover completely without paralysis.

PARALYTIC STAGE. The paralytic stage is usually preceded by meningeal irritation, but occasionally occurs with little, if any, systemic disturbance. Fever and malaise often disappear with the onset of paralysis, but may continue for a week or two. The paralysis itself is sometimes preceded by tremulousness of the limb and by tenderness in muscles which are about to be affected. Generally speaking, maximum paralysis occurs within 36 hours of the first appearance of weakness. It is usually most marked in the legs, but there are many exceptions. Sometimes paralysis ascends rapidly from the legs to involve the trunk, arms, bulb, and brainstem; this type is often fatal.

The paralysis varies in extent. It may occur in only one or two muscles, or may implicate all four limbs and the trunk. The muscles are flaccid and tender, and the appropriate tendon reflexes are abolished. Occasionally a transient extensor response is found, probably due to edema of the cord, and retention of urine lasting for a day or two is not uncommon in cases of extensive involvement of the lower dorsal and upper lumbar segments. The affected muscles begin to waste in the course of one to two weeks, and fasciculation may appear in some. The paralyzed limbs are cool and somewhat cyanotic. Contractures are likely to follow, especially in neglected cases.

Respiratory failure can be caused by paralysis of the intercostal muscles and diaphragm from involvement of the anterior horn cells, but it also occurs as the result of spread of the disease to the medulla; this causes irregularity of respiratory rhythm, with periods of apnea. Sometimes there is a transient rise of both systolic and diastolic blood pressures, and this can be followed by circulatory collapse. Nonspecific EKG changes may be found in such cases. Another, but very much rarer, cause of respiratory embarrassment is bilateral abductor paralysis of the vocal cords. This requires immediate tracheostomy.

Bulbar poliomyelitis, sometimes called polioencephalitis, can occur with or without evidence of spinal cord involvement.[10, 75] The motor fifth, sixth, seventh, ninth, tenth, eleventh, and twelfth cranial nerves may be involved unilaterally or bilaterally. Sometimes, however, paralysis is confined to a single cranial nerve, such as the facial. Nystagmus is a common but transient sign. When there is severe infection of the reticular formation, drowsiness and coma are seen, together with the respiratory and cardiovascular features referred to previously. Papilledema sometimes occurs as a result of respiratory embarrassment or (possibly) from elevation of the protein content of the cerebrospinal fluid.

A "cerebral" form is sometimes described. It usually occurs during epidemics, and is marked by focal seizures and hemiparesis. Cases of cerebellar ataxia have also been attributed to poliomyelitis, but as in the cerebral form, there is always doubt whether they are due to poliomyelitis or not.

In children, painful swellings may occur in one or more joints during the acute paralytic stage. Large joints are more affected than small, and the condition subsides without permanent disability. It can be misleading, because pseudoparalysis or unwillingness to move a limb is seen in small children suffering from any painful condition in or around the joints, such as rheumatic fever, epiphysitis, and scurvy.

Laboratory Data. There is usually a polymorphonuclear leukocytosis in the blood during the febrile prodromal phase. The pressure in the cerebrospinal fluid is normal or slightly increased, and the fluid itself is usually clear and colorless. In the meningeal stage and at the beginning of the paralytic phase, there is an increase of 10 to 300 cells/cu. mm.; as many as half of these may be polymorphs, but lymphocytes predominate from then on. Cell counts of less than 10 cells/cu. mm. are occasionally encountered. There seems to be no correlation between the extent of paralysis and the cellular content of the cerebrospinal fluid. The cells rapidly disappear after paralysis has developed. The protein is often normal or only slightly increased in the early stages, but may rise as high as 150 mg. per cent in about three weeks. This elevation can persist for some time. The sugar content of the fluid is normal, as are the chlorides. Cultures are sterile.

The infection can be confirmed by serological tests, but they take too long to be of use in immediate diagnosis; they are useful retrospectively.

Diagnosis. The disease is to be suspected in the preparalytic stage, especially in epidemics, and particularly if there is an increase of lymphocytes in the spinal fluid, without a fall of glucose or chlorides. This combination merely suggests the presence of a viral infection of some type, and lymphocytic choriomeningitis must be remembered in this context. Tuberculous meningitis develops more gradually, and there is reduction of sugar and chlorides in the spinal fluid. Coxsackie viruses may closely simulate poliomyelitis, especially under epidemic conditions, but muscular weakness is usually mild and transient. In some cases, a dual infection is present as judged by serological tests.[84]

The bulbar form is difficult to distinguish in the early phase from acute encephalitis, but the rapid appearance of patchy localized muscular weakness and the frequent presence of paralysis of muscles elsewhere in the body usually serve to differentiate the condition.[10, 75] Acute infective polyneuritis (one variety of the Guillain-Barré syndrome) can simulate the rapidly ascending form of poliomyelitis, but paresthesias and sensory impairment are usually present and there is eventually a rise of protein in the spinal fluid without any increase in the cell content. Localized weakness of rapid onset in the shoulder girdle or arm due to neuralgic amyotrophy (paralytic brachial neuritis) can simulate poliomyelitis, but there are no constitutional or meningeal symptoms, severe local pain in the shoulder is usually present for 24 hours to 14 days before paralysis appears, and there may be slight sensory impairment over the shoulder girdle; the spinal fluid is normal. Pseudoparalysis of a limb in infants suffering from disease of the bone or joints has been mentioned previously (p. 291).

Prognosis. The outlook as regards life varies greatly in different epidemics, but the mortality averages about 8 per cent. It may be lower or considerably higher. Fatalities are usually due to respiratory failure or aspiration pneumonia; persistent hypotension is of dire significance in bulbar cases. The mortality is highest—about 50 per cent—in bulbar cases and is higher in adults than in children.

The prognosis as regards the return of function in affected muscles depends on the number of motor cells involved and whether they are destroyed or merely damaged. If cellular recovery is going to take place, it usually takes two or three months to do so, and it is therefore difficult to estimate the prognosis in terms of function before this period has elapsed. Muscles showing some return of function in the first few weeks will probably re-cover, and those still totally paralyzed by the sixth month are unlikely to improve. Muscles with partial restoration of function may continue to improve in strength over a period of three to four years, especially in the young. Some 2 per cent of all patients are completely and permanently disabled, and an additional 20 per cent require the use of braces or reconstructive surgery. Severe paralysis of a limb in childhood leads to shortening of that limb, often complicated by contractures. Paralysis of the erector spinae on one side leads to scoliosis. Second attacks of the disease are rare, but do occur, and since a high degree of type-specific immunity is conferred by an attack, second attacks are presumably due to infection by a different strain.

Treatment. Prophylactic immunization by oral (Sabin) or parenteral (Salk) vaccine has proved effective, but booster doses at intervals, comparable to revaccination against smallpox, are likely to be a continuing necessity. There is no specific treatment for the disease. There is evidence that complete bed rest in the preparalytic stage may limit the extent and degree of paralysis, so it is undesirable for patients with a pyrexial illness and muscular aches to try to "fight it off"; they should go to bed. Barbiturates and valium can be used for irritability. The repeated application of moist hot packs to aching muscles is soothing and beneficial. Fluid balance must be maintained either by mouth or by venous infusion. Paralyzed or weakened muscles should be supported in a position which avoids stretching them, but rigid splintage should be avoided if possible. The legs should be protected from the pressure of heavy bed covers by a cradle or foot board. The optimal position is with the feet dorsiflexed, the knees slightly flexed, and the arms slightly abducted and externally rotated. If the deltoid is paralyzed, the arm should be supported in the abducted position, while wrist drop requires a lightweight cock-up splint. The joints should be moved passively through a complete range twice a day.

Massage and active movements, *short of fatigue*, are important during convalescence, and muscle re-education is desirable. Gentle active exercise in a swimming pool is useful. Braces may be necessary, and later on, when all possibility of further recovery is deemed impossible, orthopedic measures may be required to correct deformities and to stabilize flail joints.

Respiratory failure is a common cause of death. Weakness of the intercostal muscles and diaphragm reduces respiratory efficiency, and the situation is aggravated by the patient's inability to expel secretions. Furthermore, in bulbar cases there may be inability to keep swallowed material out of the trachea. Consequent hypoxia and accumulation of CO_2 add greatly to the patient's distress and restlessness and may produce central effects which reduce the chances of recovery. It follows that it is not enough to put the patient into a positive-pressure respirator at the earliest suggestion of respiratory failure, though this is indeed essential; tracheostomy and feeding via a nasal catheter should also be instituted early rather than late. A broad-spectrum antibiotic is desirable in the presence of respiratory difficulty. When respiratory failure is due to bulbar involvement, death usually occurs whether a respirator is used or not, but when it is caused by intercostal and diaphragmatic paralysis, the outlook for life is improved. To save such a life is sometimes to condemn the patient to spend the rest of it in a respirator, but many patients can subsequently be weaned from the "respirator life" once active infection has subsided. It is not possible to foretell at the onset whether respiratory paralysis is going to be permanent or transient.

Viral Encephalitis

The term "encephalitis" is usually used to denote infection, "encephalopathy" being employed for noninfective inflammatory and degenerative reactions of the brain, and it is desirable to use definitive adjectives, e.g., viral encephalitis, suppurative encephalitis, leptospiral encephalitis, etc. In a significant number of cases, however, the identity of the virus, or other agent, is not established during life, and at autopsy the antemortem diagnosis of "viral encephalitis" is often disproved.

Etiology. Ticks and mosquitoes can transfer neurotropic viruses from intermediate hosts to man.[76] The virus of the tick-borne encephalitides is transmitted through the eggs from one generation of ticks to another. The most important of these *tick-borne* infections is Russian spring-summer encephalitis, which is found throughout the USSR and in Central Europe. Louping ill is a disease of lambs and yearlings in Scotland and Northern England which is transmitted by ticks; the virus has caused a few cases of encephalitis in laboratory workers and others. *Mosquito-borne viruses* give rise to encephalitis in many parts of the world, e.g., Western, Eastern, and Venezuelan equine encephalitis, St. Louis encephalitis, Japanese B encephalitis, Murray Valley encephalitis in Australia, and the widely distributed West Nile encephalitis. An important fact about the arthropod-borne viruses is that although human infection may be extremely widespread as judged by serological tests, only a few of the infected individuals show clinical evidence of encephalitis.

The number of viruses identified as responsible for encephalitis is constantly increasing, but it not uncommon to encounter cases in which both the clinical and microscopic findings suggest a viral origin, but in which serological confirmation is lacking and attempts to transmit the disease to laboratory animals fail. It seems likely that in these a virus is responsible and that failure to demonstrate it reflects the limitations of existing laboratory techniques.

Pathology. In the most acute forms of encephalitis, the initial cellular infiltrate is chiefly polymorphonuclear, but this is soon replaced by lymphocytes, mononuclear cells, plasma cells, and large mononuclear phagocytes. Cuffs of lymphocytes collect around blood vessels, and lymphocytes also wander into the tissue away from the vessels. Morular cells which stand out as prominent purple mulberry-like masses are sometimes seen in subacute and chronic forms of encephalitis when stained with phosphotungstic acid hematoxylin. Proliferation of microglia is usual and may be diffuse or focal; they collect around dying nerve cells, and star-shaped formations of 10 or more hypertrophied microglial cells are sometimes found related to small vessels.

Damage to nerve cells is patchy and diffuse, only a small proportion of the cells in a given area being involved. They show varying changes; there is often a loss of Nissl granules and a shift of the cell nucleus to the periphery. In encephalitis lethargica, which is assumed to be of viral origin, most of the cells in the substantia nigra may be destroyed.

The extent to which the white matter is involved varies from case to case and from virus to virus. In some, such as Western equine encephalitis and herpes simplex encephalitis, inflammation spreads from the cortex to the white matter, producing softening, necrosis, and cyst formation. In subacute inclusion encephalomyelitis, which is due to a virus, there is a slowly progressive demyelination of the white matter.

The vessels are not always affected in encephalitis, but vasculitis occurs in equine encephalomyelitis. The vessel walls are invaded by neutrophil leukocytes, and there may be necrosis of the walls with deposition of fibrin; in some cases, thrombosis occurs, producing small infarcts.

INCLUSION BODIES. Acidophil inclusion bodies are sometimes present in neurons, astrocytes, and oligodendroglia; they have also been seen in the endothelium of small blood vessels in cytomegalic inclusion disease. Type A inclusion bodies are spherical, amorphous, or granular, occupy the greater part of the nucleus, and are surrounded by a clear halo. They were once regarded as conglomerations of viruses but are now thought to represent a specific type of degeneration caused by viruses. They are found in herpes simplex encephalitis, subacute inclusion encephalitis, and cytomegalic inclusion disease. The Negri bodies in rabies, which are in the cytoplasm, are acidophilic, have a definite internal structure, and are compatible with the continued life of the cell in which they are found. Unlike Type A intranuclear inclusions, Type B intranuclear inclusions are small and often multiple; they are seen typically in the anterior horn cells in the recovery stage of poliomyelitis, and closely resemble the acidophilic inclusions which are normally found in the substantia nigra, in old people especially.

General Clinical Features. The clinical spectrum is broad, as regards both the severity and the type of the symptoms and signs.[2] It varies from virus to virus, and from one epidemic to another. The onset is usually acute or subacute with headache, signs of meningeal irritation, and fever. The disease may be so mild as to simulate influenza, clearing up in a week or 10 days. On the other hand, in fulminating cases, patients may pass into coma within 24 hours and die in three to five days. Usually, however, the course lasts two or three weeks, with gradual recovery.

Brain function is disturbed in a variety of ways, depending on the severity and distribution of the lesions, but in most cases there is some disturbance of consciousness, ranging from confusion and blunting of attention through delirium to stupor or coma. This global defect makes it difficult to identify evidence of focal damage such as aphasia, diplopia, and minor degrees of muscular weakness. Although the pathological process is not limited to the motor system, the neurological signs are predominantly motor, involvement of somatic sensation and the special senses being relatively uncommon. Cranial nerve palsies, paralysis of limbs, involuntary movements, and seizures may occur.

When focal signs are present, they are usually more consistent with scattered small lesions than with one large one, but occasionally—as in some cases of herpes simplex encephalitis—the main impact of the disease is somewhat localized, as for instance in the temporal lobe. Although cerebral edema causes a moderate rise of intracranial pressure in some cases, papilledema is rare.

There is usually a mild lymphocytic pleocytosis and even a few polymorphs in the spinal fluid; the protein may be slightly raised, but the glucose content is normal. Other laboratory studies, notably the complement fixation test, virus neutralization tests, and animal inoculation, will sometimes identify the virus, but these methods are time-consuming and the results are seldom available when they are most needed, i.e., in the acute phase of the disease. Furthermore, in a rather large number of cases the results of viral studies are negative, and the diagnosis of viral encephalitis is therefore presumptive.

SEQUELAE. The death rate varies from epidemic to epidemic but is usually in the range of 10 to 35 per cent. Transient or permanent sequelae in the form of mental disturbance, alteration of personality, and paresis of one or more limbs are not uncommon in Eastern equine encephalitis, Japanese B encephalitis, and Russian and European spring-summer encephalitis. The most notable example of postencephalitic sequelae is parkinsonism following encephalitis lethargica (which has yet to be proved to be of viral origin).

Equine Encephalitis

Several strains of virus give rise to subacute encephalomyelitis in horses; birds act as a reservoir for the virus, and mosquitoes transmit it to horses and to man. Thus far, four types of human infection have been recognized: Eastern and Western American encephalitis, Venezuelan encephalitis, and Moscow type II encephalitis. The disease occurs in small regionally limited epidemics, usually in summer.

WESTERN EQUINE ENCEPHALITIS

Western equine encephalitis[9] is less severe than the Eastern variety. It usually occurs in adults, but can also affect infants and children. Pathologically, the brain may appear grossly normal or it may be intensely congested, and the lesions are disseminated throughout both the gray and white matter. Perivascular cuffing with both polymorphs and mononuclear cells is prominent, and collections of cells are also found throughout the brain away from the blood vessels. There is often vasculitis, and the lumina of small vessels may be clogged with neutrophils. Patchy demyelination is present. The same changes are found in milder form in the spinal cord. In some severe, "chronic" cases, the brain has been found to contain multiple glia-lined cavities which are probably the result of vascular occlusions.

Clinical Features. The onset is sudden, with fever, malaise, and headache. After a few days the headache becomes worse, and there is photophobia, stiffness of the neck, and *lethargy*. Vertigo is not uncommon, but seizures and signs of focal damage are rare. After about 10 days the symptoms usually subside, but in a few cases the lethargy progresses to coma, the temperature rises, and death ensues. The spinal fluid contains an excess of cells; in early stages, as many as 50 per cent may be polymorphs, but later on, monocytes predominate. The glucose content remains normal.

Mild sequelae in the form of irritability, liability to fatigue, and irregular headaches are not at all uncommon in adults and may last for months. Infants under the age of two months are more vulnerable. Finley and his associates[44] found permanent sequelae in 16 out of 29 children who contracted the disease before the age of one month. These children were liable to seizures, mental retardation, and motor deficits of pyramidal, extrapyramidal, or cerebellar type. In some cases, these deficits appear gradually over the years, not because the disease is getting worse, but because the nervous system fails to develop normally.

EASTERN EQUINE ENCEPHALITIS

Eastern equine encephalitis is distributed over the Eastern United States and Canada, Mexico, Cuba, and Brazil.[43] Recently, it has been spreading westward, cases having been reported in Michigan, Alabama, and Texas.

Pathological Features. The pathological features are more severe than in the Western type. The brain shows marked congestion and is softer than usual. Both perivascular and disseminated collections of neutrophils and histiocytes are prominent in the leptomeninges, cerebral cortex, and white matter. There is widespread involvement of nerve cells varying from early nuclear changes to complete disintegration. These changes are also found in the basal nuclei and in the cells of the brainstem, but the cerebellum and spinal cord are usually spared. Destruction of myelin is not prominent except in the immediate neighborhood of cellular infiltrations.

Clinical Features. The clinical features are more dramatic than in the Western type. The onset is abrupt, with high fever, malaise, lethargy, vomiting, and stiffness of the neck. Seizures are common, as are cranial nerve palsies, hemiplegia, and other signs of focal damage to the brain. The cerebrospinal fluid pressure may be raised, and there is pleocytosis, polymorphonuclears often predominating in the early stages of the disease.

The mortality has amounted to 65 per cent in some epidemics, and survivors show a high incidence of residual neurological defects, such as mental retardation, hemiparesis, partial deafness, speech disorders, and emotional instability. However, subclinical infection is not uncommon. After the New Jersey outbreak of 1959, positive complement fixation tests were found in a number of persons who were unaware of having been ill.

There is no specific treatment for the disease.

ST. LOUIS ENCEPHALITIS

In 1933, there was an outbreak of mosquito-borne encephalitis in and around St. Louis. In 1130 cases reported, the mortality was 20 per cent. A virus was identified as the cause of the disease, and since then there have been repeated outbreaks over an ever-widening area of the Middle West. Serum neutralization tests have shown that the disease sometimes occurs during epidemics of Western and Eastern equine encephalitis.[83]

Pathology. The morbid anatomy is that of typical nonsuppurative encephalitis with intense vascular congestion, perivascular and diffuse cellular infiltration of the meninges and the brain, and widespread nerve cell damage. The most intense lesions occur within the basal nuclei, notably the thalamus and substantia nigra, and the white matter is relatively spared.

Clinical Features. The illness may vary from an influenza-like incident to a fulminating encephalitis. Fever, somnolence, and repeated vomiting may be the sole expressions of the disease. In other cases, the patient remains alert, and has only headache, vomiting, or minimal signs of meningeal irritation. In the more typical, severe cases, the onset is abrupt with a rapid rise of temperature, headache, photophobia, stiffness of the neck, and a positive Kernig's sign. Within a few days, there is mild confusion and disorientation which may go on to severe delirium and coma. Ocular manifestations and other signs of focal lesions are uncommon and usually transient. After a week to 10 days, the temperature usually falls and the general condition of the patient improves. In the most extreme cases, death occurs within a few days of the onset.

The blood often shows polymorphonuclear leukocytosis in the early stages.

The spinal fluid reveals anything from 10 to 300 cells in the majority of cases; polymorphs may be present at the onset, but later mononuclear cells predominate. Diagnosis can be confirmed retrospectively by serum neutralization tests. As in other types of viral encephalitis, the sugar content of the spinal fluid is normal.

Prognosis. The disease is an acute one in most cases, with death or recovery ensuing within two or three weeks. Both the morbidity and the mortality increase steadily with age. Many patients complain of fatigability, headaches, irritability, and insomnia for months after the illness, as in other forms of encephalitis. Persistent cranial nerve palsies, hemiplegia, and other focal signs are present in a small percentage of cases. There is nothing to suggest that parkinsonism or other sequelae of encephalitis lethargica follow this form of encephalitis.

There is no specific treatment for the disease.

JAPANESE B ENCEPHALITIS

From time to time since 1891, epidemics of summer encephalitis have occurred in Japan. There were 1362 cases with a mortality rate of 30 per cent in the Tokyo epidemic of 1935. The same virus has been responsible for encephalitis on the coast of China, in Eastern Russia, and over a wide area of Southeast Asia.

The disease is transmitted by a mosquito, and it is thought that birds and animals act as a reservoir of infection. A curious feature is its tendency to appear in widely separated districts almost simultaneously.

Pathology. The pathological features are those of nonsuppurative encephalitis.[35, 56] There is mild lymphocytic leptomeningitis, intracerebral perivascular cuffing, and widespread damage to nerve cells. Glial nodules composed of large mononuclear cells and a few cells with pleomorphic nuclei are found in the areas of cell damage. The white matter is less severely affected. The name Japanese B encephalitis was coined to distinguish this disease from encephalitis lethargica, and does not imply the presence of Type B inclusion bodies; no inclusion bodies of any type have been found in this form of encephalitis.

Clinical Features. Prodromata in the form of malaise, anorexia, and slight headache are not uncommon. There is a sudden rise of temperature, often to an alarming height, within 24 to 72 hours. Signs of meningeal irritation are present, headache and vomiting may be very severe, and evidence of brain involvement soon appears in the form of disorientation, delirium, stupor, or coma. Evidence of focal cerebral involvement is less often seen, but aphasia, nystagmus, diplopia, facial paralysis, weakness of one or more limbs, and extrapyramidal rigidity have been reported.

Within seven to 10 days, the temperature begins to fall and there is a gradual resolution of symptoms; occasionally the disease lingers on in subacute form for a month or two.[35] In fatal cases, the patient passes into coma and dies in a few days.

The spinal fluid shows the usual features of viral encephalitis—pleocytosis and normal sugar content. The protein may be slightly raised.

In some epidemics, the mortality rate has been as high as 60 per cent, possibly because only the most severe cases are admitted to hospital. Late effects are not uncommon,[102] including mental retardation, hemiparesis, changes of personality in children, and the usual postencephalitic picture of headaches, fatigability, irritability, and slight impairment of memory.

RUSSIAN SPRING-SUMMER ENCEPHALITIS

Russian spring-summer encephalitis—"RSSE"—is conveyed by a wood tick. Central European encephalitis is the same disease. It has a maximum incidence in May and June. The virus produces the usual pathological features of encephalitis, and in addition, it often localizes in the spinal cord, causing extensive cell damage. Clinically, the disease is marked by fever, signs of meningeal irritation, varying degrees of impaired consciousness, monoplegia or hemiplegia, and in some cases, atrophic paralysis of muscles in the neck, shoulders, and upper limbs; the distribution of these paralyses has been attributed to the fact that the tick often bites the arm, shoulder, or neck. There is lymphocytic pleocytosis in the spinal fluid, and the virus can sometimes be isolated from the blood during the acute illness. The mortality in identified cases is between 10 and 30 per cent, and neurological or psychological sequelae have been described in 20 per cent of the survivors.

LOUPING ILL

Louping ill is a tick-borne viral disease of sheep in Scotland and Northern England, and is occasionally transmitted to man. In both sheep and man there is an initial febrile disorder followed shortly by a second and more serious elevation of temperature which is accompanied, in man, by meningeal and encephalitic signs. Headache may be severe. The neck is stiff, and there may be severe vomiting and profound prostration. Diplopia, vertigo, and cerebellar ataxia are not uncommon, and delirium or stupor occurs in severe cases. There is lymphocytic pleocytosis in the cerebrospinal fluid. There have been no fatalities in man, and no permanent sequelae have been described.

DENGUE FEVER ENCEPHALITIS

Dengue fever is a common virus disease in subtropical and tropical countries throughout the world. It is transmitted by mosquitoes, notably *Aedes aegypti*. The virus usually causes a febrile disorder characterized by intense headache, backache, and pain in the limbs—symptoms which led to the colloquial name "breakbone fever." However, the virus may also produce disturbances of the cardiovascular system, gastrointestinal tract, and adrenals. The temperature chart shows a saddle-backed curve, the temperature dropping after the third or fourth day and then rising again a day or so later. The second bout of fever may be accompanied by a petechial rash on the skin and in the mouth. Involvement of the nervous system is quite common, and may take the form of encephalitis, myelitis, or polyneuritis. The cerebrospinal fluid sometimes shows moderate lymphocytic pleocytosis. It is a self-limited disease, and permanent sequelae are rare, though seizures have been reported during convalescence.

CAT-SCRATCH DISEASE

The disease is thought to be viral in origin.[27] There is a history of being bitten or scratched by a cat a few days before the onset of illness. The lesion becomes inflamed, and there is fever, a macular rash on the limbs, lymphadenopathy, and sometimes splenomegaly. Granulomatous conjunctivitis may occur, and thrombocytopenic purpura has been described. Meningoencephalitis may appear from three to 20 days after the onset of the symptoms. There is high fever, mild signs of meningeal irritation, and a wide spectrum of neurological symptoms which include convulsions, delirium, coma, diplopia, transient paralyses, myoclonic twitches, and spasticity of the limbs. There is moderate lymphocytic pleocytosis in the cerebrospinal fluid. Complete recovery is usual. In some cases, the diagnosis can be verified by a positive skin test using cat-scratch antigen.

OTHER REGIONAL TYPES OF ENCEPHALITIS

A series of outbreaks of encephalitis occurred in the Murray Valley, Australia, between 1917 and 1951. The disease is probably transmitted to man by mosquito bites, birds and domestic chickens being the reservoir. About 50 per cent of cases occurred in children under five years old and the mortality rate in the first two epidemics was over 70 per cent. The disease is marked by fever, evidence of meningeal irritation, and a high incidence of convulsions, which may be related to the fact that so many children are affected. The mental condition is one of drowsiness or stupor, which may alternate with delirium. In fulminating cases, death can occur in 24 hours, but most fatal cases terminate in 4 to 6 days, and in nonfatal cases recovery commences after two weeks. Intellectual impairment and personality disorders have been reported.

West Nile encephalitis is widely distributed over the Middle East, the Nile Valley, Uganda (where the virus was first isolated), and India. The virus can produce encephalomyelitis when transmitted to monkeys. Clinically, there is fever, meningism, malaise, drowsiness or stupor, and sometimes a generalized lymphadenopathy. The cerebrospinal fluid shows a lymphocytic pleocytosis, and neutralizing antibodies are present in the serum. Since these antibodies are widely distributed in the population, care has to be exercised in interpreting their significance in suspected cases of encephalitis.

Rift Valley fever is endemic to East Africa. Normally a disease of sheep and other animals, it can be transmitted to man by mosquitoes, causing fever, meningeal irritation, and pain in the muscles and joints. Impairment of vision due to a retinitis has been described.

Encephalomyocarditis (Mengo encephalomyelitis) is due to a virus which has been isolated from monkeys and cotton rats. It has a worldwide distribution. The virus has a predilection for the brain and, in experimental animals, for the myocardium. It is an occasional cause of mild lymphocytic meningitis or meningoencephalitis in man.

RABIES (HYDROPHOBIA, LYSSA)

Definition. Rabies is an acute viral disease of the central nervous system which is transmitted to man by the bite of a rabid animal. It is characterized by a variable but usually prolonged incubation period, extreme excitability to all peripheral stimuli, muscular spasms, and spasmodic contractions of the pharynx and larynx; it progresses to generalized paralysis and death from paralysis of respiration.

Incidence. About 100 deaths occur annually in the United States. The virus is present in the saliva of infected animals and is transmitted to man through a bite or by contamination of a fresh wound with the animal's saliva. Dogs are the common vectors, but the disease can be harbored by cats, skunks, bats, foxes, wolves, jackals, goats, camels, deer, cows, and poultry. In South America, the vampire bat carries the virus and is a source of infection in cattle and occasionally in man; the virus is present in the bat's urine.

The incidence of the disease is very low in countries with stringent public health rules for the admission of animals; it is virtually unknown in Britain, for instance. The disease develops in less than 10 per cent of those bitten by rabid dogs. The danger of contracting it is said to be highest when wounds are severe and near the head. If the bite is inflicted through clothing, saliva has less chance of contaminating the wound, and the chances of contracting the disease are comparatively low.

Pathology. There is diffuse perivascular infiltration of the brain and spinal cord with lymphocytes and a few polymorph leukocytes and plasma cells. Degeneration of neurons occurs diffusely. In the great majority of cases coming to autopsy, there are a large number of acidophilic inclusion bodies (Negri bodies) in the neurons of the cerebral cortex, the hippocampus, and the cerebellum, as well as in the spinal ganglia (Fig. 14–4). They vary in size from 1 to 20 μ, are spherical or oval in shape, and stain readily with basic fuchsin; with differential staining they exhibit an inner mass of granules surrounded by a nonstaining halo. Microglia proliferate, forming small nodules.

Clinical Features. The incubation varies between 20 days and one year, with an average of 30 to 70 days after exposure. Experimentally, the length of incubation varies inversely with the quantity and virulence of the virus intro-

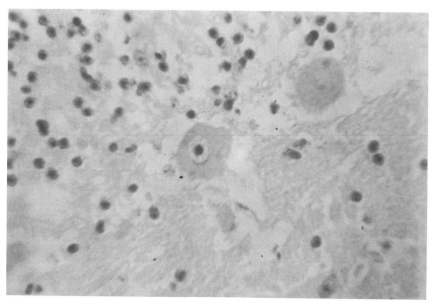

Figure 14–4.   Negri bodies in rabies. (Courtesy of Department of Neuropathology, Philadelphia General Hospital.)

duced, without relation to the site of inoculation. The earliest symptom is a change in the patient's disposition; he becomes irritable, overexcitable, and complains of malaise, headache, and discomfort at the site of the bite. Over the next few days, he becomes more restless, agitated, and apprehensive, and in patients old enough to appreciate their predicament, it can be difficult to distinguish between the organic and the functional.

A few days later, reflex spasms of the throat muscles develop. They are intensely painful and are apt to occur when an attempt is made to drink. There is often profuse salivation and vomiting, and there may be involuntary spasms of the trunk and limbs. Violent convulsions are one of the most distressing features of severe cases because consciousness is unimpaired; alternating with these periods there are intervals of quiet, during which the patient lies in bed, alert and terrified. After two or three days of this truly agonizing condition, the patient lapses into a coma and dies within the next 24 hours. The temperature commonly rises steeply toward the end.

Occasionally, a paralytic form occurs. Paresthesias in the limbs are followed by weakness and finally paralysis of scat-

tered muscle groups as a result of patchy myelitis. This paralysis may start at the feet and ascend rapidly in the manner of Landry's syndrome. Some paralyzed patients experience a few terminal spasms of the throat muscles.

Laboratory Data.   The cerebrospinal fluid is under normal pressure; there is sometimes lymphocytic pleocytosis with a moderate increase of protein. The brain of the vector, commonly a dog, will show Negri bodies, and if brain emulsion is injected intracerebrally into a mouse, these inclusion bodies appear by the sixth day and the animal dies by the tenth day.

Diagnosis.   The only condition which bears even a superficial resemblance to rabies is tetanus, in which the incubation period is between seven and 20 days. There is almost always constant trismus and persistent boarding of the abdominal muscles. The painful laryngeal and pharyngeal spasms with profuse salivation, which are so characteristic of rabies, do not appear.

Treatment.   The disease is fatal. However, if an individual has been bitten by an animal that is known or presumed to be rabid, prophylactic treatment can be given. Antirabies serum of equine origin should be injected locally into the wounds and given intramuscularly in a dose of 1000 I.U. per 20 kg. body weight, and this should be followed by a course of duck-embryo vaccine. The physician should be prepared to treat anaphylactic reaction to the horse serum.

Antirabic treatment is occasionally followed by neuroparalytic complications involving the brain and spinal cord, and (occasionally) the peripheral nerves.[20] Symptoms appear after about eight injections, but can also occur as long as two months after completion of therapy. Pathologically, there are wide areas of demyelination similar to the encephalomyelitis which sometimes follows vaccination for smallpox. The clinical presentations include acute transverse myelitis, ascending "myelitis" with eventual respiratory paralysis, or polyneuropathy involving both the peripheral and cranial nerves. Rarely, the brain alone is involved by an encephalitis. The prognosis is good except in the acute ascending type of myelopathy.

INFECTIOUS MONONUCLEOSIS (GLANDULAR FEVER)

Infectious mononucleosis is a common disease, but neurological complications are rare.[92] Of those that do occur, lymphocytic meningitis is most frequent. Encephalitis may occur and can give rise to stupor, convulsions, hemiplegia, choreiform movements, cranial nerve palsies, and cerebellar ataxia. Transverse myelitis has been recorded. Polyneuritis, associated with an elevated protein in the spinal fluid, may be mild or severe. When severe, it may resemble the Guillain-Barré syndrome, and it can be fatal. Paralysis of one or more cranial nerves may occur in the absence of the usual symptoms and signs of encephalitis.

The neurological symptoms are usually accompanied by fever, adenopathy, splenomegaly, mononucleosis, and a positive heterophile antibody test. Even in the absence of obvious involvement of the nervous system, the disease is often followed by depression and profound physical and mental fatigability, which may last for months.

MUMPS MENINGITIS AND ENCEPHALOMYELITIS

Etiology. The virus of mumps has a predilection for the salivary glands, the pancreas, the mature gonads, the breasts, and the nervous system. It can give rise to meningitis, encephalitis, encephalomyelitis, polyneuritis, and unilateral or bilateral nerve deafness.[67] Holden (1946) found that 33 of 1000 consecutive cases of mumps showed clinical signs of neurological damage. Even in cases without such signs, lymphocytosis is often present in the spinal fluid. Neurological complications usually occur from the third to the fourteenth day after the onset of parotid swelling, but can precede the parotitis. Often there is no parotitis at all, in which event diagnosis is difficult unless there is a history of exposure.

Pathology. Few pathological studies have been reported. There is lymphocytic infiltration of the meninges, lymphocytic perivascular collections in the brain, perivascular hemorrhages, perivenous demyelination, and glial proliferation.

Clinical Features. Mumps meningitis presents the usual features of meningeal irritation: headache, photophobia, neck stiffness, a positive Kernig sign, and pyrexia.[67] After a few days, this recedes and recovery is complete. However, the symptoms of meningeal irritation may be followed by signs of encephalitis with delirium, somnolence, and coma. Seizures are uncommon. A wide spectrum of neurological signs can develop, including hemiplegia, monoplegia, sensory loss on one side of the body, aphasia, choreiform movements, ataxia, and facial or bulbar palsy. Optic atrophy with blindness, and transverse myelitis have been reported. A few cases of symmetrical peripheral polyneuropathy have occurred, usually two to three weeks after the onset of the illness, i.e., during the patient's convalescence, and these have had the features of acute infective polyneuritis, which, in some cases, has swept up to involve the cranial nerves. Complete and permanent unilateral or bilateral nerve deafness can occur during the acute stage of the disease, and in a few cases this has happened in the absence of any other signs of meningoencephalitis in persons who have been in contact with mumps.

The cerebrospinal fluid shows lymphocytic pleocytosis, slight increase of protein, and normal sugar and chlorides. A rising titer of serum antibodies as judged by the complement fixation test is a useful diagnostic aid in doubtful cases. The virus may be recovered from the saliva and from the cerebrospinal fluid.

Most patients recover completely from the neurological complications of mumps. Deafness, however, is usually permanent.

INFECTIOUS HEPATITIS

Infectious hepatitis is probably caused by at least two viruses. One is spread by droplet infection and is responsible for occasional cases of viral encephalitis and encephalomyelitis. The other causes hepatitis after injections of blood or serum but does not produce neurological symptoms other than anosmia.

If encephalitis occurs, it does so four to five days before the jaundice and is thereby distinguished from the encephalopathy caused by hepatic failure. The pathological changes are those of viral encephalitis plus an unusual tendency to petechiae. In fatal cases, massive hemorrhages may occur; these are probably caused by a fall of prothrombin due to liver failure.

Clinically, the onset is with fever, gastrointestinal disturbances, photophobia, headache, and pains in the neck and back. There may be acute vertigo. The neck is usually stiff and Kernig's sign may be positive. These early features suggest meningitis rather than encephalitis, and in some cases, specific evidence of cerebral involvement never occurs at all. Jaundice usually appears later, but in some cases it is so slight that it is not recognized and the whole episode may terminate without overt evidence of hepatitis. In others, lethargy,

delirium, and coma supervene, and there may be evidence of focal damage in the form of hemiparesis, parkinsonian rigidity, transverse myelitis, or polyneuritis of varying degrees of severity. Seizures may occur.

Permanent neurological sequelae have not been described. A combination of cerebral symptoms and jaundice is also seen in cerebral malaria, leptospiral meningitis, yellow fever, hepatic failure, and (in infants) erythroblastosis.

HERPES ZOSTER
(SHINGLES)

Definition. Herpes zoster is caused by a virus which produces inflammatory changes in the posterior ganglia and sensory nerves and sometimes spreads to involve the meninges, the motor roots, and the central nervous system.[34, 105]

Etiology. The virus is closely related to that of chickenpox; contacts of one disease may develop the other. It is most common in middle or later life and occurs in patients of any age debilitated by other diseases (notably Hodgkin's disease), but the conventional doctrine that the site of zoster is often determined by the presence of disease of the vertebra, spinal cord, or nerve roots at that level is untrue of the majority of cases.

Pathology. The pathological changes are usually more widespread than the clinical features would suggest.[34] The virus attacks one or more sensory ganglia, usually on one side of the body but sometimes on both. The affected ganglia are swollen and inflamed, and there is intense lymphocytic infiltration of the ganglionic capsule and pericapsular fat. A few plasma cells may be observed. Similar infiltrates are to be found in the related peripheral nerve or nerves—a true neuritis (Fig. 14–5).[105] The inflammatory process can extend inward toward the meninges and into the root entry zone, and there may be perivascular cuffing in the ventral horns and adjacent white matter. There may be chromatolysis of both anterior and posterior horn cells and

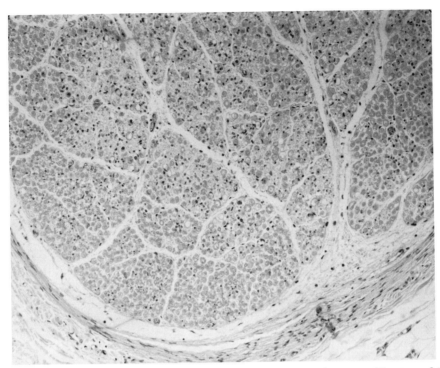

Figure 14–5. Herpes zoster. Acute inflammatory cells are present in the nerve. (Courtesy of Ayer Laboratory, Pennsylvania Hospital, Philadelphia.)

mild lymphocytic meningitis surrounding the dorsal part of the cord. Perivascular lymphocytic collections are sometimes found in the brainstem, cerebellum, and cerebral hemispheres. In rare cases encephalitis or myelitis may develop. The process of recovery is accompanied by progressive scarring of the affected peripheral nerves (Fig. 14–6).[105] The large A fibers suffer more than the small C fibers, and this imbalance may be responsible for persistent pain (p. 9).

Clinical Features. The most prominent feature is pain, often of great severity. It is in the cutaneous distribution of the affected root ganglia, and is described as continuous, burning, or shooting in character. Sometimes it is restricted to a small area, e.g., on the back or front of the chest, or in the axillary line. After two to four days a rash appears in the painful area. The skin reddens, and clusters of vesicles appear within the area supplied by the affected ganglia. In severe cases, the vesicles coalesce and become infected, and there may be su-

perficial necrosis. There is often swelling of the regional lymph nodes. Within 10 to 30 days the skin lesions start to heal, but the affected area remains red and sensitive for weeks or months. Ultimately the skin returns to normal, except for the presence of small, irregular, white scars.

In severe cases there is considerable malaise and a high temperature. The disease may spread to the meninges, and signs of meningeal irritation may be present. There is confusion and delirium if encephalitis occurs, but this is uncommon. Transverse myelitis is very rare.[78]

The most common situation for herpes zoster is on the chest wall; when the lower cervical or the lumbar ganglia are involved, the rash occurs on the limbs. Occasionally it is confined to the lower sacral segments, and the eruption is found in the perianal region. In this event, sphincter disturbances may occur, and the diagnosis will be missed unless this region is inspected.

The neurological signs are usually

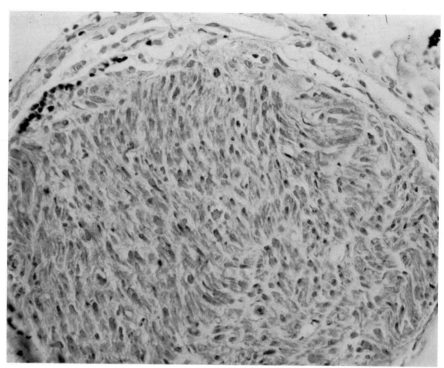

Figure 14–6. Fibrosis of a peripheral nerve, the result of herpes. (Courtesy of Ayer Laboratory, Pennsylvania Hospital, Philadelphia.)

confined to superficial sensory changes. During the acute phase of the disease there is extreme hyperesthesia of the skin in the affected dermatome(s); the patient cannot bear to have the area touched by clothing, and this hyperesthesia may persist for many months. As it disappears, it is possible to detect some impairment to touch and pinprick. If the disease has spread to the anterior horns, there will be weakness or paralysis, which is usually but not always within the area of the rash.[78] It is seldom obvious in the intercostal muscles, but significant degrees of lower motor neuron weakness of radicular distribution are occasionally found in the arm or the leg when the cervical or lumbar enlargements are affected; unilateral paralysis of the diaphragm may occur.

OPHTHALMIC ZOSTER. With involvement of the gasserian ganglion, the pain and rash are *usually* confined to the ophthalmic division. Vesicles appear on the forehead, conjunctiva, and cornea, and along the bridge of the nose in the dis-

tribution of the nasociliary nerve. The disease runs through the same stages as shingles elsewhere, but there is a special danger to the eye, which may become secondarily infected by bacteria. This can lead to panophthalmitis and even if this does not occur, corneal opacities or glaucoma can result from the herpes. Following an attack of zoster in this region, there is often some scarring of the forehead, and there may be loss of hair within the area of scalp involved. Sometimes the pupil on the affected side does not constrict to light but reacts well on convergence. Partial third nerve palsies and primary optic atrophy have been described following herpes ophthalmicus.

GENICULATE HERPES. This was first described by Hunt. It is due to infection of the otic and geniculate ganglia and starts with pain in the ear, mastoid, and tonsillar fossa.[34, 85] The pinna and external auditory meatus become inflamed, and a few vesicles will usually be found there and on the anterior pillar of the fauces. In the course of two or three days, a lower motor neuron facial palsy develops rapidly, often with loss of taste on the anterior two-thirds of the tongue on the affected side. Sometimes vertigo, tinnitus, and loss of hearing occur. The facial paralysis usually recovers completely in from one to four months. The distinction from Bell's palsy is made through the presence of severe pain and the eruption.

POSTHERPETIC NEURALGIA. This is a troublesome sequel to herpes, especially when it has affected the intercostal nerves or the ophthalmic division of the trigeminal nerve. The pain is very persistent and is often aggravated by emotion and by fatigue. It occurs by day and by night. The skin is sensitive to touch in the early phases, but after a year or two this may disappear. The burning, tearing quality of the pain is sometimes reminiscent of causalgia, and may be due to the intense scarring and fibrosis of the nerve which have been found in some of these cases.[105] It occurs in some 50 per cent of patients over the age of 60, but is rare in young subjects.

Laboratory Data. The spinal fluid may be normal, or there may be moderate lymphocytic pleocytosis. The protein content is usually normal but can be slightly raised, and the sugar is normal.

Diagnosis. In the pre-eruptive stage, the pain can lead to a mistaken diagnosis of thoracic or abdominal disease. The possibility of herpes should be considered in all cases with thoracic or abdominal pain of relatively sudden onset and for which no other cause can be found. Rarely, the eruption is so slight that it is missed, and since this happens in some patients reporting with an abrupt onset of muscular weakness of segmental distribution accompanied by fever for a few days, it is easy to make an erroneous diagnosis of poliomyelitis.

Treatment. The writer has found that large doses of steroids (60 mg. of Prednisone a day for a week, 30 mg. per day for a further week, and 15 mg. for the third week) usually abolishes pain within 48 hours, expedites recovery, and prevents postherpetic neuralgia.[40] It also promotes rapid recovery of facial paralysis in cases of geniculate herpes. Steroids should not be given to patients whose resistance has been reduced by Hodgkin's disease, carcinomatosis, or irradiation because this may lead to a dissemination of the infection. An alkali should be taken between meals and before going to bed, especially in patients with a history of peptic ulceration. *It is essential to start treatment within the first 4 or 5 days of appearance of the rash* and to use full doses of steroids if postherpetic neuralgia is to be prevented. Scheie reported favorably on the use of systemic steroids and ACTH for ophthalmic herpes zoster.

The treatment of *postherpetic neuralgia* is unsatisfactory. Mild analgesics and sedatives are seldom effective, and since the condition is likely to last a long time, a wise physician hesitates to use stronger agents with habit-producing properties. Deep x-ray treatment, alcohol injection of the affected roots, division of sensory roots, and ultrasound have all been proved unreliable. Occasionally, undercutting the area of skin involved by the scar tissue has produced a measure of permanent relief, but this has failed in more cases than it has helped. Frontal leukotomy, a desperate measure, has been used with success, but such success is usually temporary. Attempts to abolish the pain by stereotaxic operation in the intracerebral pain projection pathways are under study at the present time.

HERPES SIMPLEX ENCEPHALITIS

Etiology. The virus of herpes simplex, which resembles the viruses of chickenpox and of cytomegalic inclusion disease morphologically, is thought to persist in the human host as a latent infection, erupting from time to time as a vesicular eruption in association with other febrile diseases. In such cases, the cutaneous lesions show Type A inclusion bodies; similar intranuclear inclusion bodies have been found in the brain from certain cases of encephalitis, and be-

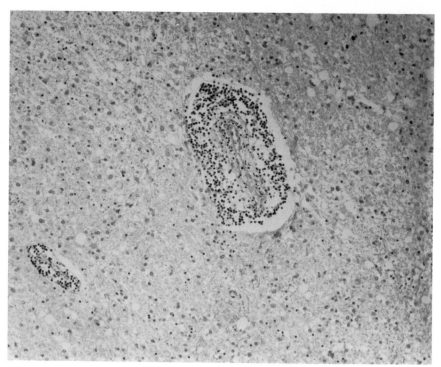

Figure 14–7. Perivascular cuffing in a patient with herpes simplex encephalitis. (Courtesy of Ayer Laboratory, Pennsylvania Hospital, Philadelphia.)

cause some of these cases have shown a rise in antibody titer in the spinal fluid and the virus has been cultivated from the brain, it is concluded that herpes simplex is the responsible agent, though it is difficult to explain why such a drastic illness can be caused by a virus which is present most of the time in an almost inert form. Herpes simplex encephalitis is uncommon, but can occur at any age from infancy to old age.

Pathology. The brain shows the usual features of a viral encephalitis. There is lymphocytic invasion of the meninges; in the brain there are perivascular collections of lymphocytes and histiocytes, proliferation of microglia, and foci of necrotic softening, especially on the orbital surface of the frontal lobes and on the medial surface of the temporal lobes (Fig. 14–7). The inflammatory reactions in these areas can be sufficient to give a positive scan with radioactive isotopes. Type A inclusion bodies—large eosinophilic intranuclear masses surrounded by a halo—are seen in nerve and glial cells.

Clinical Features. Herpes simplex encephalitis is an acute disease characterized by fever, headache, meningeal irritation, marked disturbances of memory and behavior, focal or generalized seizures, and a lymphocytic response in the cerebrospinal fluid. A herpetiform eruption is occasionally present. Mild cases may present the features of simple lymphocytic meningitis.

The onset of the disease is often marked by confusion and aberrations of behavior which may last for several days before other symptoms appear, and which may closely simulate a primary psychosis. The behavioral disturbance is partly related to disorientation for time and place, itself the result of a loss of recent memory, and it may be associated with hallucinations and confabulation, a condition reminiscent of Korsakoff's psychosis. These symptoms are probably related to infection of the temporal lobe and limbic system. This stage slowly gives place to increasing somnolence or coma, but before this happens, focal or generalized seizures may occur. Evidence of focal neurological deficits may be found: loss of taste, unilateral or bilateral pyramidal signs, aphasia, incontinence, and extrapyramidal rigidity.

Laboratory Aids. The cerebrospinal fluid shows an increase in lymphocytes and a modest increase in protein; some authors have reported the presence of red cells and xanthochromia. The serum shows a rising antibody titer; a figure of 1:64 is regarded as conclusive evidence of an active infection. Only a rise in titer can be regarded as significant since about 75 per cent of normal people have antibody in their blood.

Course and Prognosis. A considerable number of persons succumb to the disease. Survivors may be free of symptoms but may suffer from a protracted loss of memory; others have suffered a temporary global dementia.

Differential Diagnosis. Herpes simplex encephalitis has to be distinguished from other viral encephalitides. Early amnesia and confusion are suggestive, but the diagnosis can be established with certainty only by serological studies. The headache, disturbance of memory, and increase in the lymphocytic content of the spinal fluid may suggest a temporal lobe abscess, but there is no evidence of local or peripheral suppuration, and both the clinical signs and electroencephalography point to bilateral disease. Occasionally, however, a brain scan will demonstrate what appears to be a single locus of disease, notably in the temporal lobe. This can be mistaken for a cerebral abscess or tumor. Subdural hematoma is more gradual in onset, there is no fever, the stage of consciousness fluctuates markedly, and there is no lymphocytic increase in the spinal fluid. Hallucinations with amnesia may suggest Korsakoff's psychosis at first, but the appearance of focal neurological deficits and the presence of lymphocytes in the spinal fluid help to exclude it.

Treatment. There is no specific treatment, but large doses of steroids may help to reduce cerebral edema.

Acute Lymphocytic Choriomeningitis

Acute lymphocytic choriomeningitis is a specific virus infection of the meninges and choroid plexus, characterized by a clinically benign meningitis with lymphocytic pleocytosis in the cerebrospinal fluid.[42]

Etiology. The disease is due to a specific neurotropic virus, the Armstrong virus, but several related viruses including the organism responsible for pseudolymphocytic choriomeningitis can produce a similar clinical picture. The Armstrong virus has been cultivated from mice, and there is some evidence that transmission from mice to man can occur. Infection without symptomatic involvement of the meninges is probably common since neutralizing antibodies are often found in the sera of apparently healthy people. Acute lymphocytic choriomeningitis is most common between the ages of 15 and 40, is worldwide in distribution, and usually occurs in the spring and autumn.

Pathology. In infected monkeys and mice, there is an intense lymphocytic infiltration of the choroid plexus and leptomeninges. Human patients seldom die, and in the few postmortem reports available, confirmatory viral studies are lacking. There is infiltration of the meninges and choroid plexus, perivascular infiltration within the brain and spinal cord, and scattered degeneration in neurons. It has been suggested that the virus may be one of the causes of adhesive arachnoiditis.

Clinical Features. The onset is marked by malaise, headache, muscle pains, pyrexia, and upper respiratory catarrh; these symptoms may last for one to three weeks. There may then be a brief period of apparent recovery before the meningeal symptoms appear, but this is by no means the rule. The meningitic stage is characterized by severe headache, photophobia, neck stiffness, and a positive Kernig sign. It lasts for a week or 10 days, and is followed by recovery. In a minority of cases, there are signs of encephalitis in the form of excessive drowsiness and facial or ocular motor palsies. Rarely, transverse myelitis occurs. In the encephalitic forms, convalescence is apt to be protracted, and is marked by headaches, failure of recent memory, defects of concentration, and both mental and physical fatigability. This may last a year or more.

There is polymorph leukocytosis in the blood at the commencement. The spinal fluid is under somewhat increased pressure, and may be either clear or turbid, depending on the number of cells present; they vary from 50 to 3000 cells/cu. mm., of which 95 per cent are lymphocytes, and pleocytosis may persist for some weeks after the clinical symptoms have subsided. The protein content is usually slightly raised, but the sugar and chlorides are normal.

Diagnosis. The diagnosis can only be established by serological tests. Signs of meningeal irritation combined with fever and lymphocytic pleocytosis in the spinal fluid are found in a number of diseases. Of these, tuberculous meningitis is the most important; the differential diagnosis is considered on page 272. In poliomyelitis, the diagnosis usually becomes obvious with the development of paralysis, but in abortive cases, without muscular involvement, there is no way of distinguishing the two conditions except by viral studies. The ECHO and coxsackie groups of viruses, which occasionally give rise to paralysis of muscles, have been identified as a cause of localized outbreaks of lymphocytic meningitis.[84] Syphilitic meningitis, in the secondary stage of the disease, produces lymphocytic spinal fluid, headache, and pyrexia. It follows that in every case of suspected lymphocytic meningitis, serological tests for syphilis should be carried out. Some cases of mumps and infectious mononucleosis give rise to lymphocytic meningitis, which may precede the other features of these diseases. In mononucleosis, enlargement of lymph nodes, changes in the blood, and a positive serological test will *usually* appear in 10 to 20 days. Other conditions producing lymphocytic meningitis include herpes zoster, leptospirosis, and infectious hepatitis.

Treatment. There is no specific treatment for this disease.

Coxsackie Viruses

Coxsackie virus,[84] named after the village of Coxsackie, New York, where it was first identified, is worldwide in distribution, and has been isolated from sewage and flies. It is easily transmitted to suckling mice and hamsters, which rapidly develop paralyses. Man seems to be the primary natural host, and dissemination occurs chiefly by contact with infected sewage or water. Infection is more common than symptomatic disease. It is therefore necessary to exercise caution in attributing symptoms or signs to Coxsackie virus which may be present.

At the present time, there are 30 known types. They are divided into two groups. Group A viruses are responsible for herpangina and occasional cases of meningoencephalitis, while Group B is responsible for Bornholm disease and is the usual cause of Coxsackie meningitis and meningoencephalitis.

The onset may be acute or subacute, with fever, headaches, malaise, gastrointestinal symptoms, and stiffness in the neck. The virus can produce a picture similar to that of anterior poliomyelitis, but when flaccid paresis of muscles occurs in the course of Coxsackie infection, a search should also be made for serological evidence of poliomyelitis. The cerebrospinal pressure is normal or slightly raised, and there is moderate pleocytosis; from 10 to 15 per cent may be polymorphonuclear cells. The protein content is normal or slightly raised, and the sugar is normal. The diagnosis is confirmed by recovering the virus from the feces or from the pharynx, and by the demonstration of an increase in neutralizing antibodies in the serum. The disease is self-limited, and there are no aftereffects.

ECHO Viruses

The enteric cytopathogenic human orphan (ECHO) viruses, 16 or more in number, have a wide distribution. They occasionally produce benign meningitis or meningoencephalitis in man. Children are more frequently affected than adults and the clinical picture is that of a systemic infection with meningeal signs. A rubella-like rash is sometimes present. There may be considerable lethargy and irritability and even slight generalized muscular weakness. Cerebellar ataxia has been described in children, but it has not persisted. The spinal fluid shows pleocytosis, and in the early phases, polymorphonuclear leukocytes predominate. The protein content is slightly elevated or normal, and the sugar is normal. Diagnosis is established by recovery of the virus from the stool or cerebrospinal fluid and by the demonstration of a rising titer of neutralizing antibodies in the serum a week after the onset of the illness. The disease is benign and terminates within one to two weeks, without aftereffects.

Yellow Fever

Yellow fever is an acute infectious hepatitis caused by a virus which is transmitted from man to man by the mosquito *Aëdes aegypti*. The essential lesions are found in the liver, but in most cases there is also mild meningeal infiltration with lymphocytes, diffuse involvement of ganglion cells, and perivascular demyelination; gliosis may give rise to actual granulomas in the gray matter of the brainstem. The onset of yellow fever is with malaise, chills, and pyrexia. Headache, muscle pain, and vomiting may be severe, and jaundice usually appears on the fourth or fifth day. Bleeding from the gums and the gastrointestinal tract is common. Severe prostration is usual, and it is difficult to know how much of this is due to the systemic components of the disease and how much to

encephalitis. Confusion, delirium, ocular palsies, hiccough, paralysis of the vocal cords, and hemiparesis have been described. Acute hallucinosis may occur. The cerebrospinal fluid contains an excess of cells which may be lymphocytic or polymorphonuclear in type. The protein content is slightly raised. *Vaccination* against yellow fever occasionally causes headache, stiffness of the neck, and somnolence or delirium; the outlook is always favorable, though headache and a general sense of prostration may persist for weeks.

Psittacosis

Psittacosis is a virus disease which is usually transmitted to man from diseased parrots, but person-to-person infection can also occur. It commonly occurs in small epidemics as an influenzal or typhoid-like illness associated with pneumonitis. Involvement of the central nervous system usually takes the form of lymphocytic meningitis [101] with headache, nuchal stiffness, and lymphocytic pleocytosis in the spinal fluid, but in more severe cases, there is somnolence, delirium, or even deep stupor. Transient focal disturbances such as weakness or ataxia may occur, but survivors show no residual neurological defects. The virus can be isolated from the blood or sputum and complement fixing antibodies appear in the serum in four to seven days after the onset of symptoms.

Cytomegalic Inclusion Disease

The virus of this disease causes an enlargement of cells, which contain intranuclear and sometimes cytoplasmic inclusions. Inclusions are seen in astrocytes, and in the epithelium of the salivary and pancreatic ducts, in the convoluted tubules of the kidney, the bile duct epithelium, the alveolar cells of the lungs, and the endothelium of small vessels (Fig. 14–8 and 14–9).

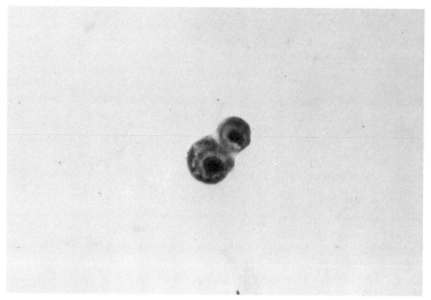

Figure 14–8. Cytomegalic inclusion body from the urine. (Courtesy of Children's Hospital of Philadelphia.)

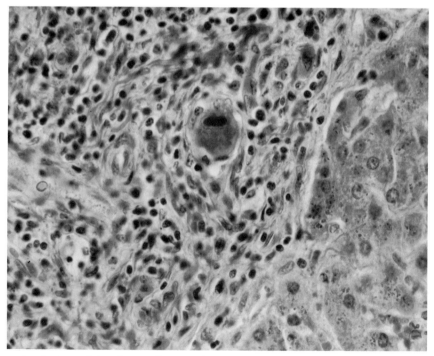

Figure 14–9. Cytomegalic inclusion disease, showing a large cell with inclusion body, in the liver. (Courtesy of Ayer Laboratory, Pennsylvania Hospital, Philadelphia.)

Intrauterine infection of the fetus by this virus has been held responsible for about 2 per cent of all neonatal deaths. It can also give rise to a number of congenital defects, including hydrocephalus, microcephaly, and mental retardation. It is one cause of intracranial calcification in mentally retarded children.[55] Prenatal infection can give rise to a serious febrile disease in the neonatal period, characterized by a hemorrhagic rash, jaundice, diarrhea, melena, and enlargement of the spleen and liver. Asymptomatic invasion of the nervous system has been found in young adults who have died following renal transplantation, the infection being presumably a by-product of immunosuppressive therapy.

Progressive Multifocal Leukoencephalopathy

This rare condition occurs in association with the lymphomas, chronic leukemia, carcinoma, tuberculosis, and other debilitating stages.[82]

Pathology. The disease is characterized by multiple areas of demyelination in the brain and spinal cord. The lesions vary in size from microscopic foci to massive areas of myelin destruction with relative preservation of axis cylinders. The largest lesions are found in the cerebral hemispheres, but the brainstem and cerebrum may be severely affected, and smaller lesions are sometimes found in the spinal cord. Oligodendrocytes at the periphery of the lesions show conspicuous changes, including the presence of inclusions which have been shown to contain particles resembling a Papova virus.[109] There is still some doubt as to whether the virus is the primary cause of the condition or is a secondary invader.

Clinical Features. The disease is subacute, with a course of from three to six months. As is to be expected from the widespread dissemination of the lesions, there are considerable case-to-case differences with respect to neuro-

logical symptoms. There may be aphasia, a confusional state, dementia, paralysis of one or more limbs, ataxia, dysarthria, visual field defects, and blindness. Seizures are uncommon. The disease progresses relentlessly to a terminal coma.

The spinal fluid is usually normal and the electroencephalogram shows nonspecific abnormalities. Contrast studies, including brain scans, are usually negative.

There is no treatment for the disease.

Jakob-Creutzfeldt Disease (Spastic Pseudosclerosis, Cortico-striato-spinal Degeneration)

This rare disease [49, 50] is characterized clinically by an insidious onset, in middle life, of progressive pyramidal and extrapyramidal symptoms, myoclonus, and organic dementia; in some few cases, muscular wasting and weakness indicate involvement of lower motor neurons.

Pathology. The changes found are those of parenchymal degeneration with atrophy and disappearance of the ganglion cells of the frontoparietal cortex, striatum, ventral and medial nuclei of the thalamus, subthalamic nucleus, and—in some cases—of the bulbar motor nuclei and the ventral horns of the spinal cord. The corticospinal tracts degenerate. The disease is considered to be due to infection by a slow virus, and it has been produced in chimpanzees from 12 to 14 months after the inoculation of suspensions of brain from human patients. Chimpanzee-to-chimpanzee transmission has also been effected.

Clinical Features. Mental disturbances either precede or follow somatic symptoms. Starting with anxiety of depression, they may progress to the intellectual loss and personality changes of an advanced organic psychosis, and if these symptoms are predominant an erroneous diagnosis of Alzheimer's or Pick's presenile dementia may be made. Somatic symptoms usually start with stiffness and weakness of the limbs, both pyramidal and extrapyramidal features being present. There may be evidence of parkinsonism. Tremor, athetosis, and spastic dysarthria may occur. In a few cases, there has been muscular wasting and fasciculation which, in the presence of pyramidal symptoms, may falsely suggest a diagnosis of amyotrophic lateral sclerosis in cases in which mental deterioration is not conspicuous.

There is no treatment for the condition, and death occurs in from one to three years.

Subacute Sclerosing Panencephalitis

In 1934, Dawson described subacute encephalitis associated with Cowdry Type A intranuclear inclusions.[33] Some years later, VanBogaert[97] reported what is now known to be the same disease under the title of "subacute sclerosing leukoencephalitis," and Pette and Doring described a similar disease, which they called "panencephalitis." There is little doubt that these conditions are similar and that case-to-case variations in terms of clinical features and pathological findings are the result of differences in the intensity and localization of the lesions.[23] The disease has been reported in individuals between the ages of two and 28 years.

Etiology. At present, the disease is thought to be due to infection by an agent similar to the measles virus.[46, 51] This is supported by the morphology and histochemistry of the inclusions, by the presence of high titers of measles virus antibody in the serum and cerebrospinal fluid, and by the fact that Katz and his colleagues have reported transmission and passage of an encephalitogenic agent by central cerebral inoculation of brain biopsy material derived from affected children.[62]

Pathology. In fatal cases there is widespread destruction of neurons and glial cells throughout the cortical matter[68]; it is sometimes most marked in the temporal and parietal regions. Similar but less severe changes are found in the basal ganglia, cerebellum, pons, and spinal cord, but there is considerable case variation in the effects of the disease on these subcortical structures. Slight demyelination is found in the subcortical white matter, notably in the temporal lobe. Intranuclear Type A inclusions are present in both neurons and oligodendroglia; they are sometimes absent in biopsy specimens, owing perhaps to the statistical hazards of sampling.

Clinical Features. The disease is gradual in onset, and the first symptoms are usually those of mild mental impairment. This is progressive and is followed by the appearance of incoordination of the limbs and periodic myoclonic jerks of the muscles of the face, trunk, and extremities. Scattered cranial nerve palsies occur in some cases. Seizures may occur from time to time. Ultimately, the limbs become rigid and there are bilateral grasp reflexes, bilateral hyperreflexia, a sucking reflex, and bilateral extensor plantar responses. The terminal phase is usually marked by decorticate rigidity and coma. Hyponatremia was present in three of seven cases described by Glaser and his colleagues. It is probably due to inappropriate excretion of an antidiuretic hormone, and it is possible that such hyponatremia may modify the clinical picture unless it is corrected by appropriate therapy.

The spinal fluid is usually normal, but the cell count may be markedly increased. The total protein content is usually normal, but a first zone colloidal gold curve is common. There is a high titer of measles antibody in the serum and spinal fluid. The electroencephalogram shows widespread abnormalities in the shape of bursts of 2 to 3 cycles per second waves and spike complexes, some of which may be synchronous with the myoclonic jerks.

The disease usually terminates fatally in from two to 12 months, but it may become arrested and a few patients that have been thought to be suffering from this disease have made a spontaneous recovery. There is no effective treatment.

Encephalitis Lethargica (Epidemic Encephalitis, Sleeping Sickness, von Economo's Disease)

An epidemic of encephalitis with a 50 per cent mortality occurred in Vienna in 1916–1917 and spread thence to the rest of Western Europe, England, and the United States.[98] It is possible that earlier epidemics such as the Tubingen sleeping sickness of 1712 and the epidemic of Nona which occurred in Italy in 1890–1891 were the same disease. Clinically, the early cases were characterized by marked somnolence and ocular motor palsies, but in the early 1920's there were more frequent reports of myoclonus and other involuntary movements. A notable feature of the disease was its capacity to produce progressive and long-lasting sequelae, notably parkinsonism in adults and disorders of personality in children. The disease is usually thought to have died out, but since this is uncertain, this section is written in the present tense.

Etiology. Encephalitis lethargica is thought to be due to a virus, but proof is lacking.

Pathology. There is congestion of the meninges, and a few petechiae are to be found on the cut surface of the brain. In acute cases, there is perivascular cuffing with lymphocytes and damage to neurons in the basal ganglia, substantia nigra, oculomotor nuclei, and tegmentum. Cellular damage varies between chromatolysis and complete destruction. In chronic cases there is some loss of pigment from the substantia nigra and a variable degree of cellular loss in the pallidus, hypothalamus, and substantia nigra. Some thickening of the adventitia of the arteries is common. Intracytoplasmic and intranuclear inclusion bodies have been found, especially in the substantia nigra.

Clinical Features. Mild cases show slight fever, upper respiratory symptoms, headache, and drowsiness, with or without transient diplopia, the whole illness lasting only a few days. More severely affected patients rapidly pass into stupor or coma, which often gives place to delirium and restlessness at night. Clonic and choreiform movements may occur, and uncontrollable hiccough is not infrequent. Seizures and evidence of pyramidal tract damage are inconspicuous. In acute cases, the face may become immobile and the limbs rigid, but the cogwheel element seen in chronic parkinsonism is usually absent. A severe degree of facial seborrhea, together with excessive salivation, is seen in some acute cases and may persist for months or years.

Fever is usually present at the onset, but sometimes does not develop until the terminal stages; in fatal cases it may rise to 105° F. or higher.

The cerebrospinal fluid is often normal, but modest lymphocytic pleocytosis and a slight increase of protein are found in some cases. The sugar content remains normal.

Course and Prognosis. The mortality varied between 10 and 50 per cent in different localities and at different times during the 1917–1926 epidemic. At first it was thought that if the patient survived the acute illness, he would make a complete recovery, but it soon became obvious that a considerable number of the survivors were to develop serious sequelae. These included parkinsonism, which is the most common, and a type of dystonia musculorum deformans. In children, disturbances of character and personality, always for the worse, were not uncommon, but mental retardation was never prominent. Other sequelae include oculogyric crises, weakness of convergence, postencephalitic psychoses, narcolepsy, obesity, diabetes insipidus, and respiratory tics.

THE POSTENCEPHALITIS PARKINSONIAN SYNDROME. This may follow directly after the acute phase, or its onset may be delayed for months or years. It often occurs in one limb at first, taking the form of mild cogwheel rigidity and a disinclination to use the limb. Voluntary movements are slow, and the patient's calligraphy deteriorates. Tremor may be present or absent, and when present it is apt to have a wider amplitude than that of paralysis agitans. Rigidity and akinesia slowly invade the rest of the musculature, and the face takes on the fixity of parkinsonism. The affected limbs adopt an attitude of flexion. These symptoms may be accompanied by intermittent spasmodic contractions of muscles, including oculogyric crises, spasmodic torticollis, or sudden flexion or extension movements of the spine.

Oculogyric crises may be the sole result of an acute attack. They consist of involuntary forced conjugate movements of the eyes, usually upward or to the side, lasting from a few seconds to an hour or two. The attacks are sometimes accompanied by compulsive thoughts and anxiety. Respiratory tics in the form of sudden gasping or grunting respirations are not uncommon. Oculogyric crises and other "forced movements" are also produced by phenothiazine tranquilizers.

Mental symptoms are common in children. There is little or no intellectual deterioration, but the previously well-behaved child becomes destructive, uncontrollable, and abnormally sadistic; reproof has no effect, although the child is usually contrite after an outburst. This change is likely to be permanent.

Involvement of the hypothalamus can lead to narcolepsy, either in association with parkinsonism or without it. Diabetes insipidus and obesity have occasionally occurred following the acute disease.

Treatment. There is no specific treatment. The treatment of postencephalitic parkinsonism is the same as for paralysis agitans (p. 234).

"Brainstem Encephalitis"

In 1951 Bickerstaff and Cloake described three patients who, following a short period of malaise and pyrexia, developed severe and widespread disturbances of brainstem function without respiratory or cardiac embarrassment, and who experienced complete recovery. Since then, further cases have been described; the condition is by no means uncommon in children and young adolescents.[18]

Pathology. Little is known about the pathology. Bickerstaff described widespread swelling and ballooning of myelin sheaths in the brainstem, hyperplasia of astrocytes, and minimal changes in ganglion cells. There was diffuse loss of purkinje cells and slight perivascular lymphocytic cuffing.

Clinical Features. Following an upper respiratory infection or slight general malaise with mild fever and photophobia, there is a rapid, though not abrupt, development of headache, drowsiness, double vision, and dysarthria. After a few days, the condition progresses, some cases showing profound stupor, paralysis of all the motor cranial nerves, and anarthria, with or without evidence of pyramidal disorder. Recovery can take weeks or months, and some patients have developed temporary extrapyramidal rigidity and parkinsonian tremor during the period of recovery. Aggressive and violent behavior has been noted. In one case, a boy of 10 exhibited rapidly oncoming headache, projectile vomiting, nystagmus, dysarthria, cerebellar ataxia of the limbs, papilledema, and moderate lymphocytic pleocytosis of the spinal fluid. There were no signs of damage to the long tracts, and he made a complete and uncomplicated recovery within 10 days of the onset. In most of the published cases the cerebrospinal pressure has been normal but there has been lymphocytic pleocytosis and a moderate increase of the protein content. Electroencephalography in two of Bickerstaff's adult cases showed widespread bursts of delta and theta activity in all leads.

SPIROCHETAL INFECTIONS

Neurosyphilis

There has been a great decline in the incidence of neurosyphilis in countries in which penicillin is readily available for the treatment of the primary and secondary stages of the syphilitic infection. In prepenicillin days, in the United

States, the nervous system came to be involved in about 30 per cent of all cases but today the medical students and physicians see so few examples of this subtle and many-sided disease that they have come to rely to an excessive extent on the results of serological tests. These can be misleading in two ways. They are occasionally negative in the presence of syphilitic disease, and secondly, even if neurosyphilis is present (with appropriate serological reactions) it is not always or necessarily the sole cause of the patient's symptoms. Therefore, despite the comparative rarity of neurosyphilis in countries with a highly developed medical service, it is still desirable to be familiar with the broad spectrum of its clinical features.

There is no entirely satisfactory method of classifying neurosyphilis. The brunt of the disease may fall on the leptomeninges, the blood vessels, or the parenchyma, but all these elements are involved to some extent in every case. Moreover, the disease may be acute, subacute, or chronic, and acute incidents of vascular origin can interrupt the more chronic forms. The result of this pathological versatility is an almost unlimited number of clinical presentations.

Serological Tests for Syphilis. Of the many tests for syphilis, the Kolmer and Wassermann reactions are usually sufficient but in doubtful cases, the Treponema pallidum immobilization (T.P.I.) test may be used, and even greater sensitivity is shown by the fluorescent treponemal antibody absorption (FTA-ABS) test, especially in very early cases, and in syphilis of long duration. The FTA-ABS test can be positive in patients with neither historical nor clinical evidence of syphilis. This can occur in conditions in which abnormal globulins are found—rheumatoid arthritis, alcoholic cirrhosis, etc. Whether such reactions represent old syphilis or false positive reactions is unsettled. It is sound practice to treat the patient for syphilis if a positive FTA-ABS test is present and if the patient's symptoms and signs *could* be syphilitic in origin.

Classification. The clinical syndromes caused by the entry of *T. pallidum* into the nervous system are difficult to classify because mixed and intermediate forms are common.

1. Congenital neurosyphilis
2. Acquired neurosyphilis
   a. Asymptomatic
   b. Meningovascular (cerebral)
      (1) Acute meningitis
      (2) Chronic meningitis
      (3) Cerebral thrombosis
      (4) Retrobulbar neuritis
      (5) Gumma
   c. Meningovascular (spinal) neurosyphilis
      (1) Acute meningomyelitis
      (2) Chronic meningomyelitis
      (3) Hypertrophic pachymeningitis
      (4) Thrombosis of spinal arteries
      (5) Gumma of the cord
      (6) Erb's syphilitic spastic paraplegia
   d. Parenchymatous neurosyphilis
      (1) General paresis (dementia paralytica)
      (2) Tabes dorsalis
      (3) Taboparesis
      (4) Optic atrophy

Pathogenesis. Although the spirochete invades the central nervous system within weeks of the primary infection, producing lymphocytosis in the spinal fluid in many cases, clinical evidence of disease seldom appears until two or more years have elapsed; exceptionally, acute meningeal or vascular symptoms appear in the secondary stage. It is not known why some infected individuals develop neurosyphilis while others do not, nor why white races are more affected than colored, nor why males are more prone to the parenchymatous forms than females. Thorough and early treatment greatly reduces the incidence of subsequent neurosyphilis, but inadequate treatment increases it. Acute fevers during the asymptomatic stage can prevent neurosyphilis, an observation which led Wagner-Jauregg to introduce fever therapy for general paresis in 1917.

ASYMPTOMATIC NEUROSYPHILIS

There are no symptoms or objective clinical signs of disease in the nervous system in asymptomatic neurosyphilis, but there is lymphocytic pleocytosis and usually a rise of protein in the spinal fluid, and the serological tests are positive in both blood and spinal fluid. It occurs in some 60 per cent of infected persons who have not received treatment. The incidence rises in the first two years of infection and then declines. Treatment is by the administration of 1,000,000 units of penicillin intramuscularly each day for 20 days. If the spinal fluid is still abnormal six months later, the course is repeated, and the spinal fluid is re-examined after six months. If the spinal fluid abnormality is detected more than three years after the date of infection, the response—as judged by the spinal fluid—is slow, and there is a greater likelihood of parenchymatous neurosyphilis developing later on. If the patient is sensitive to penicillin, Aureomycin, Terramycin, or erythromycin can be used.

MENINGOVASCULAR SYPHILIS

Meningovascular syphilis [73] can occur at any time after infection, but most commonly appears within five years; it can also complicate the parenchymatous forms of the disease later on. Generally speaking, its impact is either mainly intracranial or mainly spinal, and in each case both the meninges and the blood vessels are affected, albeit in varying proportions. The symptoms may be acute, subacute, or chronic, and appear in a profusion of clinical combinations.

Pathology. The earliest changes are in the leptomeninges, which are infiltrated with lymphocytes and plasma cells; polymorphs are sometimes present in acute cases. The infiltration is patchy in distribution and is more marked at the base than over the cerebral hemispheres. The acute inflammatory response ultimately gives place to varying degrees of fibrous hyperplasia which can block the circulation of cerebrospinal fluid, thereby producing hydrocephalus, and can involve cranial nerves and spinal nerve roots. Syphilitic arteritis (Heubner's arteritis) affects the larger vessels; all the coats of the vessel are involved by an inflammatory process which narrows the lumen and can cause thrombosis. Gummas are common in meningeal syphilis but are usually small; exceptionally, they attain a considerable size and by compressing the brain or spinal cord give rise to the features of a rapidly developing tumor.

Clinical Features

INTRACRANIAL. *Acute syphilitic meningitis* is uncommon, occurring in the secondary stage and occasionally in the tertiary stage in the case of patients who have been inadequately treated. Severe headaches, vomiting, and stiffness of the neck appear, and may be accompanied by seizures. Papilledema and cranial nerve palsies are common, and the spinal fluid is found to be under increased pressure and to contain a lymphocytic pleocytosis and a few polymorphs. The serology is positive in the spinal fluid, but the sugar content is normal.

Chronic syphilitic meningitis is illnamed because the traditional features of meningitis are commonly lacking. There may be headache, but signs of meningeal irritation are usually absent. The most frequent presentation is a partial third nerve palsy. The fourth, fifth, and sixth nerves may also be involved, but the lower cranial nerves are seldom affected. Narcolepsy and diabetes insipidus may occur, and if the egress of spinal fluid from the posterior fossa is blocked, symptoms of raised intracranial pressure will supervene. Sometimes the condition extends over the convexity of the hemispheres, producing seizures, focal cerebral symptoms from the associated arteritis, and mental symptoms of organic complexion which may amount to dementia.

Syphilitic retrobulbar neuritis, a rare condition, is characterized by a rather sudden impairment of vision which is usually, but not necessarily, limited to one eye. Edema of the disc may be present. There is enlargement of the blind spot, concentric contraction of the smaller isopters, and central or paracentral scotomas. The spinal fluid may be normal, but the blood serology is positive. Vision improves rapidly following antisyphilitic treatment.

Syphilitic cerebral thrombosis usually occurs without clinical evidence of meningitis. Any of the larger cerebral or brainstem arteries may be involved, and the symptoms and signs are those of cerebral thrombosis. Syphilis should always be considered in cases of cerebral infarction in young or middle-aged persons. There is usually lymphocytosis in the spinal fluid. The blood serology is positive but in some cases that of the spinal fluid is negative.

Cerebral gumma occasionally produces the signs of a tumor, but this is so rare that the presence of a positive serology in a patient with an expanding intracranial lesion should not be taken to mean that the symptoms are necessarily syphilitic in origin.

SPINAL SYPHILIS. *Acute syphilitic meningomyelitis* can give rise to root pains and girdle sensations, followed by the rapid development of a transverse lesion of the cord, usually in the thoracic region. The result is paralysis and sensory loss below the level of the lesion, loss of sphincter control, and extensor plantar responses. There is sometimes a zone of hyperalgesia over a segment or two above the lesion. The damage to the cord is the result of arterial thrombosis.

Chronic meningomyelitis of syphilitic origin is a rare condition which comes on many years after infection. There is inflammatory thickening of the leptomeninges and diffuse arteritis of the vessels supplying the cord. In some cases, the pyramidal tracts show degenerative changes; in others, the anterior horn cells are mainly involved. There is usually degeneration of the white matter on the periphery of the cord. Weakness and wasting of the muscles appear in the shoulder girdle, arms, and hands, or the legs may be involved below the knees. The weakness may be accompanied by pain and paresthesias, and in the course of time pyramidal signs, sensory impairment, and sphincter disturbances appear.

Hypertrophic pachymeningitis is a rare condition in which the dura is involved as well as the leptomeninges. It commonly occurs in the cervical region and results in compression of the cord and symptoms from involvement of the motor and sensory roots as they pass to the intervertebral foramina. Consequently, root pains, sensory impairment, and atrophic weakness of the upper limbs are combined with spastic weakness of the legs and impairment of sensation in the lower part of the trunk and legs. The condition can mimic the effects of spondylosis and extramedullary tumors.

Gumma of the spinal cord is very uncommon, and presents the features of a rapidly developing cord compression.

Erb's syphilitic spastic paraplegia is an uncommon condition characterized by slowly progressive spastic weakness of the legs, with increased reflexes, extensor plantar responses, and urgency of micturition or overflow incontinence. There is no sensory loss. The arms are seldom affected. In some cases, the symptoms are almost entirely confined to the bladder, with minimal signs of pyramidal disturbance in the legs. The spinal fluid usually shows pleocytosis, an increase of protein, and positive serological reactions. There is no evidence of subarachnoid block.

The pathological basis of the condition is a demyelination of the lateral columns and the superficial white matter of the cord, and it is regarded as the result of a chronic meningomyelitis accompanied by arteritis of the circumferential vessels of the cord.

Treatment is usually unsatisfactory because irreparable damage has been done by the time symptoms appear.

The Spinal Fluid in Meningovascular Syphilis. Serological tests are positive in the blood and spinal fluid in more than 90 per cent of all cases. The pressure of the spinal fluid is raised in acute syphilitic meningitis and in the presence of internal hydrocephalus or a large cerebral gumma. Evidence of spinal block will eventually be present in compression of the cord by pachymeningitis or gumma.

The number of cells in the spinal fluid is a measure of the meningeal inflammation. The response is predominantly lymphocytic. In the more chronic forms of meningovascular syphilis, the cell count may be normal. The protein content is usually raised to a modest degree, and the globulin is disproportionately high; it is this which gives rise to the disturbance in the colloidal gold curve which in meningovascular syphilis may be either paretic or luetic in character; in some cases no precipitation occurs. The sugar and chloride contents of the spinal fluid are normal, with the exception of a modest reduction of the former in some cases of acute syphilitic meningitis.

Treatment. On the whole, meningovascular syphilis can be effectively treated,[32, 90] but once irreparable damage has occurred—as a result of cerebral thrombosis or transverse myelitis, for instance—the objective of therapy is to prevent further progress of the disease. Penicillin is the drug of choice. It is given intramuscularly; intrathecal administration is unnecessary. It is wise to start with a small dose to avoid a Herxheimer reaction. Five thousand units are given on the first day, and 10,000 on the second day; if there has been no untoward response, 1,000,000 units are given daily for 20 days; some authorities prefer a larger dose over a shorter period. The effect of treatment may not be apparent in the spinal fluid for several months, and lumbar puncture should be repeated six months later. If the fluid is still abnormal, another course of penicillin is necessary, and the spinal fluid is again examined six months later.

If the patient is sensitive to penicillin, oxytetracycline hydrochloride (Terramycin), a tetracycline (Achromycin), or erythromycin can be used in doses of from 2 to 4 gm. daily, but it must be emphasized that these drugs are less effective than penicillin for the treatment of *early* syphilis and that they give rise to

a large number of side effects. For these reasons, it is better to attempt to continue penicillin despite mild allergic reactions; these can usually be controlled by the administration of antihistamines and steroids.

It is worth noting that in days gone by remarkably good results were obtained by treating meningovascular syphilis with large doses of oral potassium iodide and daily inunctions of mercury or by combining iodides with intramuscular injections of a suspension of bismuth oxychloride containing 0.2 gm. of the metal. Such a course would consist of 10 injections at weekly intervals. Better results can be obtained with arsenical preparations such as Neosalvarsan and Mapharside, the latter being given intravenously in doses of from 30 to 60 mg. weekly.

TABES DORSALIS

Tabes dorsalis, once called locomotor ataxia, is characterized pathologically by degenerative changes in the posterior roots and posterior columns of the spinal cord and brainstem, and clinically by progressive sensory ataxia, lightning pains, loss of tendon reflexes, impairment of sensation, and sphincter disorders. It is uncommon nowadays, but it used to develop in approximately 10 per cent of all infected persons and accounted for about 25 per cent of all cases of neurosyphilis. Males are affected more often than females (in a ratio of four to one), and the disease develops in from four to 30 years after infection, with an average of about 15 years. Consequently, the age of onset usually lies between 35 and 55. Tabes dorsalis can occur in congenital syphilis, in which event it occurs before the age of 12.

Pathogenesis and Pathology. Macroscopically, there is atrophy of the dorsal spinal roots, especially in the lower thoracic and lumbosacral regions, and the posterior columns of the cord are flat and shrunken, whence the name "tabes dorsalis," meaning dorsal wasting (Fig.

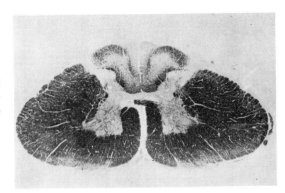

Figure 14–10. Tabes dorsalis, cervical spinal cord. (From Robbins, S. L.: *A Textbook of Pathology.* 2nd Ed. W. B. Saunders Co., Philadelphia, 1962.)

14–10). Microscopically, there is degeneration of the posterior roots, but the dorsal root ganglion cells are seldom affected. Since the lower thoracic and the lumbosacral roots are most seriously involved, it is the fasciculus gracilis of the posterior columns which suffers most severely, but the more laterally placed fasciculus cuneatus is also involved in advanced stages of the disease. Mild neurological proliferation is seen in the affected areas. Rarely, there is degeneration of anterior horn cells. The leptomeninges are cloudy and slightly thickened, and even in advanced cases there may be evidence of active inflammation in the form of slight infiltration with lymphocytes and plasma cells. Similar inflammatory processes are seen at times in and around the posterior nerve roots, and there may be mild endarteritis of the meningeal vessels. The inflammatory changes in the leptomeninges have been blamed for the changes in the posterior roots and posterior columns, but this does not explain why the motor roots escape. An alternative theory is that tabes is due to primary degeneration of the exogenous fibers within the cord. Be that as it may, there is a notable absence of spirochetes in the meninges and cord even in patients whose condition is steadily worsening.

Visual impairment from optic atrophy is common in tabes, and may be the presenting symptom. In some cases, it results from chronic low-grade syphilitic meningitis around the optic nerves. In others, inflammatory changes are less obvious, and there appears to be primary parenchymatous degeneration of the optic nerve fibers.

The arthropathy which occurs in tabes was first described by Charcot; it consists of initial hyperplasia of the cartilage followed by destruction of the joint surface, erosion of the epiphyses, and the development of osteophytes. The synovial fluid is increased and the surrounding ligaments are relaxed and may rupture, giving rise to subluxation of the affected joint. A considerable degree of bone absorption is seen in long-standing cases.

Clinical Features. Tabes usually starts insidiously, but in rare cases ataxia may become severe in a few months. Occasionally symptoms are first noted after an accident or an unrelated illness, and the patient is apt to blame the illness or accident for his condition, but neurological examination will usually reveal abnormal physical signs which must have been present for some time.

The symptoms and signs are the result of degeneration of the sensory nerve roots and posterior columns. The patient has pain, paresthesias, sensory impairment, and loss of tendon reflexes. Ataxia is caused by loss of sensory information from joints and muscles which normally passes to the cerebral cortex via the posterior columns and to the cerebellum via the spinocerebellar tracts and posterior columns. Sphincter disturbances and impotence occur from the interruption of autonomic fibers in the posterior roots. Trophic disturbances are the result of repeated minor traumas to tissues which have lost their sensory innervation.

A variety of symptoms may first bring the patient to the doctor. They include pain in the limbs, girdle sensations, unsteadiness of gait, attacks of vomiting, disturbances of micturition, failing vision, diplopia, Charcot's arthropathy, and perforating ulcers of the foot. In some cases, the condition is observed for the first time during a routine physical examination, the patient being unaware that anything is wrong. In taboparesis mental failure can be the presenting symptom.

SENSORY SYMPTOMS. Lightning pains are the most characteristic symptoms of tabes, and occur in no other condition if they fulfill certain criteria; they occur in bouts with intervals of freedom, and are felt as brief repetitive stabs of pain as if a knife were being driven in; less often the pain seems to shoot down the leg. The site can vary from one paroxysm to another, and the skin of the affected spot may become sensitive and pink; this is very unusual, but the local erythema is reminiscent of the flush which develops in the foot pad of the cat as the result of electrical stimulation of the peripheral end of the cut posterior roots. Lightning pains are more common in the legs than in the arms, and are rare in the face. Burning discomfort and tearing pain in the feet are sometimes complained of, but they are not peculiar to tabes. Girdle sensations around the trunk and band-like sensations around the legs are not uncommon, but these occur in other types of spinal cord disease as well.

Paresthesias of the feet are not uncommon. The patient complains that the feet feel numb or that the floor feels as if it is covered with wool. Visceral sensory impairment causes inability to know when the bladder is full; this may be the first clinical symptom of the disease.

The earliest objective sensory *signs* are impairment of vibration and joint sensibility at the periphery of the limbs; the foot is usually affected before the hand. Loss of pain on deep pressure (as on squeezing the tendo Achillis, calf muscles, or testicles) precedes and is usually more marked than impairment of cutaneous sensibility. Hypalgesia to pinprick is patchy in distribution. It is said to be most common on the side of the nose, the front of the chest, the ulnar side of the forearms, the perianal area, and the front of the legs below the knees, but in the author's experience, sensory impairment in these traditional sites is the exception rather than the rule in present-day tabetics. Sometimes there is delayed appreciation of pinprick, the stimulus being felt a second or two after it has been delivered, or it may be felt on the opposite side of the body, but these aberrations are not peculiar to tabes. Ultimately, light touch and temperature sensibility may be impaired over the legs, arms, and trunk.

MOTOR SYMPTOMS. Weakness and wasting do not usually appear until late in the disease but ataxia is prominent. The afferent input to the motor cortex and cerebellum is impaired, and motor performance is correspondingly clumsy. The feet are raised too high and put down too forcibly. Balance is upset, and the patient has to walk and stand on a wide base. Closing the eyes on attempting to stand aggravates the ataxia (rombergism). In some cases, the ataxia and imbalance are out of proportion to the loss of conscious postural sensation, presumably because the sensory input to the cerebellum is more reduced than "conscious" sensation. Ataxia is present when the patient is lying down; the heel-knee test is poorly performed, and voluntary movement against resistance is carried out jerkily. In extreme cases, the patient may not be able to sit up without swaying. Ataxia is less common in the upper limbs, but fine movements may be clumsily performed. Muscle tone is reduced, and the joints of the limbs can be placed in exaggerated positions; this can contribute to the production of Charcot's arthropathy.

The tendon reflexes disappear because of degeneration of the afferent pathways in the posterior roots, and since the lumbosacral cord is affected sooner than the cervical, the ankle and knee jerks are lost before the reflexes in the arms. The plantar responses remain flexor except in taboparesis. The abdominal reflexes are either normal or brisk in tabes.

Bladder function is often disturbed late in the disease; exceptionally, retention is an early symptom, but it is usually accompanied by objective signs of tabes even if other symptoms are absent or slight. Typically, the bladder is distended, its wall is trabeculated, and infection is present. Constipation is usual, but if the anal sphincters are affected, fecal incontinence will result if the feces are fluid. Impotence may be early, late, or absent.

Cranial nerve palsies occur in some cases. Optic atrophy, pupillary abnormalities, and partial third nerve paralysis are the most common.

The pupillary reactions are disturbed in the majority of tabetics. The classic features described by Argyll Robertson in 1869 are pathognomonic of neurosyphilis[6]; the pupils are small, do not react to light, respond normally to convergence, and dilate slowly and incompletely with atropine. It is considered to be the result of a combination of miosis from interruption of sympathetic fibers to the pupil and interruption of the reflex pathway running between the external geniculate body and the third nerve nucleus. *Large* pupils which respond to convergence but not to light can be found in both syphilitic and nonsyphilitic lesions of the midbrain (tumors, head injuries, encephalitis), and bilateral abnormalities of this type are also seen in some oculomotor nerve lesions and after herpes ophthalmicus. In early tabes it is common to find only a reduced and ill-sustained reaction to light. In some cases the pupillary reactions are normal.

Slight bilateral ptosis, which the patient counteracts by elevating the eyebrows, is fairly common and is probably due to disease of the sympathetic fibers to the smooth muscle of the upper lid. Diplopia from third, fourth, or sixth nerve palsy (usually incomplete) is not uncommon in advanced cases.

Optic atrophy can occur by itself or in association with other signs of tabes. When it appears early in the disease, ataxia tends to be slight, and the other symptoms of tabes may not develop. It is usually bilateral, but one eye may be affected before the other. Optic atrophy is characterized by a very slow and painless impairment of vision; there is general depression of visual acuity, and peripheral constriction of the fields which affects some sectors more than others, so that the field loss may bear a superficial resemblance to incomplete quadrantic or bitemporal hemianopia. A central scotoma is rare, and when present tends to expand slowly to involve the whole visual field. Argyll Robertson pupils are usually present, but the impairment of the response to light is more severe than is justified by the degree of visual impairment. The optic discs are pale, with clear-cut margins and a normal physiological cup.

Other cranial nerves are occasionally involved. The symptoms include anosmia, loss of taste, impairment of sensation over the central part of the face, deafness, vertigo, laryngeal paralysis, and unilateral weakness of the tongue.

TABETIC CRISES. A gastric crisis consists of a bout of abdominal pain and vomiting lasting from hours to days. There is tenderness of the abdominal wall, but rigidity is absent. The situation is easily mistaken for a surgical abdominal emergency, and in this context it is worth mentioning that in advanced tabes, abdominal disease is sometimes unaccompanied by pain or rigidity. A rectal crises consist of attacks of cough, dyspnea, and stridor, caused by adduction of tenesmus which may last for several days. In vesical crises, there is pain in the bladder and strangury. Laryngeal crises consist of attacks of cough, dyspnea, and stridor, caused by adduction of the vocal cords (i.e., weakness of the abductors).

TROPHIC CHANGES. The most common is Charcot's arthropathy, which is usually seen in the knees or hips but may occur in the shoulders, ankles, small joints of the hands and feet, or spine. The swollen joint contains fluid, and is abnormally mobile and painless. There is usually some generalized decalcification of bone in advanced tabes, and pathological fractures may occur.

Trophic ulceration occurs under the metatarsal bone of the great toe and at other pressure points in the feet. The skin thickens and then sloughs away, leaving an indolent ulcer which may ultimately penetrate to the bone and cause necrosis. Ulceration can be started by overzealous chiropody.

Dementia paralytica may supervene in tabes. Rarely, meningovascular syphilis complicates the situation; for example, in the form of a cerebral thrombosis.

Laboratory Aids. The serological reactions are usually positive in the blood and spinal fluid in the early stages, but as the disease advances, the blood serology and the cerebrospinal fluid may revert to normal, even in untreated cases. Lymphocytic pleocytosis accompanied by a rise of protein and globulin is usually present *when the disease is active.* A midzone colloidal gold curve is present if the globulin content of the spinal fluid is raised. Eventually, in both treated and untreated cases, the spinal fluid may become normal even if optic atrophy and ataxia continue to grow worse.

Diagnosis. Difficulties can arise in the early phase of the disease. The patient may present with bladder symptoms, an epigastric crisis, pain in the limbs, or girdle pain, but careful physical examination will usually disclose the characteristic signs of tabes in the eyes and limbs. In alcoholic peripheral neuropathy, the pupils may be sluggish, the legs painful and ataxic, the ankle jerks absent, and proprioception impaired, but the muscles are weak and *tender.* The Holmes-Adie syndrome can be a source of difficulty.[3] It occurs in otherwise healthy individuals, is almost confined to women, and is characterized by a very slow "tonic" response to light and to convergence and reduction or absence of some of the tendon reflexes (usually the ankle and knee jerks). The pupils are usually large, and the slow but ultimately full contraction in response to convergence is pathognomonic.

If a patient is known to be a tabetic, it is only too easy to attribute abdominal pain to the disease, and it has to be kept in mind that tabetics are by no means immune to peptic ulcer, carcinoma of the stomach, and other abdominal maladies. Thoracic pain may be due to an aortic aneurysm. Not all bladder symptoms in tabetics are due to the tabes.

Course and Prognosis. Tabes is extremely variable in its rate of progress and its response to treatment, but in general it tends to become worse over a number of years and then comes to a halt. Some cases deteriorate rapidly despite treatment. Charcot's arthropathy is inevitably progressive, but trophic ulcers can heal. Sphincter symptoms can improve, and impotence is not necessarily permanent. Progression is rapid if general paresis supervenes and is untreated. Death is usually due to genitourinary infection or cardiovascular disease.

Treatment. Specific treatment is the same as for meningovascular syphilis, but there is no need for it if the spinal fluid is normal and there is no clinical evidence of progression. The persistence of lightning pains and visceral crises does not necessarily signify progression in the pathological sense, and antisyphilitic treatment has no effect on these symptoms, or on Charcot's arthropathy.

Lightning pains are aggravated by constipation and by retention of urine, and these should therefore be avoided. Analgesics of the coal-tar series combined with codeine are fairly effective, but cordotomy may have to be resorted to in extreme cases. Gastric crises are difficult to treat. Sometimes they respond to intravenous Thorazine (50 mg. in 500 ml. glucose saline) and a bland diet. Sedation can also be achieved by administering sodium bromide and chloral hydrate per rectum, or by intravenous phenobarbitone. If a rectal crisis is persistent and severe, it can be interrupted by the administration of a spinal anesthetic. The inhalation of amyl nitrite is said to be beneficial in laryngeal crises.

Urinary symptoms are usually due to distention of the bladder and cystitis.

The patient should be told to micturate at regular intervals, whether he feels like it or not, and urinary infections must be dealt with by appropriate medication. In males, prostatic obstruction must be looked for and treated. A plastic urinal strapped to the thigh is necessary for male patients with dribbling incontinence. Charcot's arthropathy may require the use of calipers to stabilize the joint, and ataxia of gait can be helped by reeducational walking exercises.

DEMENTIA PARALYTICA

Dementia paralytica is characterized pathologically by a chronic syphilitic meningoencephalitis and clinically by progressive dementia followed by the gradual appearance of bilateral weakness of pyramidal origin. It usually starts about 10 to 15 years after infection; in congenital cases, it commonly appears between the ages of 10 and 20. It is more common in men than in women.

Pathology. The dura is adherent to the skull, and the thickened leptomeninges adhere to the cortex. In advanced cases the brain is shrunken and the gyri are atrophied, particularly in the frontal and temporal lobes. Occasionally, there is selective atrophy of one or both parietal lobes (the Lissauer type of the disease [74]). The ventricles are slightly enlarged, and the ependyma is granular. Microscopically, evidence of the disease is found in the meninges, the brain, and the blood vessels. The leptomeninges are infiltrated with lymphocytes and plasma cells. The ordinary arrangement of the cells in the cortex is disturbed, and they are reduced in numbers. There is demyelination in the tangential fibers of the cortex and in the pyramidal tracts in both the brain and spinal cord. The microglia enlarge and appear as "rod" cells, and a reactive astrocytic gliosis is present. Spirochetes are often present in the cortex and basal ganglia of untreated cases. Iron pigment, in the form of spicules, is found in glial cells and in the endothelium of the capillaries. Perivascular infiltration with lymphocytes and plasma cells is present in both white and gray matter, but the panarteritis of meningovascular syphilis is rarely seen.

Clinical Features. The onset is usually so insidious that it is difficult to determine when the symptoms started, but occasionally it is abrupt—with convulsions, or an acute psychotic episode, or transient hemiparesis. It is possible that vascular occlusion plays a part in such cases. Sometimes the symptoms are first noticed after a head injury, an alcoholic bout, or following delirium tremens.

The first mental symptoms may be vague. Forgetfulness, difficulty in concentration, fatigability, and anxiety may suggest a fatigue state or a neurosis, and sometimes a true anxiety state develops in the individual who has sufficient insight to realize that he is becoming inefficient because of failing mental powers. In others there is unexplained depression and irritability, or unusual restlessness and euphoria. A change of character may appear in the form of lying, discourtesy, sexual excesses, slovenliness in dress, or boastfulness. Reduced tolerance for alcohol is seen, as in other organic diseases of the brain.

When the disease is well established, the diagnosis is obvious. The simple dementing form is the commonest and is characterized by inability to concentrate, impairment of memory, difficulty in calculation, loss of judgment and insight, and a dissolution of the social sense which is evident in a general deterioration of manners and a disregard for the niceties of social intercourse. Delusions may appear.

The mood may be elevated or depressed, and the disturbance may be sufficiently severe to overshadow the underlying dementia. An expansive euphoria is occasionally encountered; the patient has splendid illusions of wealth, power, and personal importance, and his mood is appropriately genial, but he sees no incongruity between his delusions of grandeur and his deteriorating condition. Rarely, intellectual deterioration is comparatively mild, and the physical symptoms of paresis preponderate.

Signs of motor impairment are inconspicuous in the early stages of the disease, but sooner or later speech becomes slurred and slightly tremulous, and there is action tremor of the tongue, lips, face, and hands. The pupils may be normal in all respects; more often they are large and react poorly to light and briskly to convergence. The Argyll Robertson pupil is found in less than half of all cases, and it is usually late in appearing; consequently, this sign is by no means a sine qua non for the early diagnosis of general paresis. Optic atrophy and ocular palsies are uncommon except in taboparesis.

At first, there is no persistent weakness of the limbs, but mono- or hemiparesis may occur transiently from time to time, with or without an antecedent seizure. Evidence of pyramidal disease ultimately appears in the form of progressive weakness, increased tendon reflexes, and extensor plantar responses.

The sensory system is usually intact except in taboparesis and the Lissauer type of general paresis with atrophy of the parietal lobe and consequent sensory loss of cortical type.[74]

Sphincter symptoms appear late. Libido and potency occasionally appear to be increased in the early stages, but are soon lost.

Laboratory Aids. The serological reactions for syphilis are positive in the blood in practically all cases. The spinal fluid pressure is normal, but in untreated cases there is invariably moderate lymphocytic pleocytosis, increase of protein, and a positive globulin reaction. An abnormal colloidal gold curve, usually of the first-zone type, is common. If the serological tests are negative, and all the other evidence points to neurosyphilis, antisyphilis treatment should be given a trial. The electroencephalogram usually shows diffuse bilateral, high voltage slow waves; with treatment it can revert to normal or near normal.

Diagnosis. There is no great problem in recognizing an advanced case. Acute general paresis can be simulated by meningovascular syphilis, but this matters little since the treatment is the same.

Chronic alcoholism can give rise to mental impairment, social dilapidation, slurring of speech, tremor of the tongue and hands, and impaired pupillary responses to light. Progressive cerebral arteriosclerotic dementia, the presenile dementias of Alzheimer and Pick, tumors of the parietal and temporal lobes and of the corpus callosum, and chronic bromide poisoning may cause diagnostic difficulty, but examination of the spinal fluid will settle the matter once and for all.

Greater difficulty surrounds early diagnosis because of the vagueness of the patient's complaints and their similarity to those of a psychoneurosis. This is especially true when general paresis occurs in somebody with a past history of mental or emotional illness, and the greatest care has to be exercised in establishing the presence of intellectual deterioration of organic origin. Psychometric tests and electroencephalography can help, but there is nothing so convincing as the examination of the spinal fluid.

General paresis is one of the conditions which must be excluded in persons who develop seizures for the first time in adult life, or who suffer from transient hemiparetic attacks (which can simulate the effects of carotid insufficiency), and it is prudent to remember that evidence of dementia is not always obvious in the early stages of dementia paralytica.

Clinical Course. The untreated disease is usually fatal in from one to five years. Spontaneous remissions or periods of comparative standstill are sometimes seen and may last for as long as a year, but as a rule the patient's condition deteriorates steadily unless treatment is given.

To be effective, treatment must be given at an early stage of the disease, and it must be thorough. As mentioned above, the blood serology and spinal fluid should be examined at intervals after the initial course of treatment, to see whether further therapy is needed or not. Thorough treatment, thus defined and given early, can be expected to produce cure in about 50 per cent of all cases. In the remaining 50 per cent, the patient will be left with permanent residuals and in some cases will develop new neurological disabilities. A recent follow-up of 100 patients with general paresis who had survived at least 10 years after initial treatment revealed that no less than 31 developed new signs of neurological disease subsequent to treatment.[103] These developments included tabes dorsalis, optic atrophy, amyotrophy, hemiparesis, paraplegia, and ocular motor palsy. Of course, not all neurological disease occurring in a previously treated syphilitic is necessarily syphilitic in origin; most of these patients belong to an age group which is liable to atherosclerosis and its complications, spinal compression from spondylosis, and other chronic diseases of the nervous system.

The cerebrospinal fluid changes lag behind the clinical condition during and after treatment and may continue to improve 18 months after treatment is stopped. The serological reaction may never revert to normal, and the colloidal gold reaction tends to revert to normal much later than the increase of cells and protein. It is generally believed that clinical recurrences are preceded by the appearance of new signs of activity in the spinal fluid.

Treatment. Penicillin is the treatment of choice. A suitable course is two million units a day for 20 days. The cerebrospinal fluid should be examined at the end of the course and again six months later and at yearly intervals for an additional four years, in order to detect the changes in the cerebrospinal fluid which usually precede clinical relapse.

It is of more than historical interest to recall that in prepenicillin days good results were obtained by the use of fever therapy, either by infecting the patient with malaria or by using a heating cabinet. *Plasmodium vivax*, the organism of tertian malaria, was commonly used. *Plasmodium malariae* was advised for black patients, who are often immune to *P. vivax*. These strains of malaria are usually obtainable through the Public Health Service. Some experienced syphilologists believe that the best results are obtained by using penicillin and fever therapy concurrently, but fever therapy is contraindicated in patients with cardiac, pulmonary, renal and hepatic diseases.

CONGENITAL NEUROSYPHILIS

Infection of the fetus occurs during pregnancy, and the pathological changes it produces in the nervous system are similar to those which occur in the acquired form of the disease, although the symptoms to which it gives rise are slightly different. The infant with neurosyphilis may or may not exhibit cutaneous and other evidence of the infection, but even if it appears normal from the clinical point of view the spinal fluid will reveal that the infection is present. The condition corresponds to asymptomatic neurosyphilis in the adult. Meningitis, vascular accidents, dementia paralytica, tabes dorsalis, and optic atrophy can develop thereafter. If the spinal fluid serological test is negative in a child born of a syphilitic mother, congenital neurosyphilis is unlikely to develop.

Meningitis often provides the earliest clinical evidence of the disease in the nervous system, usually when the infant is four to five months old. The disease is marked by irritability, convulsions, rigidity of the neck, and bulging of the fontanelles. Cranial nerve palsies and papilledema progressing to optic atrophy may occur. The head may enlarge if hydrocephalus is caused by obstruction to the circulation of the cerebrospinal fluid in the basal cisterns. The basal leptomeningeal inflammation can also give rise to facial paralysis, diplopia, and deafness.

Cerebral thrombosis and even cerebral hemorrhage occasionally occur, usually within the second year.

Congenital dementia paralytica is uncommon and seldom appears before the tenth year. It resembles the acquired disease in the adult in some particulars, but for obvious reasons the behavioral results of increasing dementia are different at this age. There is progressive deterioration of mind and behavior, tremor of the lips, tongue, and fingers, dysarthria, occasional convulsions, and increasing evidence of pyramidal involvement on both sides of the body. The pupils are usually large and do not react to light, but the classic Argyll Robertson pupil is unusual. Syphilitic choroidoretinopathy may be present. In some cases, the course of the untreated disease is rather longer than is usual in the adult form.

Juvenile tabes dorsalis is rare. It usually starts at the age of 10 or 12 years, and the symptomatology resembles that of the acquired disease, except that lightning pains, visceral crises and Charcot joints are unusual, while urinary disturbances and optic atrophy are common. Physical retardation is usually obvious. Optic atrophy can occur by itself, without any evidence of dementia or tabes dorsalis.

When idiocy with or without microcephaly is present in a syphilitic child, it is unwise to assume that the two conditions are necessarily related, but congenital syphilis used to be considered responsible for about 3 per cent of all mental defectives.

Treatment. Syphilitic meningitis responds well to treatment with penicillin; if hydrocephalus is present, it may or may not improve. Congenital dementia paralytica and congenital tabes respond to penicillin. Infants should receive a total dose of 100,000 units of penicillin/kg. body weight. A suitable preparation is procaine penicillin G in oil with 2 per cent aluminum monostearate, in doses of 150,000 to 300,000 units every two days. In older children, penicillin is given by daily injections of half a million units for 20 days. The spinal fluid should be reexamined every six months; if treatment has been efficacious, the white cell count will have returned to normal within three to six months after treatment. The total protein may remain elevated for as long as 18 months, and the Wassermann reaction in the spinal fluid may remain positive for several years. It is wise to continue therapy intermittently until the cells and protein are normal.

Leptospiral Meningitis

Lymphocytic meningitis may complicate Weil's disease, but it can also occur in the absence of jaundice, hemorrhagic symptoms or renal damage.[15] Leptospiral meningitis starts suddenly with headache, photophobia, vomiting, pyrexia, and the usual signs of meningeal irritation. The diagnosis is suggested by a history of bathing in rivers or canals, or working in rat-infested surroundings, and by the presence of reddening of the conjunctiva. The spinal fluid contains a large number of lymphocytes and a few polymorphs; the glucose content is unchanged. The diagnosis is confirmed by the presence of a rising titer of agglutination against suspensions of the organism. Complete recovery usually occurs in two to three weeks, but severe involvement of the liver may lead to a fatal issue in the second week of the disease.

Penicillin and the tetracyclines appear to be effective against *Leptospira icterohaemorrhagica* and help to shorten the course of the disease.

Other Spirochetal Diseases of the Nervous System

A lymphocytic meningitis can be caused by swineherd's disease (*Leptospira pomona*), by relapsing fever (*Borrelia recurrentis* in Europe, *B. duttonii* in Central Africa, and *B. novyi* in America) and by rat-bite fever (*Spirillum minus*). In rat-bite fever, severe encephalitis may occur and may be fatal. These infections respond to penicillin and to the tetracyclines.

Rickettsial Diseases

TYPHUS FEVER

Etiology. The agent of epidemic typhus is *Rickettsia prowazeki*, which is spread by the body louse. A milder and nonepidemic form of the same disease is called Brill-Zinsser disease. A second type of typhus is caused by *R. mooseri*, the murine variety, a disease of rats which is spread by the rat flea and is occasionally transmitted to man.

Pathology. *Rickettsia rickettsiae* invade the endothelial cells of small arteries, capillaries, and venules. The vessels are surrounded by perivascular accumulations of phagocytic cells. Thrombosis leads to multiple microinfarcts throughout the body, notably in the skin, the brain, and the heart muscle. In fatal cases, the brain is edematous and is studded with petechial hemorrhages. There are multiple "typhus nodules," small collections of microglia, lymphocytes, and endothelial cells related to the smaller blood vessels throughout the nervous system.

Clinical Features. After an incubation period of 10 to 14 days, there is an abrupt onset, with fever, muscle aches, and malaise. A pink, macular rash appears from the third day onward, but headaches, stiffness of the neck, and delirium may appear before the rash. Untreated, the patient becomes confused and this may lead in turn to coma and death. Convulsive seizures and signs of focal damage to the brain and spinal cord occur as the result of multiple microinfarcts.

Severe arterial hypotension is common, and this is followed by evidence of renal insufficiency with a drop in urea clearance and a rise in blood urea nitrogen.

Adequate immunization by rickettsial vaccine greatly lessens the severity of the illness and has reduced the mortality practically to zero.

Laboratory Aids. Agglutinins and antibodies appear in the serum after a few days, and the Weil-Felix reaction becomes positive from the fifth to the eighth day. Diagnosis can also be made by inoculation of blood into laboratory animals or chick embryos. Meningococcal septicemia can simulate typhus, but it can be identified by finding the organism in the spinal fluid and by blood culture.

Course and Prognosis. Untreated, the case mortality rate in epidemic typhus is less than 10 per cent in children, but it is 60 per cent or more in nonimmunized patients over the age of 50. In the absence of treatment, renal insufficiency and hypotension are serious, as is gangrene of the skin.

Treatment. The tetracyclines and chloramphenicol are effective, if administered early and in adequate dosage. The initial dose for adults is 3 gr. in the first three hours, followed by 0.5 gr. every six hours until the temperature is normal. The dose is then reduced by half and is continued for two or three days. Sulfonamides are believed to have a harmful effect in typhus and should not be given.

Supportive treatment is important, notably for patients with arterial hypotension, hyperpyrexia, and pneumonia.

ROCKY MOUNTAIN SPOTTED FEVER

This disease, also known as spotted fever, tic fever, and tic typhus, is an acute infective arteritis of the smaller blood vessels caused by Rickettsia. It is transmitted by the bite of *Dermacentor andersoni* in the Western states and by the dog tick, *Dermacentor variabilis*, in the Southern and Eastern states. Related diseases, South African tick-bite fever, Kenya tick typhus, Indian tick typhus, and Marseilles fever, are caused by infection with *Rickettsia conori*, and *Rickettsia sibiricus* causes Northern Asian tick-borne Rickettsiosis. *Rickettsia australis* is responsible for Queensland tick typhus.

Pathology. The lesions in the nervous system are similar to those in typhus—a patchy vasculitis with small areas of necrosis, and glial nodules consisting of microglia, lymphocytes, and endothelial cells.

Clinical Features. The onset is marked by chills, fever, and severe malaise. A measles-like rash appears on the third or fourth day and is soon replaced by red maculopapular lesions, which appear first on the ankles and wrists and then spread to the palms and soles, the arms and legs, and the trunk. In some cases, the rash becomes hemorrhagic. The muscles are painful and tender. Delirium is common, and coarse tremors and seizures occur in severe cases. There may be deafness, slurring of speech, hemiparesis, or paraplegia.[16a] Retinal venous engorgement, retinal exudates, and papilledema have been reported. The liver and spleen are slightly enlarged and interstitial pneumonitis and myocardial involvement have been described.

Laboratory Aids. The spinal fluid is often normal in all respects, but it may contain an excess of leukocytes. The protein and glucose content remain normal. Hyponatremia and hypochloremia are common even in the absence of severe vomiting. Specific complement fixation tests and the Weil-Felix reaction become positive in the second week of the disease.

Course and Prognosis. In mild cases, the temperature falls after lysis in two or three weeks. The mortality rate is about 20 per cent in nonvaccinated and untreated patients, but it is much higher in debilitated subjects. Evidence of damage to the nervous system may persist for months.

Treatment. In areas in which the disease is endemic, care should be taken to search for and remove ticks from the body and clothing; high boots should be worn when walking through brush. Vaccination is recommended in areas where ticks abound. Both tetracycline and chloramphenicol are effective. Sulfa drugs should be avoided since they are thought to enhance the severity of the disease.

SCRUB TYPHUS

This is a self-limited, febrile disease caused by *R. tsutsugamushi*, which is transmitted by mites. It is widely distributed in the Pacific and Far East. As in other rickettsial diseases, the organism causes disseminated focal vasculitis. Acute myocarditis, encephalitic lesions, and an interstitial pneumonitis are found in almost all fatal cases.

Clinical Features. After an incubation period of six to 18 days, the illness begins suddenly with headache, chills, and fever. The conjunctivae are injected and there is a generalized lymphadenopathy. In Caucasian patients, the site of attachment of the mite is visibly inflamed. After the fifth day, a macular rash appears on the trunk and may extend to the limbs. In Asiatic patients, both the rash and the eschar at the site of the bite may be less obvious. Neurological symptoms include delirium, stupor, and muscular twitching, but on the whole the disease is relatively mild, and permanent neurological or cardiac sequelae are rare.

Diagnosis. A history of recent exposure to chiggers, in a geographical area in which the disease is endemic, points to the possibility of the disease. Agglutinins against the Ox-K strain of *Proteus vulgaris* appear in the serum of the patient, and *R. tsutsugamushi* can sometimes be recovered from the blood.

Treatment. Tetracyclines and chloramphenicol are effective and are administered as for typhus and Rocky Mountain spotted fever.

Mycotic Infections

With the exception of *Actinomyces bovis*, fungi seldom attack man, but in recent years, there has been an increase in the incidence and severity of this type of infection.[104] This increase can be attributed to three factors. Modern antimicrobial agents destroy some of the normal nonpathogenic bacterial flora which prevent the growth of fungi, and improper use of such agents for the "treatment" of minor bacterial and viral infections appears to be the determining factor in some cases of fungal infection. Second, the widespread use of corticosteroids reduces resistance to fungi. Third, the legitimate use of radiation therapy for neoplasms will sometimes open the way for fungal infection by depressing immunological mechanisms.

In view of the increasing incidence of these infections, it is appropriate to keep them in mind when faced with atypical cases of subacute meningitis, space-occupying lesions of the brain or spinal cord, and organic psychosis, all of which can be mimicked.

Actinomycosis

Actinomyces bovis occasionally invades the brain[12]; the related *Nocardia asteroides* is less often responsible. Cerebral infection is usually the result[29] of hematogenous spread from a focus elsewhere in the body, usually in the lung, ileocecal region, or the head and neck. The primary focus is usually but not always obvious. Infection can give rise to one[12] or more abscesses, meningitis, dural sinus thrombosis, or a tumor-like picture caused by a large inflammatory mass.

There is usually polymorph pleocytosis in the spinal fluid. The course of the disease is characterized by a relative absence of toxicity and by spontaneous but temporary remissions. Drugs used successfully include penicillin, streptomycin, Aureomycin, and chloramphenicol.

Coccidioidomycosis

Infection by *Coccidioides immitis* is endemic in Southern California, parts of Arizona, Mexico, Argentina, and Hawaii.[29] The organism enters the body through the skin or lungs and is disseminated thence throughout the body. The generalized infection gives rise to fever, chills, pain in the back and joints, and pleurisy. Lesions appear in the bones, joints, lungs, and elsewhere. Subacute meningitis may develop, and both the pathological and clinical features strongly resemble those of tuberculous meningitis; leptomeningeal adhesions at the base can cause internal hydrocephalus. Brain abscess may also occur, and involvement of the spinal leptomeninges by granulomatous meningitis can produce the features of spinal compression.

In the cerebral form, the pressure of the spinal fluid is increased, and there is lymphocytic pleocytosis, a raised protein level, and reduced sugar and chloride levels. The organism can sometimes be identified in smears, and it can be cultured on Sabouraud's medium. The skin test is positive except in very early cases or in the presence of an overwhelming infection.

Treatment. Amphotericin B should be given both intravenously and by intrathecal injection. For the latter, 0.5 to 1.0 mg. is dissolved in 1 ml. of glucose saline, diluted with 5 to 10 ml. of cerebrospinal fluid, and injected very slowly. The intravenous dosage is as for cryptococcosis.

Mucormycosis

Certain fungi, notably *Rhizopus*, which are not normally pathogenic to man, may prove so in the presence of diabetes, leukemia, or lymphoma, and in patients who have been treated for a long time with antibiotics and steroids. The organism can give rise to acute sinusitis and orbital cellulitis, and can spread to produce infective thrombosis of the ophthalmic and internal carotid arteries, meningitis, and encephalitis.[72, 81] It can also give rise to pulmonary and intestinal forms of the disease.

Diagnosis is made by examination of the spinal fluid which contains an excess of lymphocytes, a low sugar, and the fungus. Care has to be exercised in interpreting the significance of fungi and yeasts in cerebrospinal fluid which has been left standing for some time, since they are common laboratory contaminants.

The disease is rapidly fatal if untreated, but there is evidence that Amphotericin B is effective.

Cryptococcal Meningitis (Torulosis)

The *Cryptococcus neoformans*, a saprophyte in nature, is inhaled in dust and its primary focus is established in

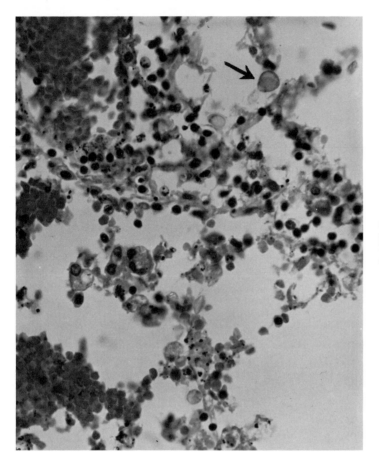

Figure 14–11. Torula meningitis, showing the organism. (Courtesy of Ayer Laboratory, Pennsylvania Hospital, Philadelphia.)

the lungs. This is often neither clinically nor radiologically apparent. The histopathological reaction to infection is a granuloma, and this is usually the end of it, but the disease can spread by the bloodstream from the lung to distant organs, including the meninges. This is apt to occur in people debilitated by other disease, such as leukemia, aplastic anemia, and Hodgkin's disease, but sometimes the central nervous system is invaded in a seemingly healthy individual.[104]

Pathology. The organisms give rise to subacute or chronic meningoencephalitis with a slimy, gelatinous exudate at the base and over the convexity of the brain. The meninges are studded with small grayish granulomatous nodules in which the organisms can be demonstrated. The infection invades the brain, both on the surface and via the ventri-

cles. Rarely, a comparatively large granuloma (toruloma) is found, without generalized meningitis, in the brain or in the spinal cord.[93]

Clinical Features. The onset is usually insidious. The presenting symptoms of 51 patients reported by Utz and his colleagues[26] were, in descending order of frequency: moderate to severe headache, significant mental changes, impairment of vision, nausea or vomiting, fever and chills, pain or stiffness of the neck, loss of balance, lethargy and fatigue, aphasia or dysarthria, and paresthesias. Less commonly encountered were seizures, paresis, incontinence, retention of urine, tinnitus, and dizziness. In 6 cases, there was no clinical suggestion of meningitis.

The symptoms may be progressive or intermittent. The course is extremely variable, as may be judged by the fact that in the cases reported by Utz and his colleagues, the period which elapsed between the onset of symptoms and the diagnosis varied from one to 72 months. DeLamater has recorded a case of a woman who had intermittent cryptococcal meningitis for over 18 years. The disease can simulate tuberculous meningitis, tumor of the brain, encephalitis, or a primary psychosis.

The cerebrospinal fluid commonly shows a modest elevation of protein, a reduction of glucose, and a lymphocytic pleocytosis. The organism can often be identified in the cerebrospinal fluid, using the India ink method. It can be cultured on Sabouraud's medium; occasionally as much as 30 to 40 ml. of spinal fluid has to be inoculated into the culture medium before the organism can be cultured.

Treatment. Prior to the use of Amphotericin B, cryptococcal meningitis was always fatal. The initial dose should be 1 mg. dissolved in 500 ml. of a 5 per cent glucose solution; dosage should then be increased by daily increments of 5 to 10 mg. until approximately 1.0 mg./kg. body weight is given daily. Alternatively, 1.5 mg./kg. body weight may be given every other day. Each infusion should be administered over a period of 2 to 6 hours. A total of at least 3 gm. of drug should be given by the intravenous route. Some authorities advise intrathecal therapy, as well, as outlined for coccidioidomycosis.

The drug is effective but is toxic to the kidney. The appearance of albumin and casts in the urine and a rise in blood urea are indications to withhold the drug temporarily.

Histoplasmosis

Histoplasma capsulatum can give rise to a low grade meningitis,[96] without the typical clinical picture of severe disseminated histoplasmosis—fever, wasting, enlargement of the liver and spleen, and oral or gastrointestinal lesions. As in cryptococcal meningitis, the onset is insidious and it may be months or years before the diagnosis is made in the simple meningeal form. There may be intermittent headaches and a little fever. Mental changes are not uncommon. Generalized weakness and unsteadiness of gait may be present from time to time.

There is an elevation of lymphocytes and protein in the spinal fluid, and the glucose content is commonly depressed. Diagnosis depends upon the isolation of the organism from the cerebrospinal fluid; it can also be obtained from the sputum and blood. The electroencephalogram shows nonspecific bilateral 3 to 6 per second waves or it may be normal.

Treatment. Amphotericin B is the treatment of choice, in the same doses as are given for cryptococcal meningitis.

PROTOZOAL DISEASES

Amebiasis

Amebic dysentery is caused by *Entamoeba histolytica*. It is most common in the tropics, but does occur in temperate zones. The organism first attacks the intestine and then spreads to the liver. Occasionally it produces purulent encephalitis or a brain abscess. The cerebral symptoms are usually preceded by evidence of bowel and liver involvement, and sometimes follow operations for amebic abscess of the liver. The cerebral signs are those of a cerebral abscess, and diagnostic measures and treatment are the same as for any cerebral abscess, together with the administration of appropriate chemotherapy for amebiasis.

Malaria

The term cerebral malaria is applied to all the nervous manifestations of infection by *Plasmodium falciparum*, whether they are cerebral, cerebellar, meningeal, or spinal. The disease is usually encountered in the tropics, but sporadic cases occur in temperate zones among travelers and, exceptionally, in drug addicts or others infected from syringes which have been used on a malarious subject. Malaria occurs in both sexes and at any age. Cerebral involvement occurs in about 2 per cent of all cases of falciparum malaria.

Pathology. The brain and meninges have a leaden hue due to the presence of malarial pigment. The vessels of the brain and cord are congested, and the capillaries are packed with parasites. There is thickening of the endothelium, and some degree of perivascular necrosis. The ganglion cells of the cerebrum and cerebellum undergo piecemeal degeneration, and may also be involved in small areas of infarction. The meninges are infiltrated with lymphocytes and plasma cells. There is often, but not invariably, an increase in the cellular and protein content of the spinal fluid.

Clinical Features. The onset of neurological symptoms may be abrupt, or the symptoms may be preceded by headache, pain about the body, and an irregular fever—a condition so unlike the classic onset of malaria that it is often mistaken for influenza. As is to be expected from the pathology, the nervous symptoms take many forms, but they are all characteristically swift in onset and rapid in development. Among the more common manifestations are convulsions, delirium or acute confusion,[5] sudden coma, hemiplegia, monoplegia, paraplegia, aphasia, cerebellar ataxia, choreiform and myoclonic movements, hyperpyrexia, and a condition of meningism so severe as to resemble acute meningitis. Paraplegia may be either cerebral or spinal in origin, the latter presenting as acute transverse myelitis. Seizures are very common in children, and may either dominate the illness throughout or give place to any of the forms mentioned. Mental symptoms may mimic any type of acute psychosis.[5] Some instances of persons "running amok" have been examples of cerebral malaria. A combination of mental confusion with slight ataxia can be mistaken for intoxication by alcohol or drugs. Patients with signs of

focal damage to the brain—dysphasia, apraxia, hemiplegia, paraplegia, hemianopia, amaurosis, cerebellar ataxia, etc.— almost always show additional features such as confusion, delirium, meningism, or multiplicity of focal signs. Hyperpyrexia may occur alone or with other signs; the temperature rises rapidly and death ensues if it is not brought down promptly. Ocular complications include dendritic ulcers, retinal hemorrhages, occlusion of the central artery by parasites, spasm of retinal arteries (from quinine, giving rise to transient or permanent visual impairment), and palsy of the third, fourth, or sixth nerve. Deafness can occur, either as a result of the malaria or from quinine intoxication.

The general condition deteriorates by reason of toxemia, increasing anemia, and a progressive fall of blood pressure. The spleen may or may not be palpable. There is polymorph leukopenia with increase of lymphocytes and monocytes. The pressure of the spinal fluid may be normal or raised, and there is often a moderate rise of lymphocytes and protein; the sugar content is normal.

Course and Prognosis. Untreated patients usually die in 12 to 72 hours, but full recovery occurs in the majority of cases if vigorous treatment is started early. Focal signs may take days, weeks, or months to clear up. Patients in whom coma or delirium has been prolonged are sometimes left with a liability to headache, poor memory, defective powers of concentration, irritability, and great asthenia of mind and body. Psychotic and psychoneurotic states have been known to follow cerebral malaria, but whether they are due to the malaria or are merely uncovered thereby it is often difficult to say.[5] Polyneuritis can occur as a result of prolonged malaria, but does not seem to be especially linked with the cerebral form of the disease.

Diagnosis. Any acute mental or neurological illness in a person who could have been exposed to malaria should be regarded as malarious until otherwise proved. The diagnosis is made by identifying the parasites in the blood, preferably using the thick film technique since they may be missed in thin films, and by the therapeutic effect of quinine and other agents. The second point is important because patients with malarial parasites in the blood are just as liable as anybody else to develop other psychological or neurological diseases, and there is a danger of ascribing too much to the malaria.

Coma or stupor with a rising temperature may be due to malaria, heat stroke, subarachnoid or pontine hemorrhage, meningitis, or encephalitis. Marked impairment or cessation of sweating when the ambient temperature is high suggests heat stroke. It should be noted that mental symptoms can occur in malaria other than the cerebral form,[5] whether from toxemia, exhaustion, severe anemia, or coincident cerebral disease such as arteriosclerosis or neurosyphilis. Psychotic symptoms have also been known to follow the use of Atabrine by intramuscular injections for the control of tertian or quartan malaria.

Treatment

GENERAL MEASURES. Cerebral malaria is a medical emergency. The patient should be nursed in Fowler's position. The fluid intake must be maintained by mouth, nasal catheter, rectal drip, or parenteral methods; the total intake depends on the size of the patient, the severity of sweating, and the climate, and is best controlled by the amount and specific gravity of the urine. Five per cent glucose-saline is the best medium by any route. If there is retention of urine, catheterization must be carried out twice daily. Pyrexia in excess of 104° F. requires the prompt application of ice packs or a hypothermic blanket; alternatively, the patient is covered by a wet sheet and placed under a fan until the rectal temperature falls to 102° F. If the hemoglobin level of the blood is under 50 per cent of normal, a slowly given blood transfusion is indicated. If the cerebrospinal fluid pressure is high, it should be reduced by repeated spinal tap. Sedation is needed for restlessness and for involuntary movements.

SPECIFIC TREATMENT.[17] Chloroquine is given intramuscularly. The initial dose for an adult is 0.375 gm. in 7.5 ml. of sterile distilled water, and half this amount is repeated every six hours until a total of 1.5 gm. has been given. The dose for a child is proportionately less. Alternatively, quinine dihydrochloride can be given intravenously in doses not exceeding 0.6 gm. in 10 ml. of saline, repeated every six hours up to a total of 1.8 gm. in 24 hours; for a child, the dose is one-twentieth the adult dose for each year of age. Intravenous quinine should be injected very slowly to avoid a fall of blood pressure. When the crisis has subsided, medication is continued by mouth. Failure to respond to adequate therapy may mean that the patient is suffering from something in addition to malaria, or that the organism is resistant. Chloroquine-resistant strains can be effectively treated by one or more doses of sulfalene (0.75 gm.) and trimethoprim (0.5 gm.), which depress folic acid metabolism; protozoa are more sensitive to folic acid deficiency than is man.[17]

Toxoplasmosis

Infection by the protozoon *Toxoplasma* is rare.[64] It can affect any age group, but commonly occurs in infants to whom it has been transmitted *in utero*. The organism is found in great numbers in the endothelial cells of blood vessels, and is also seen lying freely in the tissues (Fig. 14–12); it gives rise to small granulomas throughout the meninges and central nervous system, together with a more diffuse inflammatory reaction. Larger granulomas, up to 3 cm. in diameter, also occur, and it is in these that calcification is sometimes seen. The organism also invades the eye, the choroid especially, producing small granulomas with subsequent scarring. Other viscera may also be involved.

Clinical Features. In the congenital form, the features of meningoencephalitis appear at birth or shortly after; there

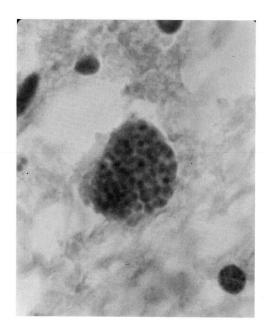

Figure 14–12. Toxoplasmosis (Courtesy of Department of Neuropathology, Philadelphia General Hospital.)

may be convulsions, spasticity of the limbs, ocular palsy, and retraction of the head. This may go on to hydrocephalus as a result of basal meningitis, or, if much damage is done to the brain, microcephaly may follow. Choroidoretinitis is common, and can lead to optic atrophy. The liver and spleen may be enlarged, and jaundice is not uncommon.

The acquired form of the disease occurs in children and adults. As in the case of fungal infections, the disease tends to appear in individuals whose immunologic responses have been reduced by therapeutic irradiation, steroids, and other forms of immunosuppressive therapy. The lymph glands, lungs, and skin are primarily involved, but the infection can also give rise to acute or chronic meningitis, acute or chronic encephalitis, and acute focal lesions of the brain, which can mimic a cerebral abscess and polymyositis.

The pressure of the cerebrospinal fluid may be normal or raised. There is usually a pleocytosis, and the protein content is elevated. Diagnosis can be confirmed by complement fixation and skin tests. Intracranial calcification in the form of small, rounded shadows, 1 to 3 mm. in diameter, have been present in about 50 per cent of published cases. Larger calcified lesions may appear in the lungs.

Prognosis. More than 50 per cent of patients with congenital cases die within a few weeks, and there is a high incidence of mental retardation and neurologic deficits in the survivors. Mortality is also high when acute brain lesions occur in children and adults. It is particularly desirable to make a positive diagnosis of this disease in the congenital neonatal forms because parents can then be reassured as to the prognosis for subsequent pregnancies.

Treatment. Sulfadiazine and sulfamethazine, used in conjunction with pyrimethamine, are of proven value in protecting experimental animals from toxoplasmosis, and there are reports of favorable results in the human disease.

Trypanosomiasis (Sleeping Sickness)

The African variety of trypanosomiasis is caused by *T. gambiense* and *T. rhodesiense*, which are transmitted to man from infected animals and from other men by the bite of the tsetse fly. It is a common disease in Africa between the

results from the presence of one or more cysts in the fourth ventricle. The blood vessels exhibit a characteristic arteritis which may play a part in the production of the focal neurological defects and the localized cortical atrophy which have been found at operation in some cases.

Clinical Features. Symptoms can arise at any time from a few months to many years after infection; the average is about five years. There are three main clinical types—seizures from cortical or subcortical cysts, cranial nerve palsies from basal arachnoiditis, and a tumor syndrome.[77] Three cases of diffuse enlargement of the muscles have been described, a pseudohypertrophic myopathy.

Seizures may be of any type: generalized convulsions, jacksonian attacks, or temporal lobe epilepsy. Leptomeningeal fibrosis can lead to loss of vision, diplopia, deafness, and vertigo. A tumor may be simulated by a mass of cysts confined to one area of the brain or by hydrocephalus induced by the presence of cysts within the fourth ventricle. Mental symptoms in the form of an acute organic psychosis occasionally occur in the invasive stage. Cysts are sometimes found in the tongue and subcutaneous tissue.

Laboratory Aids. The most certain means of diagnosis is the discovery of calcified cysts in the brain and muscles but it seldom occurs sooner than 10 years after infection, and is present in only about one-third of all cases; it may appear in muscles and not in the brain. Arteriography is useful in cases simulating symptoms of a brain tumor. The spinal fluid is often normal when the symptoms are confined to seizures, but in cases with extensive leptomeningeal infestation there is lymphocytic or eosinophilic pleocytosis, a rise of protein, and a fall of glucose. Complement fixation tests are positive in the spinal fluid in these cases.

Treatment. Seizures are treated in the usual way. If electroencephalography discloses a single discharging focus, surgical extirpation of the lesion can reduce or abolish the seizures, but the fact that the disease is usually generalized throughout the brain is discouraging from the surgical point of view. At the present time, there is no specific therapy for cysticercosis, other than surgical removal when the cysts are concentrated in a surgically accessible area of the brain.

Paragonimiasis

The fluke *Paralichthys westermani* is present in Japan, China, South America, and parts of Africa. The larvae migrate through the intestinal wall and usually develop in the lungs, but can invade the meninges and brain where they become encysted in a capsule which may ultimately calcify. The symptoms may be those of subacute meningitis or a brain tumor, or they may mimic a slowly developing cerebral thrombosis. There is usually eosinophilia. A complement fixation test is available to confirm the diagnosis.

Schistosomiasis

Although schistosomiasis is common in China, Japan, Formosa, the Philippines, Central Africa, and South America, it is an uncommon cause of neurological symptoms. Asymptomatic infestation of the brain appears to be quite common; Gelfand (in Rhodesia) found the parasite in the brains of 28 of 50 cases of bilharziasis, only one of which had shown neurological symptoms.[48]

The organism is found within small granulomas, which are most numerous in the cortex, basal ganglia, and white matter. *Schistosoma japonicum* usually localizes in the brain, while S. *haematobium* and S. *mansoni* show a predilection for the cord.[99] The granulomas are usually widely scattered, but in some cases they form massive conglomerations which can simulate a cerebral or spinal tumor.

Clinical Features. Symptoms can arise shortly after infestation, in which event the diagnosis is aided by a history of exposure to infected water in an endemic area and the presence of fever, cough, gastrointestinal symptoms, loss of weight, urticaria, enlargement of the liver, and cystitis. In some cases, however, a period of months elapses between the systemic manifestations and subsequent neurological symptoms.

The clinical manifestations are varied and include acute or subacute generalized encephalitis, a condition simulating a cerebral tumor, sudden hemiplegia or monoplegia with or without focal or generalized seizures, transverse "myelitis," and compression of the spinal cord by a granuloma.[99]

Laboratory Aids. Ova can usually be found in the stools or urine. The cerebrospinal fluid is often normal, but the protein may be elevated and there may be an eosinophilic leukocytosis. The blood usually contains an excess of eosinophils. Electroencephalography can be of localizing value in supratemporal lesions: A focal abnormality corresponding to the main site of disease was found in eight of 10 cases in one series. Angiography can help in cases simulating a tumor.

Treatment by the intravenous administration of antimony potassium tartrate is effective; most authorities advise 8 ml. of freshly prepared 0.5 per cent solution on the first day followed by doses of 12, 16, 20, 24, and 28 ml. on alternate days thereafter. The total dose should not exceed 2.22 gm. The prognosis as regards life is good, but neurological defects may persist.

Trichinosis

Infection by *Trichinella spiralis* comes from eating insufficiently cooked pork, usually in the form of sausages. The organisms are disseminated widely throughout the body and sometimes invade the meninges and brain, giving rise to subacute meningoencephalitis. As in other parasitic infestations, the inflammatory reaction takes the form of multiple small granulomas, accompanied by local and generalized eosinophilia.

Clinical Features. The nervous system is invaded in only about one in five cases, but there is usually widespread involvement of the muscles, which gives rise to profound weakness and loss of reflexes. If there is also diplopia and ptosis, the clinical picture may superficially resemble that of acute myasthenia gravis. There is often swelling of the eyelids and orbital contents, and the temperature is raised. It is against this background that meningeal and encephalitic symptoms occur. Meningitis gives rise to headache, stiffness of the neck, and lymphocytosis or eosinophilic leukocytosis in the spinal fluid. Encephalitis causes clouding of the mind, delirium, or the symptoms of a frank organic psychosis, and may also produce focal or generalized seizures and evidence of local damage in the form of aphasia, hemiparesis, or visual impairment.

The disease can be fatal within four to five weeks, and although complete recovery is usual, some survivors continue to suffer from disorientation, confusion, and diplopia for some months after the acute symptoms have passed. Seizures may persist.

Laboratory Aids. The combination of pyrexia and eosinophilia in the blood and spinal fluid indicates a parasitic infection. The organism can sometimes be found in the spinal fluid and in muscle biopsies. The skin reaction to trichinella allergen becomes positive after the third week, so this is of little value in the immediate diagnosis.

There is no specific treatment for the condition, but symptomatic improvement follows the use of steroids.

Hydatid Cysts

Etiology. The hydatid cyst is the larval form of *Taenia echinococcus*, which is prevalent in some parts of South America, Africa, and Eastern Europe. Formerly prevalent in Australia and New Zealand, it has been largely eradicated in recent years. The disease is common in countries where sheep raising is practiced, dogs are numerous, and hygiene is defective. The immediate host becomes infected by ingesting eggs in contaminated food or water; man is an intermediate host. The cysts may attain a considerable size in the brain, and are surrounded by a very thin membrane unless they are in contact with the meninges, in which case a fibrous capsule develops. There is some edema around the cyst or cysts. The local inflammatory reaction in the brain can be marked, with lymphocytes, eosinophils, and plasma cells in large numbers. A cyst can erode the skull, or by pressing upon the ventricular system can cause internal hydrocephalus. Hydatid cysts are more commonly found in the cerebrum than in the posterior fossa or spinal cord.

Clinical Features. Children are more affected than adults. The symptoms are those of raised intracranial pressure, together with localizing signs which depend on the situation of the cyst.[8, 52] As in some other intracranial space-taking lesions, the symptoms fluctuate a good deal from time to time. Straight x-rays are commonly negative except in the occasional case with calcification of the cyst wall. Arteriography discloses large rounded masses of characteristic appearance. The spinal fluid may be entirely normal, but occasionally eosinophils have been present. There is not always eosinophilia in the blood; it depends on whether the disease is active or not. The Casoni test is often negative. Secondary infection of the cyst with formation of a brain abscess is not uncommon and is very likely to follow exploratory puncture. There may be evidence of hydatid disease elsewhere, including the spinal cord, in which situation cysts are usually found in the epidural space. Surgical treatment is unsatisfactory because the intraspinal cyst often communicates with other cysts in the spine, ribs, and pleura.

MISCELLANEOUS CONDITIONS

Neurological Sequelae of Spinal Tap and Spinal Anesthesia

Neurological complications following spinal anesthesia, apart from low pressure headache, have become uncommon over the years, owing largely to improvements in technique and in the preparation and storage of anesthetic solutions. In a prospective study by Dripps and Vandamm, only one of 8460 patients developed incapacitating neurological symptoms following administration of anesthetic, and this was found to be due to an unsuspected spinal cord meningioma. Sixty-six patients complained of paresthesias in the lower limb or perineum, and in 23 of these there was sensory impairment; two other patients had temporary unilateral foot drop. Marinacci examined the records of 542 patients with neurological deficits attributed to spinal anesthesia and found a possible causal relationship in only four, of which two were doubtful.

Nevertheless, a variety of disabilities have been reported following this procedure, and they continue to occur at rare intervals.[65, 88] Before attributing symptoms and signs to spinal anesthesia, it is desirable to rule out other possibilities. In the first place, the anesthetic may have brought into prominence a hitherto unsuspected disease. Second, a distinction must be made between disabilities caused by the anesthetic and those resulting from the operative procedure itself. Third, a pressure palsy can be caused by improper placement of the lower limbs during anesthesia, too tight a plaster cast, or tourniquet paralysis.

Infection can be carried into the subarachnoid space by contaminated material or equipment, in which event a bacterial meningitis makes its appearance within 24 hours. In other cases, evidence of meningeal irritation is milder and the cerebrospinal fluid is found to contain an excess of polymorphs and lymphocytes but is and remains sterile on culture.[65]

Cranial nerve palsies have been described following spinal anesthesia, the abducens being most frequently involved. It is usually associated with postspinal postural headache, and both symptoms are of short duration.

Cerebrovascular accidents, arising as a result of hypotension induced by spinal anesthesia, can occur, especially if there is stenosis of the carotid, vertebral, or basilar artery. However, since it is usually possible to detect and combat hypotensive episodes at once, rapid recovery usually takes place. Needless to say, hypotension occurring during surgery under spinal anesthesia is not necessarily due to the anesthetic.

Arachnoiditis and arachnoiditis with myelopathy are the most serious complications of spinal anesthesia. Schwarz and Bevilacqua[88] have reported a case and have culled 31 cases with postmortem findings from the literature. Pathological changes include diffuse arachnoidal adhesions, demyelination in the spinal roots and cauda equina, and damage to the spinal cord. The latter consists of spotty or diffuse demyelination, focal necrosis, or widespread softening, and secondary demyelination of the posterior columns is seen above the major area of destruction in the lower portion of the spinal cord. An important feature is diffuse involvement of the small vessels of the roots, leptomeninges, and cord. Small arteries show thickening of the intima, duplication of the elastica, destruction of the media, and fibrosis of the adventitia.

Clinically, the symptoms appear immediately and consist of varying degrees of weakness of the legs—a flaccid paraplegia if the cauda equina is involved, and a spastic paraplegia if the main impact is above the conus. Sensory loss and sphincter paralysis have been present in many cases. Milder examples of what is presumed to be the same condition present with paresthesias, sphincter symptoms, and loss of the tendon reflexes in the legs. Some of these patients lose their symptoms after a period of several months.

There is a second group of cases, also small, in which a chronic adhesive arachnoiditis develops slowly in the lumbar region and may progress upwards until it involves the thoracic and cervical regions. Symptoms develop slowly and insidiously, with a gradual appearance of signs of cord compression and root involvement at multiple sites in the same patient. These developments may or may not be preceded by the symptoms and signs of aseptic meningitis. The condition can also be encountered in patients who have never had a spinal anesthetic. The symptoms tend to fluctuate in severity. The spinal fluid is normal as to contents, unless the subarachnoid space is completely blocked. Myelography either discloses a complete block, or the opaque medium may be seen threading its way through areas of adhesions. The treatment of arachnoiditis is unsatisfactory; the adhesions cannot be peeled from the cord without considerable risk of aggravating the condition. Single large cystic collections can be opened, but in the author's experience, any relief brought about by this procedure is only temporary.

Arachnoiditis

Etiology. Thickening and adhesions of the leptomeninges are usually the result of previous meningitis, neurosyphilis, injury, tumors, subarachnoid hemorrhage, or the injection of spinal anesthetics or radiopaque oils contaminated by antiseptics or detergents. In a few cases, however, there is no evidence of any such factor.

Clinical Features. Adhesions between the meninges and the cortex are usually the result of a head injury, and can be responsible for post-traumatic seizures. Pneumoencephalography may show dilatation of the lateral ventricle on the affected side together with pooling of air over the cicatrix, but when the adhesions are dense, there can be no local cortical collection of air because the subarachnoid space is obliterated over the affected area.

Arachnoiditis around the chiasm is an occasional source of intermittently progressive loss of vision in both eyes.[36] The visual fields may take almost any form and the condition can be diagnosed with certainty only at operation; surgical removal of the adhesions is of doubtful value.

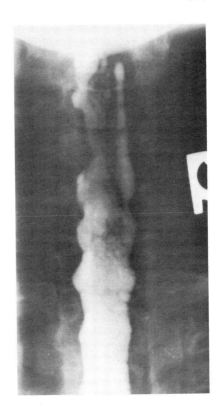

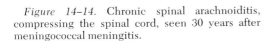
Figure 14–14. Chronic spinal arachnoiditis, compressing the spinal cord, seen 30 years after meningococcal meningitis.

Adhesions around the tentorium can obstruct the upward flow of the cerebrospinal fluid over the cerebral hemispheres, thus causing hydrocephalus (p. 207). Adhesions around the fourth ventricle may obstruct the outflow of cerebrospinal fluid, with consequent internal hydrocephalus (the Dandy-Walker syndrome). This gives rise to papilledema, with or without mild ataxia of gait. Ventriculography shows a characteristically ballooned appearance of the fourth ventricle, in contradistinction to the obliteration or distortion of the ventricle seen in intraventricular tumors. Relief can be obtained by surgery.

Spinal arachnoid adhesions can be localized or diffuse[11]; in some cases, they are associated with encysted collections of cerebrospinal fluid (meningitis serosa circumscripta).[39] Such collections can compress the cord (Fig. 14–14), but in other cases it would seem that root pains, weakness, and sensory loss in the legs occur without actual compression and the symptoms are then attributed to impairment of the blood supply to the cord. Manometric tests usually show complete or incomplete block, and myelography gives rise to a very characteristic picture, the opaque medium threading its way into the area of adhesions. Surgical removal of an encysted collection can produce some improvement, but any attempt to peel the adhesions off the cord is liable to aggravate matters.

Behçet's Disease

Behçet's disease[16] is rare, is suspected to be of viral origin, and is characterized by recurrent attacks of stomatitis, scrotal and vulval inflammation, indolent ulcers of the skin, and inflammation of the eye — conjunctivitis, uveitis, keratitis, or retinitis. In a few cases, recurrent neurological disturbances have developed, the brain showing perivascular cellular infiltrations in the white matter, together with multiple small softenings, apparently related to thrombosis of small vessels.[16, 19]

The neurological symptoms may take the form of headache, stiffness of the neck, lethargy, and symptoms suggestive of multiple small lesions of the brainstem —vertigo, diplopia, dysphagia, and weakness of one or more limbs.[41] Retrobulbar neuritis has been reported. There may be progressive dementia, with or without a previous history of intermittent neurological incidents reminiscent of multiple sclerosis. In acute attacks, the spinal fluid shows an excess of lymphocytes and sometimes a raised protein content. The course is usually remittent, with either complete or incomplete recovery between attacks. Of 20 patients reported in the literature, eight have died within three years of the appearance of the initial neurological symptoms.

Benign Myalgic Encephalomyelitis

Sometimes called Icelandic disease,[1] or epidemic neuromyositis, this condition occurred in small epidemics in Iceland (1948), London (1955), Washington, D.C. (1957), Newcastle-on-Tyne (1961), and Greenville, Illinois (1963). Sporadic cases are occasionally seen. It usually occurs in residential institutions, is much more common in women than in men, and is characterized by a marked discrepancy between the severity of symptoms and the paucity of objective signs. This discrepancy, coupled with the circumstance that the disorder tends to produce depression and hysterical reactions in patients whose premorbid personality is unstable, is apt to lead the unwary to conclude that the disorder is entirely psychosomatic. While it is possible that some of the cases seen in institutional epidemics may result from suggestion, not all physicians who have encountered these cases subscribe to the psychogenic theory.

The pathology is not known because the disease is not fatal. At the onset, there is often a mild upper respiratory infection, sometimes associated with gastrointestinal symptoms, slight pyrexia, and lymphadenopathy. There may be difficulty in focusing. Muscular pain in the neck is an early symptom, and it spreads to involve the trunk and limbs. The painful muscles are tender and there is focal or generalized weakness. In addition, there is a severe asthenia. Weakness of the muscles of respiration, hemiparesis, and paraplegia have been recorded. A curious feature about the neurological symptoms is that, although there may be profound weakness, the tendon reflexes are often conserved and the plantar responses are usually flexor. Sensory loss is usually minimal or absent, but paresthesias may be prominent and may have an irregular distribution.

The cerebrospinal fluid is usually normal, but a lymphocytic leukocytosis has been seen in a few cases. In some cases, electromyography has disclosed groups of spike action potentials with silent intervals between the groups. Creatinuria has been reported. In contrast to polymyositis, the sedimentation rate is normal.

Course and Prognosis. The course of the illness is remittent, with periods of improvement and deterioration, but ultimate recovery is usual within the year. However, the patient tends to remain extremely fatigable for many months and in some cases there have been relapses over several years after the original attack.

Diagnosis. It is difficult to identify this disease when it occurs sporadically. It may mimic the early stages of dermatomyositis and polymyalgia rheumatica, and the fact that the sedimentation rate may be within normal limits in the early stages of these conditions complicates the issue. The administration of steroids gives symptomatic relief, but the same applies to polymyalgia rheumatica and other forms of myositis.

Treatment. Steroids deserve a trial. In the author's limited experience, prednisone (10 mg. three times a day, tapering off to 5 mg. twice daily) has provided partial relief. Depression has to be countered by appropriate psychotropic drugs.

Chorea
(Sydenham's Chorea, St. Vitus's Dance, Rheumatic Chorea)

Chorea, an acute disease of children and adolescents, is characterized by widespread choreiform movements, hypotonia, and a high incidence of chronic rheumatic heart disease at a later date.

Etiology. The disease is unknown under the age of three, has a maximum incidence between 10 and 15 years, and is rare thereafter except when associated with pregnancy. It is closely linked with rheumatic fever and rheumatic carditis in that there is often a previous history of growing pains, rheumatic fever, recurrent tonsillitis, scarlet fever, or erythema nodosum, while chorea itself may have been the sole "rheumatic" manifestation in the previous history of patients with rheumatic heart disease. It may occur in the early months of pregnancy, with or without a previous history of rheumatic disease. Both rheumatic fever and chorea have been becoming progressively less common over the past four decades in communities with a high standard of living.

Pathology. The lesions are slight and difficult to demonstrate. Degeneration of neurons is found in the cortex, basal ganglia, substantia nigra, and dentate nucleus of the cerebellum. There may be very slight inflammatory change in the pia, and a mild degree of lymphocytic perivascular cuffing may be found. Endarteritis may be present in the smaller vessels. Evidence of rheumatic carditis has been found in 90 per cent of cases coming to autopsy, and the brain may show small infarcts, probably of embolic origin.

Clinical Features. These are determined by the location of the lesions in the cortex (weakness of muscles, irritability, excitement), basal ganglia (involuntary movements), and cerebellum (hypotonia and incoordination). The onset is usually insidious, with apathy or irritability, and some clumsiness of gait; objects may be dropped for no apparent reason, and admonition tends to aggravate the disability to such an extent that parents or schoolteachers may attribute the symptoms to "nerves." At this early stage, however, careful observation will often reveal fleeting grimaces or brief twitches of the fingers. The movements rapidly increase in number and vigor until there is no longer any doubt as to the nature of the disease. They are rapid and jerky, and exhibit an ever-changing distribution which is quite unlike the stereotyped movements of a psychogenic tic. Involuntary movements of the tongue, lips, palate, and muscles of respiration produce dysarthria and may embarrass swallowing. Ocular movements are rarely affected, but the lids may screw up suddenly, or the eyebrows may twitch upward. The head may jerk from side to side, and the abdominal wall is frequently involved. The upper limbs are more seriously affected than the lower. The fingers suddenly flex, extend, or adduct, and involuntary movements of the elbow and shoulder vary from slight twitches to violent displacements which may cause painful bruises from collisions with surrounding objects. Voluntary movements are also interfered with by hypotonia, incoordination, and true muscular weakness. The grip fluctuates in strength from moment to moment, and the outstretched hand assumes a characteristic posture, with flexion of the wrists and hyperextension of the metacarpophalangeal joints; the forearm is often pronated. If the arms are raised above the head, the palms turn outward. The gait is clumsy, and falls are frequent. Occasionally the involuntary movements are confined to one side (hemichorea). Some degree of weakness is always present, and in certain instances it is extreme, the child lying limply with the head lolling to one side (limp chorea); this is a benign form.

There is no disorder of the special senses or of somatic sensation. Tendon reflexes are sluggish. If the legs are allowed to hang over the side of the bed, a tap on the ligamentum patellae elicits a sluggish reflex, and the leg goes on swinging for a few seconds thereafter—a pendular knee jerk. In other cases, however, the reflex contraction of the quadriceps may be unduly sustained for a fragment of a second owing to the occurrence of a simultaneous choreiform contraction of the muscle. The abdominal and plantar reflexes are usually normal; exceptionally, an extensor response bears witness to pyramidal involvement.

Emotional instability is almost the rule and may be the presenting symptom. Excitement bordering on delirium occurs in severe cases, and both it and the choreiform movements are much aggravated by surrounding noise and movement. Mania, depression, and hallucinations occasionally occur, especially in young adults and in chorea gravidarum.

Constitutional symptoms are slight or absent. There is no fever in mild cases, but hyperpyrexia can be a terminal event. Pallor of the skin and moderate hypochromic anemia are frequently observed, and if carditis is present, the erythrocyte sedimentation rate is usually increased. Other manifestations of rheumatic infection may be present, notably rheumatic arthritis, subcutaneous nodules, erythema nodosum, or tonsillitis, but they are more likely to appear in the past history than to accompany the chorea.

Diagnosis. Choreiform movements are pleomorphic, in contrast to the stereotyped movement which is characteristic of psychogenic tics. Congenital and "senile" chorea cannot cause confusion in diagnosis. Acute epidemic encephalitis may include choreiform movements in its symptomatology, but could be identified by the presence of lethargy, ocular palsies, and fever during the epidemic of 1915–1920. Huntington's chorea occurs in the second half of life. Patients who have had chorea in adolescence sometimes reproduce the symptoms in mild degree many years later as a manifestation of conversion hysteria. However, chorea itself recurs in mild forms in 20 to 30 per cent of all cases during the year or two following the initial attack.

Course and Prognosis. Chorea can last from three to 10 weeks but sometimes persists for many months. It is difficult to know when it is finally cured because convalescence may be interrupted by occasional movements, clumsiness, or attacks of emotional instability. Death occurs in less than 2 per cent of all cases. Hyperpyrexia and severe delirium are of serious import. Chorea gravidarum carries a somewhat higher death rate if untreated (by therapeutic abortion), and there may be recurrences with subsequent pregnancies. Rheumatic carditis is seldom fatal in the acute stage of the disease, but whether it has been present or not during the attack of chorea, chronic rheumatic valvular disease is likely to appear in later life.

Treatment. There is no specific treatment. Bed rest is essential. If movements are violent, the sides of the cot should be padded to prevent injury. The child should be isolated from others in order to avoid exciting factors which increase the severity of the movements. Meals should be small, frequent, and of high caloric value, and should be supplemented by vitamins. Tube feedings should be resorted to at once if there is difficulty in swallowing. Restlessness can be treated by use of phenobarbitone or chlorpromazine in doses appropriate to the child's age. It is usual to give calcium aspirin for its supposed antirheumatic effect, and for its sedative value in children. If sleeplessness cannot otherwise be controlled and is causing exhaustion, hyoscine hydrobromide is a useful soporific. Chorea gravidarum can be terminated by removal of the fetus. In mild cases, however, it will disappear at term.

Mollaret's Meningitis

Mollaret's meningitis, which may be a syndrome rather than a disease, has been reported repeatedly in the European literature.[25] It is a benign recurrent meningitis, characterized by attacks of headache, neck rigidity, and a positive Kernig sign, together with fever, general malaise, muscular pains, vomiting, and occasionally a convulsive seizure. There are no signs of focal neurological damage. The attacks come on abruptly and last only two or three days, *but are apt to recur* at intervals of weeks or months. During the attack, there is a sharp rise in the white cell count of the spinal fluid, with a predominance of lymphocytes and large monocytes. There is a moderate rise of protein, but the sugar content remains normal.

Sarcoidosis

Boeck's sarcoid causes a chronic relapsing inflammatory disease which is sometimes interrupted by subacute exacerbations, and which is characterized by the presence of multiple granulomas in the viscera, skin, and bones. Of 537 cases studied by James and his colleagues,[60] there was intrathoracic involvement in 82 per cent, ocular disease in 58 per cent, cutaneous lesions in 29 per cent, lymphadenopathy in 26 per cent, splenomegaly in 10 per cent, neurological disease in 7 per cent, enlargement of the parotid gland in 1 per cent, and of the lacrimal gland in two cases. Asymptomatic involvement of muscles is not uncommon, but in rare instances it gives rise to a slowly progressive proximal myopathy.[100] The liver and the small bones of the hands and feet are often involved.

Etiology. The cause is unknown. Many of these patients used to die of tuberculosis and it was thought that the two diseases were related. This suspicion was fortified by the circumstance that in sarcoidosis, the tuberculin reaction is often negative, but it has been found that this anergy applies to other antigens as well. The disease can occur at any age and in either sex. In the United States, it is more common in blacks than in whites, but in South Africa, it is more common in the white population.

Pathology. In the nervous system, the disease commonly occurs as a chronic, patchy granulomatous leptomeningitis, which causes paralysis of one or more cranial nerves and may also give rise to an obstructive hydrocephalus.[61] Massive granulomas may occur within the brain substance. Peripheral neuritis is not uncommon. The muscles, including the heart, are often invaded. An unexplained hypercalcemia occurs in some cases, and this can lead to renal insufficiency from nephrocalcinosis. Extreme involvement of the lung parenchyma can produce cor pulmonale.

Clinical Features. Sarcoidosis is often accompanied by malaise, and a low-grade fever may persist for months. There is often enlargement of the spleen, liver, and lymph glands, and there may be localized osteoporosis of the phalanges and other small bones of the hands and feet. The lungs and hilar glands are frequently affected. However, systemic involvement may be inconspicuous in patients with involvement of the nervous system. Uveitis is the most common ocular manifestation, but nodular conjunctivitis, keratitis, and retinopathy are not rare. Optic neuritis is not uncommon and may progress to optic atrophy. Papilledema is occasionally encountered as a result of hydrocephalus. Diabetes insipidus and hypersomnia have been reported.

Involvement of the brain[60, 61] causes seizures, or a tumor syndrome with symptoms appropriate to its situation. The most common neurological presentation is paralysis of one or more cranial nerves. The facial nerves are most often involved, but diplopia, deafness, vertigo, and unilateral paralysis of the palate or tongue are not rare. Uveoparotid polyneuritis is a relatively acute form, characterized by fever, swelling of the parotid glands, bilateral facial palsy, and polyneuritis. Leptomeningitis can give rise to obstructive hydrocephalus with headache, stiffness of the neck, papilledema and an excess of cells in the cerebrospinal fluid. Lesions of the spinal cord are rare. The peripheral nerves can be involved singly, or in the form of a more or less symmetrical polyneuritis. A slowly progressive proximal myopathy can occur.[100]

Laboratory Aids. Secondary anemia with moderate leukocytosis is not uncommon and the serum globulin is elevated in about 50 per cent of all cases.

Hypercalcemia can occur. The tuberculin test is negative in about 50 per cent of all cases. The spinal fluid may be normal even when the nervous system is involved, but in some cases there is a moderate pleocytosis and excess of protein, the glucose content remaining normal. The Kveim test (production of a skin nodule by intradermal injection of sarcoid material) is positive in some cases but not in all. Diagnostic assistance is often obtained as a result of biopsy from skin, muscle, lymph nodes, or spleen. X-ray changes in the lung and small bones of the hands and feet can be of diagnostic assistance.

Course and Prognosis. Sarcoidosis is a benign but persistent disease. Intermissions, remissions, and exacerbations are not uncommon. Spontaneous recovery is usual, but death can occur from sarcoidal involvement of the cardiac conducting system, from heart failure due to cor pulmonale, and from renal failure.

Treatment. Long-term administration of steroids (for example, 5 mg. of prednisone four times a day) can help to control the disease. Satisfactory results have also been obtained from oxyphenbutazone, 100 mg. four times a day.[59] If tuberculosis develops in the course of the disease, it can be treated successfully by appropriate methods.

REFERENCES

1. Acheson, E. D.: The clinical syndrome variously called benign myelitis, Iceland disease and epidemic neuro-myasthenia. *Amer. J. Med.* 26:569, 1959.
2. Adams, R. D., and Weinstein, L.: Clinical and pathological aspects of encephalitis. *New Eng. J. Med.* 239:865, 1948.
3. Adie, W. J.: Tonic pupils and absent tendon reflexes. *Brain* 55:98, 1932.
4. Altrocchi, T. H.: Acute spinal epidural abscess vs. acute transverse myelopathy. *Arch. Neurol.* 9:18, 1963.
5. Anderson, W. K.: *Malarial Psychoses and Neuroses.* Oxford Medical Publications, New York, 1927.
6. Argyll Robertson, D.: Four cases of spinal miosis, with remarks on the action of light on the pupil. *Edinburgh Med. J.* 15:487, 1869.
7. Asenjo, A., Valladares, H., and Fierro, J.: Tuberculomas of the brain. *Arch. Neurol. Psychiat.* 65:146, 1951.
8. Ayres, C. M., Davey, L. M., and German, W. J.: Cerebral hydatidosis. *J. Neurosurg.* 20:371, 1963.
9. Baker, A. B., and Noran, H. H.: Western Variety of equine encephalitis in man. *Arch. Neurol. Psychiat.* 47:565, 1942.
10. Baker, A. B., Matzke, H. A., and Brown, J. R.: Bulbar poliomyelitis: a study of medullary function. *Arch. Neurol. Psychiat.* 63:257, 1950.
11. Barker, L. F., and Ford, F. R.: Chronic arachnoiditis obliterating the spinal subarachnoid space. *J.A.M.A.* 109:785, 1937.
12. Barter, A. P., and Falconer, M. A.: Actinomycosis of the brain. *Guy. Hosp. Rep.* 104:35, 1955.
13. Batson, O. V.: The role of the vertebral veins in metastatic processes. *Ann. Int. Med.* 16:38, 1942.
14. Baylis, J. H.: The effect of transection on the ascent of tetanus toxin in the rabbit's spinal cord. *J. Path. Bact.* 64:47, 1952.
15. Beeson, P. B., and Hankey, D. D.: Leptospiral meningitis. *Arch. Int. Med.* 89:575, 1952.
16. Behçet, H.: Some observations on the clinical features of the so-called triple symptom complex. *Determatologica* 81:73, 1940.
16a. Bell, W. E., and Lascari, A. D.: Rocky Mountain spotted fever: Neurological symptoms in the acute phase. Neurology 20:841, 1970.
17. Berman, S. J.: Therapy of *Plasmodium falciparum malaria. J.A.M.A.* 207:128, 1969.
18. Bickerstaff, E. R.: Brainstem encephalitis: Further observations on a grave syndrome with a benign prognosis. *Brit. Med. J.* 1:1384, 1957.
19. Bienenstock, H., and Margulies, M. E.: Behçet's syndrome: Report of a case with extensive neurologic manifestations. *New Eng. J. Med.* 264:1342, 1961.
20. Blatt, N. H., and Lepper, M. H.: Reactions following antirabies prophylaxis. *Amer. J. Dis. Child.* 80:395, 1953.
21. Botulism in the United States, U.S. Department of Health, Education, and Welfare, Review of Cases, 1899–1967.
22. Bowers, V. M., and Danforth, D. N.: The significance of poliomyelitis during pregnancy. *Amer. J. Obstet. Gynec.* 65:34, 1953.
23. Brain, W. R., Greenfield, J. G., and Russell, O. S.: Subacute inclusion encephalitis (Dawson Type). *Brain* 71:365, 1948.
24. Browne, S. G.: Some less common neurological findings in leprosy. *J. Neurol. Sci.* 2:253, 1965.
25. Bruyn, G. W., Straathof, L. J. A., and Raymakers, G.: Mollaret's meningitis. *Neurology* 12:745, 1962.
26. Butler, W. T., Alling, T. W., Spickard, A., and Utz, J. P.: Diagnostic and prognostic value of clinical and laboratory findings in cryptococcal meningitis. *New Eng. J. Med.* 270:59, 1964.
27. Carithers, H. A., Carithers, C. M., and Edwards, R. O.: Cat scratch disease. *J.A.M.A.* 207:312, 1969.

28. Cochrane, R. G.: *Leprosy in Theory and Practice.* John Wright, Bristol, England, 1959.
29. Conant, N. F., Martin, D. S., Smith, D. T., Baker, R. D., and Callaway, J. L.: *Manual of Clinical Mycology.* 2nd Ed., W. B. Saunders Co., Philadelphia, 1954.
30. Connolly, J. H., Allen, I. V., Hurwitz, L. J., and Millar, J. H. D.: Subacute sclerosing panencephalitis. *Brain* 59:625, 1968.
31. Courville, C. B., and Rosenvold, L. K.: Intracranial complications of infections of nasal cavities and accessory sinuses: A survey of lesions observed in a series of 15,000 autopsies. *Arch. Otolaryng.* 27:692, 1938.
32. Dattner, B., Thomas, E. W., and Wexler, G.: *The Management of Neurosyphilis.* Grune and Stratton, Inc., New York, 1944.
33. Dawson, J. R.: Cellular inclusions in cerebral lesions of epidemic encephalitis. *Arch. Neurol. Psychiat.* 31:685, 1934.
34. Denny-Brown, D., Adams, R. D., and Fitz-Gerald, P. J.: Pathological features of herpes zoster. *Arch. Neurol. Psychiat.* 5:216, 1944.
35. Dickerson, R. B., Newton, J. R., and Hansem, J. E.: Diagnosis and immediate prognosis of Japanese B encephalitis. *Amer. J. Med.* 12:277, 1952.
36. Dickman, G. H., Cramer, F. K., and Kaplan, A. D.: Optochiasmatic arachnoiditis: Surgical treatment and results. *J. Neurosurg.* 8:355, 1951.
37. Dixon, H. B., and Hargreaves, W. H.: Cysticercosis (*Taenia solium*). *Quart. J. Med.* 13:107, 1944.
38. Dutton, J. E. M., and Alexander, G. L.: Intramedullary spinal abscess. *J. Neurol. Neurosurg. Psychiat.* 17:303, 1954.
39. Elkington, J. St.C.: Meningitis serosa circumscripta spinalis. *Brain* 59:181, 1936.
40. Elliott, F. A.: The treatment of herpes zoster with high doses of prednisone. *Lancet* 2:610, 1964.
41. Evans, A. D., Pallis, C. A., and Spillane, J. D.: Involvement of the nervous system in Behçet's syndrome. *Lancet* 2:349, 1957.
42. Farmer, T. W., and Janeway, C. A.: Infections with the virus of lymphocytic choriomeningitis. *Medicine* 21:1, 1942.
43. Feemster, R. F.: Eastern equine encephalitis. *Neurology* 8:882, 1958.
44. Finley, K. H., *et al.*: Western encephalitis and cerebral ontogenesis. *Arch. Neurol.* 16:140, 1967.
45. Forbes, G. B., and Auld, M.: The management of tetanus. *Amer. J. Med.* 18:947, 1955.
46. Freeman, J. M., Magoffin, R. L., Lennette, E. H., and Herndon, R. M.: Additional evidence of the relation between subacute inclusion-body encephalitis and measles virus. *Lancet* 2:129, 1967.
47. Gajdusek, C.: Discussion on kuru, scrapie, and experimental kuru-like syndrome in chimpanzees. *Current Topics in Microbiology and Immunology* 40:59, 1967.
48. Gelfand, M.: *Schistosomiasis in South Central Africa.* Juta and Co., Ltd., Cape Town, South Africa, 1950.
49. Gibbs, C. J.: Infectious etiology in chronic and subacute degenerative diseases. *Current Topics in Microbiology and Immunology* 40:44, 1967.
50. Gibbs, C. J., and Gajdusek, C.: Infection as the etiology of spongiform encephalopathy (Creutzfeldt-Jakob disease). *Science* 165:1023, 1969.
51. Glaser, G. H., Solitare, G. B., and Manuelides, E. E.: Acute and subacute inclusion encephalitis. *Res. Pub. Ass. Nerv. Ment. Dis.* 44:178, 1964.
52. Goinard, P., and Descuns, P.: Echinococcus cysts of the nervous system. *Rev. Neurol.* 86:369, 1952.
53. Greene, N. M.: Neurological sequelae of spinal anesthesia. *Anesthesiology* 22:682, 1961.
54. Hadlow, W. J.: Scrapie and kuru. *Lancet* 2:289, 1959.
55. Haymaker, W., Girdany, B. R., Stevens, J., Lillie, R. D., and Felterman, G. H.: Cerebral involvement and periventricular calcification in generalized cytomegalic inclusion disease. *J. Neuropath. Exp. Neurol.* 13:562, 1954.
56. Haymaker, W., and Sabin, A. B.: Topographic distribution of lesions in the central nervous system in Japanese B encephalitis. *Arch. Neurol. Psychiat.* 57:673, 1947.
57. Heusner, A. P.: Non-tuberculous spinal epidural infections. *New Eng. J. Med.* 239:845, 1948.
58. Hurst, E. W.: Acute hemorrhagic leuco-encephalitis: A previously undefined entity. *Med. J. Austral.* 2:1, 1941.
59. James, D. G., Carstairs, L. S., Trowell, J., and Sharma, O. R.: Treatment of sarcoidosis. *Lancet* 2:526, 1967.
60. James, D. G., and Sharma, O. R.: Neurological complications of sarcoidosis. *Proc. Roy. Soc. Med.* 60:1169, 1967.
61. Jefferson, M.: Sarcoidosis in the nervous system. *Brain* 80:540, 1957.
62. Katz, M., Rorke, L. B., Masland, W. S., Koprowski, H., and Tucker, S. H.: Transmission of an encephalitogenic agent from brains of patients with subacute sclerosing panencephalitis to ferrets. *New Eng. J. Med.* 279:793, 1968.
63. Kloetzel, K.: Clinical patterns in severe tetanus. *J.A.M.A.* 185:559, 1963.
64. Koppisch, E.: *Protozoal and Helminthic Infection in Pathology.* Edited by Anderson, W. A. D., Henry Kimpton, London, 1953.
65. Kremer, M.: Meningitis after spinal anesthesia. *Brit. Med. J.* 2:4418, 1945.
66. Loeser, E., and Scheinberg, L.: Brain abscess, a review of 99 cases. *Neurology* 7:601, 1957.
67. Macrae, J., and Campbell, A. M. G.: Neurological complications of mumps. *Brit. Med. J.* 2:259, 1949.
68. Malamud, N., Haymaker, W., and Pinkerton, H.: Inclusion encephalitis. *Amer. J. Path.* 26:133, 1950.
69. Margolis, G., and Kilham, L.: Virus induced cerebellar hypoplasia. *Res. Pub. Assoc. Nerv. Ment. Dis.* 44:113, 1964.
70. Martins, A. M., Kempe, L. G., and Hayes, G.H.: Acute haemorrhagic leucoencephalitis

(Hurst) with concurrent primary herpes simplex infection. *J. Neurol. Neurosurg. Psychiat.* 27:493, 1964.

71. Meade, R. H.: Treatment of meningitis. *J.A.M.A.* 185:1023, 1963.

72. Merriam, J. C., and Tedeschi, C. G.: Cerebral mucormycosis. *Neurology* 7:510, 1957.

73. Merritt, H. H., Adams, R. D., and Solomon, H. C.: *Neurosyphilis.* Oxford University Press, New York, 1946.

74. Merritt, H. H., and Springlova, M.: Lissauer's dementia paralytica. *Arch. Neurol. Psychiat.* 27:987, 1932.

75. Minnesota Poliomyelitis Research Commission, Minneapolis: Bulbar form of poliomyelitis: Diagnosis and correlation of clinical with physiologic and pathologic manifestations. *J.A.M.A.* 134;757, 1947.

76. Neal, J. B.: *Encephalitis: A Clinical Study.* Grune and Stratton, Inc., New York, 1942.

77. Obrador, S.: Clinical aspects of cerebral cysticercosis. *Arch. Neurol. Psychiat.* 59:457, 1948.

78. Parkinson, T.: Rare manifestations of herpes zoster. *Brit. Med. J.* 1:8, 1948.

79. Pawan, J. L.: Paralysis as manifestation of human rabies. *Ann. Trop. Med.* 33:21, 1937.

80. Plum, F.: Poliomyelitis. *Clinical Neurology.* Edited by Baker, A. B., Paul B. Hoeber Medical Div., Harper and Row, New York, 1962, Vol. 3.

81. Prockop, L. D., and Silva-Hutner, M.: Cephalic mucormycosis. *Arch. Neurol.* 17:379, 1967.

82. Richardson, E. P.: Progressive multifocal leucoencephalopathy. *New Eng. J. Med.* 265:815, 1961.

83. Riggs, S., Smith, D. L., and Phillips, C. A.: St. Louis encephalitis in adults during the 1964 Houston epidemic. *J.A.M.A.* 193:284, 1965.

84. Rubin, H., Lehan, P. H., Doto, I. L., Chin, T. D., Heeren, R. H., Johnson, O., Wenner, H. A., and Fercolow, M. L.: Epidemic infection with Coxsackie virus Group B, Type 5, clinical and epidemiological aspects. *New Eng. J. Med.* 258:255, 1958.

85. Sachs, E., and House, R. K.: The Ramsey-Hunt syndrome: Geniculate herpes, *Neurology* 6:262, 1956.

86. Sahs, A. L., and Joynt, R. J.: Meningitis. *Clinical Neurology.* Edited by Baker, A. B., Paul B. Hoeber Medical Div., Harper and Row, New York, 1962, pp. 717–773.

87. Schiller, F., and Shadle, O. W.: Extrathecal and intrathecal suppuration. *Arch. Neurol.* 7:331, 1962.

88. Schwarz, G. A., and Bevilacqua, J. E.: Paraplegia following spinal anaesthesia: Clinico-pathologic report and review of literature. *Arch. Neurol.* 10:308, 1964.

89. Shaw, C. M., and Alond, E. C.: Cava septi pellucidi et vergae: Their normal and pathological states. *Brain* 92:213, 1969.

90. Short, D. H., Knox, J. M., Glicksman, J.: Neuro-

syphilis, the search for adequate treatment. *Arch. Dermat.* 93:87, 1966.

91. Smith, A. C.: The treatment of severe tetanus by paralyzing drugs and intermittent pressure respiration. *Proc. Roy. Soc. Med.* 51: 1006, 1958.

92. Smith, P. C.: Neurological complications of glandular fever (infectious mononucleosis). *Brain* 88:323, 1965.

93. Swanson, H. S., and Smith, W. A.: Torular granuloma simulating cerebral tumor. *Arch. Neurol. Psychiat.* 51:426, 1944.

94. Swinburne, G.: The surgical pathology of brain abscess. *Med. J. Austral.* 2:169, 1948.

95. Turner, J. W. A.: Spinal cord lesions in cerebrospinal fever. *Lancet* 1:398, 1948.

96. Tymes, B. S., Crutcher, J. C., and Utz, G. P.: Histoplasma meningitis. *Ann. Int. Med.* 59:615, 1963.

97. VanBogaert, L.: Sur une leucoencephalite sclerosante subaigue. *J. Neurol. Neurosurg. Psychiat.* 8:101, 1945.

98. Von Economo, C.: *Encephalitis Lethargica: Its Sequelae and Treatment.* Oxford University Press, New York, 1921.

99. Wakefield, G. S., Carroll, J. D., and Speed, D. E.: Schistosomiasis of the spinal cord. *Brain* 85:535, 1962.

100. Wallace, S. L., Lattes, R., Malia, J. P., and Ragan, C.: Muscle involvement in Boeck's sarcoid. *Ann. Int. Med.* 48:497, 1958.

101. Walton, K. W.: The pathology of a fatal case of psittacosis. showing intracytoplasmic inclusions in the meninges. *J. Path. Bact.* 68:565, 1954.

102. Weaver, O. M., Pieper, S., and Kurland, R.: Japanese encephalitis sequelae. *Neurology* 8:888, 1958.

103. Wilner, E., and Brody, J. A.: Prognosis of general paresis after treatment. *Lancet* 2:1370, 1968.

104. Wolstenholme, G. E. W., and Porter, R. (eds.): *Systemic Mycoses.* Little, Brown and Co., Boston, 1968.

105. Zacks, S. I., Langfitt, T. W., and Elliott, F. A.: Post-herpetic neuritis. A light and electron-microscopic study. *Neurology* 14:744, 1964.

106. Zacks, S. I., Metzger, J. F., Smith, C. W., and Blumberg, J. M.: Localization of ferritin labelled botulinus toxin in the neuromuscular junction of the mouse. *J. Neuropath. Exp. Neurol.* 21:610, 1962.

107. Zacks, S. I., Rhoades, M. Y., and Sheff, M. F.: The localization of botulinum A toxin in the mouse, *J. Exp. Molec. Path.* 9:77, 1968.

108. Zacks, S. I., and Sheff, M. F.: Tetanism: Pathobiological aspects of tetanal toxin in the nervous system and skeletal muscle. Academic Press, Inc., New York, *Neurosciences Research*, 3:209, 1970.

109. Zu Rhein, G. M., and Chou, S.: Particles resembling papova virus in human demyelinating disease. *Science* 148:1477, 1965.

CHAPTER FIFTEEN

Vascular Disease of the Brain and Spinal Cord

THE APPLIED ANATOMY OF THE CEREBROVASCULAR SYSTEM

The Carotid Artery

The right common carotid begins at the bifurcation of the innominate artery behind the sternoclavicular joint, and the left springs from the arch of the aorta beyond the origin of the innominate artery. The usual site for atheromatous stenosis of the internal carotid is just above the bifurcation of the common carotid, in the region of the carotid sinus, but it can occur both above and below this level. Each internal carotid artery enters the cranial cavity through the carotid canal, passing anteriorly through the cavernous sinus in which it lies medial to the third, fourth, sixth, and first and second divisions of the fifth cranial nerve; these nerves can be involved singly or together by saccular aneurysms within the sinus; leakage from an aneurysm in this situation gives rise to caroticocavernous fistula (p. 394). Emerging from the cavernous sinus, it gives off the posterior communicating branch. From the phylogenetic point of view, this is really the proximal part of the *posterior cerebral artery,* but it is often small or vestigial. It is a common site for aneurysms which arise from its origin from the carotid and can give rise to diplopia from involvement of the third or fourth cranial nerve, or both.

The *anterior choroidal artery* rises from the carotid trunk above the posterior communicating artery; sometimes its place is taken by a group of small vessels. It supplies the amygdala, the hippocampus, the tail of the caudate nucleus, the medial part of the globus pallidus, the ventrolateral thalamus, the lateral geniculate body, and the choroid plexus of the temporal horn of the lateral ventricle. Occlusion of this artery can produce symptoms similar to those of middle cerebral artery occlusion, notably hemiparesis, hemianesthesia, and hemianopia, together with some disturbance of memory as a result of hippocampal infarction, but since many of these symptoms may fail to develop

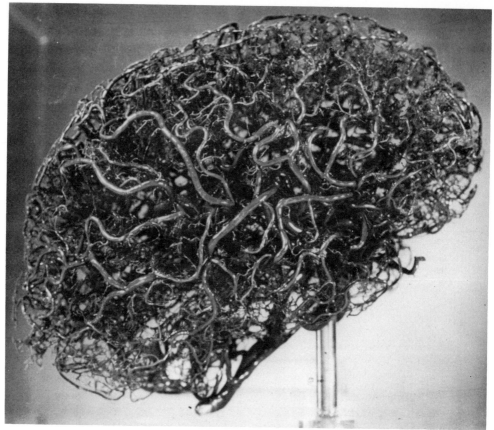

Figure 15–1.   Plastic cast of the intracranial blood vessels. (Prepared by Dr. David Tomsett. Courtesy of Royal College of Surgeons.)

following ligation of the artery, it is apparent that its territory of supply varies from case to case.

Middle Cerebral Artery

The vessel passes laterally across the olfactory trigone, hooks around the insula, and runs backward in the sylvian fissure. Branches arising from the main trunk enter the anterior perforated substance to supply the internal capsule, the corpus striatum, and the anterior part of the thalamus. One artery of this group is larger than the rest and was termed by Charcot "the artery of cerebral hemorrhage" because of its supposed involvement in the massive hemorrhages which are common in this area. The cortical branches of the middle cerebral artery supply the lateral part of the orbital surface of the frontal lobe, the precentral, lower, and middle frontal gyri, and the parietal lobe, with the exception of the upper rim of the hemisphere which is supplied by the anterior cerebral artery. Two or three temporal branches are distributed to the lateral surface of the temporal lobe. From this it will be seen that occlusion of the middle cerebral artery near its origin will lead to infarction of the internal capsule, basal ganglia, and large areas of the frontal, parietal, and temporal lobes. If occlusion occurs distal to the points of origin of the perforating branches, infarction will involve the cortex and subjacent white matter only. There are many ingredients to the subsequent clinical picture, notably aphasia and apraxia of the left hand (if the dominant hemisphere is involved), bosis is limited to superficial cortical branches. The case may be cited of a woman who lost her way because she could not recognize familiar surroundings; this did not unduly disturb her, because she failed to recognize her lapse. Arteriography disclosed poor filling of the arteries in the right (nondominant) parietal lobe. Another patient was admitted to hospital because of sudden "confusion." He could see but he could not read or do simple calculations, and he had failed to recognize some of his colleagues. These symptoms of damage in the posterior temporoparietal region were gradually succeeded by the more dramatic features of complete occlusion of the middle cerebral artery about one inch from its source. Symptoms related to focal cortical ischemia of this type can also occur from vascular insufficiency when the occlusion is in the internal carotid artery in the neck.

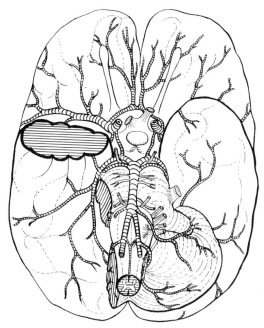

Figure 15–2. The arteries of the brain. The tip of one temporal lobe, one cerebellar hemisphere, and a portion of the pons have been removed.

contralateral weakness of the face and arm (the leg area being supplied by the anterior cerebral artery), sensory impairment in the face and arm, quadrantic hemianopia from involvement of the optic radiation in the temporal lobe, and a number of striking but variable symptoms due to involvement of the parietal lobe, which are described in Chapter 16.

Additional features sometimes encountered in middle cerebral thrombosis are: paralysis of conjugate gaze to the opposite side from involvement of the posterior end of the second frontal convolution; difficulty in using the contralateral hand because of reflex avoidance reactions (repellent kinetic apraxia); frontal "ataxia"; impairment of optokinetic nystagmus, and varying degrees of intellectual impairment. In most cases of middle cerebral thrombosis, the situation is dominated by profound hemiplegia and hemianesthesia, with or without homonymous hemianopia. The more esoteric symptoms enumerated above will escape notice, but they can occur in relative isolation when throm-

The Anterior Cerebral Artery

The artery arises from the internal carotid at the medial end of the lateral cerebral sulcus and passes forward and medially above the optic nerve to the commencement of the longitudinal fissure, at which point it is connected to its fellow by the short anterior communicating artery. Sometimes both arteries arise from a common trunk, in which event thrombosis of this vessel will lead to bilateral infarction, with paralysis of both legs. Saccular aneurysms of the anterior communicating artery and of the anterior cerebral artery are common, and are difficult to deal with surgically. The rupture of such aneurysms is apt to provoke profound coma.

The artery curves over the genu of the corpus callosum and runs backward on that structure to end in anastomoses with branches of the posterior cerebral artery. In the presence of internal hydrocephalus, the artery is pushed upward and its arc widened, as can be demonstrated by angiography.

The anterior cerebral artery supplies

the medial aspect of the undersurface of the frontal lobe, the medial aspect of the frontal and parietal lobes, and a narrow rim on the medial border of the hemisphere. Heubner's artery originates either immediately above or just below the anterior communicating artery and passes through the anterior perforated space to supply the anterior part of the internal capsule, the head of the caudate nucleus, and the putamen. Occlusion of the anterior cerebral artery proximal to the origin of Heubner's artery therefore produces weakness of the face and arm as the result of capsular infarction, together with weakness of the leg from damage to the "leg" area of the motor cortex. The result is hemiplegia. If occlusion develops distal to Heubner's artery, only the leg is affected; in both instances some sensory impairment of the lower limb is to be expected. Heubner's artery also supplies the white matter underneath the insula so that motor aphasia can be added to the symptomatology of thrombosis in the proximal portion of the anterior cerebral artery.

The anterior cerebral supplies the paracentral lobule which is concerned, inter alia, with the regulation of sphincter function; either retention or incontinence can occur from lesions in this area. The artery also supplies the cingulate gyrus. Bilateral cingulate softening has been recorded as the result of thrombotic disease, giving rise to akinetic mutism. The patient appears to be awake but lies with eyes open, neither speaking nor moving, and not responding to external stimuli. The condition can occur with lesions elsewhere in the brain (p. 26), but when it is the result of anterior cerebral infarction, pyramidal signs will usually be present in the legs.

When the branches to the medial aspect of the frontal lobe are affected, a grasp reflex may be obtained contralaterally, and the patient may exhibit the phenomenon of Gegenhalten or counterpull—an involuntary resistance to passive movement. Motor perseveration may be present.

The Vertebral Artery

The vertebral artery arises from the first portion of the subclavian and ascends through the foramina in the transverse processes of the upper six cervical vertebrae; in this part of its course, it lies immediately lateral to the intervertebral discs and can be displaced by protruded discs if spondylosis is present.[52, 90] It winds behind the lateral mass of the atlas and passes into the skull through the foramen magnum; at the lower border of the pons, it unites with its fellow from the opposite side to form the basilar artery. Stenosis of the subclavian proximal to its origin can lead to reversal of blood flow in the vertebral artery when the arm on that side is used, and this can bring about symptoms of brainstem insufficiency.[75] Atheromatous stenosis of the artery can occur at any part of its course and can become a serious source of vascular insufficiency when, as often happens, the opposite vertebral artery is congenitally small. Another source of transient insufficiency in elderly people with spondylosis is head turning, which can temporarily obstruct blood flow in the artery.[90]

The posterior spinal artery may originate from the vertebral artery at the side of the medulla, but more often it arises from the posterior inferior cerebellar artery and passes backward before descending as two branches, one in front and the other behind the posterior roots of the spinal nerves. These are reinforced by a succession of twigs arising from the vertebral, posterior intercostal, and lumbar arteries. Thus, the two posterior spinal arteries are continued to the lower part of the spinal cord into the cauda equina. The anterior spinal artery arises near the termination of the vertebral artery and descends in front of the medulla to unite with its fellow from the opposite side at the level of the olive. The trunk thus formed descends on the front of the spinal cord and is reinforced by a succession of small branches which enter the vertebral canal through the in-

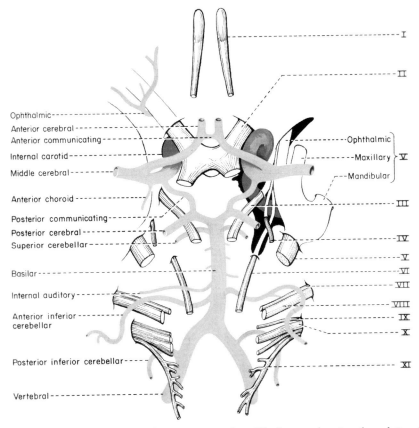

Ophthalmic
Anterior cerebral
Anterior communicating
Internal carotid
Middle cerebral
Anterior choroid
Posterior communicating
Posterior cerebral
Superior cerebellar
Basilar
Internal auditory
Anterior inferior cerebellar
Posterior inferior cerebellar
Vertebral

I
II
Ophthalmic
Maxillary ⎱ V
Mandibular ⎰
III
IV
V
VI
VII
VIII
IX
X
XI

Figure 15–3. Arterial connections in the posterior and middle fossae, showing the relationship of the cranial nerves to the arteries. (After Brock, S.: *Basis of Clinical Neurology*. Williams & Wilkins Co., Baltimore, 1953.)

tervertebral foramina. The vessel lies in the pia along the anterior median fissure and supplies the anterior two-thirds of the cord.[86]

The *posterior inferior cerebellar artery* can be small, large, or absent. It winds backward around the lower end of the olive and ascends behind the roots of the glossopharyngeal and vagus nerves to the lower border of the pons, and then runs laterally to the cerebellum. The trunk of the artery supplies branches to the lateral portion of the medulla oblongata, and its terminal branches supply the ipsilateral cerebellar hemisphere and the inferior vermis. Occlusion of this vessel is a common lesion, giving rise to Wallenberg's syndrome or, more often, to an incomplete syndrome. Dysphagia is caused by involvement of the nucleus ambiguus of the tenth nerve. There is impairment of pain and temperature sense on the ipsilateral side of the face through implication of the descending root and tract of the trigeminal nerve, and similar sensory impairment on the contralateral side of the body if the medial lemniscus is affected. There are ipsilateral cerebellar signs in the arm and leg, nystagmus, and cerebellar dysarthria. Horner's syndrome may occur on the side of the lesion. In some cases, the tongue is paralyzed on the affected side. Consciousness is seldom lost, and the prognosis for recovery is surprisingly good.

The Basilar Artery

The vessel is formed by the junction of the two vertebral arteries, and lies in a shallow median groove on the ventral surface of the pons. It is placed between the two abducens nerves below and the two oculomotor nerves above. It divides into the two posterior cerebral arteries at the upper border of the pons.

The basilar artery gives rise to a large number of small penetrating branches to the pons, and to the internal auditory and the superior cerebellar arteries. The former accompanies the facial and auditory nerves into the internal auditory meatus, and supplies the internal ear. At its termination, it divides into two branches, one going to the labyrinth and the other to the cochlea. Thrombosis of the main trunk of the artery gives rise to sudden unilateral deafness together with vertigo and loss of labyrinthine function on that side, while occlusion of either branch alone produces appropriate defects.

The anterior inferior cerebellar artery curves backward to supply the undersurface of the cerebellum and also gives some twigs to the lateral portion of the lower pons and medulla.

The *superior cerebellar artery* arises near the termination of the basilar, and passes laterally below the oculomotor nerve to wind around the peduncle and supply the superior aspect of the cerebellum; it also supplies important branches to the pons and the pineal region. Thrombosis of this vessel produces vertigo, severe ipsilateral cerebellar ataxia, and impairment of sensibility in the contralateral limbs.[60] Consciousness may be lost at the outset. It should be noted that massive cerebellar infarction can constitute a surgical emergency[37]; edema of the cerebellum causes acute intimal hydrocephalus from which the patient may die unless suboccipital decompression is carried out.

Atheromatous stenosis of the basilar artery itself is common, and can reach an advanced degree without producing symptoms if the carotid circulation and the circle of Willis are adequate. The symptoms of basilar insufficiency are described on page 378, but it is worth repeating that because the basilar artery

divides into the two posterior cerebral arteries which supply important areas of the midbrain, temporal lobe, and occipital lobe, simultaneous bilateral lesions of the cerebral hemispheres can follow basilar stenosis. For instance, cortical blindness from bilateral infarction of the striate area is commonly the result of basilar disease.

Large aneurysms can occur on the vertebral and basilar arteries; these are described on page 393.

Massive infarction of the pons from thrombotic occlusion of the basilar artery or its branches induces immediate loss of consciousness. The pupils may be widely dilated or pinpointed, hyperpyrexia is common, and the patient lies in the position of decerebrate rigidity. Few recover, though a tenuous hold on life may be established by the use of hypothermia and assisted respiration. In the few survivors, the subsequent dysarthria, dysphagia, and quadriplegia impose a severe burden on patient and nurses alike (see p. 26).

The Posterior Cerebral Artery

The posterior cerebral artery is an important vessel, which passes laterally from its origin in the basilar artery and receives the posterior communicating branch of the internal carotid, which is extremely variable in size and may be absent. The artery so formed winds around the cerebral peduncle and reaches the tentorial surface of the cerebrum, where it breaks up into branches for the supply of the temporal and occipital lobes. The artery can be compressed by a tentorial pressure cone as it ascends into the superior compartment between the brainstem and the edge of the tentorium. Perforating branches supply important structures. Some pierce the posterior perforated substance to supply the anterior part of the thalamus, the lateral wall of the third ventricle, and the globus pallidus. Others supply the lateral geniculate body, the posterior end of the thalamus, and the choroid plexus of the third and lateral ventricles. A few twigs are given to the fornix. Yet other branches supply the cerebral peduncle (containing the pyramidal tract), the posterior part of the thalamus, the pineal, and the quadrigeminal and medial geniculate bodies. Cortical branches are distributed to the undersurface of the temporal lobe, the hippocampal gyrus, the medial aspect of the occipital lobe, and the occipital pole. It will be observed from the disposition of these arteries that thrombosis or embolism of the posterior cerebral artery can produce contralateral hemiplegia, hemianesthesia, and homonymous hemianopia; consequently, it may be very difficult to distinguish between this situation and the results of middle cerebral artery occlusion. The difficulty is compounded by the circumstance that posterior cerebral artery insufficiency or embolism can give rise to severe memory defect for life's experiences, apparently due to a lesion of the hippocampal gyrus; disorders of memory are also seen in middle cerebral thrombosis. Infarction of the thalamus can produce a thalamic syndrome in both middle and posterior cerebral artery occlusion, but some help is obtained from the fact that a third nerve palsy is often present on the side of the lesion if the latter vessel is at fault. Third nerve palsy and contralateral hemiplegia from infarction of the peduncle constitute Weber's syndrome. Weakness of vertical eye movements, ptosis, sluggish pupillary responses and (rarely) retraction nystagmus are features of midbrain involvement which are not seen when the stroke is due to middle cerebral artery occlusion. Decerebrate attacks, as mentioned above, occur when the basilar artery is involved.

The brainstem comprises important structures, and they are supplied by a large number of small arteries derived from the vertebral, the basilar, the posterior cerebral, and the posterior communicating arteries. It is therefore not surprising that symptoms occur in all sorts of combinations. These are too numerous to be discussed here, but are well described by Fisher.[41] However, a few symptoms deserve special mention. Persistent hiccup is seen in lesions of the medulla. Hemiballismus—gross, violent, irregular, and usually unilateral movements of the arm or leg or both—is commonly the result of a lesion of the subthalamic nucleus of Luys; it can be cured by thalamotomy. Thirdly, paralysis of conjugate gaze to the side of the lesion, which is sometimes seen in acute frontal lesions, also occurs in pontine lesions near the sixth nucleus. Internuclear paralysis of ocular movements is discussed on page 91. Palatal nystagmus or palatal myoclonus, which is often accompanied by synchronous movements of the lower face, tongue, and diaphragm, is sometimes seen in vascular lesions involving the olivary system.

Anastomoses

For practical purposes, there are no anastomoses between the terminal arteries within the substance of the central nervous system, but there are considerable connections on the surface of the brain and between extracranial vessels.

The circle of Willis connects the anterior, middle, and posterior cerebral arteries on the two sides. Imperfect development of this system is common, and there is a higher incidence of cerebral infarction in such cases than in persons with a normal circle.[3]

Second, there are anastomoses between the cortical branches of the anterior, middle, and posterior cerebral arteries, and between the cortical branches of the cerebellar arteries; the latter may extend across the midline. The anastomoses between the three cerebral arteries are found mainly in the depths of the sulci and usually involve vessels from 50 to 120 μ, though sometimes vessels from 300 to 500 μ anastomose. Infarctions are not uncommon in these border zones, despite the anastomoses, probably because under conditions of

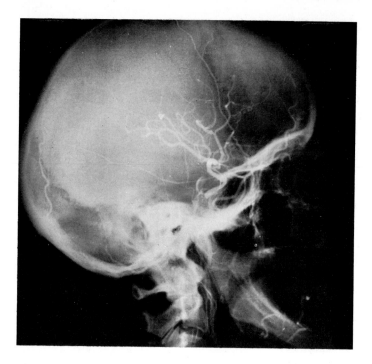

Figure 15–4. Gross stenosis of the right internal carotid artery, with retrograde filling of the intracranial vessels via the ophthalmic artery.

reduced perfusion, flow in the most distal branches will fall to a critical level before that in the proximal branches. This principle of the "distal field" is supported by the fact that the parietal region is the most vulnerable and the first to be affected, while the more proximal orbital-frontal and sylvian regions are less often involved. These cortical infarctions occur as a result of profound systemic hypotension (e.g., open-heart operations, coronary thrombosis) and in association with stenosis of large intracranial or extracranial arteries. The combination of systemic hypotension and carotid or vertebral basilar stenosis may be expected, on theoretical grounds, to provide a double threat to border-zone areas.

There are also anastomoses between the external and internal carotid systems by way of the ophthalmic artery (Fig. 15–4), the meningeal branches of the internal carotid, and the middle meningeal arteries. Furthermore, when the common carotid is obstructed, blood can be diverted into the internal carotid by back-flow from the external carotid, which in turn derives blood from the opposite external carotid and occipital arteries via the scalp vessels. These anastomoses have great practical significance since they can develop so successfully in the face of slowly progressive stenosis of major vessels that symptoms of vascular insufficiency may not appear at all. Thus, it is possible for a subject to function normally with complete occlusion of one internal carotid and partial occlusion of the other, but such individuals are vulnerable to sudden thrombotic occlusion at the sites of the stenoses, and to the effects of hypotension and hypoglycemia. The latter can have a preferential impact on an area of brain supplied by a narrowed artery.

CEREBROVASCULAR DISEASE

Incidence. Analyses by Wylie [102] and by Riishede [85] have shown that there has been both a relative and an absolute increase in the incidence of strokes in the United States, Western Europe, and the British Isles in recent years, though there has been a leveling off of deaths from cerebral hemorrhage. In 1958, the number of deaths attributed to stroke was 175,000, and in 1963, it was over 200,000. The incidence rate varies not only from country to country, but from area to area within the same country. Thus, the incidence rate and the mortality rate are both far higher in the southeastern and the far western states than in the central and mountain regions in the United States.

Even more important than the mortality statistics is the fact that some 80 per cent of all cases of cerebral infarction survive the first incident. Some recover completely, but many suffer permanent impairment, and about 50 per cent of the survivors die somewhere between four and five years after the initial incident, usually from a recurrent stroke or from a heart attack. There are no accurate figures as to the number of physically disabled survivors leading restricted lives as a result of a stroke. Also lacking is a reliable figure as to the incidence of organic psychoses due to vascular disease. In 1920, the rate of first admissions to the New York State Hospitals with this diagnosis was 21.3 per 100,000 population over the age of 45, and by 1950 it had risen to 62.2, during which period the increase of first admissions from all causes was only 37 per cent.[64] However, cerebral arteriosclerosis is often used as an alibi for organic psychoses of undetermined origin in elderly persons, although it is unwise to ascribe to arterial disease any smoothly progressive organic brain syndrome. A history of one or more "incidents" of abrupt onset is a *sine qua non* for diagnosis.

Nondegenerative forms of cerebrovascular disease are far less common than the atherosclerotic variety, but they are sufficiently numerous to justify careful appraisal of every case of stroke, especially in the younger age groups.[39] Scrutiny of the causes of cerebrovascular accidents listed in Table 15–1 will disclose a number of conditions for which treatment is available.

Etiology. Degenerative arterial disease is the usual cause of the common stroke. Though atheroma usually starts in the second or third decade and increases steadily until old age, there are exceptions. It can reach an advanced degree, sufficient to cause coronary thrombosis or a stroke, in children suffering from premature senility[5] (progeria), while it can be minimal in individuals reaching the ninth decade. It is often present in the aorta in the second or third decade; the coronary arteries can be affected in the third decade and the intracranial vessels are usually involved much later. The carotid arteries can be involved in the fourth decade. It is influenced by sex in the sense that vascular catastrophes are less common in women of the same age, before the menopause, than in men, whereas the incidence is approximately equal thereafter. After removal of both ovaries in young women, the incidence of atherosclerosis and vascular catastrophes is approximately the same as in males. Liability to vascular disease is apt to run in families.

Although the cause of atherosclerosis is unknown, there is clinical and experimental evidence that its progress can be accelerated by a number of factors, notably arterial hypertension, diabetes, diets rich in animal fats and refined sugar (overeating), the polycythemias, hypothyroidism and chronic infections (e.g., urinary infection). There is also persuasive evidence that excessive cigarette smoking can aggravate coronary and peripheral vascular disease. Liability to arterial thrombosis can be increased by rare conditions such as sickle-cell anemia, macroglobulinemia, and thrombotic thrombocytopenic purpura. The polycythemias and macroglobulinemias do not affect blood flow through major arteries but are capable of compromising flow through the microvasculature, and a question still to be answered is whether the impact of these diseases on large arteries could be caused by compromise of the vasa vasorum, which nourish not only the adventitia and outer media in normal arteries but also help to sustain the nutrition of living atheromatous plaques.

*Table 15–1.   Classification of Cerebrovascular Disease.**

I. Cerebral Infarction (Pale, Red [Hemorrhagic] and Mixed Types)
  A. Thrombosis with Atherosclerosis
  B. Cerebral Embolism
    1. Of cardiac origin
      (a). Atrial fibrillation and other arrhythmias (with rheumatic, atherosclerotic, hypertensive, or congenital heart disease)
      (b). Myocardial infarction with mural thrombus
      (c). Acute and subacute bacterial endocarditis
      (d). Heart disease without arrhythmia or mural thrombus
      (e). *Complications of cardiac surgery*
      (f). *Nonbacterial thrombotic ("marantic") endocardial vegetations*
      (g). *Paradoxical embolism with congenital heart disease*
    2. Of noncardiac origin
      (a). Atherosclerosis of aorta and carotid arteries (mural thrombus, atheromatous material)
      (b). From sites of cerebral artery thrombosis
      (c). Thrombus in pulmonary veins
      (d). *Fat*
      (e). *Tumor*
      (f). *Air*
      (g). *Complications of neck and thoracic surgery*
      (h). *Miscellaneous: Rare types*
      (i). *Of undetermined origin*
  C. Other Conditions Causing Cerebral Infarction
    1. Cerebral venous thrombosis
    2. Systemic hypotension
    3. Complications of arteriography
    4. Arteritis
    5. Hematologic disorders (polycythemia, thrombocytosis, sickle-cell disease, thrombotic thrombopenia, etc.)
    6. *Dissecting aortic aneurysm*
    7. *Trauma to carotid*
    8. *Anoxia*
    9. *Radioactive or x-ray radiation*
    10. *With tentorial, foramen magnum, and subfalcial herniations*
    11. *Miscellaneous: Rare types*
  D. Cerebral Infarction of Undetermined Cause
II. Transient Cerebral Ischemia Without Infarction
  A. Recurrent Focal Cerebral Ischemic Attacks (previously called vasospasm, usually associated with thrombosis and atherosclerosis)
  B. Systemic Hypotension ("simple faint," acute blood loss, myocardial infarction, Stokes–Adams syndrome, traumatic and surgical shock, sensitive carotid sinus, severe postural hypotension)
    1. With focal neurologic deficit
    2. With syncope
  C. Migraine
III. Intracranial Hemorrhage (including intracerebral, subarachnoid, ventricular, rarely subdural)
  A. Hypertensive Intracerebral Hemorrhage
  B. Ruptured Saccular Aneurysm (if unruptured, see *IV, A*)
  C. Angioma (if unruptured, see *IV, B*)
  D. Trauma
  E. Hemorrhagic Disorders (leukemia, aplastic anemia, thrombopenic purpura, liver disease, complication of anticoagulant therapy, etc.)

---

*Rare conditions are indicated by italics.

Table 15–1   (Continued)

F.   Of Undetermined Cause (normal blood pressure and no angioma)
G.   *Hemorrhage into Primary and Secondary Brain Tumors*
H.   *Septic Embolism with Mycotic Aneurysm*
I.   *With Hemorrhagic Infarction, Arterial or Venous* (see under *I* and *VII*)
J.   *Secondary Brainstem Hemorrhage (temporal lobe herniation)*
K.   *Hypertensive Encephalopathy*
L.   *Idiopathic Brain Purpura*
M.   *With Inflammatory Disease of Arteries and Veins* (see under *VI, VII*)
N.   *Miscellaneous: Rare types*
IV. Vascular Malformations and Developmental Abnormalities
A.   Aneurysm: Saccular, Fusiform, Globular, Diffuse (if ruptured, see *III*, B)
B.   Angioma (including familial telangiectasis, trigeminal encephalo-angiomatosis [Sturge-Weber-Dimitri], retinal-pontine hemangiomas); (if ruptured, see *III, C)
C.   Absence, Hypoplasia, or Other Abnormality of Vessels (including variations in pattern of circle of Willis)
V. Inflammatory Diseases of Arteries
A.   Infections and Infestations
1.   Meningovascular syphilis
2.   Septic embolism
3.   *Arteritis secondary to pyogenic and tuberculous meningitis*
4.   *Rare types (typhus, schistosomiasis mansoni, malaria, trichinosis, etc.)*
B.   Diseases of Undetermined Origin
1.   *Lupus erythematosus*
2.   *Rheumatic arteritis*
3.   *Polyarteritis nodosa (necrotizing and granulomatous forms)*
4.   *Cranial arteritis (temporal)*
5.   *Idiopathic granulomatous arteritis of aorta and its major branches*
VI. Vascular Diseases Without Changes in the Brain
A.   Atherosclerosis
B.   Hypertensive Arterio- and Arteriolosclerosis
C.   *Hyaline Arterio- and Arteriolosclerosis*
D.   *Calcification and Ferruginization of Vessels*
E.   *Capillary Sclerosis, etc.*
VII. Hypertensive Encephalopathy
A.   Malignant Hypertension (*essential, chronic renal disease, pheochromocytoma, etc.*)
B.   Acute Glomerulonephritis
C.   Eclampsia
VIII. Dural Sinus and Cerebral Venous Thrombosis
A.   Secondary to Infection of Ear, Paranasal Sinus, Face, or Other Cranial Structures
B.   With Meningitis and Subdural Empyema
C.   *Debilitating States (Marantic)*
D.   *Postpartum*
E.   *Postoperative*
F.   *Hematologic Disease (polycythemia, sickle-cell disease)*
G.   *Cardiac Failure and Congestive Heart Disease*
H.   *Miscellaneous: Rare Types*
I.   *Of Undetermined Cause*
IX. Strokes of Undetermined Origin

Aside from atherosclerosis, with its tendency to produce occlusion of the carotid, vertebral, basilar, and cerebral arteries, the penetrating vessels of the brain are often the seat of a different process marked by the appearance of miliary aneurysms of the small arteries and arterioles. These aneurysms, first described by Charcot and subsequently forgotten, have been reestablished as a pathological entity by Russell[88] and others. So far as is known at the present time, they do not involve small arteries in the other viscera, perhaps because the anterior, middle, and posterior cerebral arteries have exceptionally thin walls and are poorly endowed with muscle, elastic tissue, and adventitia. This may explain their tendency to rupture under the influence of arterial hypertension.

Strokes can occur as a result of inflammatory changes in the arteries, as in syphilitic endarteritis, the collagen diseases, septicemia, and bacteremia.

Cerebral embolism can occur whether the intracranial vessels are normal or not. Emboli arise in the heart or great vessels. The more common causes of embolism are listed in Table 15–1.

Atherosclerosis is the usual cause of transient ischemic attacks. These are marked by abrupt and transient cerebral dysfunction, the clinical features of which depend upon the site of the arterial insufficiency. In some cases, they result from the impaction of small emboli derived from atheromatous plaques in the large vessels, or from mural thrombi in the heart. Occasionally, they are due to the combined effects of episodic systemic hypotension and atheromatous stenosis of the vessels in the neck. Rarely, they are due to hypoglycemia— commonly from an overdose of insulin— in combination with atheromatous stenosis of arteries in the neck or within the head; the hypoglycemia will have its maximum effect in areas of the brain which are already compromised by arterial insufficiency. The effects of hypotension are most felt in the inappropriately named watershed areas, where the peripheral branches of the anterior, middle, and posterior cerebral arteries meet within the cerebral cortex. The infarctions which result from systemic hypotension occur in the most distal areas supplied by these vessels, just as gangrene is apt to appear first in the toes from insufficiency of the iliac or femoral artery.

The role of arterial spasm is still under debate. It is now recognized that transient ischemic attacks, whether from embolism or from hypotension in the presence of arterial stenosis, account for many of the phenomena formerly attributed to arterial spasm. Nevertheless, there is abundant clinical and experimental evidence that the lodgment of an embolus can promote local spasm, and that slowly developing arterial "constriction" involving not only one hemisphere but both can occur following experimental trauma to a cerebral artery,[92] or rupture of an aneurysm. Furthermore, in hypertensive encephalopathy, focal or generalized arterial constriction may affect the cerebral vessels as well as the peripheral circulation.

Spasm of cerebral vessels has also been invoked to explain the prodromal neurological symptoms of migraine and the occasional occurrence of persistent neurological deficit following such attacks.

Focal vascular lesions can also occur as a result of thrombosis of the dural sinus and cerebral veins.[54, 93] These events are sometimes classified as strokes, but the circumstances under which they occur are very different. They usually occur in young people or in the middle-aged, commonly in debilitating states, after parturition, or in the presence of gross hematological disease or congestive heart failure. Dural sinus thrombosis can also occur in healthy young women who are taking oral contraceptive agents[6] and in persons suffering from paroxysmal nocturnal hemoglobinuria.

Cerebral incidents which occur in women using contraceptive pills are uncommon, and it has been argued that death or disability is no more frequent in users of "The Pill" than in those who do not employ this form of contraception. This problem is unresolved from the statistical standpoint, but the author has been impressed not so much by the number of vascular accidents occurring in these cases as by the bizarre quality of the symptoms and signs. Leaving aside the increased incidence of venous thrombosis and thromboembolic phenomena—which is to be expected in a state of real or spurious pregnancy—these cerebral incidents are dramatic but short-lived, and therefore do not usually impinge on *mortality* statistics. Moreover, when the patient stops taking the agent, all evidence of vascular disease commonly disappears, whereas if the medication is resumed, further accidents can occur. The incidence of these minor or major disasters is extremely small in relation to the large number of women taking contraceptive pills.

Vascular accidents in the brain, brainstem, and spinal cord sometimes occur as a result of ruptured angiomatous malformations, particularly in young women. Similar disasters occur, very rarely, in children. The abrupt onset, with or without blood in the spinal fluid, and the subsequent improvement leave no reasonable doubt that the symptoms are due to a vascular accident. In most of the cases that the author has encountered, there has been cutaneous evidence of neurofibromatosis or telangiectases. The latter are usually most obvious at the time of the menses. The disaster can occur in late adolescence or early adult life.

The most rare of all cerebral vascular catastrophes is that caused by a dissecting aneurysm of the aortic arch. The onset is dramatic, with precordial pain and shock, suggesting severe myocardial ischemia. Cerebral symptoms resulting from cutting off the blood supply to the innominate artery or the left carotid and subclavian arteries (or both) dominate the picture, and the cerebral symptoms arise immediately.

Trauma to the neck can cause carotid artery thrombosis, and head injuries are occasionally followed within a few days by either carotid or middle cerebral artery thrombosis. Trauma to the head can also be followed after a week or so by intracerebral hemorrhage.

The physician is sometimes confronted by a patient who develops what appears to be a cerebral infarct, but who presents no collateral evidence of degenerative arterial disease or of any of the conditions which predispose thereto. The blood pressure is normal, the lipid profile is within normal limits, there is nothing to suggest a blood dyscrasia, diabetes is absent, there is no history of injury, histological tests for syphilis are negative, there is no evidence of heart disease, arteriography fails to reveal signs of vascular disease or angiomatous malformation, there is nothing to suggest a collagen disease, and the subsequent course of the case excludes the possibility of a cerebral tumor or of the cerebral embolism which occasionally occurs as the result of vegetations on the heart valves in the presence of visceral carcinoma. These rare cases usually end up with clear-cut evidence of atherosclerosis in the head, neck, heart, kidney, or peripheral vessels.

Classification

The classification of cerebrovascular disease found in Table 15–1 has been proposed by the Advisory Council of the National Institute of Neurological Diseases and Blindness, United States Public Health Service.

CEREBRAL HEMORRHAGE

Hemorrhage into the substance of the brain occurs as the result of a variety of disorders, of which by far the most common is the combination of hypertension with atherosclerosis.

Incidence. The precise incidence of hypertensive cerebral hemorrhage is difficult to estimate. In the United States and Western Europe, it is less common than cerebral infarction as a cause of stroke, but as Fisher[41] has pointed out, evidence of small, nonfatal hemorrhage is not uncommonly found in autopsies of persons who have died from other causes, and it is often difficult to distinguish with certainty between cerebral infarction and cerebral hemorrhage during life. The incidence of cerebral hemorrhage varies with sex, age, and race. Although the incidence of coronary artery disease and cerebral infarction rises with age, fatal cerebral hemorrhage in white males, Negro males, and Negro females tends to decline from the age of 50 onwards. In white females, the incidence increases to the age of 65 and then declines slightly. Negroes of both sexes are more liable to cerebral hemorrhage than whites, and it occurs at an earlier age. There is evidence that in recent years there has been a relative drop in the incidence of cerebral hemorrhage, probably because of the increasing use of hypotensive agents for the control of arterial hypertension. It is important to emphasize that asymptomatic and therefore unsuspected arterial hypertension can cause fatal intracerebral hemorrhage in individuals under the age of 40.

Etiology. Common and uncommon causes of cerebral hemorrhage are listed on page 358. The great majority are due to hypertension and atherosclerosis. Saccular aneurysms usually rupture into the subarachnoid space but may do so into the brain itself. Angiomas within the brain substance have usually given evidence of their presence before the occurrence of a major hemorrhage, but this is not always the case.[61] Severe head injuries are occasionally followed within about 10 days by massive bleeding into the brain (late traumatic apoplexy). Blood diseases, notably the leukemias and aplastic anemia, often terminate with cerebral hemorrhage, but this is rarely a presenting symptom.

Hemorrhage into primary cranial tumors is rare; it occurred in only nine of 461 autopsies in cases of intracranial hemorrhage reported by Russell.[87] Small hemorrhages in the brainstem are not uncommon in the presence of an acute intracranial space-occupying lesion[18] (including cerebral hemorrhage) which has given place to a tentorial pressure cone, but these appear to be venous in origin and are attributed to interference with venous drainage into the system of Galen. On the other hand, primary intrapontine hemorrhage is usually encountered in the malignant and nephritic forms of hypertension.

Pathology. The classical site for hypertensive hemorrhage is in the region of the basal ganglia, which is supplied by the long, thin-walled perforating branches of the middle cerebral artery. In a recent survey of 393 cases of fatal intracerebral hematoma, Freytag[43] found 42 per cent in the area of the striate body, 16 per cent in the pons, 15 per cent in the thalamus, 12 per cent in the cerebellum, and 12 per cent in the cerebral white matter. Seventy-five per cent of the hematomas in this series ruptured into the ventricles, and 15 per cent extended through the cortex into the subarachnoid space. Six per cent spread through the arachnoid into the subdural space. Secondary hemorrhages in the midbrain or pons were present in 54 per cent of the cases of supratentorial hematomas.

Hemorrhages in the region of the basal

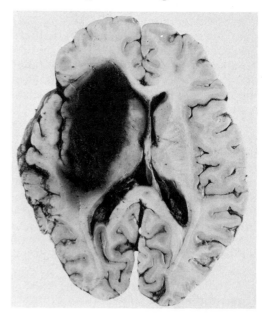

Figure 15–5. Cerebral hemorrhage. (Courtesy of Ayer Laboratory, Pennsylvania Hospital, Philadelphia.)

ganglia may be situated laterally or medially (Fig. 15–5). The medial type, which is usually fatal, arises medial to the putamen and usually destroys the thalamus and ruptures into the ventricle. The more laterally placed hemorrhages arise in the putamen, external capsule, or claustrum, and the chances of survival are better. Hemorrhages into the pons, midbrain, and cerebellum are usually fatal.

Fresh blood clot is found in the center, and when the clot is removed it leaves a ragged cavity into which small vessels are often found projecting; some of these are thrombosed and necrotic. The surrounding white matter is edematous and soft and may be dotted with small ring and ball hemorrhages around capillaries. In the surrounding tissue, astrocytes are swollen and increased in number and there is phagocytosis of hemosiderin and dead tissue. The mass of the hematoma itself, together with edema of the surrounding brain, causes the displacement of other cerebral structures, and this can lead to a pressure cone.

Multiple hemorrhages are occasionally seen in the hemisphere, and in some cases there are petechial or massive hemorrhages in other viscera, even in the absence of obvious hemorrhagic disease. Such visceral hemorrhages were found in 22 per cent of 135 cases of cerebral hemorrhage recorded by Mutlu and his colleagues.[73]

The large vessels at the base of the brain are usually atheromatous, and the arterioles show diffuse hyperplastic sclerosis and fibrinoid degeneration,[40] in varying combinations. Tiny miliary aneurysms may be found along deep penetrating vessels in areas not destroyed by the hematoma. Described long ago by Charcot, they have been re-established as a true pathological entity by Russell[88] and others. Using a radiographic technique on 100 brains from hypertensive subjects and another 100 brains from normotensive patients, Yates found intracerebral arterial aneurysms in 46 per cent of the hypertensives and 7 per cent

of the controls. There is some evidence that these aneurysms become more common as age advances.

Primary Cerebral Hemorrhage

Clinical Features. Cerebral hemorrhage may occur with or without premonitory signs. There is sometimes evidence that the patient felt unwell for a day or two or for some hours before the ictus; there may have been headache, lightheadedness, or a sense of general malaise; similar symptoms sometimes precede cerebral thrombosis or embolism. The explanation of such premonitory symptoms is not known. Severe emotional stress sometimes precedes hemorrhage, perhaps because of elevation of an already high blood pressure.

In many cases of cerebral hemorrhage the onset is abrupt; in a minority, it is gradual. Consciousness is lost immediately in only about half of all cases. The following figures are derived from McKissock's experience with 232 surgically verified cases of primary intracerebral hemorrhage in which the mode of onset was known.[66]

1. Sudden onset without loss of consciousness, 89 cases.

2. Sudden onset with loss of consciousness, 117 cases.

3. Gradual onset without loss of consciousness, 23 cases.

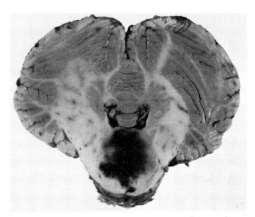

Figure 15–6. Spontaneous pontine hemorrhage. (Courtesy of Ayer Laboratory, Pennsylvania Hospital, Philadelphia.)

4. Gradual onset with later loss of consciousness, 3 cases.

It will be observed that almost half these patients were not unconscious at any time. Of those conscious at the onset, 26 later became unconscious, 19 of them within 48 hours and seven within three to five days. Of those rendered unconscious initially, 21 regained consciousness, 18 within 48 hours and 3 in three to five days. These facts demonstrate how difficult it is to differentiate between thrombosis and hemorrhage by clinical progression alone.

In the most severe type of case, involving the basal ganglia, often with rupture into the third ventricle, the onset is abrupt and the patient becomes deeply unconscious within a minute or two. There may be one or more seizures. The head and eyes may be deviated to the opposite side. The pulse is full and bounding, the face flushed, and breathing soon becomes stertorous. The limbs are flaccid, and it may be impossible to detect neurological signs of lateralizing value, while in others unilateral flaccidity of the limbs and asymmetry of the mouth indicate the side of the lesion. In pontine hemorrhage,[35] coma usually supervenes within minutes of the onset (Fig. 15–6). There is impairment or loss of conjugate lateral eye movements in response to head rotation and caloric stimulation. The pupils are usually small and nonreactive. Bilateral extensor spasms may occur, and bilateral pyramidal signs may be evident. Intermittent spasms of irregular downward movements of the eyes (ocular dance) are occasionally seen. Hyperpyrexia is common.

Irregularities of the pulse are not uncommon as the result of rapidly increasing intracranial pressure and the development of a pressure cone. The blood pressure is commonly raised, and it may be difficult to know how much of this is due to preceding hypertension and how much to the intracranial lesion. A rise of intracranial pressure can cause a secondary rise of blood pressure, but in addition to this, there can be an acute rise of both systolic and diastolic pressures as a result of small lesions in the brainstem. It is of some practical importance to remember that hypertension originating thus may respond dramatically to minute doses of reserpine and other hypotensive agents which, if given in conventional doses, can provoke a catastrophic fall in blood pressure.

If blood has escaped into the spinal fluid, or if the expanding hemorrhagic lesion in the cerebral hemisphere has produced a pressure cone, the neck may be stiff. Papilledema is unlikely to appear unless the patient has survived for more than a day, but hypertensive retinopathy or subhyaloid hemorrhages may be present. When the initial state of shock passes off, the reflexes return and localizing signs emerge. In milder cases with a less severe onset, localizing signs appear early and gradually become more pronounced, only to be lost to view as stupor gives place to coma. A dire prognosis is implied by a rising pulse rate, rising temperature, and Cheyne-Stokes or ataxic respiration; hyperpyrexia is common when the hypothalamus is involved or when a pontine hemorrhage has occurred.

Some patients start to improve after a day or two, and are left with residual defects, such as aphasia, hemiparesis, hemianopia, or change of personality. Patients who survive laterally placed lesions in the cerebral hemisphere or a cerebellar hemorrhage sometimes achieve an unexpectedly satisfactory degree of recovery.

Hemorrhage into the cerebellum is relatively uncommon; for instance, in one series, only 15 instances occurred in 421 autopsied cases of apoplexy[30]; in 12 of these, the initial symptoms were severe and the course rapidly fatal, but in three others, the onset was gradual, permitting a clinical diagnosis of a cerebellar lesion to be made, and it is in these that prompt evacuation of the clot can save life.[67] Similar symptoms can arise from a large infarct of the cerebellum, and decompression is urgently called for.[37]

Cerebellar hemorrhage is usually rapid

in onset, with intense dizziness, vomiting, and unsteadiness of gait. Headache may be prominent but is sometimes absent. The patient is confused and may be drowsy. Speech is slurred. The limbs on the affected side show incoordination. There is sometimes paralysis of conjugate gaze towards the side of the lesion, and there may be forced deviation of the eyes to the opposite side. Horizontal nystagmus is present, with the quick phase to the side of the lesion. The plantar responses are usually extensor. Nuchal rigidity may be present or absent.

Laboratory Aids. The only unequivocal laboratory evidence of an intracerebral hemorrhage is blood in the spinal fluid, but it is absent in about one in five cases because the blood has not gained access to the subarachnoid space. A tap done immediately after the onset of hemorrhage may be clear, but the fluid may be bloody some hours later. A moderate amount of blood is occasionally found in the presence of a hemorrhagic infarct caused by embolism. The white cell count is usually high in proportion to the red cells, a curious situation which is best explained by the presence of a leukocytic response in the edge of a hematoma which has not ruptured into the ventricles or subarachnoid space. If in such a case the onset has been slow rather than abrupt, unjustified suspicions of cerebral abscess may be entertained. The protein of the spinal fluid is raised in the presence of blood.

Focal or generalized abnormalities of the electroencephalogram are common in patients with cerebral hemorrhage, as they are in other acute vascular lesions.

Abnormalities in the electrocardiogram (EKG) fall into two classes—those which can be interpreted on the basis of electrolyte imbalance or preexisting heart disease, and those which cannot be so interpreted. The latter types, which may mimic the effects of myocardial infarction (among other things), are seen after acute intracranial vascular insults and head injuries. In such cases, the lesions responsible for the abnormal EKG are found in the hypothalamus or in the medial part of the temporal lobes. Explanations which have been advanced for the EKG changes are vagal overactivity, sympathetic overactivity, a combination of the two, or an excessive release of catecholamines. There is experimental evidence to favor all four of these propositions, but in addition, Connor[22] has directed attention to the presence of myocardial damage in the form of patchy myocytolysis, which he found in 18 of 231 hearts examined. Thirteen of the patients had died of intracranial hemorrhage, two from intracranial infection, and one each from trauma, tumor, and cerebral infarction. Myocytolysis has also been encountered in poliomyelitis, insulin shock, and other conditions. The fact that structural change can occur in the heart following acute intracranial incidents may help to explain some cases of cardiac arrhythmia, cardiac arrest, and acute pulmonary edema, all of which can occur unexpectedly following acute insults to the brain.

Albuminuria, with or without casts, may be present in any acute vascular accident, whatever its nature, and the same is true of hyperglycemia and glycosuria. Ketones may appear in small quantities in the urine if the patient has been without food for a day or two.

Arteriography, surprisingly, disclosed an intracerebral hematoma in only 114 of 167 cases reported by McKissock,[66] but this is a useful procedure in selected cases.

Echoencephalography will disclose a shift of midline structures (Fig. 15–7). Brain scanning will often show increased vascularity around the hematoma from about the sixth day onwards.

Differential Diagnosis. See page 379.

Prognosis. Large hemorrhages deeply situated within the hemisphere in grossly hypertensive patients are usually fatal, and the same applies to primary pontine hemorrhage. The outlook is always poor when coma is present. However, small, nonfatal hemorrhages are not uncommon. McKissock and his colleagues studied 180 unselected cases of cerebral hemorrhage, 91 of which were treated conserv-

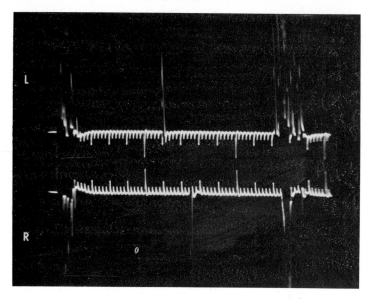

Figure 15-7. Echoencephalograph of massive right-sided cerebral hemorrhage.

atively and 89 by surgery. Forty-nine per cent of patients survived conservative treatment, and 35 per cent of the surgically treated patients lived. On the other hand, a recent study from the Mayo Clinic[98a] disclosed that 80 per cent of patients with intracerebral hemorrhage had died by the tenth day. The discrepancy between these two sets of figures is difficult to explain. In the author's experience, survivors of a cerebral hemorrhage fare less well than patients with cerebral infarction, and this is confirmed by the fact that only 6 per cent of the Mayo Clinic series with cerebral hemorrhage survived for a period of four years.

Treatment. The fact that some patients survive the initial stroke emphasizes the importance of good nursing care from the very outset. The patient should be propped up in bed to reduce venous pressure inside the head and to ease respiration. If this is not practicable, he should be nursed on his side. Mucus must be aspirated from the pharynx, and tracheostomy is essential in comatose patients. Frequent changes of position and attention to the skin of the back are desirable from the beginning. Feeding via a nasogastric tube should be started if the patient survives the first 24 hours. Catheterization is necessary if retention

occurs; the use of a plastic urinal is desirable in male patients who are incontinent. Repeated spinal puncture for relief of intracranial pressure is dangerous inasmuch as it may precipitate a tentorial pressure cone. Hypertension should be controlled by hypotensive agents[69]; as mentioned, these patients are sometimes very sensitive to such agents. The administration of antibiotics helps to prevent the bronchopneumonia which so often proves fatal in untreated cases. In some instances, electrolyte disturbances occur, and these must be adjusted by appropriate therapy. The criteria for surgical intervention cannot be regarded as fully established at the present time, but there is evidence that nothing is to be expected from operating on the deeply comatose patient with a large, deeply placed hemorrhage, whereas it can be worthwhile in patients whose progression has been slow and who are not yet in coma.[66, 67]

Cerebral Thrombosis

Etiology. The great majority of cerebral thromboses occur after middle age as a complication of atherosclerosis and hypertension. This is the setting, but

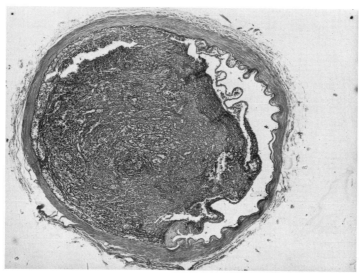

Figure 15–8. Dissecting aneurysm of the middle cerebral artery. (Courtesy of Dr. L. Wolman.)

little is known of the mechanisms which determine the development of a thrombus at a particular spot and at a particular moment in a patient's history. Nor is it clear why a thrombus will form on one atheromatous plaque and not on another, or why thrombi are occasionally found in arteries which appear to be healthy. The answers to these and other questions concerning the pathogenesis of degenerative vascular disease and its complications lie in the future. All that can be said at the present time is that statistical and experimental studies indicate that atherosclerosis and thrombosis appear to be influenced by certain factors, notably heredity, hypertension, cardiac disease,[89] stress, diets rich in animal fat, familial hypercholesterolemia, hyperlipemia, obesity, diabetes mellitus, polycythemia, thrombocythemia, and infection.

Thrombotic infarction is often associated with stenosis of extracranial vessels. Atheromatous plaques in the latter can be responsible for embolic infarctions within the brain, in which event the symptoms come on abruptly and achieve their maximum development at once. In other cases, thrombosis of an intracranial artery is the source of an infarct, and the relevance of this event to stenosis in a large feeding vessel is

often difficult to define. The present trend, based on autopsy evidence, is to attribute an increasingly large number of cases of "cerebral thrombosis" to embolism from extracranial sources, notably the heart and great vessels in the neck. It seems likely that cerebral infarction resulting from a combination of arterial stenosis and episodic hypotension is relatively uncommon.

Thrombosis also occurs in syphilitic endarteritis, septic arteritis in the course of generalized and localized infections, the arteritis of collagen diseases (including rheumatic fever),[27, 72] congestive heart failure,[89] following closed injuries to the head and neck, dissecting aneurysm, certain blood disorders (polycythemia, thrombocythemia, and sickle cell disease), and following radiation. It is not certain whether thromboangiitis obliterans should be included; if it occurs in the brain at all, it must be very rare.

Strokes occasionally occur in young women who are taking contraceptive hormones, but the incidence is very low. Little is known about the pathology, since most cases recover completely. The clinical course may suggest arterial thrombosis or embolism, but venous occlusion is another possibility which has to be entertained in the light of the fact

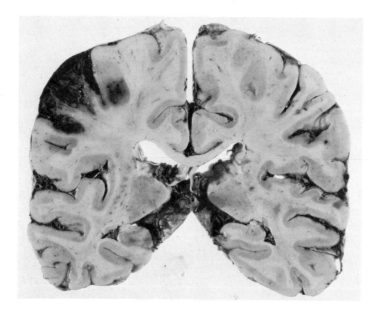

Figure 15–9. Hemorrhagic infarct. (Courtesy of Ayer Laboratory, Pennsylvania Hospital, Philadelphia.)

that thrombosis of the dural venous sinuses has been found in cases coming to autopsy.[6]

Pathology. When a thrombus develops it may (1) break up into fragments under the influence of plasma fibrinolysin or because it lacks tensile strength, thus giving rise to emboli, (2) become covered with endothelium from the surrounding intima, so giving rise to one form of subintimal atheromatous plaque as described by Duguid,[33] or (3) grow in size until it occludes the arterial lumen, with subsequent recanalization or conversion of the artery into a fibrous cord.

Whether or not the thrombus produces an infarct depends on the degree of occlusion and on the adequacy or inadequacy of the anastomotic channels distal to the obstruction; since arteries have virtually no anastomosis once they have penetrated the white matter, occlusion beyond this point necessarily produces an infarct (Fig. 15–9). Whether or not an infarct will produce symptoms depends on its size and situation. A pea-sized infarct in the caudate nucleus, for instance, may pass unnoticed, but a similar lesion in the middle of the internal capsule or in the optic radiation is likely to make its presence known.

Infarcted brain is usually pale and bloodless, with marginal congestion and petechiae; if gray matter is involved, it is more likely to be hemorrhagic. If infarction is complete there is destruction of all tissues within it, but if it is incomplete the nerve cells and myelinated fibers are chiefly involved, blood vessels and supporting elements remaining relatively intact. If the infarct is large, there is usually a considerable amount of edematous swelling of the brain, and this can lead to uncal herniation. Destroyed tissue is scavenged by phagocytes, and the parenchyma is replaced by cystic spaces filled with fluid and lined by astrocytes and astrocytic fibers; the margin between old infarcts and the surrounding brain is sharp.

In large, fresh infarcts, the site of arterial occlusion can often be found by diligent search, but this is not so in the case of small or old lesions, possibly because by the time the patient comes to autopsy, the thrombus has disappeared as a result of fibrinolytic activity, recanalization, or incorporation of the clot within the vessel wall. Infarction often occurs without local thrombosis or embolism, as for instance when hypotension occurs in a patient with severe stenosis of a major vessel in the neck.

Clinical Features. The majority of all cases of cerebral thrombosis occur as a complication of atherosclerosis and hypertension and therefore usually occur in those over 40 years of age. A raised blood pressure is almost as usual as it is in cerebral hemorrhage, but the latter is more likely to take place when the diastolic pressure is very high.

Premonitory symptoms in the shape of headache, dizziness, confusion of mind, and focal incapacity occur in rare instances. Sometimes there is a feeling of general malaise and fatigue which the patient may relate to a preceding period of overwork or stress. When fleeting premonitory focal symptoms occur, in the form of aphasia, numbness or weakness of the limbs, unsteady gait, etc., they probably represent a temporary failure of the blood flow during the growth of a mural thrombus or result from emboli which break off from the growing clot.

The onset is rapid rather than abrupt, and incapacity may increase rapidly and smoothly or with a steplike progression (cerebral hemorrhage sometimes behaves in the same fashion, but embolism does not). Headache may be absent, slight, or severe, and may be either generalized or localized over the area of skull adjacent to the infarct. Seizures, either focal or generalized, may occur, but they are infrequent, presumably because few thrombotic infarcts involve the cortex. There is little disturbance of pulse or respiration with small lesions, but changes appropriate to a rapidly increasing mass within the skull are sometimes encountered in massive infarcts accompanied by edema. Early loss of consciousness is common in cases coming to autopsy—that is to say, in the more serious cases, but in less severe examples consciousness is often preserved or is but lightly depressed. Loss of consciousness depends on the suddenness of the catastrophe and on the site and size of the infarct.

Focal incapacity may appear immediately or within hours of the onset, and its character will depend not only on the identity of the obstructed vessel (pp. 349 to 355) but also upon the efficiency of the anastomotic system in the case of thrombosis in extracerebral vessels. If the anastomotic vessels are also involved by atheromatous stenosis or thrombosis, the effect will be so much the greater. For example, a slowly evolving thrombotic occlusion of the internal carotid artery in the neck may produce minimal symptoms if the opposite carotid is patent and the circle of Willis is normal, whereas even partial occlusion of one carotid can give rise to widespread dysfunction if the collateral circulation is already compromised, or if for any reason the systemic blood pressure falls below a critical level. Another factor which influences the focal symptomatology of a single infarct is the existence of previous damage in the same or opposite hemisphere. Thus, whereas a middle cerebral thrombosis will not ordinarily cause persistent dysarthria or dysphagia, it will do so if the opposite corticobulbar pathway has already been damaged by previous involvement of the pyramidal system in the cerebrum or brainstem, even if the previous incident did not produce bulbar symptoms at the time. Again, a slight disturbance of mind and mood induced by a unilateral lesion will be compounded by pre-existent infarcts of the opposite hemisphere, even when the latter have given no overt signs of their presence. These circumstances are some of the reasons for apparent case-to-case variability in what appear to be comparable infarctions as seen at autopsy.

Changes in the vital signs—pulse, blood pressure, and respiration—may be absent, slight, or considerable. A small infarct in the orbital region of the frontal lobe, the hypothalamus, or the brainstem can cause a sharp rise of blood pressure whether or not the patient was formerly hypertensive. Such hypertension is sometimes extremely sensitive to reserpine and other hypotensive agents, and it is therefore desirable before prescribing hypotensive agents to determine from the history and from a consideration of the heart size and the retinal vessels whether the patient was hypertensive prior to the ictus. A second cause of hypertension is massive edema of the brain surrounding a large infarct in the cerebrum or cerebellum. Ectopic rhythms and inversion of the T wave in the electrocardiogram can occur under similar circumstances, leading to an erroneous diagnosis of coronary occlusion, but in general, the characteristics of the EKG changes and the absence of hypotension will prevent this mistake. Since cerebral infarction can occur as a result of a coronary occlusion (whether from immediate hypotension or, later on, from emboli derived from intracardiac thrombi), the distinction is of practical importance.

Laboratory Aids. The pressure of the spinal fluid is commonly normal, but pressures above 250 mm. Hg are sometimes seen in large infarcts complicated by cerebral edema. The protein content and cell counts may be normal or slightly elevated, depending on whether or not the infarct reaches the surface of the brain or ventricles; a few polymorphs may appear. Xanthochromia may be present in patients with a hemorrhagic infarction. A test for syphilis should be carried out routinely.

Brain scanning can provide useful information if the lesion is supratentorial. If performed within the first week after the onset of symptoms, the probability of a positive scan is about 20 per cent, but as time goes on the percentage of positives increases because of the vascular response around the infarct. If the scan is positive within the first 24 hours, a tumor or a cerebral hemorrhage is to be suspected.

The electroencephalogram has comparatively little to offer. Focal abnormalities are found in most cases with vascular disease of one hemisphere, and the abnormality tends to decrease as time goes on, even if the neurological signs do not improve. The most common EEG finding in occlusion of an internal carotid or middle cerebral artery is a slow wave focus in the middle sylvian area, with a frequency between the theta and delta ranges. There is often a depression of voltage on the same side. Occlusions may be present without any change in the EEG.

Arteriography [16] can supply a great deal of information as to the state of the extracranial and intracranial vessels, but it is not always easy to decide when to use it and when to refrain, and there are no hard and fast rules on the subject. An arteriogram will occasionally disclose not cerebral infarction but a glioblastoma, or a subdural hematoma, or an angiomatous malformation. Four-vessel arteriography is ultimately necessary before any attempt is made to correct extracranial arterial stenosis, which is often responsible for cerebral thrombosis and cerebral embolism. It is perhaps possible for all to agree on one rule, viz., that elderly, debilitated patients with advanced cerebral vascular disease should not be put to the discomfort and expense of arteriography which is carried out only for the satisfaction of academic curiosity.

Estimations of fasting blood sugar, of cholesterol, triglycerides, and uric acid levels, and of hematocrit values should be done as a routine, so that deviations from the normal may be identified and treated. The Framingham study has demonstrated that there is an increased risk of stroke in patients with comparatively modest elevations in hematocrit levels, which may fall within the upper limit of what is usually considered normal (47 per cent for women and 54 per cent for men). Similar modest elevations are also found in some patients with coronary disease and peripheral vascular disease.

Electrocardiography, combined with radiological assessment of the heart size and careful examination for evidence of decompensation, are desirable in all cases. The EKG abnormalities which occur in cerebral hemorrhage (p. 365) can also occur in large cerebral infarcts.

Course and Prognosis. Generally speaking, the outlook is better than for hemorrhage and worse than for embolism. About eight of 10 patients with cerebral hemorrhage die within a month, whereas about 80 per cent of all patients with cerebral infarction survive for a month or more.[19] The immediate prognosis for survival is poor when there is a large, deep infarct, and in the presence of prolonged unconsciousness, high blood pressure, ischemic heart disease, diabetes, and old age. Patients with a blood fibrinogen level of over 500 mg. per cent do badly, presumably because the fibrinogen level reflects the amount of brain damage.[34]

The long-term prognosis for those who survive an initial cerebral infarct depends on many factors, including race, sex, age, geography, and the control of hypertension, diabetes, hypercholesterolemia, the polycythemias and other diseases which aggravate the underlying condition. Several surveys[1, 7, 19, 45, 61a, 85, 98a, 102] have been carried out on the long-term prognosis of strokes in general or of cerebral thrombosis in particular. Almost all of them show that there is a relatively high mortality in the first year or two, compared with subsequent years, and that by the end of five years, about 50 per cent of the patients have died, usually from another stroke or from ischemic heart disease. Patients over 60 years of age fare less well than younger individuals, and those who are left with severe physical incapacity as the result of the stroke do badly. Thus, Adams and Merrett[1] found that 50 per cent of their patients below the age of 65 who recovered from a stroke survived at least six years, compared with a 20 per cent survival rate for those who remained incapacitated, and all of Carter's[19] bedridden patients died within five years. The chances for survival are vitiated by ischemic heart disease, hypertension, the presence of bilateral cerebral lesions, and diabetes.[61a] It is probable that the hyperlipidemias and the polycythemias have a similar effect, and it is reasonable to suppose that the chances for survival would be improved by appropriate treatment of all the factors known to accelerate arterial degeneration and to promote thrombosis.

Differential Diagnosis. See page 379.

Treatment. In the mildest cases with minimal signs, a few days of bed rest is all that is required. At the other end of the scale is the deeply unconscious patient. In this case, the head and shoulders should be elevated and attention should be paid from the very beginning to the care of the skin over pressure points. Frequent changes of position are desirable—no easy task in the case of heavy patients. The mouth must be kept clean and the pharynx clear of mucus. The provision of a good airway is essential, and tracheostomy may be necessary to secure it. Fluid balance and nutrition can be maintained by mouth, by nasal catheter, or by intravenous infusion. Catheterization is necessary to avoid retention of urine, and it is important that this be carried out early, because overdistention favors the development of urinary infections.

Anticoagulants should be reserved for normotensive subjects below the age of 70 who have had recurrent transient ischemic attacks. They have no place in the treatment of the completed stroke. The drugs are contraindicated in the elderly diabetics, and in those with severe hypertension because of the danger of inducing hemorrhage into the infarcted area. Such hemorrhages can occur even when the prothrombin time is maintained within acceptable limits.

Fibrinolytic agents have been successful in the dissolution of thrombi in experimental animals, but their use in man has been disappointing, except in the treatment of thrombophlebitis by urokinase.

Stellate block does not increase cerebral blood flow or reduce vasoconstriction, and has proved of no value in cerebral thromboembolism.

Vasodilator agents, such as nicotinic acid and isoxsuprine hydrochloride (Vasodilan) are of doubtful value except as a convincing placebo. Hexobendine, given intravenously, increases cerebral blood flow and decreases vascular resistance in patients with cerebral vascular disease, without causing systemic hypotension. It remains to be seen whether an effective vasodilator such as this does the patient any good or merely steals blood away from the infarcted area. Five per cent carbon dioxide is a highly effective cerebral vasodilator, but clinical trials have failed to achieve useful therapeutic effects in patients with thromboembolism.

Factors which produce vascular disease and thrombosis must be attended to. They include uncontrolled hypertension, diabetes, polycythemia, thrombocythemia, hypercholesterolemia, and overeating. There is nothing to indicate that small quantities of alcohol are harmful. Cigarette smoking should be discouraged because of its effect on the heart and peripheral arteries. Once the patient has had symptoms of vascular origin, whether in the brain or elsewhere, his habits should be reorganized to avoid excessive stress, to encourage physical exercise short of fatigue, and to prevent overeating.

Physiotherapy should be started as early as possible. At first, it suffices for the nurse or a relative to put the joints of the paralyzed limbs through a complete range of movements at least three times a day in order to avoid periarticular adhesions. This is particularly important at the shoulder. Later on, the patient must be encouraged to try to use the weakened limbs himself. Much can be done by enthusiastic and skillful physiotherapy, but therapists must be cautioned against inducing fatigue by overlong sessions; physical and mental fatigability is often considerable in cerebrovascular disease. In cases of aphasia, re-education by a speech therapist is usually advised, but it is a long and arduous process, and its effectiveness is difficult to evaluate.

Cerebral Embolism

Etiology. Cerebral embolism is commonly caused by disease of the heart (coronary thrombosis, auricular fibrillation, changes of rhythm, rheumatic heart disease, congenital heart disease, bacterial endocarditis, marasmic endocarditis). Emboli can also arise from atheromatous plaques in the aorta and great vessels in the neck, and they may originate in thrombi within pulmonary veins. Rarely, a thrombus starting in the right subclavian artery will spread proximally to the point of origin of the common carotid artery and thus produce emboli within the carotid circulation. Minute emboli composed either of platelets or of cholesterol crystals may break off from atheromatous plaques to impact in the cerebral or retinal circulation; in the latter, they can cause transient blurring of vision. Small thrombi from systemic sources can reach the brain by bypassing the lungs through a patent foramen ovale. Emboli are often multiple, but the symptoms are commonly attributable to a single large fragment. On the other hand, in fat and air embolism, multiple small obstructions are the rule.

In a study of 4558 autopsies by Kane and his colleagues,[55] in patients 16 years of age or older, embolic lesions were twice as common in the female as in the male, regardless of age, race, the presence or absence of diabetes, the nutritional state, or the size of the heart.

Pathology. Embolic infarcts demonstrate a predilection for cerebral and cerebellar cortical locations via long circumferential arteries, and they tend to spare the parasagittal perforating branches supplying the brainstem and diencephalic structures.

In some instances, the clot first lodges in a large vessel and then breaks up into fragments, which come to rest high up in the arterial tree. The area of brain supplied by the affected vessel becomes infarcted and the subsequent pathological changes are the same as in thrombotic occlusion, except that the infarct is more likely to be hemorrhagic and the cortex is more often involved. If the embolus is infected, it may give rise to local septic arteritis, which can cause a mycotic aneurysm, and this in turn may lead to hemorrhage; septic arteritis can also give rise to cerebral abscess, but the embolic incident which precedes brain abscess and pyemia seldom causes recognizable neurological deficit at the time of impaction because the embolus is too small to do so.

Clinical Features. Premonitory symptoms, notably headache, sometimes occur days or hours beforehand, perhaps because of the liberation of minute emboli before the main attack. The latter is characterized by an abrupt onset, maximum disability occurring at once. Headache may or may not be present; it is not as severe as in subarachnoid hemorrhage. Consciousness is often retained, and seizures are not infrequent. Focal signs are demonstrable at once (unless obscured by deep coma), and are consistent with the site of the infarct. In some cases, there is rapid improvement, with a narrowing down of the area of apparent damage as judged by clinical examination. This may be due to relaxation of arterial spasm in collateral branches; the impaction of solid emboli in the cerebral vessels of experimental animals is followed in some instances by widespread contraction of cerebral arterioles, dilatation of veins, and local slowing of blood flow; similarly, widespread vasoconstriction sometimes accompanies embolism in human limbs.[20]

Differential Diagnosis. See page 379.

Course and Prognosis. Embolism is rarely fatal. If a fatal issue is going to occur it usually takes place in one to 14 days after the ictus, and is caused not by the infarct itself but by pulmonary complications or by the disease which gave rise to the emboli. The prognosis as regards focal disability is better in young people than in old, but because the middle cerebral artery is so often the one involved, many patients are left with hemiparesis, with or without aphasia, hemianopia, or liability to seizures.[84]

Treatment. There is doubt as to the efficacy of procedures and drugs designed to promote vasodilatation, such as stellate block, the inhalation of 5 per cent carbon dioxide, and the rapid intravenous injection of 50 mg. of Priscoline or papaverine. Carefully controlled studies have failed to prove that these methods consistently influence the overall mortality or morbidity, but the abrupt improvement which occasionally follows the early administration of Priscoline or papaverine is, in the author's experience, too dramatic to be ignored or attributed to coincidence; however, such responses are uncommon. The effect of intravenous Hexobendine is being evaluated at the time of writing.

General supportive treatment is given, as for other forms of stroke. Statistical evidence suggests that long-term anticoagulants reduce the frequency of further incidents when the underlying lesion is likely to continue serving as a source for emboli, as in cardiac disease and atheromatous ulcers on the great vessels in the neck.

DECOMPRESSION SICKNESS, AIR EMBOLISM, AND DYSBARISM

In caisson sickness ("the bends"), the symptoms are the result of a too-rapid reduction of the ambient pressure after exposure to high atmospheric pressure. Bubbles of nitrogen appear in the blood stream, leading to multiple small hemorrhagic infarcts. The patient experiences acute pain in muscles and joints, headache, vertigo, difficulty in breathing ("the chokes"), pain in the chest, and symptoms referable to the central nervous system, which can include confusion, seizures, paraplegia, and loss of consciousness. Recovery from the somatic and cerebral symptoms is usual if the patient is rapidly put back into the compression chamber and is supplied with oxygen at increased partial pressure, but when embolic ischemia has occurred in the spinal cord, the consequent paraplegia, sensory loss, and bladder paralysis may not recover.

Air embolism occurs occasionally in the course of operations on the chest and great vessels, including the superior sagittal sinus, and can be a complication of obstetrical procedures. The symptoms are those of pulmonary, coronary, or cerebral infarction.

Dysbarism is the name given to what was formerly known as aeroembolism.[97] Bubbles of gas are formed in the tissues and not in the blood stream, as the result of flying at altitudes above 30,000 ft. in an unpressurized cabin. The symptoms are more sudden in onset than the effects of anoxia. They include pain in the joints and muscles, dyspnea, pain in the chest, confusion, amnesia, aphasia, cerebral paralysis of one or more limbs, spinal paraplegia, sensory loss, visual impairment, seizures, migraine-like headaches, etc.[97]

Fat Embolism

The origin of the fat emboli is a controversial subject.[36] While it is possible that fat may get into vascular channels after trauma or the injection of medications suspended in oil, recent studies have shown that an alteration of the normal plasma colloidal dispersion of chylomicrons occurs, with the result that they coalesce into larger fat droplets. There is also evidence that a lipid mobilizing hormone is activated by trauma, resulting in an increase in the blood lipid concentration.

Symptoms may occur within a few hours of trauma, or they may be delayed for as much as four days. The symptoms begin suddenly, as is appropriate in embolism. Impaction in the lungs produces dyspnea and cyanosis; petechiae appear around the neck, upper part of the trunk, and proximal portions of the limbs. Involvement of the brain produces drowsiness, restlessness, and delirium; the kidneys often escape, but oliguria can occur.

The temperature is elevated and there is usually sinus tachycardia and an increase in the rate of respiration. Free fat is found in the urine in about 50 per cent of the patients within the first three days after injury, and there is an increase in serum lipase in some patients. X-rays of the chest may show a "snowstorm" appearance. A drop in hemoglobin is common.

The differential diagnosis can include delirium tremens following an accident, epidural and subdural hematoma, and late traumatic apoplexy.

Treatment is symptomatic.[82] It ha been claimed that the mortality rate (which ordinarily is about 5 per cent) i reduced by the intravenous administra tion of 200 ml. of 20 per cent decholir sodium, which is given with the objec of reducing the size of the circulating fat globules. It is also claimed tha Dextran 40, given in doses of 500 ml every 12 hours, is useful insofar as i reduces intravascular aggregation o red cells and thereby improves capillary flow.

Hypertensive Encephalopathy

Definition. The term "hypertensive encephalopathy" was introduced by Oppenheimer and Fishberg in 1928 to describe the seizures and stupor which sometimes occur in the course of eclamp sia, glomerulonephritis, malignant hy pertension, and lead poisoning.[79]

Etiology and Pathogenesis. Byrom found that experimental hypertension induced in rats caused arteriolar spasm in cortical vessels; the spasm disappeared with reduction of blood pressure, but i it was maintained, it gave rise to multi ple cystic infarcts in the cortex. Aboli tion of the hypertension usually resulted in dramatic relief of the spasm. This ex perimental model precisely reflects the events in hypertensive encephalopathy in man, including the relief of symptoms as the result of hypotensive agents.[7] Moreover, episodic pallor of the skin and narrowing of retinal arterioles which accompany the attacks bear witness to the presence of vasoconstriction.

Pathology. It is only the more severe cases which come to autopsy as a result of an encephalopathic attack. There is usually considerable cerebral edema, with flattening of the convolutions, microinfarcts of the cortex, and, occasionally, massive intracranial hemorrhage. The kidney, heart, and blood vessels show changes appropriate to the condition causing the hypertension.

Clinical Features. Headache, confusion, and—oddly enough—itchiness of the nose may herald a seizure, and there may also be a sense of constriction in the chest. If the blood pressure is lowered at this stage, convulsions may be averted. If not, typically epileptiform seizures occur, with tonic and clonic phases, incontinence, and tongue biting. There may be a succession of seizures as in eclampsia, or there may be recurrent attacks from time to time over several months, as in malignant hypertension. Some of the seizures start in a focal manner and become generalized, while others are generalized throughout. Persistent focal neurological deficits such as hemiplegia, aphasia, or hemianopia are attributed to cerebral infarction or small hemorrhages. The blood pressure soars above its previous high level, and cardiac failure with both pulmonary and systemic congestion may supervene. The cerebrospinal fluid pressure is increased between convulsions, and papilledema is often present. Hypertensive retinopathy is usually present in cases of nephritis and malignant hypertension. The urine contains casts and albumin, and the blood urea is raised. The spinal fluid protein may be increased to as much as 200 mg. per cent, but the cell count is usually normal.

The hypertensive encephalopathy of lead poisoning must be distinguished from lead encephalopathy in which the blood pressure may be normal or slightly raised, and in which the symptoms are due to the direct effect of lead on the brain.

Prognosis. Hypertensive encephalopathy is of dire import in malignant hypertension and renal hypertension, but if an eclamptic recovers, no other trouble need be anticipated unless the woman is allowed to become pregnant again. In this event, eclampsia may or may not recur. If it does, persistent renal damage may supervene.

Treatment. Blood pressure must be reduced by bed rest and the use of hypotensive agents, but caution must be exercised to avoid too drastic a drop of pressure, e.g., below 100/70, because of the danger of precipitating cerebral or myocardial infarction. Seizures can be controlled with intravenous Dilantin or Valium.

Arterial Stenosis

Etiology. Atherosclerotic plaques are seen in arteries ranging in size from the carotid to vessels measuring 0.6 mm. in diameter; smaller branches are less often affected, except in the presence of severe hypertension, hypercholesterolemia, and diabetes. The degeneration of the elastic and muscular elements of the arterial wall which constitutes arteriosclerosis in aging subjects gives rise to dilatation rather than obstruction. Narrowing is usually due either to a large atheromatous plaque which juts into the lumen or to fibrous organization of a thrombus, but occasionally it occurs as a result of open or closed injuries. A thrombus may form on a necrotic atheromatous plaque, still further narrowing the lumen

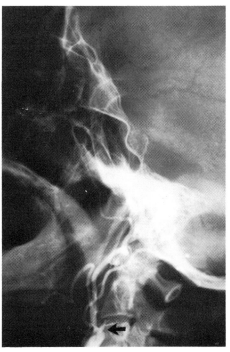

Figure 15–10. Complete occlusion of the internal carotid artery at its origin from the common carotid.

and serving as a source of emboli, including small collections of platelets and cholesterol crystals.

If occlusion develops slowly over a period of months or longer, the collateral circulation may suffice to prevent symptoms of cerebral ischemia, but if the obstruction develops suddenly, or if it cannot be short-circuited in this fashion, evidence of focal dysfunction will eventually appear.

The abrupt appearance of symptoms in such a case can be caused in several ways: (1) The ischemia may have passed a critical point with respect to the metabolic requirements of the affected portion of brain. (2) A fall of systemic blood pressure from any cause will reduce the blood flow through the stenosed vessel and its anastomotic allies. This occurs in hemorrhagic shock, coronary thrombosis (which may be overshadowed by the cerebral symptoms, and therefore escape notice), traumatic shock, abuse of hypotensive agents, lumbar sympathectomy, postural hypotension, hypersensitive carotid sinus, cardiac arrhythmias, steam baths, high spinal anesthesia, and overdosage of barbi-

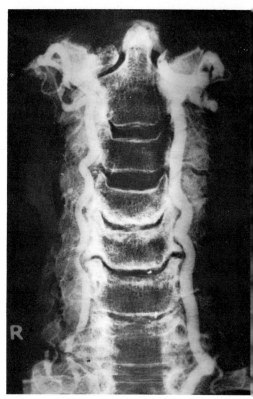

Figure 15–12. The effect of spondylosis on the vertebral arteries. (Courtesy of Drs. E. C. Hutchinson and P. O. Yates, and the editor of *Brain.*)

turates and tranquilizers. (3) Hypoglycemia. (4) Emboli from a thrombus on an atheromatous plaque in the stenotic zone can break off and pass upward to impact in a distal branch. (5) Cerebral hemorrhage within the territory supplied by the stenosed vessel. (6) Thrombosis of a *branch* of the stenosed artery. (7) In the presence of stenosis of the carotid or vertebral artery or both, turning the head to either side can temporarily obstruct the circulation to the brain, leading to dizziness, syncope, or sudden falls without loss of consciousness. Distortion of the vertebral arteries by the bony changes of cervical spondylosis may play a part in the production of symptoms induced by movements of the head (Fig. 15–12).[52, 90] (8) If stenosis of the subclavian artery occurs proximal to the origin of the vertebral artery, use of the arm on the affected side can "steal" blood from the vertebral artery, in which

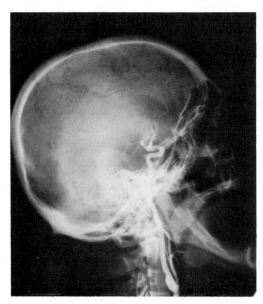

Figure 15–11. Carotid insufficiency. Angiogram showing small indentation of internal carotid just above its origin. Later films showed good filling of intracranial branches.

the direction of blood flow is reversed, with consequent reduction of blood supply to the brainstem and the appearance of symptoms of basilar-vertebral insufficiency.[75, 83]

CAROTID STENOSIS

The most commonly affected site is just distal to the point of origin of the internal carotid artery from the common carotid (Fig. 15–13). Flow through the external carotid may increase, with discernible increase in pulsation of the arteries of the face and temple, and increased perfusion of the face and scalp can be disclosed by thermography or by directly comparing the skin temperature of the two sides (thermometry). The increased vascularity may be the cause of the unilateral headache which is sometimes encountered in these cases. In many instances there are no neurological symptoms at all and diagnosis is made by the accidental discovery of a harsh systolic bruit over the internal carotid artery. When symptoms do occur, they usually take the form of transient ischemic attacks,[63] but occasionally a catastrophic thrombosis of the internal carotid artery is the first symptom. If the thrombus extends to the point of origin of the internal ophthalmic artery, there is blindness on the side of the thrombosis, with a contralateral hemiplegia and hemianesthesia.

Ischemic ocular inflammation sometimes occurs on the affected side.[56] It is essentially a uveitis, and the symptoms include amaurosis fugax, pain in the eye, and impairment of vision from corneal edema. There is a diffuse episcleral injection, neovascularization and atrophy of the iris, and irregularity of the pupil. Small hemorrhages are to be found in the periphery of the retina, and the retinal arteries are usually narrowed.

Ophthalmodynamometry will disclose lowered systolic and diastolic pressures in the retinal arteries on the side of the carotid stenosis, in many cases.

The most satisfactory way of demonstrating the site and degree of arterial stenosis is by arteriography, and this should include both carotids and both vertebral arteries if surgical correction is under consideration. The carotid compression test is sometimes used: With complete or partial occlusion of one carotid in the neck, compression of the contralateral normal artery may result in syncope. Similarly, syncope may result from compression of either carotid artery if there is vertebral basilar insufficiency. Carotid compression is not without its dangers; it can cause cardiac standstill in the presence of a hyperactive carotid reflex and may produce hemiplegia, presumably from dislodgment of the thrombus or portion of the plaque. It is questionable whether the information supplied by this procedure justifies these risks.

Treatment. The treatment of carotid stenosis is still controversial. In assessing either medical or surgical treatment, it is necessary to remember that any patient with considerable stenosis of one or both carotid arteries may remain free from symptoms for many years and even when intermittent symptoms do develop, they may pass off for long periods without any treatment whatsoever. There is statistical evidence that anticoagulants diminish transient ischemic attacks. Surgical efforts to restore blood flow can be worthwhile, but since atherosclerosis is a progressive disease, surgery should be followed by measures to control factors which are known to accelerate its development or which are thought to promote thrombosis. There is no doubt

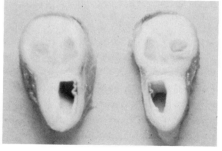

Figure 15–13. Occlusion of the internal carotid with patency of the external carotid. (Courtesy of Department of Neuropathology, Philadelphia General Hospital.)

that atherosclerotic stenosis can recur after endarterectomy. In general, it is probably wise to attempt to restore blood flow in cases with severe stenosis of one carotid artery provided that there is satisfactory flow in the other carotid and in the vertebral-basilar circulation.

VERTEBRAL-BASILAR STENOSIS

The vertebral arteries may be narrowed at their origins from the subclavian artery or there may be multiple stenoses in their course, or in the basilar artery. Congenital hypoplasia of one vertebral artery can aggravate the effects of atheromatous stenosis in the other. Symptoms may be induced by turning the head to one side, thereby reducing flow in an already compromised artery. Reference has already been made to the effect of stenosis of the subclavian artery proximal to the origin of the vertebral artery in promoting reversal of flow within the latter and consequent arterial insufficiency in the brainstem[75] (p. 376). Vertebral-basilar insufficiency is characterized by transient ischemic attacks, as will be described below.

TRANSIENT ISCHEMIC ATTACKS

This term is applied to brief attacks of cerebral dysfunction of vascular origin, which are not followed by persistent neurological deficit. The symptoms last from a few minutes to hours. As ordinarily understood, the term does not include brief spells of inadequate cerebral blood flow secondary to failure of the systemic circulation such as occurs in fainting, severe hemorrhage, myocardial infarction, Stokes-Adams syndrome, tussive syncope, carotid sinus sensitivity, or severe postural hypotension.

Most cases of transient cerebral ischemia are associated with occlusive vascular disease. It is thought that minute fragments of blood clot, small masses of fused platelets, and atheromatous material break off from atheromatous plaques and are swept upwards to impact in small intracranial vessels,

from which they are removed by normal fibrinolytic mechanisms. Studies of regional cerebral blood flow in patients following transient hemiparesis have disclosed focal areas of ischemia, and hyperemia with focal vasoparalysis, during the first three or four days after the attack, following which cerebral blood flow returns to normal. Rarely, a sudden fall of blood pressure can cause ischemia in the distribution of a stenosed artery, in which event the ischemic attack may be cut short either by recovery of the blood pressure or by an arterial input from the collateral circulation. Emboli from the heart (mural thrombi, vegetations on the valves) may also cause transient ischemic attacks (notably amaurosis fugax in patients with rheumatic heart disease) but are more important as a source of massive embolic infarction.

The clinical features of transient ischemic episodes in the *carotid system* include unilateral weakness or numbness on one side of the body (or a portion of it), disturbances of speech and thinking, monocular blurring of vision, brief impairment of memory, disorientation in time and place, and—perhaps—focal epileptic seizures.

When the vertebral-basilar system is involved, symptoms are more diverse. They include vertigo, diplopia, transient paralysis of gaze, blurred vision, hemianopia, cortical blindness, scintillating visual hallucinations, memory lapses (including global amnesia), numbness down one side of the body or in the face, bilateral weakness, alternating weakness on the two sides of the body, dysarthria, dysphagia, impaired hearing in one ear, vertigo, staggering, sudden drop attacks without unconsciousness, and a curious sense of lightheadedness without vertigo which the patient finds difficult to describe. Between attacks, patients with vertebral-basilar insufficiency sometimes complain of vertigo and staggering when they rise suddenly from a chair or from bed. Symptoms may also occur on turning the head to one side, thereby compressing one of the vertebral or carotid arteries.

Most transient ischemic attacks last from a few minutes to three or four hours; some authors accept a disability lasting 24 hours as falling within the permitted range, provided there is complete recovery at the end.

Course and Prognosis. Between 5 and 10 per cent of persons with transient ischemic attacks will have a stroke within the following 12 months, but such strokes are not necessarily severe. In a series of 79 patients studied by Baker and his colleagues[7] for an average period of 41 months, only 15 per cent subsequently developed major strokes, but in a *fifteen year* follow-up of patients with transient ischemic attacks conducted at the Mayo Clinic,[43b] 50 per cent died of cardiac disease and 36 per cent died of stroke. The morbidity and mortality rates are adversely affected by increasing age, the presence of hypertension, and occult or obvious heart disease.

Treatment. Long-term treatment with anticoagulants is probably effective in reducing the number and severity of transient ischemic attacks, but in assessing the effects of such treatment it is prudent to recognize that many patients cease having these attacks spontaneously. Anticoagulants are contraindicated in the very elderly, in diabetes, and in uncontrolled hypertension.

If the hematocrit level is elevated above 50 per cent, it should be reduced by repeated phlebotomy. The Framingham study has shown that individuals with a modest elevation of hematocrit values are twice as liable to stroke as those with normal levels.

Surgical correction of extracranial arterial stenosis should be carried out if preliminary studies, including four-vessel arteriography, indicate the need for it. The criteria, however, are still being debated. Whether surgery is carried out or not, care must be exercised to control all those factors which are known to accelerate the development of atherosclerosis or to promote thrombosis, notably hypertension, diabetes, hyperlipidemia, and polycythemia. Cigarette smoking should be stopped because of its effect on the coronary arteries, and the patient should be protected from domestic and professional stress so far as this is possible.

Differential Diagnosis of Cerebrovascular Accidents

Differential diagnosis requires answers to two questions: Are the symptoms due to a cerebrovascular accident? If so, what kind of stroke is it? The first is often easier than the second, because in the majority of cases the onset is more abrupt than in any other disease of the nervous system, but the problem becomes difficult when the onset is gradual rather than abrupt, or when the patient is unconscious and no information is available as to the past history or mode of onset.

A gradual onset can occur in both cerebral hemorrhage and thrombosis, but is more common in the latter. Such a history, together with the appearance of progressively increasing evidence of focal neurological disturbance, also occurs in subdural hematoma, delayed epidural venous hemorrhage following trauma, glioblastoma, and cerebral abscess.

Epidural and subdural hematomas cannot be excluded with certainty without the aid of angiography, which may also disclose thrombotic occlusion of a major or a minor artery. It may or may not demonstrate an abscess or intracerebral hemorrhage. The former will usually be accompanied by fever and polymorph pleocytosis in the spinal fluid, and the latter will commonly show blood in the fluid. However, blood is absent in about one in six cases of cerebral hemorrhage. In syphilitic thrombosis, the spinal fluid may or may not show pleocytosis, increase of globulin, and positive serological reactions; the blood serology will always be positive, but the report on this is not likely to be available immediately, and even if it is positive, it is not proof that the patient's present illness is necessarily due to syphilis.

The problem of the stuporous or comatose patient whose medical history is not known is too large a subject to be discussed here, but priority should be given to the investigations required for the identification of diseases in which immediate treatment is essential to save life—subdural and extradural hemorrhage, diabetic coma, hypoglycemia, exogenous poisons, fulminating meningitis, cerebral abscess, cerebral malaria, adrenal cortical failure, hypothyroidism, eclampsia, heat stroke, etc. Uremia qualifies for inclusion in this group if facilities for hemodialysis are available. Cerebrovascular accidents account for coma in the great majority of middle-aged and elderly patients, and since clinical examination will often reveal evidence of unilateral focal neurological signs, together with hypertension and atherosclerosis, a presumptive diagnosis of stroke is often justified.

The distinction between primary cerebral hemorrhage, subarachnoid hemorrhage, cerebral thrombosis, cerebral embolism, and cerebrovascular insufficiency can be made in many cases by the history, physical signs, and examination of the spinal fluid, but it is difficult to distinguish between cerebral thrombosis and those cases of cerebral hemorrhage which come on slowly and are unaccompanied by blood in the spinal fluid, Atheroma, hypertension, and focal neurological signs are present in both groups. Arteriography is the most useful means of differentiation, for it may disclose occlusion of an artery or displacement of vessels by hematoma or tumor, but even in experienced hands, it may fail to reveal hemorrhage (e.g., in 30 per cent of McKissock's series of surgically verified cases).[66] The presence of glomerulonephritis, hypertension, and raised blood urea favors a diagnosis of hemorrhage, rather than thrombosis, but there are many exceptions to this. Electroencephalography cannot distinguish with any certainty between hemorrhage, thrombosis, and embolism, and the same applies to echoencephalography, thermography, thermometry, and brain scans.

PSEUDOBULBAR PALSY

The clinical effects of repeated vascular insults to the brain are variable. There may be diverse combinations of focal neurological deficits, some of which have started abruptly as an easily recognizable vascular accident while others have appeared to creep up on the patient. In the presence of bilateral infarcts involving the corticobulbar tracts, the resulting clinical syndrome is characterized by weakness and spasticity of the muscles which control talking, movements of the lips and tongue, and swallowing. This is known as pseudobulbar palsy. It may be associated with a variety of other defects, including supranuclear ocular palsies, spasticity of the limbs, and parkinsonism.[24, 96]

Pathogenesis. Two clinical varieties of pseudobulbar palsy are seen in cerebrovascular disease. The common form results from multiple, discrete and easily recognized vascular accidents involving the cerebral hemispheres or the brainstem. In such cases, the bulbar symptoms are usually part of a double hemiplegia, and the condition is not progressive unless further vascular accidents occur. In the second type, which is rare, major strokes are unusual but although a casually taken history may suggest that the clinical course has been smoothly progressive, careful interrogation of relatives and friends will bring out a story of slight but abrupt "worsenings" or obvious transient ischemic attacks. The reason for assuming a vascular pathology in this group is the presence of multiple small scars and lacunae within the territory of the penetrating arteries supplying the basal ganglia, midbrain, and pons.[41, 96] A single brain may contain as many as 50 of these lacunae. There is degeneration of both association and projection fiber systems, and in elderly subjects there may also be cellular degeneration in the gray matter of the cortex and basal ganglia, senile plaques, and other changes of senescence. In addition to lacunae, larger areas of infarction may be present, especially in the "watershed" areas of the cortex. The blood vessels show atheroma and arteriosclerosis.

Clinical Features. The number, distribution, and size of the lesions are variable, so the clinical features show a correspondingly wide spectrum.[96] The onset is often marked by a transient ischemic attack—for instance, vertigo, dysarthria, diplopia, or a brief confusional state.

In the fully developed syndrome, speech is slurred and there may be spastic dysphagia. The voice loses its modulation, and speech is further disturbed by a lack of coordination between articulation and respiration. In an advanced case, the patient takes a breath and then proceeds to say as much as possible while it lasts, so that his words tumble out in an explosive rush and then trail off to an inaudible whisper toward the end of expiration. Words are telescoped into each other, and between breaths, the lips may continue in soundless speech. Palilalia is sometimes present. Swallowing may or may not be disturbed; the first difficulty is usually with fluids, which cause choking, but solids give rise to the greatest difficulty when the problem is one of weakness rather than rigidity.

The face becomes masklike[24] and this may be mistaken for parkinsonism. Pursing the lips and shutting the eyes voluntarily become difficult, but the eyes will close in sleep and laughter, and grief will throw the face into the customary corrugations. In advanced cases, reflex sucking movements of the lips and tongue will occur when an object is introduced between the lips.

Impairment of voluntary conjugate movements of the eyes, with retention of reflex and automatic movements, is not uncommon. Weakness of upward movement is usually the first to appear, but lateral movement may be affected as well. The patient who cannot move his eyes on command may nevertheless be able to follow a slowly moving finger, and if the gaze is fixed on a stationary object and the head is passively moved, the eyes will move so as to keep the object in view. Once the patient's gaze has fixed on an object, it may be difficult for him to detach it in order to look at something else. This "spasm of fixation" renders voluntary movements difficult; if thick lenses are placed in front of the eyes to prevent fixation, ocular movements are facilitated. Yet, when the patient is daydreaming and not looking at anything in particular, his eyes may move in the direction for which purposive movement is abolished. Normally, efferents from the occipital cortex to the ocular motor nuclei of the brainstem help to maintain fixation; this mechanism is under the control of the motor cortex, but in the presence of bilateral damage to corticopontine fibers, the fixation reflex gains ascendancy. Although voluntary ocular movement may be impossible, stimulation of the labyrinth by hot or cold water will evoke conjugate movements of the eyes; unlike the response in normal subjects, caloric tests may fail to evoke vertigo or nausea. It should be emphasized that this type of supranuclear paralysis of ocular movement depends on the disposition of the lesions rather than on the nature of the disease. It can occur, for instance, in multiple sclerosis.

Patients with pseudobulbar palsy sometimes show evidence of more diffuse disease. The limbs may show extrapyramidal rigidity[24, 96] or unilateral or bilateral pyramidal signs with weakness and spasticity, or a curious type of plastic rigidity which differs from parkinsonism in that it may be barely perceptible when the patient is examined in bed, but becomes apparent when he attempts to stand or walk. The patient stands unusually erect, unlike the usual general attitude of flexion in parkinsonism. So erect, indeed, that he is in danger of falling over backward if he loses his balance. These patients exhibit a striking stillness and lack of normal fidgeting movements. Movements are slow, deliberate, and rather clumsy. Thurel[96] has described choreiform movements and athetosis. Palatal nystagmus (palatal myoclonus) may occur when the olive or its connections are involved.

Objective sensory disturbances are uncommon except as a relic of a major vascular accident. The reflexes vary according to whether the pyramidal or extrapyramidal system is chiefly involved. Frequency of micturition and occasional incontinence may occur.

The mental state varies from normal to mild dementia, depending on the situation and extent of the disease. It is sometimes surprising to find an alert intellect behind the discouraging facade presented by an expressionless face and profound dysarthria. Pathological weeping or laughter is common in pseudobulbar palsy.

Course and Prognosis. Most cases pursue a slow course of gradual deterioration over a number of years. It may be punctuated at any time by a vascular accident. As is to be expected, the prognosis is vitiated by hypertension because of increased liability to a terminal stroke or myocardial infarction.

Diagnosis. Pseudobulbar palsy has to be distinguished from the bulbar palsy of amyotrophic lateral sclerosis; in the latter, there is no disturbance of ocular movement, the mind is entirely clear, and atrophy and fasciculation will often be present. In postencephalitic parkinsonism and paralysis agitans, bulbar symptoms usually appear late, pyramidal signs are absent, and the clinical history is not punctuated by vascular accidents.

Behrman and his colleagues [10a] and others have described a condition which arises in late adult life and is characterized by progressive supranuclear palsy of eye movements, associated with slowly progressive pseudobulbar palsy, masklike face, dysequilibrium in standing and walking, and a tendency to keep the neck extended. The pathological changes are largely confined to the brainstem and cerebellum; there is swelling and degeneration of the nerve cells, many of which contain neurofibrillary tangles. Severe loss of neurons is evident in the dentate nuclei, without any significant abnormality of the cerebellar cortex. The pathological features are in-

consistent with a vascular etiology, and the existence of this condition—which s closely resembles the pseudobulba palsy of vascular origin—emphasizes th need for caution in attributing pseudo bulbar palsy of gradual onset to vascula causes.

Treatment. High blood pressure should be treated, but it must be borne ir mind that some of this group will have stenosis of the carotid or vertebral basilar arteries, or both, and that in such cases symptoms can be induced by over enthusiastic administration of hypoten sive drugs and diuretics. There is good sense in the view that a blood pressure in the region of 160/100, observed in the physician's office, is best left alone. A diet low in animal fat and refined sugar is indicated, and polycythemia should be treated if present. Diabetes should be looked for.

PROGRESSIVE SUBCORTICAL ENCEPHALOPATHY
(Binswanger's Disease)

There is some doubt whether the condition described by Binswanger in 1894 is a disease sui generis or not. It is characterized by the insidious onset in the fifth and sixth decades of progressive impairment of intellect, focal neurological deficits on one or both sides of the body, and either focal or generalized seizures.[78] Bilateral disposition of lesions within the corticobulbar tracts leads to the development of bulbar palsy. The disease is progressive, and death occurs within one or two years. Pathologically, there is patchy demyelination of the white matter, the cortex being spared. The demyelination leads to widespread destruction of nerve fibers, and there is a compensatory proliferation of glia. The ventricles may be much dilated. In Binswanger's original case, the white matter of the frontal lobes was spared. There is considerable atheroma in the circle of Willis, and the arterioles supplying the white matter are densely sclerosed. Despite these arterial changes, it is not certain that this disease is vascular in origin, though it is usually so described.

Arteriosclerotic Dementia

Arteriosclerosis is often blamed for dementia in aging persons,[64] but pathological evidence indicates that, unless there is a history of recurrent cerebral infarction, dementia from this cause is rare, and arteriosclerosis is not the usual cause of senile dementia. Of course, a single stroke involving the dominant hemisphere or the parietal lobe of the minor hemisphere can impair specific tools of the intellect and can alter personality, but it will not cause the global depression of intellectual capacity which alone justifies use of the term dementia. The fact that the demented patient presents evidence of vascular disease in the brain, heart, or lower limbs does not necessarily justify a conclusion that the mental symptoms are due to the same process, and it is necessary to exclude by appropriate diagnostic procedures conditions such as Alzheimer's disease, Pick's disease, normal pressure hydrocephalus with dementia, cerebral tumor

(midline meningiomas in particular), neurosyphilis, and so on. There is no good evidence that stenosis of one or both internal carotid arteries can cause a smoothly progressive dementia. Paulson and Perrine studied 30 demented patients with a diagnosis of "chronic brain syndrome associated with cerebral arteriosclerosis" and found only four with significant degrees of carotid artery stenosis. Moreover, patients with total bilateral occlusion of the internal carotid arteries seldom show evidence of dementia.

Cerebrovascular Accidents in Children

Cerebrovascular accidents are far less common in childhood and early adult life than in persons over 40, but they do occur (Fig. 15–14).

Generalized infections—pertussis, scarlet fever, typhoid, typhus, rheumatic fever, and others—can produce arteritis, which occasionally leads to massive infarction or hemorrhage, usually after the second week of illness. In other cases, there are multiple small hemorrhagic infarcts, which give rise to convulsions, delirium, and coma.

Acute infantile hemiplegia is a condi-

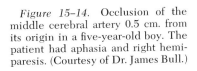

Figure 15–14. Occlusion of the middle cerebral artery 0.5 cm. from its origin in a five-year-old boy. The patient had aphasia and right hemiparesis. (Courtesy of Dr. James Bull.)

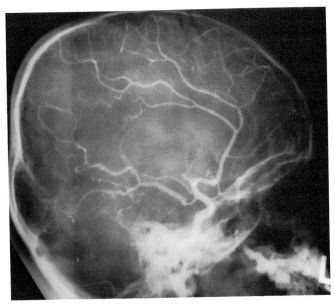

tion of obscure origin, usually occurring in children under the age of six. In some cases, autopsy has disclosed thrombosis of major arteries which show atheromatous plaques, necrosis of the media, and disintegration of the elastic laminae. In a few, venous thromboses have been found, without obvious cause; they give rise to localized cerebral edema, which can be so marked as to mimic a cerebral tumor. In both the arterial and venous types, the usual presentation is abrupt hemiplegia followed by partial recovery; seizures and athetosis may persist after convalescence, and speech may be delayed if the lesion is in the major hemisphere. A mild degree of mental deficit is not uncommon.

Dural sinus thrombosis can occur in marasmic infants and also as a result of infections in the ear and frontal sinuses. It is described on page 396.

Malignant hypertension can occur in early life, usually at about 10 years of age. It gives rise to atheroma and arteriosclerosis, as in adults. Neurologically, there may be transient focal symptoms and seizures, or persistent hemiplegia from massive thrombosis or hemorrhage. Peripheral paresis of the sixth and seventh cranial nerves has been described. Hypertensive retinopathy is the rule. It should be noted that severe hypertension in children under the age of eight can give rise to an intracranial bruit in the absence of an arteriovenous shunt or aneurysm.

Death from stroke or myocardial infarction in the first or second decade occurs in the very rare form of precocious senility known as *progeria*.[5] The hair and teeth fall out, the face is wizened and triangular, the joints are afflicted with osteoarthritis, the bones lose their calcium, and the subcutaneous fat disappears. There is extensive atheroma of the aorta and smaller vessels. Insufficient attention has been given to the implications of this disease with regard to the pathogenesis of arterial degeneration.

Polyarteritis nodosa occasionally occurs in children and can give rise to the usual wide spectrum of symptoms, including thrombosis of the centr artery of the retina, subarachnoid hen orrhage, intracerebral hemorrhage, an cerebral infarction.[72] Another collage disease, *disseminated lupus erythemate sus*, may produce neurological symptom either at the start of the disease or afte other clinical features have appeare The neurological features include su arachnoid hemorrhage, convulsion abrupt hemiplegia, confusion and con from multiple small infarcts, acute tran verse myelopathy, polyneuropathy, an myositis.

Hemorrhagic diseases, including he mophilia, hemorrhagic disease of th newborn, and thrombocytopenic pur pura, can be responsible for subaracl noid and intracerebral hemorrhage Hemophilia can also give rise to hemor rhage into the cord and peripher nerves. *Congenital heart disease* asso ciated with cyanosis and polycythemia i sometimes responsible for cerebral in farction and for dural sinus thrombosis and there is also a significant liability t brain abscess in Fallot's tetralogy. Em bolism can occur as a result of surgica operation on the heart and during car diac catheterization. *Bacterial endocar ditis* usually gives rise to multiple smal infarcts, which may be cerebral, cere bellar, or in the brainstem. The lodg ment of infected emboli can cause loca arteritis of cerebral vessels followed by the formation and rupture of a my cotic aneurysm. *Saccular aneurysms* though less common than in early adul life, are an occasional cause of sub arachnoid or intracerebral hemorrhage and angiomatous malformations have also to be considered when intracerebra hemorrhage develops with no apparen cause in a young person. In adolescence and early adult life, cerebral infarc tion from *syphilitic endarteritis* is not uncommon in communities where the incidence of syphilis is high.

Temporal Arteritis

Giant cell arteritis is a widespread vascular disorder and is not confined to the temporal or cranial arteries.[65] The larger vessels, including the aorta, the pulmonary arteries, and the coronary arteries, may be affected, but the renal arteries usually escape.[23]

Pathology. The features are those of a granulomatous arteritis. There is disintegration of the internal elastic lamina, and cellular infiltration with mononuclear and plasma cells, giant cells, and occasional eosinophils and polymorphs. Cellular infiltration may also be seen in the adventitia. The intima shows diffuse thickening, and the lumen may be very much reduced. Arterial thromboses are common, but recanalization can occur.

Clinical Features. The presenting symptom is usually headache, but in some cases this is preceded by a period of general ill health, with anorexia, loss of weight and appetite, aching pains in the muscles of the trunk and limbs, and night sweats.[28, 48] Rarely, sudden blindness is the first symptom.

The headache is commonly bilateral and the pain may spread into the face, jaw, tongue, or neck. Sometimes it is aggravated by chewing. There may be areas of considerable tenderness over the scalp, notably over the temporal arteries. These are usually swollen, nodular, and tender, with reduction or loss of pulsation. Occasionally, ulceration occurs over the swollen arteries, and patchy gangrene of the tongue has been recorded.

Meadows[65] recorded blindness in one or both eyes in more than half of his cases, and 15 per cent developed ophthalmoplegia, giving an incidence of neuro-ophthalmic complications in over 66 per cent of the series. This is higher than is usually encountered in general neurological practice. The interim between the onset of headache and the onset of blindness varies from days to months. Momentary visual symptoms consisting of obscuration of vision of one or both eyes may occur for a day or two before the onset of blindness. Visual hallucinations may occur in this early period. The onset of blindness is usually abrupt; one eye is affected first. It may stop there, or the other eye may be involved within a week or two.

Although the loss of vision is ischemic in origin, the classical features of central retinal artery occlusion are rarely seen. Usually there is pale swelling of the optic discs, with a few hemorrhages and cottonwool exudates nearby. The papilledema subsides within a few weeks and is replaced by optic atrophy.

The intracranial arteries can be involved[51] and death may occur from infarction of the brainstem. Bilateral cortical blindness due to infarction of both occipital lobes has been described. An acute organic psychosis may obscure the somatic symptoms.

The arteritis may affect the vessels of the face. There is intense pain in the face, with diffuse subcutaneous edema which can be sufficient to alter the patient's appearance by obliterating wrinkles.

The external carotid arteries are tender. The sedimentation rate is raised and there is usually a modest polymorphonuclear leukocytosis.

Course and Prognosis. Spontaneous improvement can occur in from three to 24 months, but loss of vision is permanent. Coronary thrombosis or loss of a limb from giant cell arteritis may occur.

Treatment. The most effective method is the administration of steroids, e.g., Prednisone in doses of 60 mg. per day for a week, followed by 5 mg. three times a day for as long as is necessary. This relieves headache and seems to cut short the disease in many cases. Great care must be exercised in terminating treatment by steroids. If they are abruptly withheld, the disease may flare up; for instance, the author has seen fatal coronary thrombosis, and another case in which thrombosis of the femoral artery from giant cell arteritis followed immediately upon the abrupt withdrawal of the drug. It may be necessary to continue the administration of small doses of Prednisone for a year or more. Cutting the temporal artery proximal to the point of tenderness can help to relieve headache, and for this reason, biopsy of the temporal arteries is good therapy.

Vascular Syndromes in the Spinal Cord

Vascular accidents in the spinal cord are extremely rare, and when they do occur they are commonly secondary to some other pathological process. Thus, hemorrhage into the cord is usually due to rupture of an angiomatous malformation or to spinal injury, and thrombosis is seen as a complication of meningovascular syphilis, compression of the cord, and spinal meningitis. Infarction can result from a dissecting aneurysm of the aorta, which interferes with the blood supply that the anterior spinal artery derives from the intercostal arteries.

Fieschi and his colleagues (1970) found spinal cord softenings in 5 of 10 elderly subjects with severe atherosclerosis, who had died from ischemic brain lesions. The ischemic foci were located either in the central part of the gray matter or at the base of the anterior horns. There was no clear-cut relationship between the site of the lesions and either the position of the radicular arteries or the size and degree of atherosclerotic changes in the afferent arterial loops, and there was no occlusion of the intraparenchymal arteries related to the ischemic foci.

Thrombosis of the Anterior Spinal Artery

This rare condition is usually a complication of some other disease, e.g., spinal compression, meningovascular syphilis.

The anterior spinal artery supplies the anterior two-thirds of the spinal cord. The tip of the posterior horns and the posterior columns are supplied by the two posterior spinal arteries. Thrombosis of the small penetrating branches of the anterior spinal artery to the anterior horn cells can give rise to an abrupt lower motor neuron paralysis of a muscle or a group of muscles. This is a rare event; the author has seen it occur in a patient with meningovascular syphilis, and in an elderly man with compression of the cervical cord from spondylosis.

Occlusion of the main trunk of th artery[81] causes intense pain at and belov the level of the lesion, presumably fron partial interruption of the spinothala mic tracts, together with lower moto neuron paralysis of the muscles receiv ing their innervation from the infarctee segment. Since the pyramidal tracts are also involved, there is weakness of up per motor neuron type below the leve of the infarction. Pain and temperature sense are impaired to varying degrees but proprioception is preserved since it is mediated by the posterior columns which are supplied by the posterio spinal arteries. Paralysis of the bladde is usual. The combination of intense pair and an incomplete transverse lesion o the cord is highly suggestive of throm bosis of the anterior spinal artery. I the occlusion has been created by a dis secting aneurysm of the descending aorta, there will also be evidence o renal dysfunction, and if the dissection has reached the aortic bifurcation, the pulse will be lost in one or both lowe limbs.

Thrombosis of the Posterior Spinal Arteries

Infarction of the posterior portion of the spinal cord has been reported from time to time and in some cases, but not in all, the posterior spinal arteries were found to be occluded.[95] In most cases, there was sensory loss below the level of the lesion, together with paraplegia. From the description of the physical signs, it would seem that in many cases the infarction had spread beyond what is commonly regarded as the territory supplied by these vessels.

Intracranial Aneurysms

Rupture of an intracranial aneurysm is the usual cause of primary subarachnoid hemorrhage. It accounts for less than 10 per cent of all cerebrovascular accidents, but it is the most common type of vascular catastrophe in persons under the age of 40 and is responsible for about 5 per cent of all sudden and unexpected deaths from natural causes.[32] Unruptured aneurysms can also produce symptoms of an expanding mass, or may remain silent throughout life. Symptoms can arise at any time between infancy and old age, but are most common in persons between 30 and 60 years of age.[29, 46]

Etiology and Pathology. The saccular or berry aneurysm results from a congenital weakness of the media; it is usually found at or near an arterial bifurcation, and the great majority are situated in the subarachnoid space at the base of the brain, being rare within the brain substance. Approximately half of them are situated on the internal carotid or middle cerebral artery; others arise from the anterior cerebral, the anterior communicating, the posterior communicating, the basilar, or the vertebral artery. Usually they are the size of a small pea but can be much larger (Fig. 15–15) and are sometimes multiple.[11]

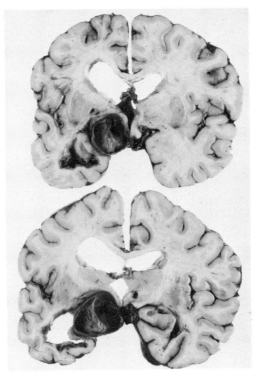

Figure 15–16.   Saccular aneurysm. (Courtesy of Ayer Laboratory, Pennsylvania Hospital, Philadelphia.)

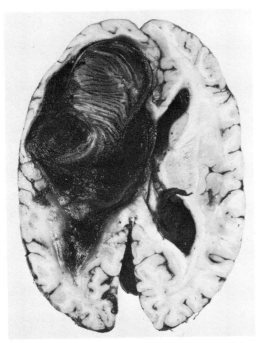

Figure 15–15.   Large aneurysm surrounded by organized clot, simulating intracranial neoplasm. (Courtesy of Dr. L. Wolman.)

The sexes are equally affected. Aneurysms are occasionally associated with other congenital malformations, notably intracranial angiomas, polycystic kidneys, and coarctation of the aorta.

The aneurysm is usually attached to its vessel of origin by a short neck. Its wall is thin and is composed of fibrous tissue, and the sac may be partly filled with an organized or organizing blood clot. Atheromatous changes may occur in its wall, and calcification may be present; exceptionally, it is visible radiologically (Fig. 15–17). Rupture usually occurs into the subarachnoid space or into the brain, or the extravasated blood may plough through the brain into the ventricles.[26] Rarely, rupture occurs into the subdural space.

Atherosclerotic aneurysms are usually seen after the age of 40 and consist of an irregular fusiform dilatation of a vessel. They usually occur on the internal carotid artery, notably within the cavernous sinus, and in the basilar artery.

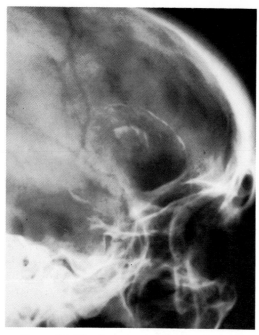

Figure 15–17. An exceptionally large saccular aneurysm, with calcification in its wall. (Courtesy of Dr. R. H. Chamberlain.)

Dissecting aneurysms are rare, but have been seen in association with saccular aneurysms, atherosclerosis (Fig. 15–8), head injury, and syphilis.[99]

Mycotic aneurysms occur when the wall of the artery, usually the middle

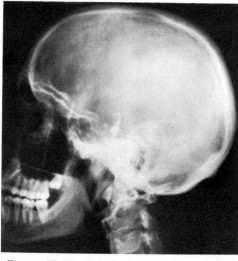

Figure 15–18. Vertebral arteriogram showing aneurysm of superior cerebellar artery. The P-A views showed that it was situated to the right of the midline.

cerebral, is weakened from within by small infective embolus, as in bacteri endocarditis or pyemia. They have b come uncommon since the introductic of antibiotics.

Multiple small aneurysms occur occ sionally in the course of polyarterit nodosa; subarachnoid hemorrhage o curred in seven of 300 cases reviewe by Malamud and Foster.

Syphilis is an extremely rare cause intracranial aneurysms; the associatic of a positive serology with an aneurysi is usually coincidental.

SPONTANEOUS SUBARACHNOID HEMORRHAGE

This term is applied to sudden blee ing into the subarachnoid space, in cor trast to conditions in which blood present in the cerebrospinal fluid as result of head injuries, hemorrhagic di ease, and primary intracerebral hemor rhage.[98]

Etiology. Spontaneous subarachnoi hemorrhage usually occurs as a resu of a rupture of a congenital or athero sclerotic intracranial aneurysm. Hemo rhage from vascular malformation an angiomatous tumors is much less com mon, and rupture of mycotic aneurysm or those of polyarteritis nodosa is rar Spontaneous spinal subarachnoid hemor rhage is a rare condition which occur from the rupture of a vascular malfor mation of the spinal cord. It can also b caused by bleeding from a metastati deposit of endometrial tissue in endo metriosis.

Pathology. Blood spreads rapidl through the basal cisterns, over the convexity of the brain, and into the spi nal subarachnoid space. In some cases it percolates into the subarachnoid space around the optic nerve, thereby block ing the venous return from the retina and giving rise to subhyaloid hemorrhages o papilledema. The blood may plough into the surrounding brain, giving rise to an intracerebral hematoma. Infarction may occur in the area of brain normally sup plied by the bleeding vessel, and dif fuse vascular spasm in the collateral circulation can also interfere with function in portions of the brain outside the territory of the bleeding vessel.

Examination of the brains of patients dying days or weeks after subarachnoid hemorrhage shows histological evidences of patchy ischemia in the cortex and edema of the white matter, which are present in both hemispheres, although they are most obvious in the territory of the vessel in which the aneurysm was situated.[26] The cerebellum and brainstem are spared, and the central gray matter is but little affected. Smith suggested that these changes may be due to diffuse arterial spasm secondary to aneurysmal rupture, and this is borne out by the experimental work of Simeone and his colleagues.[92] It is probable that these remote lesions are in part responsible for the incapacity which can follow subarachnoid hemorrhage.

It seems likely that one or more of these factors—hemorrhage into the brain, infarction, or arterial spasm—is responsible for the immediate loss of consciousness which usually accompanies spontaneous subarachnoid hemorrhage because there is no evidence that extravasation of blood in the subarachnoid space can, by itself, cause unconsciousness.

Rupture of a carotid aneurysm within the cavernous sinus bring about a caroticocavernous fistula with a loud bruit and a pulsating exophthalmus; blood is absent from the spinal fluid.

The spinal fluid is red during the first few days but soon begins to turn yellow-brown or orange. Spectroscopic tests of the supernatant reveal the presence of hemoglobin and oxyhemoglobin as well as bile pigments within a few hours after the onset of symptoms, and the red cells are crenated. After about two days, white cells appear; an initial predominance of polymorphs gives place to lymphocytes and mononuclear cells after a day or two. At the end of four or five weeks, there may still be a few lymphocytes present, but the pigment will have disappeared from the fluid unless hemorrhage has continued. If oxyhemoglobin is present a week after the clinical onset of subarachnoid hemorrhage, it suggests that bleeding is still going on.[9]

Clinical Features. In the majority of cases, the aneurysm will not have given evidence of its presence before rupture; occasionally there is a history of headache or diplopia. The onset is usually abrupt and may occur while the patient is at rest or active; physical strain is not usually a factor. The onset may be so acute that the patient thinks he has been struck on the head, or the pain may take 30 or more minutes to reach maximum severity. Early and profound unconsciousness suggests leakage from an anterior communicating aneurysm. In some cases, headache is followed by a deepening degree of confusion, which may be marked by excitement, rigidity of the neck, a positive Kernig sign, and a moderate rise of temperature. In others consciousness is retained, and the patient is able to complain of a severe headache which passes into the neck and is often associated with photophobia, double vision, or pain in the face. Vertigo occurs occasionally. Retinal and subhyaloid hemorrhages may appear, and papilledema may occur after a few days. Aphasia, monoplegia, or hemiplegia appears in about 25 per cent of all cases. Convulsions occasionally occur at the onset. *Pain may be felt first in the lower back and down the legs*, preceding the symptoms of intracranial bleeding by an hour or two.

During recovery, unconsciousness gives place to confusion, excitement, or Korsakoff's syndrome. Such symptoms may persist for weeks, but they usually pass off completely. Glycosuria with or without ketonuria can occur, and albuminuria is common.

Laboratory Data. Intracranial pressure is usually increased. The fluid is uniformly blood-stained, and the supernatant is yellow; this color fades on exposure to sunlight. There is a moderate increase of the white cell count. Straight x-rays are usually unrevealing in the case of saccular aneurysms, but sometimes they disclose an unsuspected calcified angiomatous malformation. Opinions differ as to whether arteriography should be resorted to as an emergency measure or whether it is better to wait a few days. The liability to complications, probably due to arterial spasm, seems to be somewhat higher when it is carried out immediately. In some cases, the dye will not enter the aneurysm because it is filled with blood clot; therefore, a negative result does not exclude the presence of an aneurysm. The prognosis is relatively good under these circumstances. Large aneurysms can sometimes be detected by brain scan or by echoencephalography.[42]

Abnormalities in the electrocardiogram are present in a high proportion of cases; they usually take the form of inverted T waves in the limb leads (see p. 365).

Diagnosis. The presence of glycosuria and ketonuria in a comatose patient can lead to an erroneous diagnosis of diabetic coma, but the degree of ketonuria is far less than is the case in diabetic coma. The distinction from meningitis is made by spinal tap since pyrexia, headache, nuchal rigidity, confusion, and double vision are common to both. Distinction between hemorrhage from a saccular aneurysm and from the extension into the subarachnoid space of an intracerebral hemorrhage can be difficult, but in general, a hemiplegic onset in the presence of hypertension is likely to be due to an intracerebral hemorrhage. Hemorrhagic disease (purpura, leukemia) can produce subarachnoid bleeding, but there is usually other evidence of its presence, and the diagnosis can be confirmed by examination of the blood.[91]

Course and Prognosis. Estimates of the immediate mortality rate of first hemorrhages vary between 35 and 50 per cent; an additional 15 per cent die from further bleeding within the next few weeks. The prognosis is vitiated by advancing age, hypertension, and extension of the hemorrhage into the brain. About 80 per cent of those who survive the initial hemorrhage have no recurrence for many years, and some never

have a recurrence.[12] In one case, the was a symptom-free interval of 22 yea between the first hemorrhage and tl second, fatal incident.

The clinical course in those who su vive the first several hours is variabl Sometimes the aneurysm continues leak, on and off, for one or two week while in others there may be rapid in provement which is interrupted by fresh and fatal hemorrhage. In mo cases, convalescence is marked by heac aches, dizziness on sudden changes posture, mental fatigability, irritabi ity, and photophobia—symptoms ve like the postconcussional syndrom Ocular palsies and signs of focal cere bral lesions, such as hemiparesis, usual recover completely in patients under 4(Twelve per cent of patients in a serie reported by Walton suffered from seiz ures following recovery from the acut incident.[98] Following recovery from ru; ture of an *anterior* cerebral aneurysr whether treated conservatively or surg cally, some patients exhibit personalit changes in the form of loss of initiative irresponsibility, inappropriate elevatio of mood, and a tendency to laugh or cr more readily than usual. On the othe hand, analysis of 79 such cases by Logu and his colleagues[59] disclosed nine pa tients in whom there had been an overal personality change for the better.

Treatment. The reduction of the cere brospinal fluid pressure by lumbar punc ture is sometimes followed by clinica improvement. In such cases, the punc ture should be repeated as often as i necessary to keep the pressure withir normal limits, but repeated spinal tap are dangerous when there is evidenc of a large intracerebral clot because this can act like a tumor, producing pressure cone. Therefore, spinal tap i: contraindicated in the presence of symp toms or signs indicating a pressure cone

At present, there is no method of over coming the spreading arterial "spasm' which sometimes occurs not only withir the territory of the injured artery but alsc in the opposite hemisphere. In experi mental animals, Simeone[92] has showr that such spasm can be overcome by artificially induced hypertension and it remains to be seen whether this mechanism can be applied to human beings without the risk of a further hemorrhage.

In conscious patients, headache is very troublesome. Opium and its derivatives are contraindicated in this, as in any other condition in which the respiratory center may be depressed. Unhappily, it is illegal to use the most effective drug for this type of headache—heroin—in many parts of the world. The physician has to rely on Demerol and other synthetic analgesics.

Arteriography is carried out to determine the site of an aneurysm; if it is accessible, surgery is indicated in the majority of cases. Surgical results have greatly improved in the past few years as a result of new techniques, notably the use of the dissecting microscope.

FOCAL SIGNS OF ANEURYSMS AT SPECIAL SITES

INTRACAVERNOUS PORTION OF THE INTERNAL CAROTID ARTERY. These aneurysms usually take the form of a fusiform dilatation of the artery (Fig. 15–19).[53] They seldom rupture, but if they do, the resulting carotid-cavernous fistula produces an intracranial bruit, pulsating proptosis of the ipsilateral eye, oculomotor paresis, and extreme edema of the lids, conjunctiva, and orbit. In the absence of rupture, there may be no symptoms at all, or there may be pain in and around the eye and partial or complete paralysis of the third cranial nerve. The fourth and sixth nerves may also be implicated, and there may be impairment of sensation of the skin supplied by the upper two divisions of the trigeminal nerve. Sometimes these aneurysms enlarge greatly and come to involve the optic nerve and chiasm, and they may produce proptosis. The expanding mass gives the symptoms of an intracranial tumor, and diagnosis depends on angiography.

INTRACRANIAL PORTION OF THE INTERNAL CAROTID ARTERY. The aneurysm may arise from any branch of the carotid artery, or it may be situated at the origin of the posterior communicating, anterior choroidal, or middle cerebral artery (Fig. 15–20).[46] The characteristic symptomatology is partial or complete paralysis of the third nerve, with or without pain in the distribution of the first division of the fifth nerve. In

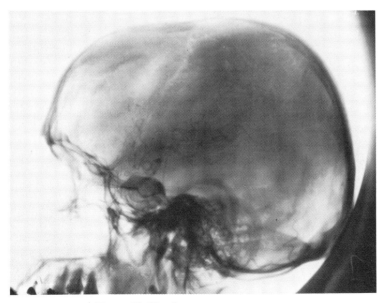

Figure 15–19. Intracavernous aneurysm.

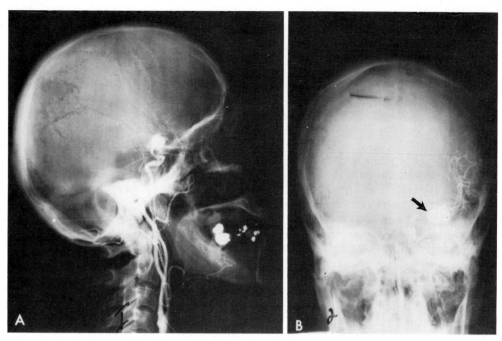

Figure 15–20.   Saccular aneurysm of the middle cerebral artery.

some cases, slow leakage gives rise to an expanding hematoma, which gives the clinical picture of an intracranial tumor. Angiography may fail to disclose a sac if the blood within it has clotted, and differentiation from tumor may be impossible without surgical exploration.

Extremely large aneurysms may occur at the base of the brain. In a series of 22 cases reported by Bull,[15] three were over 6 cm. in diameter. Most of them lay in or near the circle of Willis. The most common complaint was a disturbance of vision, and study of the visual fields made it possible for the physician to localize the lesion, if not to predict the pathology. Headache is common. Six of these patients presented with dementia. One case presented as a Brown-Séquard syndrome, caused by a large aneurysm on the vertebral artery at the foramen magnum. The diagnosis is made by arteriography, but it should be noted that owing to the presence of large clots within the aneurysm, angiography often discloses only a fraction of the aneurysm's true size. Without angiography, it is very easy to mistake an aneurysm for a tumor.

ANTERIOR CEREBRAL AND ANTERIOR COMMUNICATING ARTERIES.   These a usually of the saccular type (Fig. 15–21 The aneurysm may involve one vess but is more likely to implicate both a terior cerebrals and the anterior comm

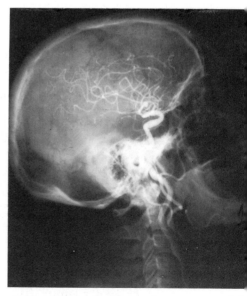

Figure 15–21.   Small saccular aneurysm of th anterior communicating artery.

nicating artery. Focal symptoms are rare, but anosmia and involvement of the optic nerve and chiasm may occur.[53b] Impairment of the circulation in the anterior cerebral artery can lead to weakness of the contralateral leg or to hemiplegia. Seizures may occur. In many cases, hemorrhage is the first indication of its presence and in this event, deep unconsciousness is likely to supervene. Until recently, the operative mortality in this group was very high, but technical advances have greatly improved the outlook.

MIDDLE CEREBRAL ARTERY. These aneurysms are usually saccular in type, but can be arteriosclerotic or mycotic in origin.[26, 68] Some disclose their presence by rupture while others increase in size and produce the symptoms of an expanding mass. Seizures and contralateral hemiparesis are common, and aphasia is likely if the circulation to the dominant hemisphere is compromised.

POSTERIOR COMMUNICATING ARTERY. Most of these occur at the junction of the posterior communicating artery and the carotid (Fig. 15–22). Consequently, paralysis of the third or fourth cranial nerve is a common presenting feature. Some reach a large size and simulate a tumor. Direct operative treatment is unsatisfactory because the area is difficult of access and there is a danger of disturbing the blood supply to the adjacent brainstem, but ligation of the internal carotid artery in the neck is fairly effective.

BASILAR AND VERTEBRAL ARTERIES. These may be saccular or atherosclerotic in origin (Fig. 15–23).[74] Those occurring low down in the posterior fossa can simulate tumor, with involvement of the lower cranial nerves. Occipital headache, occurring when the patient changes the position of his head in space, is a suggestive symptom.

PITUITARY FOSSA. Very rarely an aneurysm *within the pituitary fossa* expands the sella, and impinges on the optic chiasm. The symptoms and signs develop more rapidly than is usual in pituitary tumors; since arteriography may fail to reveal the aneurysm, the first hint of its nature may come during surgical exposure.

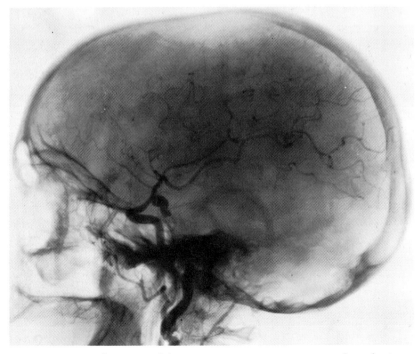

Figure 15–22. Aneurysm at the origin of the posterior communicating artery from the internal carotid.

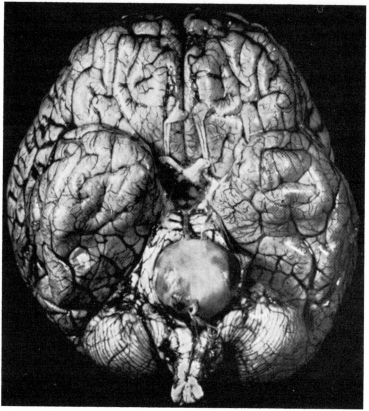

Figure 15–23. Aneurysm of the basilar artery. (From Wechsler, I.: *Clinical Neurology.* 9th Ed. W. B. Saunders Co., Philadelphia, 1963.)

Carotid Cavernous Fistula

Pathology. The fistula is usually the result of a closed head injury in elderly subjects. In most cases, the vessels involved are presumed to have been normal prior to injury, but occasionally a pre-existing aneurysm of the carotid ruptures into the cavernous sinus, while in arteriosclerotic subjects, a split in the vessel wall can be responsible for the fistula. Injury is sometimes denied, but there may be a history of unwonted exertion immediately prior to the rupture.

Clinical Features. The head injury is usually severe, with damage to the skull, accessory nasal sinuses, brain, or cranial nerves. The symptoms referable to the fistula are the result of the transmission of arterial blood pressure into the cavernous sinus and its tributaries. The patient complains of a noise in his head, diplopia, proptosis, and pain in the face.

Examination discloses protrusion and pulsation of the eye; there is intense chemosis and, in the later stages, enlargement of conjunctival and scleral vessels. Papilledema develops. Ocular movement is disturbed by paresis of the third, fourth, and sixth nerves and edema of the orbit, and the pupil is dilated and fixed. There is usually hypoalgesia in the first and second divisions of the fifth nerve. The opposite orbit may be affected, but to a lesser degree.

Auscultation discloses a systolic bruit which is heard all over the head but is louder on the affected side; it is abolished by compression of the ipsilateral carotid artery. The diagnosis is confirmed by arteriography.

Treatment. Spontaneous recovery occurs in some cases. In others, surgical correction is necessary.

THE INTRACRANIAL VENOUS SINUSES AND VEINS

Venous blood from the upper portion of the cerebral hemispheres drains into cortical veins which enter the superior sagittal (longitudinal) sinus, entering it at an angle opposite to that of the blood flow (Fig. 15–24). The sinus starts at the crista galli, where it communicates with the nasal and facial veins (a route for infection from without), and terminates at the internal occipital protuberance by turning laterally into (usually) the right lateral sinus; at this point, the torcular Herophili, it communicates with the left lateral sinus and the straight sinus. The superior sagittal sinus is also a major pathway for the absorption of cerebrospinal fluid via the many arachnoid villi and pacchionian granulations which project into it. Consequently, occlusion of the sinus by thrombosis or neoplasm can cause a rise of intracranial pressure by damming back the venous outflow, and by reducing the absorption of cerebrospinal fluid; however, owing to the profuse anastomosis between cortical veins, the rise of pressure can be compensated for to some extent by drainage into the lateral and cavernous sinuses.

Much of the lateral surface of the hemisphere is drained by veins running into the middle cerebral (sylvian) vein, which enters the cavernous sinus. The great anastomotic vein of Trolard runs into both the superior longitudinal sinus above and the sylvian vein below, while the anastomotic vein of Labbé links the sylvian vein with the transverse sinus. The inferior longitudinal sinus lies in the posterior portion of the lower border of the falx, and receives veins from the medial aspect of the cerebral hemispheres. It joins the straight sinus. Veins from the inferior aspect of the frontal, temporal, and occipital lobes drain into the cavernous and transverse sinuses.

The deep venous drainage of the cerebral hemispheres and upper midbrain is into the great cerebral vein of Galen, which joins the straight sinus. The latter usually turns to the left at the torcula to form the left lateral sinus. Venous drainage of the posterior fossa from the pons downward is into the superior and inferior petrosal sinuses, the transverse sinus, and the vertebral veins. There is often an anastomosis between the pontine veins and the basal veins which join the two internal cerebral veins to form the great vein of Galen.

The *lateral sinuses* pass laterally and

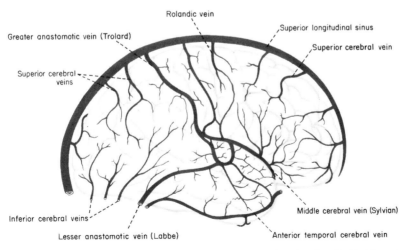

Figure 15–24. The venous system on the surface of the brain. (After Crosby, E. C., Humphrey, T., and Lauer, E. W.: *Correlative Anatomy of the Nervous System.* The Macmillan Company, New York, 1962.)

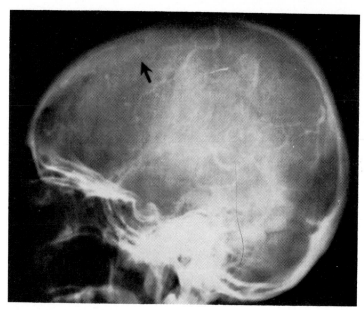

Figure 15–25.   Postpartum thrombosis of the posterior part of the superior sagittal sinus. Only the anterior half (arrow) has filled in the venous phase of a carotid arteriogram.

forward in the attached border of the tentorium and then turn downward at the sigmoid sinuses, each of which lies in a tortuous groove on the inner aspect of the mastoid — a relationship which explains the frequency of lateral sinus thrombosis in untreated mastoiditis. The sinus leaves the skull through the jugular foramen to form the internal jugular vein. Manual compression of the neck, as in Queckenstedt's test, blocks the venous outflow from the head, and the consequent rise of intracranial pressure is communicated to the spinal subarachnoid space unless there is an obstruction within that space.

The *cavernous sinuses* consist of a compact mass of plexiform veins with very thin walls which lie on either side of the sella turcica and body of the sphenoid. They are interconnected by a plexus which invests the pituitary fossa, and each receives the ophthalmic veins and the important middle cerebral (sylvian) vein. Each cavernous sinus is drained by the superior and inferior petrosal sinuses; the former joins the lateral sinus and the latter the sigmoid sinus.

The dural sinuses are directly con-nected with extracranial structures by diploic veins and by emissary veins which accompany the cranial nerves and the carotid artery. They are also con-nected with the epidural network of the vertebral canal.[10] These communi-cations explain the ease with which in-fection can enter the skull from the head, neck, or thoracic and abdominal viscera, a spread which is facilitated by the absence of valves in the intracranial and epidural venous networks.

The cavernous sinus contains the car-otid artery, lateral to which lie the third, fourth, and sixth cranial nerves, and the upper two divisions of the trigeminal nerve. One or more of these nerves is commonly involved in thrombosis of the sinus, in intracavernous carotid aneu-rysm,[53] in caroticocavernous fistula, and in rare cases of infiltration of the sinus by a pituitary tumor.

Intracranial Venous Thrombosis

Etiology.   Thrombophlebitis of dural sinuses and cerebral veins [8, 93] can occur as a result of: infection of the head and neck, notably otitis media, mastoiditis, sinusitis, and furunculosis; bacteremia and septicemia; marasmus and cachexia; closed head injuries, especially those along the course of the superior sagittal sinus; low-grade infection occurring in the puerperium[62]; invasion of the superior sagittal sinus by new growth; and congestive heart failure.[89] The use of oral contraceptive agents has been followed by fatal dural sinus thrombosis in healthy young women.[6] Paroxysmal nocturnal hemoglobinuria is a rare cause of cerebral venous thrombosis.

Pathology. The clot may occupy a portion of the sinus, the entire sinus, or one or more cortical veins. In some cases, the superior sagittal sinus is not completely obstructed, but the venous efflux into it is prevented by the presence of a thick deposit of fibrin along its walls. The brain becomes edematous, and the swollen tributary veins may be bordered by areas of hemorrhagic softening. Leakage from such areas leads to the appearance of red cells in the spinal fluid. When the process occurs acutely, intracranial pressure rises steeply as a result of venous obstruction and impaired absorption of spinal fluid into the dural sinuses. However, if the process occurs slowly, in a limited section of a single sinus, the intracranial pressure may remain normal.

Clinical Features. These vary greatly from case to case, depending on the severity, extent, and situation of the thrombus, the presence or absence of infection, and the nature of the underlying disease. Thus, a sterile thrombus limited to the anterior portion of the superior sagittal sinus or one lateral sinus may be clinically silent, whereas purulent thrombophlebitis of similar size and in the same situations will produce a high temperature, profound toxemia, and a greater tendency to focal neurological symptoms.

Cavernous sinus thrombosis gives rise to proptosis, edema of the eyelids and conjunctiva, papilledema, and diplopia from involvement of the third, fourth, and sixth nerves within the sinus. Impairment of vision, or even blindness, may occur. Pain is usually present behind the eye and over the forehead. The infection may spread to the opposite side, thus involving both eyes. There is a swinging temperature and profound toxemia if infection is present. Even with modern antibiotics the prognosis is grave, especially when *Staphylococcus aureus* is responsible.

Superior sagittal sinus thrombosis usually gives rise to headache, and pain may also be felt behind one eye. However, pain is absent in cases which develop slowly. The neck may be stiff. Seizures are common; they may be jacksonian or generalized, and when generalized, they often start in the lower limbs. Paresis of one or both legs is highly characteristic, and hemiplegia in which the leg is more affected than the arm is not uncommon. The patient may be alert, obtunded, or stuporous. If intracranial pressure is raised, papilledema will appear in a day or two, and in infants, the anterior fontanelle will be distended. Distention of the veins of the scalp has been described in long-persisting cases. Pyrexia may be high, moderate, or absent, depending on the nature of the underlying disease. The combination of high temperature, headache, and stiffness of the neck suggests a diagnosis of meningitis, but the spinal fluid will be found to contain red cells with a proportionate number of leukocytes, and organisms will not be present. Carotid arteriography will disclose a normal arterial system, but the venous phase will show partial or total occlusion of the sinus, with or without occlusion of some of the tributary veins.

Lateral and sigmoid sinus thrombosis, usually the result of mastoiditis, produces headache, pain in the ear and neck, and vomiting. In many cases, the entire picture is dominated by the presence of pyemia with swinging temperature and profound toxemia. The jugular vein may be tender or hard, but this does not necessarily mean that it is totally obstructed. If obstruction is complete, manual compression of the neck on that side will fail to cause a rise of intracranial pressure as judged by spinal manometry. If the infection spreads to the superior sagittal sinus, the straight sinus, or the opposite lateral sinus, intracranial pressure rises steeply, papilledema appears, and the patient becomes increasingly stuporous.

Prognosis. The outlook of all forms of intracranial thrombophlebitis has improved immeasurably since the introduction of chemotherapy. The use of anticoagulants is contraindicated because of the danger of hemorrhage into the brain. On theoretical grounds, treatment with fibrinolytic agents is indicated. Permanent loss of function can occur following cortical venous thrombosis, and the possibility of subsequent epilepsy has to be borne in mind.

The Veins of the Spinal Cord

The posterior half of the spinal cord is drained by radially disposed veins which join the posterior part of the coronal plexus on the surface of the cord; this in turn joins the posterior medullary veins which accompany the posterior

roots to the intervertebral foramen where they join the anterior medullary veins (and veins from the epidural plexus) to form the intervertebral vein.[43a]

The anterior half of the cord has a dual venous drainage. The lateral quadrants are served by radially disposed veins which join the anterior portion of the coronal plexus on the surface of the cord. The median quadrants, including most of the anterior horns, are supplied with veins which join the anterior median spinal vein in the anterior fissure. The anterior medullary veins leave the anterior median spinal vein, are joined by radicles from the anteromedial column of white matter, and then pass laterally along the anterior spinal root.

Intersegmental veins unite the intermedullary or intrinsic veins of adjacent segments, and the same applies to the coronal plexus. A large vein, the great anterior medullary vein, leaves the lumbar enlargement along the first or second lumbar root, usually on the left.

Gillilan[43a] has pointed out that venous lesions, whether thrombotic or due to compression of the cord, have their

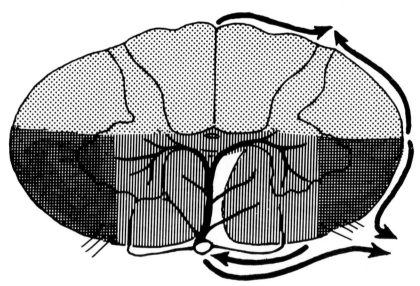

Figure 15–26. Diagram illustrating the intrinsic venous drainage path of the spinal cord. Posterior half (stippled) is drained through the coronary plexus into the posterior medullary veins. The anterior half (vertical lines and cross hatching) is drained by way of the anterior medullary veins. The medial portion drains through the central vein system into the anterior median spinal vein. Arrows indicate the direction of flow of venous blood. (Reproduced by the courtesy of Dr. Lois A. Gillilan and the editors of *Neurology.*)

greatest impact on the posterior horns and the lateral half of each side of the cord, and cites the disposition of the lesions in subacute necrotic myelitis in support of this contention (Fig. 15–26).

SUBACUTE NECROTIC MYELITIS

In 1926, Foix and Alajouanine described a form of spinal cord disease with distinctive pathological and clinical features. The latter took the form of weakness of the legs with sensory impairment and sphincter disturbances.

Etiology. The cause of this curious and uncommon disease is unknown. Because of the pathological features to be described, and because some cases have been associated with thrombophlebitis of the legs or of the inferior vena cava, the consensus is that it is the result of thrombophlebitis of the spinal veins.

Pathology. There are patchy fibrous and hyalin changes in the small arteries and veins of the lower half of the spinal cord. Surface veins may be large and tortuous, but there is no evidence of angiomatosis or arteritis. There may be considerable hypertrophy of the walls of the intramedullary arteries and veins, without reduction of the lumen. Recanalization of venous thrombi may be seen. The lumbar and lower thoracic segments are the site of extensive degeneration or necrosis of the white matter of the cord, with a variable degree of involvement of the gray matter. The lesions are patchy, and within the affected segments there is destruction of myelin and axis cylinders, and large numbers of phagocytic cells may be present in acute cases.

Clinical Features. The disease is usually insidious in its onset, but a few acute cases have been described. In these, there was a rapid development of flaccid weakness in the legs with loss of reflexes, objective sensory loss below the level of the lesion, and sphincter disturbances. These all occurred within a few weeks of the onset, and the spinal fluid revealed an increase of protein without pleocyto-

sis or a subarachnoid block. Such cases could easily be mistaken, on clinical grounds, for the necrotizing myelopathy which occurs in association with visceral carcinoma.

In the subacute form,[44] which is the more usual type, the presenting symptom is weakness of the legs which gradually increases and is sometimes associated with pain. Signs of both upper and lower motor neuron involvement appear; there is some increase of tone, extensor plantar responses, increased or diminished reflexes, and atrophy and fasciculation of the leg muscles. Sensory changes appear later, usually starting in the sacral dermatomes and gradually ascending to the lumbar and lower thoracic segments. The sensory loss involves both proprioception and cutaneous sensibility, but sometimes pain and temperature sensation are relatively unaffected. Sometimes the muscles are tender. As in the acute cases, there is usually an increase of the cerebrospinal fluid protein, and there may or may not be a lymphocytic pleocytosis.

The disease is steadily progressive, death usually occurring from urinary infection or intercurrent disease in the course of one or two years. This protracted course helps to distinguish these cases from the necrotizing myelopathy associated with occult or obvious visceral carcinoma, which is fatal in from one to two months.

VASCULAR MALFORMATIONS OF THE NERVOUS SYSTEM

For practical purposes, the group can be divided into vascular anomalies and vascular tumors, although the dividing line between the two is sometimes indistinct. Vascular anomalies consist of abnormal vessels, venous, arterial, or capillary. The symptoms they produce are due to hemorrhage or thrombosis rather than to pressure. Vascular tumors arise from primitive vascular tissue, and produce signs and symptoms similar to those of other types of intracranial or spinal neoplasms.

Vascular Malformations of the Cerebral Hemispheres

Pathology. The *venous angioma* is composed of abnormal venous channels, and may appear as a single large vessel, a small knot of vessels, or a racemose mass of veins covering a wide area. The angioma may be on the surface of the brain or cord, or it may be buried within a sulcus, but even when it appears to lie on the surface, abnormal venous channels may penetrate deeply into the brain.[13] Vascular malformations are more common in Indians and Asiatics than in Caucasians.

The malformation usually lies within the territory of the middle cerebral artery, and less often on the surface of the midbrain and pons. Occasionally the overlying dura may be involved.

In the spinal cord, venous angiomas are often extensive, running down from the thoracic region to the cauda equina.

They occur at all ages, though the onset of symptoms commonly occurs in adult life. Their occasional occurrence in early life and the presence of other malformations suggest a congenital origin.

Arteriovenous angiomas are composed of arterial and venous channels, with few capillaries and many arteriovenous shunts. Involvement of the meninges is common, and vessels of the scalp may be included in the complex. The angiographic appearance may be dramatic, with huge tortuous arterial and venous channels (Figs. 15–27, 15–28), but this picture is misleading because the angioma itself is usually quite small, much of the mass being composed of feeding vessels which may return to their normal size when the angioma is removed.

Angiomas in the brainstem tend to be extensive, and in some instances there is a strand of arteriovenous tissue extending all the way from the orbit to the lower brainstem.[100] In the spinal cord, they are usually more extensive than the venous angiomas, and occur at any level.

Clinical Features. Hemisphere malformations occur at all ages and give rise

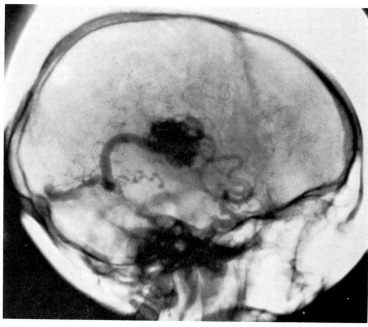

Figure 15–27. Common carotid angiogram showing angioma with feeding arteries and a large venous channel draining into the lateral sinus. (Courtesy of Dr. Brodie Hughes.)

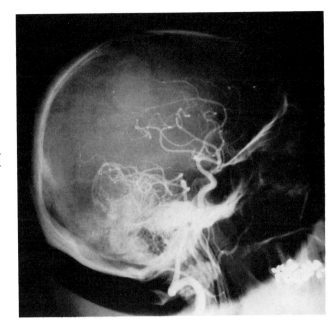

Figure 15–28. Arteriovenous malformation supplied by the superior cerebellar arteries.

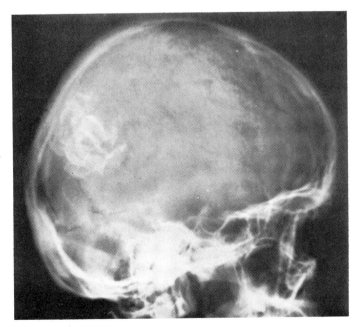

Figure 15–29. Calcified angiomatous malformation.

to symptoms by progressive impairment of the blood supply to surrounding brain and by vascular accidents.

There is often slight underdevelopment of the affected region of the brain, and the limbs may be noticeably smaller on the opposite side of the body. A slight degree of mental deficit may or may not be present, but severe deficiency is rare. Focal seizures are frequent. A bout of almost continuous focal attacks may bring the patient to the doctor for the first time. Temporal lobe seizures in the absence of neurological deficit may be due to small angiomas in the temporal lobe which are too small to be identified by angiography.

Progressive impairment of the blood supply to the surrounding brain gives rise to increasing hemiparesis, and motor recovery after a seizure is often incomplete, each attack leaving behind more disturbance of function than was present before. On occasion, sudden severe hemiplegia can be the presenting feature; it is sometimes preceded by severe headache on the side of the angioma. These events are attributed to thrombosis or to intracerebral hemorrhage.[61] Rupture of vessels may also declare itself as a subarachnoid hemorrhage.

In the *arteriovenous form*, the common carotid artery and the vessels of the scalp may be enlarged. Examination of the fundi may show angiomatosis in the retina, and red arterial blood may be seen in the retinal veins.

The only clinical sign which distinguishes an arteriovenous angioma from a venous angioma is the presence of an intracranial bruit. It is best heard over the site of the angioma, but may be detected all over the head and neck. A thrill can sometimes be felt. The bruit varies from time to time, may alter with posture, and is not always noticed by the patient.

Diagnosis. There is often evidence of increased vascularity in the skull in the form of a widening of diploic channels. The foramina for emissary veins may be enlarged, especially in the parietal re-

gion, and basal views may demonstrate an enlarged carotid canal. Calcification can be seen in some venous angiomas.

The diagnosis can be made with certainty only by angiography, which will demonstrate the site of the angioma and outline its feeding and draining vessels, thus providing information which is essential for rational operative treatment.

Ventriculography and pneumoencephalography are not helpful and may be misleading. Usually the films are normal; but if thrombosis has occurred with consequent brain atrophy, it may be reflected in focal dilatation of the lateral ventricle. If there has been a recent thrombosis or hemorrhage, the x-ray appearance may suggest a space-occupying lesion which is easily mistaken for an intrinsic brain tumor.

Prognosis and Treatment. Without treatment, the prognosis is poor in the arteriovenous form. In most instances, survival after the onset of symptoms is a matter of months or a few years. Focal epilepsy of increasing frequency and severity, intermittent increase of hemiparesis from repeated thrombotic episodes, and finally death from massive thrombosis or hemorrhage are usual, but the period of survival may be more prolonged in children who present with sudden severe hemiplegia.

Until recently, the treatment of choice was surgical extirpation, which can be carried out with a minimum of postoperative disability, provided that it is recognized that many of the large vessels which feed the angioma can be left in situ. Recently, cryosurgery has been used successfully to induce thrombosis within the vascular anomaly.

Angioma of the Brainstem and Cerebellum

The story is usually one of intermittent, brief episodes of dysfunction related to the cranial nerves or cerebellum. At first recovery may be complete, but later on some degree of disability remains between attacks, and the clinical story may closely resemble that of multiple sclerosis except for the abruptness of onset of each incident. Extensive angiomatosis of the brainstem is sometimes associated with retinal angiomatosis.[101]

Subarachnoid bleeding is less common than in the supratentorial variety, and the final episode is usually a brainstem thrombosis. Thrombosis or hemorrhage occasionally produces obstructive hydrocephalus. In the absence of such obstruction, air studies are usually normal, and arteriography may fail to visualize the malformation. An audible bruit may or may not be present, and evidence of increased extracranial vascularity is unusual. Because of the intimate connection between the vascular supply of the brainstem and these angiomas, surgical extirpation is impossible.

Angioma of the Spinal Cord

The usual presentation is a sudden, partial transverse lesion of the cord, which is sometimes accompanied by root pain.[4, 100] The signs often indicate that the lesion is of considerable length, and a clear-cut upper level of motor or sensory loss is seldom present. A bruit may be heard over the spinal column.

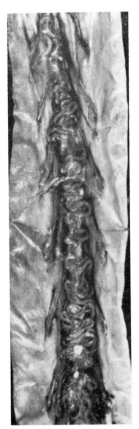

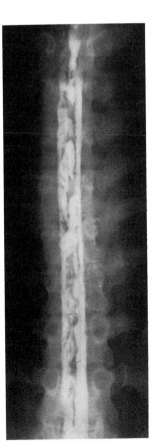

Fig. 15–30.

Fig. 15–31.

Figure 15–30. Dorsal aspect of the lower spinal cord obscured by venous malformation. (From Russell, D. S., and Rubenstein, L. J.: *Pathology of Tumors of the Nervous System.* Edward Arnold Publishers, Ltd., London, 1959.)

Figure 15–31. Venous malformation. The myelogram shows the typical "candle guttering" effect. (Courtesy of Dr. James Bull.)

Recovery from the initial episode may be surprisingly complete. but after repeated attacks, permanent defects appear in the form of spastic paraplegia, patchy sensory impairment below the level of the lesion, and sphincter disturbances. A cutaneous hemangioma is sometimes present on the back. Occasionally, the first attack leads to a complete transverse lesion of the cord from which little recovery takes place. Rarely, there are symptoms of intermittent paraparesis which bear a strong resemblance to transient ischemic attacks occurring in the brain.[94] Yet another mode of onset is with bleeding into the subarachnoid space, and this may be difficult to distinguish from intracranial subarachnoid hemorrhage, cord signs being inconspicuous.

X-rays of the spine are usually normal; occasionally an associated hemangioma of a vertebral body is to be seen. Contrast myelography will usually show incomplete block and the oil will be seen to break up into drops and streaks at the level of the lesion (Fig. 15–31). This may be difficult to distinguish from the appearances of chronic arachnoiditis — and, indeed, many cord angiomas are associated with a considerable degree of arachnoidal adhesions. Selective aortography will sometimes reveal the angioma.

In the absence of subarachnoid bleeding, the cerebrospinal fluid may be normal or even show varying degrees of protein increase and xanthochromia. Manometry may be normal or may show partial or complete block.

Encephalofacial Angiomatosis (Sturge-Weber's Disease)

In its complete form, this condition is characterized by a nevus on the forehead, buphthalmus, contralateral hemiparesis, seizures, mental defect, and radiological evidence of calcification in the cortex (Fig. 15–32).[57] There is excessive vascularity of the pia mater on the affected side, and in the subjacent cortex there are deposits of a crystalline material consisting of iron and calcium. These deposits are mainly in the outer cortical layers, but they may also be found in the deeper layers and in the subcortical white matter. In some cases,

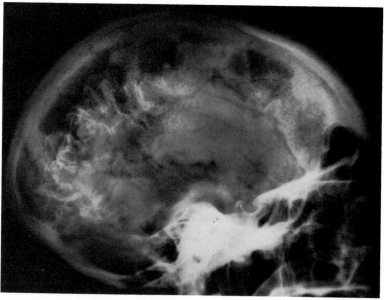

Figure 15–32. Sturge-Weber syndrome in a 19-year-old girl. Calcification outlines the convolution of the right parieto-occipital region. (Courtesy of Dr. James Bull.)

there are areas of ischemic cortical damage.

There is no record of an association between leptomeningeal angiomatosis and cortical calcification with facial nevi confined to the cheek or mandibular area.

Hereditary Hemorrhagic Telangiectasia (Rendu-Osler-Weber Syndrome)

This condition is transmitted as a simple dominant trait. There is a defect in the vessel wall leading to localized dilatation of capillaries and arterioles, and in some instances to the development of arteriovenous aneurysms.[49, 71] The lesions on the skin assume the appearance of either small violaceous hemangiomas or spider nevi. Both the skin and the mucous membranes are involved, and in addition there may be telangiectasia in the brain, spinal cord, lung, and abdominal viscera (Fig. 15–33). Though the telangiectases are present in childhood, they are found in increasing numbers and become more obvious as age advances.

Epistaxis and gastrointestinal bleeding are the most frequent symptoms and

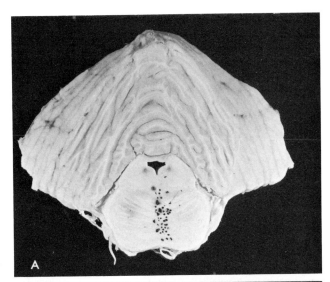

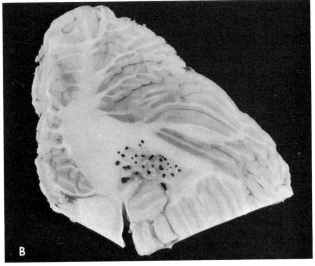

Figure 15–33. Telangiectases clustered about the midline of the pons (*A*) and in the cerebellum (*B*). (Courtesy of Drs. R. R. Heffner and G. B. Solitare.)

iron deficiency anemia is usual. Hemorrhage into the brain or spinal cord may occur spontaneously or while holding the breath during muscular efforts, such as straining at stool or lifting a heavy weight.

REFERENCES

1. Adams, G. F., and Merrett, J. D.: Prognosis and survival in the aftermath of hemiplegia. *Brit. Med. J.* 1:309, 1961.
2. Allen, N., and Mustian, V.: Origin and significance of vascular murmurs of the head and neck. *Medicine* 41:227, 1962.
3. Alpers, B. J.: Compensatory mechanisms in occlusive vascular disease of the brain. *Arch. Neurol.* 1:531, 1959.
4. Antoni, N.: Spinal vascular malformations (angiomas) and myelomalacia. *Neurology,* 12:795, 1962.
5. Atkins, L.: Progeria. Report of a case, with postmortem findings. *New Eng. J. Med.* 250:1065, 1954.
6. Atkinson, F. A., Fairburn, B., and Heathfield, K. W. G.: Intracranial venous thrombosis as complication of oral contraceptives. *Lancet* 1:914, 1970.
7. Baker, R. N., Ramseyer, J. C., and Schwartz, W. S.: Prognosis in patients with transient ischemic attacks. *Neurology* 18:1157, 1968.
8. Barnett, H. J. M., and Hyland, H. H.: Noninfective intracranial venous thrombosis. *Brain* 76:36, 1953.
9. Barrows, L. J., Hunter, F. T., and Banker, B. Q.: The nature and clinical significance of pigments in the spinal fluid. *Brain* 78:59, 1955.
10. Batson, O. V.: The function of the vertebral veins and their role in the spread of metastases. *Ann. Surg.* 112:138, 1940.
10a. Behrman, S., Carroll, J. D., Janota I., and Matthews, W. B.: Progressive supranuclear palsy—clinicopathological study of 4 cases. *Brain* 92:663, 1969.
11. Bigelow, N. J.: Multiple intracranial aneurysms. *Arch. Neurol. Psychiat.* 73:76, 1955.
12. Bjorkesten, G., and Troupp, H.: Prognosis of subarachnoid hemorrhage: A comparison between patients with verified aneurysms and patients with normal angiograms. *J. Neurosurg.* 14:434, 1957.
13. Brock, S., and Dyke, C. G.: Venous and arteriovenous angiomas of the brain. *Bull. Neurol. Inst. N.Y.* 2:247, 1932.
14. Bruetsch, W. L., and Williams, C. L.: Arteriosclerotic muscular rigidity with special reference to gait disturbances. *Amer. J. Psychiat.* 111:332, 1954.
15. Bull, J.: Massive aneurysms at the base of the brain. *Brain* 92:535, 1969.
16. Bull, J. W., Marshall, J., and Shaw, D. A.: Cerebral angiography in the diagnosis of acute stroke. *Lancet* 1:562, 1960.
17. Byrom, F. B.: The pathogenesis of hypertensive encephalopathy and its relation to the malignant phase of hypertension. *Lancet* 2:201, 1954.
18. Cannon, B. W.: Acute vascular lesions of the brainstem; a complication of supra-tentorial space-occupying lesions. *Arch. Neurol. Psychiat.* 66:687, 1951.
19. Carter, A. B.: *Cerebral infarction,* The Macmillan Company, New York, 1964.
20. Cohen, S. M.: Traumatic arterial spasm. *Lancet* 1:1, 1944.
21. Cole, F. M., and Yates, P.: Intracerebral microaneurysms and small cerebrovascular lesions. *Brain* 90:759, 1967.
22. Connor, R. C. R.: Myocardial damage secondary to brain lesions. *Amer. Heart J.* 78: 145, 1969.
23. Cooke, W. T., Cloake, P. C., Govan, A. D., and Colbeck, J. C.: Temporal arteritis: A generalized vascular disease. *Quart. J. Med.* 15:47, 1946.
24. Critchley, M.: Arteriosclerotic parkinsonism. *Brain* 52:23, 1927.
25. Critchley, M.: The neurology of old age. *Lancet* 1:1119, 1931.
26. Crompton, M. R.: The pathology of ruptured middle-cerebral aneurysm. *Lancet* 2:421, 1962.
27. Crompton, M. R.: Giant cell arteritis: General and neurological aspects. *World Neurol.* 2:237, 1961.
28. Cullen, J. F.: Occult temporal arteritis. *Trans. Ophth. Soc. U.K.* 83:725, 1963.
29. Dandy, W. E.: *Intracranial Arterial Aneurysms.* Comstock Publishing Co., Inc., New York, 1944.
30. DeFine Olivarius, B., and Bisgaard-Frantzen, C. F.: Cerebellar apoplexy. *Ugeskr. Laeg.* 118:131, 1956.
31. Deller, J., Scalettar, R., and Levens, A. J.: Pain as a manifestation of acute anterior spinal-artery thrombosis. *New Eng. J. Med.* 262:1078, 1960.
32. Dinning, T. A. R., and Falconer, M. A.: Sudden or unexpected natural death due to ruptured intracranial aneurysm. *Lancet* 2: 799, 1953.
33. Duguid, J. B.: Mural thrombosis in arteries. *Brit. Med. Bull.* 2:36, 1955.
34. Elliott, F. A., and Buckell, M.: Fibrinogen changes in relation to cerebrovascular accidents. *Neurology* 11:120, 1961.
35. Epstein, A. W.: Primary massive pontine hemorrhage. *J. Neuropath. Exp. Neurol.* 10: 426, 1951.
36. Evarts, C. M.: Diagnosis and treatment of fat embolism. *J.A.M.A.* 194:899, 1965.
37. Fairburn, B., and Oliver, L. C.: Cerebellar softening: A surgical emergency. *Brit. Med. J.* 1:1335, 1956.
38. Faris, A. A., Poser, C. M., Wilmore, D. W., and Agnew, C. H.: Radiologic visualiza-

tion of neck vessels in healthy men. *Neurology* 13:386, 1963.

39. Feigin, I., and Prose, P.: Some uncommon forms of cerebral vascular disease. *J. Mount Sinai Hosp. N.Y.* 24:838, 1957.

40. Feigin, I., and Prose, P.: Hypertensive fibrinoid arteritis of the brain and gross cerebral hemorrhage. *Arch. Neurol.* 1:98, 1959.

41. Fisher, C. M.: *Pathogenesis and Treatment of Cerebrovascular Disease.* Edited by Fields, W. S., Charles C Thomas, Springfield, Ill., 1961, Chap. 7.

42. Ford, R., and Ambrose, J.: Echoencephalography. The measurement of the position of midline structures in the skull with high frequency pulsed ultrasound. *Brain* 86:189, 1963.

43. Freytag, E.: Fatal hypertensive intracerebral hematomas. A survey of the pathological anatomy in 393 cases. *J. Neurol. Neurosurg. Psychiat.* 31:616, 1968.

43*a*. Gillilan, L. A.: Veins of the spinal cord. *Neurology* 20:860, 1970.

43*b*. Goldner, J. C., Whisnant, J. P., and Taylor, W. F.: Longterm prognosis of transient cerebral ischemic attacks. *Stroke* 2:160, 1971.

44. Greenfield, J. G., and Turner, J. W. A.: Acute and subacute necrotic myelitis. *Brain* 62:227, 1939.

45. Groch, S. N., McDevitt, E., and Wright, I. S.: A long term study of cerebral vascular disease. *Ann. Int. Med.* 55:358, 1961.

46. Hamby, W. B.: *Intracranial Aneurysms.* Charles C Thomas, Springfield, Ill., 1952.

47. Hardy, W. G., Lindner, D. W., Thomas, L. M., and Gurdjian, E. S.: Anticipated clinical course in carotid artery occlusion. *Arch. Neurol.* 6:138, 1962.

48. Harrison, M. J. G., and Bevan, A. T.: Early symptoms of temporal arteritis. *Lancet* 2:638, 1967.

49. Heffner, R., and Solitare, G. B.: Hereditary haemorrhagic telangiectasia. *J. Neurol. Neurosurg. Psychiat.* 32:604, 1969.

50. Hollenhorst, R. W.: The ocular manifestations of internal carotid arterial thrombosis. *Med. Clin. N. Amer.* 44:897, 1960.

51. Hollenhorst, R. W., Brown, J. R., Wagener, H. P., and Shick, R. M.: Neurologic aspects of temporal arteritis. *Neurology* 10:490, 1960.

52. Hutchinson, E. C., and Yates, P. O.: The cervical portion of the vertebral artery: A clinico-pathological study. *Brain* 79:319, 1956.

53*a*. Jefferson, G.: Saccular aneurysms of the internal carotid artery in the cavernous sinus. *Brit. J. Surg.* 26:267, 1938.

53*b*. Jefferson, G.: Compression of chiasma, of the optic nerves and of the optic tracts by intracranial aneurysm. *Brain* 60:444, 1937.

54. Kalbag, R. M., and Wolf, A. L.: *Cerebral Venous Thrombosis with Special Reference to Primary Aseptic Thrombosis.* Oxford University Press, London, 1967.

55. Kane, W. C., and Aronson, S. M.: Cerebrovascular disease in an autopsy population (I). *Arch. Neurol.* 20:514, 1969.

56. Knox, D. L.: Ischemic ocular inflammation. *Amer. J. Ophthal.* 60:995, 1965.

57. Krabbe, K. H.: Facial and meningeal angiomatosis associated with calcifications of the brain cortex. *Arch. Neurol. Psychiat.* 32:737, 1934.

58. Kuller, L., Lilienfeld, A., and Fisher, R.: Sudden and unexpected deaths in young adults. *J.A.M.A.* 198:248, 1966.

59. Logue, V., Durward, M., Pratt, R., Piercy, M., and Nixon, W. L.: The quality of survival after rupture of an anterior cerebral aneurysm. *Brit. J. Psychiat.* 114:137, 1968.

60. Luhan, J. A., and Pollack, S. C.: Occlusion of the superior cerebellar artery. *Neurology* 3:77, 1953.

61. Margolis, G., Odom, G. L., Woodhall, B., and Bloor, B. M.: The role of small angiomatous malformations in the production of intracerebral hematomas. *J. Neurosurg.* 8:564, 1951.

61*a*. Marquardsen, J.: The natural history of acute cerebrovascular disease. *Acta Neurol. Scand.* 45, Suppl. 38, 1969.

62. Martin, J. P., and Sheehan, H. L.: Primary thrombosis of the cerebral veins (following childbirth). *Brit. Med. J.* 1:349, 1941.

63. Martin, M. J., Whisnant, J. P., and Sayre, G. P.: Occlusive vascular disease in the extracranial cerebral circulation. *Arch. Neurol.* 3:530, 1960.

64. Marzburg, B.: Trends of mental disease in New York State, 1920–1950. *Proc. Amer. Phil. Soc.* 99:176, 1955.

65. Meadows, S. P.: Temporal or giant cell arteritis. *Proc. Roy. Soc. Med.* 59:329, 1966.

66. McKissock, W., Richardson, A., and Walsh, L.: Primary intracerebral hemorrhage. Results of surgical treatment in 244 consecutive cases. *Lancet* 2:683, 1959.

67. McKissock, W., Richardson, A., and Walsh, L.: Spontaneous cerebellar hemorrhage, a study of 34 consecutive cases treated surgically. *Brain* 83:1, 1960.

68. McKissock, W., Richardson, A., and Walsh, L.: Middle cerebral aneurysms: Further results in the controlled trial of conservative and surgical treatment of ruptured intracranial aneurysms. *Lancet* 2:417, 1962.

69. Meyer, J. S., and Bauer, R. B.: Medical treatment of spontaneous intracranial hemorrhage by the use of hypotensive drugs. *Neurology* 12:36, 1962.

70. Meyer, J. S., Waltz, A. G., and Gotoh, F.: Pathogenesis of cerebral vasospasm in hypertensive encephalopathy. *Neurology* 10:735, 1960.

71. Michael, J. C., and Levin, P. M.: Multiple telangiectases of the brain. *Arch. Neurol. Psychiat.* 36:514, 1936.

72. Miller, H. G., and Daley, R.: Clinical aspects of polyarteritis nodosa. *Quart. J. Med.* 15:255, 1946.

73. Mutlu, N., Berry, R. G., and Alpers, B. J.: Massive cerebral hemorrhage. *Arch. Neurol.* 8:644, 1963.

74. Norlen, G., and Paly, S. N.: Aneurysms of the vertebral artery. *J. Neurosurg.* 17:830, 1960.

75. North, R. R., Fields, W. S., DeBakey, M. E., and Crawford, E. S.: Brachial-basilar insufficiency syndrome. *Neurology* 12:810, 1962.

76. Olivecrona, H.: The cerebellar angioreticulomas (70 cases). *J. Neurosurg.* 9:317, 1952.

77. Olivecrona, H., and Riives, J.: Arteriovenous aneurysm of the brain. *Arch. Neurol. Psychiat.* 59:567, 1948.

78. Olszewski, J.: Subcortical arteriosclerotic encephalopathy: Review of the literature on the so-called Binswanger's disease, and presentation of two new cases. *World Neurol.* 3:359, 1962.

79. Oppenheimer, B. S., and Fishberg, A. M.: Hypertensive encephalopathy. *Arch. Int. Med.* 41:264, 1928.

80. Paterson, J. H., and McKissock, W.: A clinical survey of intracranial angiomas with special reference to their mode of progression and surgical treatment. *Brain* 79:233, 1956.

81. Peterman, A. F., Yoss, R. E., and Corbin, K. B.: The syndrome of occlusion of the anterior spinal artery. *Proc. Mayo Clin.* 33:31, 1958.

82. Pipkin, G.: The early diagnosis and treatment of fat embolism. *Clin. Orthoped.* 12:171, 1956.

83. Reivich, M., Holling, H. E., Roberts, B., and Toole, J. F.: Reversal of blood flow through the vertebral artery and its effect on the cerebral circulation. *New Eng. J. Med.* 265:878, 1961.

84. Richards, E. P., and Dodge, P. R.: Epilepsy in cerebral vascular disease. *Epilepsia* 3:49, 1954.

85. Riishede, J.: Cerebral apoplexy. Statistical considerations. *Acta Psychol. Scand.* Suppl. 108:347, 1956.

86. Romanes, G. J.: The arterial supply of the human spinal cord. *Paraplegia* 2:199, 1965.

87. Russell, D. S., Falconer, M. A., Beck, D. J. K., and McMenemey, W. H.: The pathology of spontaneous intracranial hemorrhage. *Proc. Roy. Soc. Med.* 47:689, 1954.

88. Russell, R.: Observations on intracerebral aneurysms. *Brain* 86:45, 1963.

89. Scheinker, I. M.: Cerebral vasothrombosis in cardiac diseases: A clinico-pathologic study. *Ann. Int. Med.* 42:128, 1952.

90. Sheehan, S., Bauer, R. B., and Meyer, J. S.: Vertebral artery compression in cervical spondylosis: Arteriographic demonstration during life of vertebral artery insufficiency due to rotation and extension of the neck. *Neurology* 10:968, 1960.

91. Silverstein, A.: Intracranial hemorrhage in patients with bleeding tendencies. *Neurology* 11:310, 1961.

92. Simeone, F. A., Ryan, K. G., and Cotter, J. R.: Prolonged experimental cerebral vasospasm. *J. Neurosurg.* 29:357, 1968.

93. Symonds, C. P.: Venous thrombosis in the central nervous system. *Proc. Roy. Soc. Med.* 37:387, 1944.

94. Taylor, J. R., and Van Allen, M. W.: Vascular malformations of the cord with transient ischemic attacks. *J. Neurosurg.* 31:576, 1969.

95. Trevor-Hughes, J.: Thrombosis of the posterior spinal arteries. *Neurology* 20:659, 1970.

96. Thurel, R.: Les pseudobulbaires. Thesis, Paris, 1929.

97. Vavala, D. A.: The present status of aeroembolism. *J. Aviat. Med.* 26:230, 1955.

98. Walton, J. N.: *Subarachnoid Haemorrhage.* E. & S. Livingstone, Edinburgh, 1956.

98a. Whisnant, J. P., Fitzgibbons, J. P., Kurland, L. T., and Sayre, G. P.: Natural history of stroke in Rochester, Minnesota, 1945 through 1954. *Stroke* 2:11, 1971.

99. Wolman, L.: Cerebral dissecting aneurysm. *Brain* 82:276, 1959.

100. Wyburn-Mason, R.: *The Vascular Abnormalities and Lesions of the Spinal Cord and Its Membranes.* Henry Kimpton, London, 1943.

101. Wyburn-Mason, R.: Arterio-venous aneurysm of midbrain and retina, facial nevi, and mental changes. *Brain* 66:163, 1943.

102. Wylie, C. M.: Death statistics of cerebrovascular disease. *Stroke* 1:184, 1970.

CHAPTER SIXTEEN

Tumors of the Nervous System

INTRACRANIAL NEOPLASMS

Incidence. From autopsy records, it has been estimated that between one and two per cent of all deaths are due to intracranial tumors; figures arrived at from national vital statistics are usually lower, possibly because of faulty clinical diagnoses and lack of postmortem verification. Intracranial tumors increase in frequency up to the seventh year, after which the incidence declines until a second rise starts at or about puberty and reaches a maximum in the fifth decade. No age is immune.

Classification. It is logical to classify intracranial neoplasms according to the tissue from which they arise—brain, meninges, cranial nerves, pituitary gland, pineal body, blood vessels, and congenital "cell rests." To these must be added the growths which invade the nervous system from outside. Pseudotumor cerebri has been included as a matter of convenience.

Clinical Features. The pathology and clinical characteristics of individual tumors will be dealt with seriatim, but before doing so it is useful to consider certain general principles which apply in greater or lesser degree to all intracranial space-occupying lesions.

The symptoms and signs of an intracranial tumor are due in the main to two factors: the local destructive effects of the tumor, and increasing intracranial pressure.

Local symptoms usually precede the appearance of raised intracranial pressure, but this is not always the case. A small tumor in or near the ventricular system can obstruct the flow of cerebrospinal fluid and give rise to internal hydrocephalus before it grows large enough to produce focal signs in its own right, and a tumor growing in a relatively silent area, such as the temporal lobe of the minor hemisphere, or either frontal lobe, can grow large enough to raise intracranial pressure before it produces significant neurological deficit. In the case of supratentorial tumors, generalized or focal seizures may precede both focal symptoms and raised intracranial pressure by months or years.

Although focal symptoms usually advance progressively over a period of weeks or months, they sometimes do so in stepwise fashion, with periods of arrest or improvement, a situation which can closely mimic the effects of cerebrovascular insufficiency. It is presumed that the intermittent exacerbations are related to degenerative changes within the tumor and to variations in the amount of edema in the surrounding brain. Sometimes the onset is rapid enough to suggest cerebral infarction or hemorrhage.

The cranium is able to accommodate a comparatively large mass if it grows slowly and if it does not obstruct the flow

409

of cerebrospinal fluid from the ventricular system to the areas from which it is absorbed, but any sudden expansion in the growth, or increase of edema, is apt to produce immediate symptoms.

It follows from these considerations that the presenting symptoms and subsequent course of an intracranial tumor can take several forms. They include: (1) generalized or focal seizures; (2) intermittently or steadily progressive focal symptoms and signs which point to a single area of the brain; this group includes patients in whom mental symptoms are the first to appear; (3) a rapid or even abrupt onset which may mimic a stroke; (4) symptoms of raised intracranial pressure. In the special case of pituitary and suprapituitary tumors, endocrine disturbances may be the first to appear.

Regional Symptoms of Localizing Value

Frontal Lobe. A tumor of the frontal lobe can be relatively silent for a long time, giving rise to no other indication of its presence than an occasional generalized seizure.[32] Changes of mood, personality, and behavior may give the earliest indication that something is amiss, the most characteristic symptoms being euphoria, irresponsibility, and behavior out of keeping with the patient's social and moral background. Tactlessness, childishness, slovenliness in dress, and amoral behavior are common ingredients. There may be excessive excitement in both pleasurable and discomforting situations, and explosive irritability has been recorded in tumors involving the septal area, below the rostrum of the corpus callosum.[27] There is often an incapacity to understand the total significance of a situation, which has been defined by Goldstein as "loss of the abstract attitude"; the patient fails to foresee the implications of his acts or to anticipate the repercussions of external events. It is a remarkable paradox that the general effects of a frontal tumor on

a previously normal personality are usually adverse, whereas improvement in affect and behavior often follow frontal leukotomy in patients suffering from severe psychotic or psychoneurotic disorders.

Motor aphasia may occur in tumors involving Broca's area, and is also encountered when Penfield's supplementary speech area on the medial aspect of the frontal lobe is implicated.[76] Apraxia of the left hand is occasionally seen in right-handed persons when the latter area is compressed by a parasagittal meningioma or is infiltrated by a tumor arising in the anterior portion of the corpus callosum. Facio-oral apraxia is occasionally seen in frontal tumors of the dominant hemisphere (p. 35).

In the early stages, cranial nerves are not involved. Later on, when intracranial pressure is rising, anosmia can occur from compression of the olfactory nerves, and vision may be disturbed by papilledema. Optic atrophy in one eye and papilledema in the other (the Foster-Kennedy syndrome) has been described. As intracranial pressure rises, abducens palsy and other false localizing signs may appear (p. 99).

Motor function is sometimes disturbed before the tumor reaches the motor pathways. Grasping and groping reflexes appear in the contralateral hand, and plantar flexion of the toes occurs when the sole of the foot is *lightly* stroked. Motor perseveration sometimes makes it difficult for the patient to switch from one form of manual activity to another. Paratonia (*Gegenhalten*) is sometimes present in the contralateral arm and leg.

Frontal tumors, especially large convexity meningiomas, were at one time notorious for their capacity to mimic cerebellar tumors,[26] but most of these reports appeared in the first quarter of the present century, at a time when insufficient attention was paid to the capacity of large hemisphere tumors to displace the brainstem and to produce tentorial impaction. Bruns defined two syndromes. The first, bilateral cerebellar ataxia in the terminal stages of large frontal tumors (when intracranial pressure is high), is attributed to pressure on the cerebellum and downward displacement of the brainstem. Bruns and others described a second type of ataxia which appears before the intracranial pressure is elevated. In these cases, the ataxia is contralateral to the side of the tumor, and the clinical signs include intention tremor, hypotonia, dysmetria, dysdiadochokinesia, and unsteadiness of posture and gait. These symptoms have been ascribed to interruption of the frontopontine cerebellar pathways, but this explanation is unsatisfactory since the syndrome does not occur after frontal lobe injuries, resection of the frontal lobe, or section of the frontopontine pathways. It seems likely that in the reported cases, the ataxia was due to displacement of the brainstem, which can occur without a generalized increase of intracranial pressure. The same is probably true of the cerebellar ataxia found in some parietal tumors and abscesses.[19]

Difficulty in walking is sometimes the result of an apraxia of gait. The patient finds it difficult to initiate each step and may complain that his feet seem to stick to the floor, but there is no loss of equilibrium. The apraxia can be demonstrated by asking the patient to lie on his back and simulate the movements of kicking a ball or pedaling a bicycle. He will have difficulty in carrying out these movements though power, tone, and coordination are unaffected.[65]

When a frontal tumor spreads backwards to involve the motor cortex or motor pathways, an early symptom may be palsy of the contralateral side of the face for emotional movement, as in smiling or crying, with retention of voluntary movements such as shutting the eyes or showing the teeth. At this stage, rapid alternating movements of the contralateral fingers are often defective and the outstretched arm may droop slightly when the patient closes his eyes, although neither sensory loss nor weakness can be demonstrated. Ultimately, pyramidal signs become obvious.

Incontinence of urine sometimes occurs in frontal tumors. In some cases, it is not a true incontinence but reflects the mental attitude of the patient, who has become careless of social conventions, including the disposal of excreta. In others, there is impairment of the ability to prevent the micturition reflex when the bladder is full, and there may be a similar disorder of defecation. Alternatively, there is retention of urine. According to Andrew and Nathan,[1] these symptoms occur in lesions involving the superior frontal gyrus and the anterior part of the cingulate gyrus, but in the author's experience, similar symptoms sometimes appear with tumors involving the paracentral lobule.

The Sensory-Motor Region. Motor or sensory jacksonian seizures, contralateral weakness, and slight sensory impairment occur early in infiltrative tumors in this region, but a slowly growing convexity meningioma may attain a considerable size without giving rise to any symptoms whatsoever, and when signs do appear, they are more likely to be motor than sensory. Tumors in this situation affect the face and upper limb more than the leg, and if the major hemisphere is involved, there may be expressive aphasia. As in frontal tumors, facio-oral apraxia may be present, and with it there is occasionally an apraxia for swallowing: The patient cannot swallow voluntarily, but will do so reflexly once the bolus reaches the pharynx.

Parasagittal tumors involving the sensory-motor cortex, notably meningiomas, are apt to involve both leg areas, thereby giving rise to asymmetrical spastic weakness of both legs and sphincter disturbances. This combination may falsely suggest a lesion of the spinal cord, but a sensory level is usually present in the latter. Tumors in this region can also give rise to sudden attacks of weakness in the legs, leading to unexplained falls. Such "drop attacks" are very similar to those which are encountered in basilar-vertebral insufficiency and (less frequently) in insufficiency involving the anterior cerebral arteries. Tumors in this region can also give rise to jacksonian attacks limited to the foot and ankle, and the patient usually complains that the foot feels "numb" between attacks; at this stage, cutaneous and deep sensibility are often normal, but there is slowness of toe wiggling, slight spasticity, and an equivocal plantar response on that side. Involvement of the paracentral lobule by an interhemispheric tumor can cause episodes of urinary incontinence without disturbance of consciousness or other evidence of a seizure.

Parietal Lobe. Tumors in this region are not infrequent and are often silent in the early stages of their development unless they produce sensory symptoms and signs from involvement of the sensory cortex. In this event, there may be sensory jacksonian seizure, and there is often a moderate degree of hemiparesis as well. However, even when the tumor is entirely silent in the sense of failing to produce conventional sensory and motor loss, it may give rise to the subtle sensory and motor symptoms of the "parietal lobe syndrome."[19, 20]

This syndrome is most obvious when the nondominant hemisphere is affected, but this may be due to the fact that the speech defects that often accompany lesions in the dominant hemisphere may to some extent obscure the patient's description of the symptoms.

In a fully developed case, the patient has a normal appreciation of contralateral tactile, olfactory, auditory, and visual stimuli but if presented with stimuli given simultaneously to the two sides, he will ignore those coming from the side opposite to the lesion. This "inattention" or "extinction" is thought to be the result of perceptual rivalry. It is apt to vary from hour to hour. Moreover, the patient tends to ignore the opposite side of the body. If the disease has spread to the motor cortex or pyramidal tract, with consequent paralysis, he may deny the fact that he is paralyzed (anosognosia). There may be difficulty in reading a page of print because the patient attends to only one-half of the page, or even to only one-half of a word. Instructed to draw a map of the United States, or a bicycle, he pays little attention to the portion of the drawing contralateral to the side of the lesion. There may be difficulty in copying simple figures or constructing designs with matches or building blocks; such constructural apraxia seems to be a special feature of lesions of the nondominant hemisphere. Bilateral motor apraxia may occur in lesions of the caudal part of the dominant parietal lobe. These disturbances impart a bizarre quality to many of the patient's actions, and unless they are recognized for what they are, they may be falsely attributed to psychosis or psychoneurosis.

There is often difficulty in recognizing familiar objects placed in the hand (astereognosis), though the sense of touch is normal. Cortical sensory impairment also leads to clumsiness of the contralateral upper limb, a form of sensory ataxia. When the patient is asked to hold his hands out in front of him with his eyes closed, the fingers will often execute slight involuntary "piano playing" movements. Another and rather uncommon motor effect of a parietal lesion of either hemisphere is the avoiding reaction. If the palm of the patient's hand is lightly stroked, the fingers and hands extend and the whole arm may move away from the contact. According to Denny-Brown, this is a release phenomenon which depends on the integrity of the frontal lobe.

Wasting of the contralateral limbs, the hand especially, occurs in some long-standing parietal lesions.

If a lesion involves the region of the angular gyrus of the dominant hemisphere, it may give rise to Gerstmann's syndrome — inability to judge between left and right, finger agnosia, inability to calculate, and dyslexia. Individual components of this syndrome are frequently encountered, but it is seldom seen in pure form, and may occur in parietal lesions which do not involve the angular gyrus.

In the presence of hemiparesis from an expanding lesion which also involves the parietal lobe, the disorder of motility is somewhat modified. There is greater paucity of movement than can be accounted for on the basis of paralysis, and catatonic-like postures may be adopted by the upper limb. The affected limbs may be flaccid rather than spastic, and the plantar response on the sole of the affected foot may be absent. Parietal lesions have been reported to give rise to ataxia of cerebellar type,[19] and spontaneous turning movements around the vertical axis of the body are occasionally seen when the patient attempts to walk. Although these symptoms have been attributed to involvement of parieto-vestibular-cerebellar connections, it is likely that when they occur in tumors or abscesses they are due to displacement of the brainstem and cerebellar peduncles.

Optokinetic nystagmus is reduced or absent when the drum is rotating towards the side of the lesion, whereas the response is normal when it rotates towards the normal side.

Occipital Lobe. Headache is a common early symptom of tumors in this region, and is usually occipital. Seizures occur in only about one-third of all cases and are often preceded by an aura consisting of flashes of light, unlike the more complex visual hallucinations of temporal lobe lesions. In some cases, repeated flashes of light in the contralateral visual fields occur without a convulsion.

As is to be expected, visual field defects occur at an early stage and can usually be found by perimetry, even if the patient has not noticed them. Careful examination of both the peripheral and central fields provides information which cannot be supplied by any other form of investigation. A lesion of the calcarine cortex produces homonymous and congruous field loss. Tumors situated posteriorly in the calcarine fissure will produce central defects in the upper and lower fields. Those situated anteriorly can produce monocular loss of the temporal crescent, without affecting central vision. Deeply placed tumors which involve the geniculo-calcarine pathway produce congruous homonymous field defects of the depression type, scotomata being uncommon.[46] Forward extension of a tumor in the dominant hemisphere results in dyslexia, which the patient may interpret as a difficulty in "seeing," and the true nature of the disability may therefore be missed.

Temporal Lobe. *Rapidly* developing tumors in the temporal lobe produce

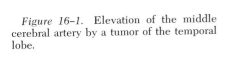

Figure 16–1. Elevation of the middle cerebral artery by a tumor of the temporal lobe.

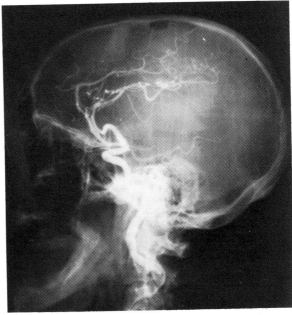

headache (often ipsilateral), generalized or temporal lobe seizures, contralateral congruous homonymous hemianopic field defects (which usually appear first in the upper quadrants), and aphasia if the dominant hemisphere is involved. Pressure on the third nerve produces appropriate oculomotor signs, and displacement of the brainstem to the opposite side can give rise to an ipsilateral hemiparesis. Mental symptoms, so prominent in slowly growing tumors of this region, tend to be overshadowed by the more dramatic features of neurological incapacity and of raised intracranial pressure.

Slowly growing tumors, on the other hand, are apt to produce a more subtle picture, which is often dominated at first by mental symptoms and uncinate or other types of temporal lobe attacks. This form of presentation is most likely to arise when the tumor lies on the inferomedial aspect of the lobe, involving the amygdaloid nucleus, the hippocampal gyrus, and the uncus. When the main impact of the tumor is on the speech area of the dominant hemisphere, sensory aphasia is likely to precede mental symptoms, and as it spreads backward towards the occipital lobe, the aphasia may be associated with dyslexia, dysgraphia, acalculia, right-left disorientation, and finger agnosia. Homonymous field cuts, which are usually congruous, appear sooner or later.

The mental symptoms are qualitatively similar to those which have been reported in tumors affecting other parts of the limbic system,[27, 63] notably the hypothalamus, the cingulate gyri, the fornix, the septum pellucidum, and the septal area. It is pertinent to recall that mental symptoms and behavioral disorders are sometimes prominent in other diseases affecting the limbic system, notably vascular lesions, subacute inclusion encephalitis, some cases of herpes simplex encephalitis, and the encephalopathy which occasionally occurs in association with visceral carcinoma. The mental state may be one of anxiety, depression or apathy, impairment of memory, or a schizophrenia-like illness. Patients with temporal lobe tumor are occasionally admitted to mental wards before the true origin of the disorder is appreciated.

Seizures are common and are often the first complaint. Any type of temporal lobe epilepsy can occur, including visual, auditory, and uncinate hallucinations, feelings of unreality, a sense of detachment, and so on (p. 130). The patient will often fail to volunteer information about these curious experiences and will not mention them unless directly questioned about them. As in non-neoplastic disease of the temporal lobe, it is possible that continuing subclinical seizure discharges may contribute to the interictal mental symptoms which these patients so often display. Generalized convulsions may occur but are sometimes preceded by a "temporal lobe" aura.

When mental symptoms or temporal lobe seizures are the first to appear, the diagnosis is difficult because at this early stage a negative result is apt to be given by brain scan, arteriography, and pneumoencephalography. Careful examination of the visual fields will sometimes disclose a depressional type of homonymous field defect, commonly in the upper quadrant. It is well known, but it is worth repeating, that the patient is usually unaware of the hemianopia.

Deafness does not occur in unilateral temporal lobe lesions, though difficulty in the localization of sounds has been reported. The caloric responses may provide diagnostic assistance; in some cases, there is directional preponderance towards the affected side in lesions of the posterior temporal region.

Corpus Callosum. The fibers of the corpus callosum unite both homologous and heterologous areas of the two hemispheres, and bundles of fibers pass from each hemisphere to the internal capsule of the opposite side. The hemispheres are also linked by the anterior, posterior, and habenular commissures, and by the massa intermedia when it is present. These subsidiary interhemispheric connections explain why it is possible to divide the corpus callosum from end to

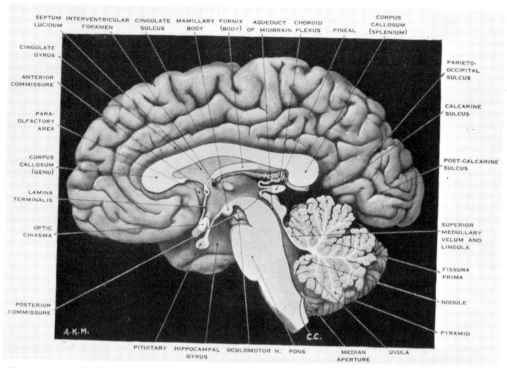

Figure 16–2. Median section of the brain, showing relationships of deep midline structures. (From Hamilton, W. J., ed.: *Textbook of Human Anatomy.* MacMillan Co., London, 1962.)

end without producing any obvious symptoms. Tumors of the corpus callosum, on the other hand, produce a variety of symptoms, both psychological and somatic, but they are due to involvement of contiguous structures.[27] A tumor starting in the rostrum and genu can spread into the septal area of the frontal lobe, or backward to involve the septum pellucidum and fornix, and it is well placed to obstruct the foramen of Monroe (Fig. 16–2). Lateral spread from the body of the corpus callosum will involve the basal ganglia, and if the tumor extends upward and laterally, it will involve the cingulate gyrus, the "leg" area of the motor and sensory cortex, and the paracentral lobule which is concerned, inter alia, with the control of the bladder and rectum. Tumors of the splenium are apt to spread to the occipital lobe, midbrain, and sylvian aqueduct, producing appropriate symptoms.

The outstanding *early* clinical feature of a callosal tumor is mental and emotional deterioration, the result of spread to the frontal lobes and cingulate gyri. The most consistently reported feature is apathy, also described as indifference, lack of interest, and "imperviousness." Apathy also occurs in bilateral cingulate lesions without involvement of the corpus callosum and is prominent in cysts of the third ventricle, tumors and other lesions of the inframedial aspect of the temporal lobe, raised intracranial pressure, and acquired hydrocephalus from any cause. In tumors of the corpus callosum, apathy is accompanied by slowness of thought, lack of initiative, poverty of ideas, and inattention, and ultimately the condition may be one of akinetic mutism. Some patients are depressed, and others, especially those with frontal lobe involvement, are euphoric. On the other hand, explosive irritability may be prominent when the rostrum and septal area are involved. Some cases exhibit delusions of persecution and olfactory, gustatory, visual, and auditory hallucinations; when these symptoms are associated with apathy and negativism, the resemblance to schizophrenia may be close, but the delusions are less systematized than in the latter. It is possible that the patient's premorbid personality influences the mental picture.

Intellectual impairment may be present. Failure of memory has been seen in posterior callosal tumors and in those invading the fornix. Sprofkin and Sciarra (1952) have reported three cases in which a Korsakoff's psychosis was the presenting symptom of a tumor involving the septum pellucidum and the corpus callosum.

Expressive aphasia has been described, perhaps from involvement of the supplementary motor area of the dominant hemisphere; it has also been seen in infarction of the medial surface of the frontal lobe from thrombosis of the anterior cerebral artery, and in parasagittal meningiomas.

The motor disturbances which eventually appear in most cases of callosal tumor can give a clue as to the site of the disease. Left-sided apraxia occurs in some 10 per cent of all cases when the lesion is in the anterior portion of the corpus callosum and has spread to involve the frontal lobes. Involvement of the medial aspect of the frontal lobe may produce contralateral grasping and groping reflexes which interfere with the voluntary use of the hand. Ataxia and apraxia of gait have been reported.

Lateral and upward spread of a callosal tumor will involve the corticospinal pathways to the lower limbs and is apt to give rise to a hemiparesis on one side, mainly affecting the leg, together with pyramidal signs on the other side. The motor signs are usually asymmetrical. Deep penetration to the corpus striatum can produce extrapyramidal signs, notably choreiform movements of parkinsonism. Sensory impairment of cortical type may be found in the lower limb below the knee.

Posteriorly situated tumors will spread into the occipital lobe or lobes, producing appropriate changes in the visual fields.

Ultimately, the clinical picture is dominated by the features of raised intracranial pressure. Occasionally, this occurs early in the course of the disease, with headache, papilledema, mental dulling, and false localizing signs. It is desirable to reiterate, however, that in many patients a rise of intracranial pres-

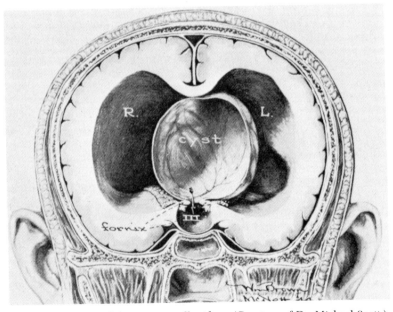

Figure 16–3.   Cyst of the septum pellucidum. (Courtesy of Dr. Michael Scott.)

sure is deferred for a long time, and the presenting symptoms are primarily psychological. Moniz (1927) emphasized the variability of the mental picture, which can resemble schizophrenia in young adults, general paresis or presenile dementia in middle-aged persons, and senile or arteriosclerotic dementia in the elderly.[27]

The Septum Pellucidum. The septum pellucidum stretches between the undersurface of the corpus callosum and the fornix and is composed of two thin layers, each consisting of nerve fibers covered by a layer of gray matter. It has connections with the hippocampus, hypothalamus, and the septal nuclei (i.e., with the limbic system). Between the two laminae, there is a space of variable extent, the cavum septi pellucidi. This space can become distended to form a cyst of considerable size, which acts like a tumor by blocking the foramen of Monroe, thereby producing internal hydro-

cephalus (Fig. 16–3). As in the case of other midline tumors, the principal symptoms take the form of mental deterioration on the one hand and symptoms due to raised intracranial pressure on the other. At first, the pressure symptoms tend to be intermittent. This is usually attributed to periodic obstruction of the foramen of Monroe, but spontaneous evacuation of the cyst's contents into the ventricles is another possibility which has to be entertained because small ragged holes in the cyst wall have been observed at autopsy in some cases.[22] Paroxysmal headache, vomiting, and stupor occur during periods of raised intracranial pressure. Mental symptoms may be present or absent between episodes of raised pressure; they range from apathy to dementia.

Tumors of the septum pellucidum are rare.[15] Astrocytomas, glioblastomas, and oligodendrogliomas have been reported (Fig. 16–4). In some cases, there is a rel-

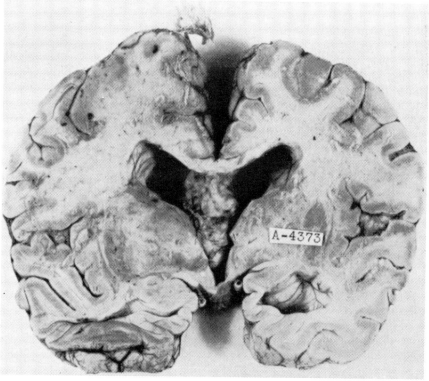

Figure 16–4. Glioblastoma of the septum pellucidum. (Courtesy of Drs. J. D. Chusid and C. D. DeGutierrez-Mahoney.)

atively acute onset of symptoms of raised intracranial pressure due to obstruction of the foramen of Monroe, in which event there are no features which direct attention specifically to the septum pellucidum, and the diagnosis will depend on contrast studies. In other cases, mental symptoms precede the development of the high pressure syndrome and are attributed to involvement of the limbic system, with spread to the frontal lobe. Ultimately, false localizing signs develop as a result of the high pressure.

Centrum Ovale. With tumors in this region, hemiparesis, deep sensory loss, and hemianopia tend to occur early because the tracts concerned with these functions come closer together as the capsular region is reached. For this reason, motor weakness tends to be distributed widely and to affect the whole of one side of the body. Symptoms and signs of striatal involvement may appear, though they are not at all common; it is rare for extrapyramidal rigidity or tremor to be the presenting sign of a cerebral tumor. Highly vascular tumors in this region, notably the glioblastoma multiforme, will occasionally mimic a stroke, the abrupt onset being due to hemorrhage within the tumor. Intermittent symptoms reminiscent of transient ischemic attacks are also encountered, but the motor and sensory symptoms do not completely clear up in the interval between the attacks. When the tumor involves the hypothalamic region, sudden and severe disturbance of consciousness may result — either an attack of short duration which may simulate ordinary sleep, or prolonged coma.

Thalamus. Primary tumors[13, 60] starting in the thalamus are estimated by McKissock and Paine to account for not more than 1 per cent of all encephalic tumors. The presenting symptoms and signs in the majority of cases are those of raised intracranial pressure. Headache, nausea and vomiting, apathy and dulling of the intellect, diplopia, and blurring of vision from papilledema are common early features. Occasionally, mental symptoms varying from apathy to dementia are prominent, before there is any evidence of raised intracranial pressure — a feature common to many lesions of deep midline structures.[27] Weakness of the contralateral limbs is common, and extrapyramidal tremors are not rare. Intention tremor and other "cerebellar" symptoms have occasionally been recorded, but it is not clear whether these are due to the effects of raised intracranial pressure or to interference with the pathways between one lobe of the cerebellum and the contralateral frontal lobe. Considering the role of the thalamus in sensory function, sensory symptoms and signs are remarkably mild. Contralateral paresthesias, sensory loss and hyperesthesia are rare, as is the fully developed "thalamic syndrome" of Déjerine-Roussy. Diplopia and inequality of the pupils are common[60]; in some cases, they appear to be due to raised intracranial pressure with displacement of the brainstem; in others, there is evidence of a downward spread of the tumor into the midbrain. Hemianopia is unusual in the early stages.

Expressive aphasia has been recorded, and it is usually assumed that this indicates the spread of the tumor into the temporal region, but this may not be the whole explanation. This symptom has been reported following stereotactic thalamotomy for Parkinson's disease,[7] and Penfield and Roberts[76] and others have seen aphasia following hemorrhage into the pulvinar of the dominant hemisphere.

Tumors of the thalamus can spread to the hypothalamus, causing hypersomnia or coma of relatively rapid onset.

The Brainstem. Gliomas of the brainstem[57, 95] are most common in childhood and early adult life. They account for some 10 per cent of the intracranial tumors encountered in childhood.

The initial symptoms and signs depend not only on whether the tumor arises in the midbrain, pons, or medulla, but also on whether it is so situated as to obstruct the outflow of cerebrospinal fluid. If so, it will produce early signs of raised intracranial pressure, but in many brainstem tumors this is a comparatively late event, and the symptomatology is confined to unilateral or bilateral involvement of the cranial nerves, the cerebellar peduncles, and the long motor and sensory tracts. Another feature of these cases is that the symptoms may be intermittent in the early stages of the disease; this is illustrated by intermittent diplopia.

Disturbances of mind, mood, and behavior sometimes occur in gliomas of the midbrain and pons; they include apathy, lethargy, temper tantrums, aggressive behavior, or progressive dementia.[57] On the other hand, children with subtentorial tumors are sometimes, in Davidoff's words, "unusually alert and cooperative, and of sweet disposition"; it is possible that in some cases this sweetness of disposition reflects a pathological docility. Mental symptoms were present in 5 of 32 cases of brainstem tumor reported by Cairns and in 8 out of 27 pontine gliomas described by Lassman and Arjona.[57] Kerschner and his associates found psychological symptoms in no less than 47 per cent of a group of 120 patients with subtentorial tumors and noted that the symptoms appeared early in the disease in 12 per cent of their cases.

There is as yet no satisfactory explanation for these mental symptoms, which can occur in the absence of internal hydrocephalus or raised intracranial pressure. Langford and Kligman have stressed the importance of personality and environmental influences, but such factors can scarcely be invoked to explain loss of memory and other features of dementia. It is pertinent to recall that marked changes of behavior occur in monkeys and cats with experimental lesions of the midbrain. Sprague and his colleagues[90] found that in cats, unilateral midbrain section of the specific sensory pathways produced not only changes of personality and behavior but also inattention to visual and auditory stimuli on the side contralateral to the lesion. Robson found that similar lesions in monkeys produced tranquility, lack of appropriate affective reactions, and an apparent inability to be alerted by, or to learn from, their environment; they, too, displayed an inattention to contralateral auditory and visual stimuli, which was reminiscent of the parietal syndrome in man. Denny-Brown's observations on monkeys with lesions in the mesencephalic tegmentum lead him to conclude that this area is "essential for the reaction which we call general awareness, for which it has an initiative function." These and other experimental studies on animals, taken in conjunction with the psychological effects of subtentorial tumors in man, emphasize how undesirable is the common practice of equating mental symptoms with supratentorial lesions alone.

Midbrain Tumors. Midbrain tumors are apt to produce paralysis of conjugate upward gaze and nerve palsies on one or both sides, with or without a rise of intracranial pressure and with or without signs of involvement of the long motor and sensory tracts. Cerebellar symptoms may occur from involvement of the superior cerebellar peduncles. Infiltration of the red nucleus can give rise to an ipsilateral third nerve palsy and a tremor of the contralateral hand and foot. Sudden and sometimes permanent loss of consciousness can occur, probably from implication of the ascending reticular formation.

Pontine Tumors. Pontine tumors usually present with signs of cranial nerve involvement, sometimes accompanied by ataxia, for weeks or months before the long tracts are affected or headache appears.[57] Ocular features include nystagmus, paralysis of conjugate lateral gaze, sixth nerve paralysis, and internuclear ophthalmoplegia. Trigeminal symptoms include paresthesias on one side of the face, and *pain* in the face, tongue, or pharynx. The seventh nerve is particularly vulnerable. In the earliest stages of bilateral facial weakness, there is sometimes a lack of facial expression, and drooling may be troublesome. Unilateral tonic facial spasm has been reported. Involvement of the long tracts may give rise to spastic weakness of one or more limbs. Hemiparesthesias are more common than sensory loss and varying degrees of ataxia are common.

Medullary Tumors. Medullary tumors[18] commonly involve the descending nucleus of the fifth nerve and the auditory and vestibular components of the eighth nerve; consequently, paresthesias in the face and tongue, unilateral tinnitus, and intermittent vertigo are common. The vertigo may be positional in character, or it may be related to movement of the head. Motor, sensory, and cerebellar signs are not unusual. Disturbances of the autonomic nervous system are common: In children particularly, attacks of effortless vomiting and diarrhea may continue for some time in the absence of all other features of an intracranial tumor and it is only too easy to mistake these symptoms for evidence of gastrointestinal disease. Elements of a Horner's syndrome may be found in both pontine and medullary tumors. Disturbances of pulse, respiration, and heat regulation are not uncommon, but they are usually obscured by the more dramatic somatic symptoms. Paralysis of the lower cranial nerves is rather unusual. Palatal nystagmus can occur as a result of implication of the olivodentate system.

Cerebellum. A distinction must be made between tumors of the lateral and medial regions of the cerebellum. In the former, disturbance of motor function is unilateral and is confined to the side of the lesion. Nystagmus is usually present on lateral gaze and consists of a slow deviation away from the point of fixation towards the midline, followed by a rapid (cortical) movement of restitution to the fixation point. It is most marked when the patient looks towards the side of the tumor. A fine nystagmus is sometimes seen on upward gaze.

Speech is slow and may be scanning in character; in acute cases, the dysarthria may be so marked as to render speech unintelligible.

Ataxia affects the upper limb more than the leg. Muscle tone is diminished and slight weakness is sometimes present. The affected limbs tire easily, droop when outstretched, and are more easily displaced than on the normal side. There is often considerable clumsiness of fine movements. Intention tremor is marked, and dysmetria is present.

There is usually a disturbance of gait, with a tendency to drift to the affected side, and the patient adopts a wide-based gait to avoid this. The arm fails to swing normally on the affected side. Owing to reduced tone, the tendon reflexes on the affected side are diminished, and a pendular knee jerk is usually present.

Midline tumors, notably the medulloblastoma of childhood,[48] commonly affect the flocculonodular lobe. Lesions in this area give rise to disturbances of equilibrium and gait. Nystagmus is usually absent and speech is unaffected. Gait is slow and staggering, and the patient is apt to fall backward or to either side. The trunk sways when the patient sits upright with the eyes closed and the arms stretched out.

Tumors of the cerebellum soon come to obstruct the fourth ventricle and aqueduct, with consequent hydrocephalus and a rise of intracranial pressure. In many cases, the tumor does not remain confined to the cerebellum and before long, evidence of pressure on, or destruction of, neighboring structures will become evident. The fifth, seventh, and eighth nerves are the most often affected; long tract signs are usually late in appearing in both lateral and midline tumors. Pressure on the brainstem can give rise to so-called cerebellar seizures, which consists of a tetanus-like opisthotonos that is regarded as an episodic form of decerebrate rigidity. This occurs in the terminal stages of cerebellar tumors.

The Chiasmal Region. Primary tumors in this area commonly involve vision before they are big enough to raise intracranial pressure by obstructing the third ventricle (Fig. 16–5). Headache can be caused, in the absence of raised intracranial pressure, by displacement of neighboring pain-sensitive structures, but it is often absent. If the situation is not relieved, the features of raised intracranial pressure ultimately supervene. Endocrine changes may precede all other symptoms in the case of pituitary tumors.

The outstanding focal signs of neoplasms in and around the chiasm are impairment of the visual fields and optic

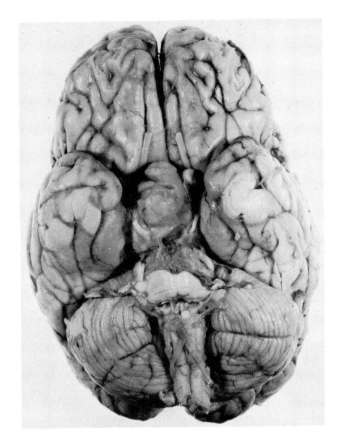

Figure 16–5. Glioma of the optic chiasm. (Courtesy of Dr. Lionel Wolman.)

atrophy.[16, 46, 49, 52] Unhappily, the patient is often unaware of them until late, when central vision comes to be affected. If the tumor arises beneath the chiasm, it will first compress nerve fibers from the inferior portions of the retinae; consequently, the upper fields will be affected first. Usually, the defect starts in the upper temporal quadrant and spreads to the lower temporal and lower nasal quadrants, in that order. Sometimes the initial change is a scotoma in each eye. This brings itself to the notice of the patient earlier than would a peripheral field loss. If the tumor comes from above, bitemporal field changes start in the lower quadrants. In some cases, one optic nerve, or the optic tract, is involved first.

Growths in the chiasmal region may spread to involve the hypothalamus; this can lead not only to hypothalamic symptoms but also to blockage of the third ventricle, with consequent internal hydrocephalus. As mentioned in the section on false localizing signs of brain tumor, bitemporal hemianopia, hypothalamic symptoms, and endocrine disturbances can also result from internal hydrocephalus due to a posterior fossa tumor, the distended third ventricle pressing down on the chiasm and pituitary gland.

Lateral extension of the tumor can involve the third nerve and temporal lobe, giving rise to diplopia, uncinate fits, generalized seizures, memory impairment, and disturbances of mood and behavior.

Craniopharyngiomas occasionally give rise to orthostatic arterial hypotension as the presenting symptom in adults.[82] In children, they can cause stunting of growth and persistent headaches, in the absence of visual impairment or other symptoms.[23]

The Cerebellopontine Angle. The most common tumor at this site is the neurinoma of the eighth nerve, but meningiomas, neurinoma of the fifth nerve, sarcomas, and epidermoid tumors may also be responsible. Occasionally a glioma of the brainstem or cerebellum extends into the lateral recess to produce somewhat similar symptoms. Any tumor expanding within the recess can involve the eighth, seventh, and fifth cranial nerves, usually in that order, and can compress the middle cerebellar peduncle and cerebellum on the same side. Later on, it can spread downwards to affect the lower cranial nerves, and it will ultimately give rise to obstructive hydrocephalus and the symptoms of increased intracranial pressure, including those of a pressure cone. Meningiomas and neurinomas in this situation usually grow extremely slowly and may attain a large size without causing a rise of intracranial pressure. Moreover, the neurological symptoms and signs in these cases may be comparatively slight,[28] amounting to no more than a moderate degree of nerve deafness, occasional vertigo, minimal facial weakness, or pain and paresthesias in the face on the affected side. When pain is present, it may take the form of a dull ache accompanied by paresthesias, or it may have most of the characteristics of tic douloureux, with or without sensory impairment. Revilla found that 5.1 per cent of a series of cases operated on for tic douloureux had tumors which were unsuspected before operation. By modern standards, this proportion is unduly high, but it is unquestionably true that symptoms indistinguishable from tic douloureux and unaccompanied by any other symptoms or signs may be caused by a tumor on the cerebellopontine angle. A tumor in this situation may mimic Meniere's disease, and the author has encountered a case in which a large meningioma gave rise to symptoms indistinguishable from those of pseudotumor cerebri.

The Third Ventricle. Invasive tumors of the third ventricle are apt to produce symptoms of hypothalamic damage: somnolence, coma, obesity, impotence, diabetes insipidus, hyperglycemia, disturbances of temperature regulation, and —very rarely—episodes of diencephalic epilepsy. Tumors involving the anterior part of the hypothalamus in infants can give rise to extreme wasting, coupled with alertness of mind and retraction of the eyelids.[96]

The symptoms of colloid cysts arising *within* the ventricle[77] are usually caused by intermittent or persistent obstructive hydrocephalus. Headache of rapid onset, sometimes induced by change of posture, may be accompanied by confusion, disorientation, excitement, or apathy, and these symptoms may be followed by akinetic mutism, hypersomnia, or coma. This train of symptoms may disappear spontaneously, only to repeat itself days or weeks later. The abrupt remission of such incidents within a day or two is highly suggestive of tumor in this situation. Mental disturbances during the acute incidents are apt to overshadow the headache, and in some cases there is progressive dementia without headache or papilledema.[79]

The Fourth Ventricle. Tumors in this region produce obstructive hydrocephalus at an early stage. When the tumor is small and pedunculated, the symptoms and signs may be intermittent, as in tumors of the third and lateral ventricles.

The symptoms resulting from the presence of an expanding mass in the fourth ventricle are sometimes referred to as the Bruns syndrome.[26] Bruns and others thought that the syndrome was characteristic of cysticercosis of the fourth ventricle, but later they came to recognize that similar symptoms could be caused by tumors. The patient experiences periodic attacks of violent vertigo, vomiting, and headache, which are often precipitated by movements of the head. He may hold his head in an abnormal posture, which is usually one of anterior flexion and slight lateral tilting. The attacks may be accompanied by blurring of vision, unformed visual hallucinations, palpitations, irregular respiration, or syncope. The symptoms appear to be due partly to an acute rise of intracranial pressure and partly to excitation of the central vestibular system brought about by movements of the head. Sooner or later additional symptoms arise from infiltration of the medulla, pons, and cerebellum, together with the features of persistent internal hydrocephalus. Ultimately, a medullary pressure cone is likely to supervene.

Episodes of headache, vomiting and mental symptoms can also occur with tumors of the third and lateral ventricles, but the head is not tilted, vertigo is less common, and mental symptoms are more prominent. Profound anorexia and failure to thrive, sometimes found in tumors of the hypothalamus,[96] have also been reported in tumors of the fourth ventricle.

RAISED INTRACRANIAL PRESSURE

In the erect posture, there is a negative pressure in the ventricles, while at the cisterna magna, the pressure is atmospheric and in the lumbar sac it is equivalent to the height of spinal fluid column between the point of measurement and the cisterna magna. With the patient horizontal, the pressure is roughly the same throughout the ventricular system and the spinal subarachnoid space, so that ventricular pressure is higher when the patient lies down than when he stands up; this may help to explain why a patient with internal hydrocephalus or tumor is usually more subject to headache when lying down than when erect. Intracranial pressure is increased by stooping, coughing, sneezing, straining at stool, and lifting heavy weights. These activities aggravate the headache of both increased and decreased intracranial pressure, but the latter is relieved by lying down.

Elevation of pCO_2 causes dilatation of intracranial blood vessels, and this greatly increases intracranial pressure—hence the need for a satisfactory airway and good pulmonary ventilation if the pressure inside the head is already elevated.

Intracranial space-occupying lesions can elevate intracranial pressure in four

ways: by their volume, by evoking edema in the surrounding brain, by obstructing the circulation and absorption of the cerebrospinal fluid, and—when the pressure is very high—by impeding the cerebral circulation and so causing generalized edema.

The effect of the mass itself depends to some extent on its rate of growth. If it enlarges slowly, it can be accommodated for some time without causing a general rise of intracranial pressure, but if it grows swiftly, the pressure rises sharply. A small tumor in the third or fourth ventricle can cause a rise of pressure which is out of proportion to its size by causing internal hydrocephalus, but here again, if the pressure rises slowly, symptoms may be minimal, whereas an acute obstruction will give rise to the immediate and dramatic symptoms of a hydrocephalic crisis.

The edema evoked by a tumor, abscess, or infarct will often spread far beyond the mass, and contributes to the rise of intracranial pressure. At a later stage, edema results from obstruction of cortical veins and dural sinuses, and finally, when intracranial pressure is high enough to impede the arterial circulation, cerebral hypoxia plays a part in producing edema of the brain as a whole.[56]

Interference with the circulation and absorption of the spinal fluid can be caused in three ways. Obstruction to the outflow pathways has already been mentioned. Secondly, a tentorial pressure cone will not only obstruct the sylvian aqueduct but will also prevent the cerebrospinal fluid from reaching the surface of the brain, from which much of it is absorbed. Thirdly, compression of the dural venous sinuses and the veins which enter them will reduce the rate at which the cerebrospinal fluid can be absorbed and will increase cerebral edema.

The relationship between intracranial blood flow and intracranial pressure is a complex subject which is not fully understood. A rapid rise of intracranial pressure evokes an immediate rise of blood pressure (the Cushing reflex), but this is less evident when intracranial pressure rises slowly. The cerebral vessels have a considerable capacity for autoregulation, which enables them to adapt to changes of blood pressure and body posture in order to maintain a constant cerebral blood flow. Kety and his colleagues found that in man cerebral blood flow does not fall until the intracranial pressure exceeds 140 mm. Hg, while Zwetnow[103] found that in dogs intracranial pressure could be raised to within 20 to 30 mm. Hg of the diastolic blood pressure without reducing blood flow. However, as the intracranial pressure continues to rise, blood flow declines, and when the pressure within the head equals the mean arterial pressure, cerebral blood flow ceases. When this occurs, opaque media injected into the carotid or vertebral arteries do not enter the intracranial vessels. Autoregulation can break down as the result of acute vascular accidents and head injury (including surgical manipulation of the brain). The brain swells abruptly because the arteries and arterioles dilate passively under the influence of the arterial blood pressure.[56]

Another and very dangerous factor is the "pressure wave" described by Lundberg and by Langfitt and his colleagues.[56] When intracranial pressure is raised by any space-occupying process, the pressure does not remain constant but is subject to certain fluctuations, the most serious of which are pressure waves in which the pressure may reach as high as 140 mm. Hg. Usually they occur spontaneously, but at times they are precipitated by hypoxia or by hypercapnia. During these episodes, headache increases, the level of consciousness is depressed, the patient may vomit, and there may be confusion, disorientation, and disturbances in respiration. When the pressure approaches 140 mm. Hg, blood flow through the brain is arrested. The cause of these waves is not fully understood. They appear to be due to episodic vasodilatation rather than to loss of autoregulation. They have been observed in patients with severe head injury, hydrocephalus, pseudotumor

cerebri, brain infarcts, spontaneous subarachnoid hemorrhage, etc. They are particularly liable to occur in the presence of mild respiratory insufficiency and can be controlled by hyperventilation or by removal of the cerebrospinal fluid from the lateral ventricle. The latter procedure has its disadvantages, including the circumstance that a pressure wave can kill the patient before there is time to insert a cannula into the lateral ventricle.

Pressure Cones

When a mass expands in the supratentorial compartment, it displaces unaffected regions of the brain.[45, 62] If laterally placed, it first pushes the surrounding brain medially, while centrally placed masses push it directly downwards. In either event, the initial impact of the pressure is on the thalamus and hypothalamus, i.e., on the diencephalon. As the pressure increases, basal structures are forced towards the only point of escape, the tentorial hiatus. When this occurs, the brainstem is displaced downward, but the extent to which it can move is limited by the attachments of cranial nerves and blood vessels and by the denticulate ligaments in the cervical canal. In consequence, the brainstem may be kinked. This downward displacement of the brainstem explains certain false localizing signs, notably unilateral or bilateral abducens paralysis.

As the supratentorial mass increases in size, it displaces the brain (Fig. 16–6) and pushes the uncus on one or both sides into the tentorial hiatus, or the hippocampal gyrus may herniate around and behind the midbrain. In either event, the latter is compressed. This is dangerous because (1) it interferes with the venous return from the upper part of the brainstem, (2) it compresses the posterior cerebral arteries, (3) it compresses the sylvian aqueduct, and (4) it obstructs the pathway of the cerebrospinal fluid to the surface of the cerebral hemispheres. This interference with the cere-

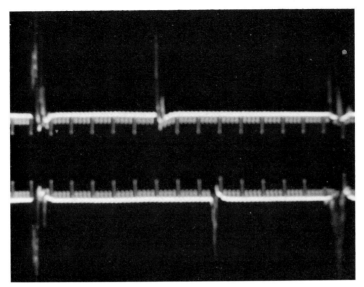

Figure 16–6. Echoencephalogram showing displacement of midline structures to the left by right-sided meningioma.

brospinal fluid circulation causes a further rise of the already elevated pressure in the superior compartment. One or more hemorrhages may occur in the brainstem, notably in the pons, and this can cause sudden death.

Ultimately, the downward displacement of the brainstem brings about impaction of the medulla and cerebellar tonsils in the foramen magnum[45]; this is the situation which Collier (1902) first described as a pressure cone.

An expanding mass in the posterior fossa will sometimes displace the anterior lobe of the cerebellum upwards into the tentorial hiatus, thereby compressing the brainstem, with or without concomitant coning in the foramen magnum. Medullary coning is especially likely to arise in individuals who have a congenital displacement of cerebellar tissue into the foramen magnum.

McNealy and Plum[62] have pointed out that in the presence of raised intracranial pressure from a supratentorial mass, there is usually an orderly progression of symptoms and signs indicating successive depression of function in the diencephalon, midbrain and upper pons, and medulla. This progression can often be observed when the process develops gradually, but when the rise of pressure

in the supratentorial department is abrupt (e.g., intracerebral hemorrhage) or rapid (e.g., epidural hematoma), the symptoms of diencephalic compression pass so rapidly into those of a tentorial herniation that they are easily missed. Nevertheless, the appearance of diencephalic symptoms should always alert the physician to the imminence of a tentorial pressure cone and to the need for immediate intervention in cases in which the underlying disease is treatable.

Clinical Features. In the following account, abnormalities in the electroencephalogram and caloric responses will be referred to, but it must be emphasized that the appearance of a tentorial pressure cone often signifies a surgical emergency which demands immediate treatment and which cannot wait upon the results of special investigation. For this reason, the diagnostician must rely primarily on the results of careful bedside examination.

Diencephalic Compression. If the patient has been conscious, he becomes torpid, confused, and eventually comatose. Breathing is normal at first, but soon Cheyne-Stokes respiration sets in. This type of periodic breathing is often but incorrectly attributed to medullary distress. The pupils tend to be small but react to light. Conjugate doll's-eye movements are more easily elicited than usual because of weakened cortical control. Caloric stimulation with cold water produces tonic deviation of both eyes towards the stimulated side, with reduction or absence of the fast cortical component. Paratonic resistance to passive movement (*Gegenhalten*) appears in the neck and in limbs not already paralyzed by the primary lesion, and decorticate posture is present bilaterally: The legs are extended and the upper limbs are flexed at the elbows, wrist, and fingers. If this posture is not apparent on the nonparalyzed side, it can often be brought out by noxious stimuli, such as muscle pinching, pressure on the supraorbital nerve, or suction of mucous from the throat. The EEG which originally disclosed unilateral slow activity or unilateral positive spikes, now shows bilateral synchronous slow waves.

Midbrain Compression. This results from uncal or hippocampal herniation on the side of the primary lesion. If the patient is conscious, headache becomes severe. The neck is usually stiff. When nuchal rigidity is present, forceful attempts at flexion of the neck can cause dilatation of both pupils, followed by sudden death if a medullary pressure cone is also present. Dilatation and fixity of the pupil on the side of the lesion is an important early sign of uncal herniation; ptosis and complete oculomotor palsy follow on one or both sides. Breathing is rapid, regular and stertorous. Pyramidal signs may appear on the side of the lesion because the opposite crus is pushed against the edge of the tentorium. The plantar responses are extensor. Decerebrate rigidity develops, with the jaws clenched, the arms extended and pronated, and the legs extended. In the early stages of brainstem compression, decerebrate posture may be present only in response to noxious stimuli. Doll's-head eye movements are disconjugate when oculomotor paralysis is present, and eventually they are difficult to elicit at all because of pressure on the vestibular-oculomotor pathways in the pons

and midbrain. The temperature rises and may swing widely, and sweating is profuse. The blood pressure is usually elevated. Stimulation of the ear by cold water causes tonic deviation of the ipsilateral eye to the stimulated side, but the opposite eye will fail to move medially if the third nerve is paralyzed as is usually the case. The EEG continues to show bilateral synchronous slow waves, and sleep-spindles and K complexes may be present. One or more hemorrhages may occur in the brainstem, in the pons especially, and if this happens, the temperature rises still further, the limbs become flaccid, and death ensues.

Medullary Compression. Medullary compression in the foramen magnum is a terminal event when it occurs as a result of a supratentorial mass. Breathing becomes shallow and irregular; this is appropriately referred to as ataxic respiration, the word *ataxia* meaning "without order." The pulse is irregular and weak and ultimately respiration ceases abruptly, often with a terminal gasp.

A medullary compression cone can occur as a result of an infratentorial mass, without tentorial impaction, and in this event the patient may be conscious. It is preceded by symptoms due to the local disease, to which may be added tinnitus, impairment of hearing, and dysphagia from traction on the vagus nerves. As coning develops, the neck becomes stiff, and since the cerebrospinal fluid cannot escape from the fourth ventricle, an acute hydrocephalic crisis develops, with headache, fleeting dimness of vision, and coma of rapid onset. Respiration is shallow and irregular and ceases abruptly at the end.

Lumbar Puncture. Spinal tap is dangerous in the presence of raised intracranial pressure *from a mass lesion*. If a cone is present, even the slight venting produced by spinal manometry can cause a fatal downward shift of the medulla. Moreover, coning may occur a day or two after spinal fluid has been removed because of continued seepage of fluid through the hole made by the needle.

Clinical Features of Raised Intracranial Pressure

Headache, vomiting, and papilledema, usually described as the classical triad of raised intracranial pressure, are found together in only about 50 per cent of all cases, and even then usually in the late stages.

Headache. Headache is due to tension on pain-sensitive structures, including the dura, large venous sinuses, basal arteries, and the cranial nerves which convey common sensation—the fifth, ninth, and tenth. Headache does not necessarily result from a generalized increase of intracranial pressure, a situation well illustrated by benign intracranial hypertension, in which pain is sometimes absent despite gross papilledema and a high pressure.

The headache of intracranial tumor is usually dull and intermittent. It is aggravated by factors which increase intracranial pressure, such as stooping, coughing, and straining, and is often most severe on waking. Headache may be generalized or localized, but its position is not a reliable guide to the site of the tumor. Occipitonuchal pain usually indicates a posterior fossa lesion, but a frontal or temporal tumor may cause occipital headache by inducing a tentorial pressure cone. Expansion of the pituitary fossa causes bitemporal pain which is not usually affected by changes of position. Pressure on the trigeminal nerve can give rise to facial pain on the affected side.

Papilledema. Papilledema is caused by obstruction to the venous return from the retina via the central retinal vein and the ophthalmic veins, which drain into the cavernous sinus. Raised intracranial pressure from any cause is transmitted to the optic nerve via the extension of the subarachnoid space which invests it, and this leads to compression of the central retinal vein, which lies within the distal part of the nerve. Papilledema can also occur from a mass in the orbit, from thrombosis of the cavernous sinus, and

from the raised intracavernous pressure which results from a caroticocavernous fistula. It occurs in malignant hypertension when the intracranial pressure is raised by cerebral edema, but coexistent hypertensive retinopathy can confuse the retinal picture. Unilateral papilledema can occur in the absence of raised intracranial pressure if the intraocular pressure in the affected eye is low.

In intracranial tumors, papilledema may appear early or late, depending on the rate at which the pressure rises and the height which it attains. If often appears in one eye before the other, but this has no lateralizing value. Rarely, when a tumor compresses one optic nerve and simultaneously raises intracranial pressure, optic atrophy appears on the side of the tumor and papilledema in the opposite eye (the Foster-Kennedy syndrome).

The earliest symptom of papilledema is amaurosis fugax—transient attacks of blurred vision in one or both eyes, often precipitated by stooping or coughing, and commonly described by the patient as a "blackout." At this stage, there is distention of retinal veins, reddening of the disc, blurring of its margins, and filling of the physiological pit by exudate. Examination of the tangent screen may reveal enlargement of the blind spot. Later, the surrounding retina becomes red and swollen, and fine, striated hemorrhages radiate from the disc; hemorrhages also occur in the macular region, and in severe cases, a macular "fan" can be seen. Macular hemorrhages may impair central vision. If the condition is unresolved, secondary atrophy of the optic nerve follows; edema and hemorrhages are absorbed, and the discs become grayish-white, with ill-defined margins; this is due to gliosis of the nerve head. The onset of visible atrophy is preceded by impairment of the peripheral fields of vision, which usually starts in the lower nasal quadrants and spreads thence to the rest of the nasal field and to the temporal fields. At first, the field for small objects is preserved (except in the presence of macular hemorrhage), but eventually it is encroached upon.[46] Once this process has started, it can develop rapidly over a period of hours or days, and since the patient is usually unaware of impairment of the peripheral fields, the true state of affairs will be missed unless perimetry is carried out. Consecutive atrophy is usually irreversible, even if the intracranial pressure is reduced, so the advantage of early perimetry is obvious. This train of events can occur with increased intracranial pressure from any cause, and it is particularly tragic when visual loss is allowed to occur as the result of benign intracranial hypertension or other remediable or self-limited conditions.

Vomiting. Vomiting is commonly due to irritation of the medulla, either by the tumor itself, or as a result of increased intracranial pressure. In some instances, the vomiting is not preceded by nausea and is forceful. Such projectile vomiting is most common in children, but it is necessary to remember that cerebral vomiting is not always projectile, nor is projectile vomiting always due to cerebral disease.

Seizures. These occur in about 30 per cent of all cases, but it is often difficult to tell whether they are due to the tumor or to the rise of intracranial pressure. Persistent focal seizures of a uniform pattern indicate a focal lesion, although not necessarily a tumor. Both generalized and localized seizures are most common in supratentorial lesions. Tonic spasms ("cerebellar seizures") which sometimes occur in the presence of posterior fossa tumors and tentorial pressure cones are not true convulsions but represent brief attacks of decerebrate rigidity caused by pressure upon the brainstem; they are frequently accompanied by cyanosis and rapid stertorous respiration, and the patient is usually unconscious.

Intellectual functions often show impairment when the pressure is high, but it may be impossible to distinguish between the effects of the pressure per se and those of a supratentorial tumor. There is sluggishness of thought, forgetfulness, difficulty in abstract thought, and slowness of perception. The patient may appear dazed or sleepy. If the pressure continues to rise, lethargy gives place to stupor and coma as a result of pressure on the ascending reticular formation.

Pulse and blood pressure are significantly affected only when there has been a steep and sudden rise of intracranial pressure. Bradycardia with ectopic beats, slowing of respiration, and slight elevation of blood pressure are common. Cheyne-Stokes respiration occurs when the diencephalon is compromised, but in elderly persons it may also occur during natural sleep.

Treatment. Surgical measures for the relief of raised intracranial pressure are ordinarily carried out by a neurosurgeon, but there are occasions when the physician is called upon to keep the patient alive until surgical assistance is available. The first thing to do is to ensure a proper airway; coughing, choking, and an obstructed airway cause a rapid elevation of intracranial pressure. The provision of a free airway and oxygen, with or without assisted respiration, will often bring about an immediate amelioration of symptoms. Second, corticosteroids should be given intravenously or by intramuscular injection. Third, intravenous Mannitol can provide immediate respite, but the effect of this treatment is short-lived, and it may be followed by increase of cerebral edema within three or four hours. If it is used in an unconscious patient, a catheter should be inserted into the bladder to cater for the extreme diuresis which is induced by Mannitol. If epidural, subdural, or intracerebral hemorrhage is suspected as the cause of raised intracranial pressure, Mannitol and other agents of this type are contraindicated because shrinkage of the brain is liable to increase the bleeding.

False Localizing Signs

The early symptoms and signs of an intracranial tumor are of greater localizing value than are those which develop late in the disease, because as the mass increases in size, it is apt to produce false localizing signs by displacing other parts of the brain.[34] Second, a small tumor can give rise to false localizing signs, not because of its own bulk, but because it produces internal hydrocephalus, the dilated lateral and third ventricles then acting as expanding "tumors."

Mental dulling is often present when intracranial pressure is elevated, but it is doubtful whether the pressure per se is responsible (except when it is sufficiently high to impede blood flow) because mental activity is normal in pseudotumor cerebri despite a considerable degree of intracranial hypertension. On the other hand, mental symptoms can occur in both supra- and infratentorial tumors when the pressure is normal, and they are particularly common in deep midline tumors involving the limbic system.[27, 63]

Anosmia can result from a rise of intracranial pressure from any cause. Vision is sometimes disturbed by papilledema; in addition, bitemporal hemianopia can result from pressure on the chiasm by a distended third ventricle in the presence of a posterior fossa tumor. Homonymous hemianopia can be caused by a tentorial pressure cone which compresses the posterior cerebral artery against the edge of the tentorium.

The most common false localizing sign is weakness or paralysis of the abducens nerve as a result of downward displacement of the brainstem. A partial third nerve palsy, unilateral or bilateral, can be caused by a tentorial pressure cone. The trochlear nerve is seldom involved. Pain and tingling on one side of the face is occasionally encountered in supratentorial tumors, probably from displacement of the brainstem. Mild facial paresis of lower motor neuron type is sometimes seen as a false localizing sign but *marked* facial weakness of peripheral type usually has true localizing value. Tinnitus may occur in both supra- and infratentorial tumors and slight bilateral high tone deafness is not uncommon in the presence of raised intracranial pressure.

A mass in one hemisphere can push the midbrain against the opposite edge of the tentorium and so give rise to an ipsilateral hemiparesis involving the face, arm, and leg, even when the tumor itself does not involve the motor pathways. A foraminal pressure cone can depress vibration and postural sensibility on both sides of the body.

The occurrence of a cerebellar type of ataxia in frontal lobe tumors has received much attention in the literature.[26, 65] This is discussed on page 410.

Internal hydrocephalus from a posterior fossa tumor can depress hypothalamic-pituitary functions and so give rise to diabetes insipidus, obesity, and (in children) failure to grow. Pituitary infarction can occur in large supratentorial tumors.

THE GLIOMAS

Gliomas account for about 50 per cent of all primary intracranial tumors. They stem from cells derived from the primitive neuroectoderm and are glial in origin. Modern classification started with Bailey and Cushing (1926), who divided the gliomas into 14 main groups in terms of the morphological stages through which the cells pass in their ontogenetic development.[6] Alternative classifications have been introduced by Cox (1933), Scherer (1935),[83] and Zülch (1956).[102] In what Russell[81] has called a "radical bid for simplicity," Kernohan and his associates[54] reduced the gliomas to five types, four of which they graded in terms of malignancy (Table 16–1). They are: astrocytomas (Grades I to IV), ependymomas (Grades I to IV), oligodendrogliomas (Grades I to IV), neuroastrocytomas (Grades I to IV), and medulloblastomas. A disadvantage in using grading systems is that sections taken from different portions of the same tumor may show varying degrees of differentiation and regression, and the histological permutations which can arise from this situation often cause difficulties in the identification of a tumor on the basis of biopsy material alone.

Table 16–1.   *Classification of the Gliomas*

Old Terminology	Kernohan et al. (1952)
Astrocytoma	Astrocytoma, Grade I
Astroblastoma	Astrocytoma, Grade II
Glioblastoma multiforme	Astrocytoma, Grades III and IV
Polar spongioblastoma	Astrocytoma
Ependymoma	Ependymoma, Grade I
Ependymoblastoma	Ependymoma, Grades II, III, and IV
Medulloepithelioma	Ependymoma, Grade IV
Oligodendroglioma	Oligodendroglioma, Grade I
Oligodendroblastoma	Oligodendroglioma, Grades II, III, and IV
Neurocytoma	Neuroastrocytoma, Grade I
Ganglioneuroma	Neuroastrocytoma, Grade I
Gangliocytoma	Neuroastrocytoma, Grade I
Ganglioglioma	Neuroastrocytoma, Grade I
Neuroblastoma	Neuroastrocytoma, Grades II, III, and IV
Spongioneuroblastoma	Neuroastrocytoma, Grades II, III, and IV
Glioblastoma	Neuroastrocytoma, Grades II, III, and IV
Medulloblastoma	Medulloblastoma

Many pathologists feel that the Kernohan classification is oversimplified. The European literature tends to follow the classification of Zülch (1965), while the Anglo-Saxon literature draws heavily on those of Zimmerman and Netsky (1956),[101] and Russell and her associates (1959).[81]

Since 1950, the nomenclature committee of the Union International Contre le Cancer (UICC) has been attempting to synthesize these classifications into an internationally acceptable form. The most recent attempt, together with commonly used synonyms, is tabulated in the second American edition of Zülch's book.

Pathology. The pathology and behavior of individual gliomas will be considered under separate headings below. Most of these tumors are locally invasive. Some of the more malignant ones appear on naked eye examination to be encapsulated, but the zone of apparent demarcation represents an area of compression of adjacent brain, and there may be infiltration beyond this. Normal brain may be found between areas of infiltration and the tumor can spread to the opposite hemisphere via the corpus callosum or basal structures. Only on the rarest occasions do gliomas metastasize outside the nervous system. On the other hand, they frequently invade the leptomeninges, from which they may enter the brain to form other deposits; the tumor cells may also be carried by the cerebrospinal fluid to the ependyma of the ventricles and to the surface of the spinal cord and cauda equina. This seeding process can give rise to neurological symptoms, notably root pains, paresthesias, and sensory impairment of radicular distribution. Rarely, compression of the spinal cord is produced in this way.

Astrocytoma (Grade I).   This type of astrocytoma accounts for more than one-third of all gliomas. It can occur anywhere in the brain and spinal cord and is usually deeply placed. It consists of either fibrillary or protoplasmic astrocytes; the latter is the more rapidly growing of the two. The center of the tumor may show cystic degeneration. Another type of cyst, which is found in the cerebellum of children, appears as a cavity in the brain with a small astrocytic tumor in its wall. Astrocytomas usually grow slowly, and localizing symptoms

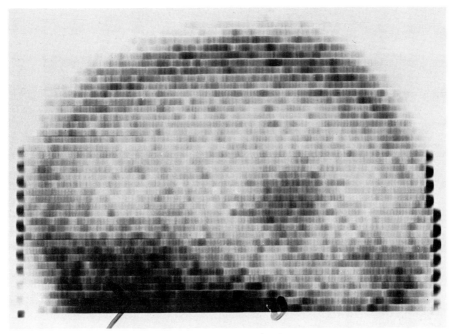

Figure 16–7. Brain scan of an astrocytoma.

may be vague; in many cases, it is the symptoms of increased intracranial pressure which induce the patient to seek medical advice.

Astroblastoma (Astrocytoma, Grade II). These tumors are rare, and are more malignant than those of Grade 1. The cells are well endowed with cytoplasm and contain two or three nuclei. They attach themselves to blood vessels by foot processes. Cystic degeneration may be present within the tumor. The astroblastoma is usually found in young adults, and occasionally in children.

Glioblastoma Multiforme (Astrocytoma, Grades III and IV). This tumor occurs in middle life and is practically always confined to the cerebral hemispheres. It appears as a soft reddish or yellowish mass, which often contains hemorrhagic cysts (Fig. 16–8). Microscopic examination shows a mixture of primitive spongioblasts, astroblasts, and astrocytes; mitotic figures are prominent. The tumor is well endowed with blood vessels, which can be demonstrated by angiography (Fig. 16–9). Glioblastomas grow rapidly, and the presenting signs may be those of raised intracranial pressure without localizing features. Alternatively, focal symptoms may develop so rapidly that a stroke may be suspected. Untreated, the clinical course seldom exceeds a few months. The treatment of choice is removal of as much of the tumor as possible, combined with deep therapy, intracavitary irradiation, or intracavitary chemotherapy. In general, the younger the patient, the better the prognosis following treatment.

Polar Spongioblastoma. This term is still used for astrocytomas composed of intersecting bundles of narrow, elongated cells arranged in parallel rows which are separated by a fine vascular stroma. Most pathologists reject the idea of a tumor derived from spongioblasts and argue that this tumor is an astrocytoma and that the shape and arrangement of the cells has been imposed by their environment. This type is most commonly found in the optic nerve, chiasm, hypothalamus, pons, or cerebellum. The degree of malignancy varies; it may be relatively benign, especially in children.

Medulloblastoma. This highly malignant growth usually occurs in children. It grows from the midline of the cere-

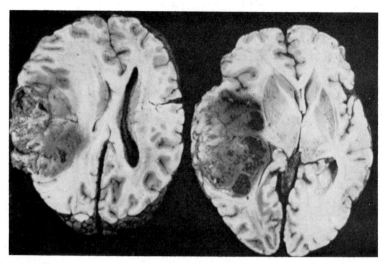

Figure 16–8. Rapidly growing glioblastoma. (From Wechsler, I.: *Clinical Neurology,* 9th Ed. W. B. Saunders Co., Philadelphia, 1963.)

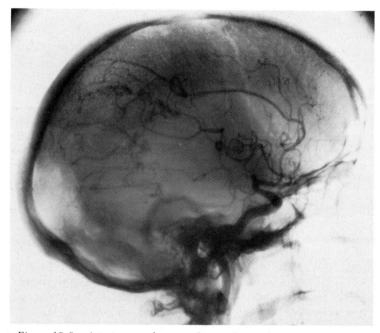

Figure 16–9. Arteriogram showing abnormal vessels in a glioblastoma.

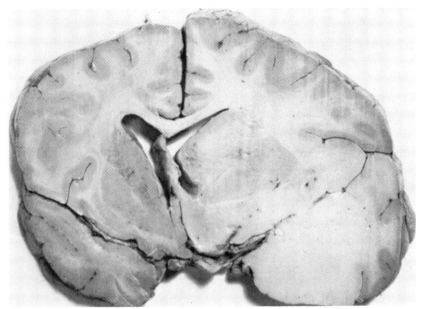

Figure 16–10. Diffuse fibrillary astrocytoma of right cerebrum. (From Russell, D. S., and Rubenstein, L. J.: *Pathology of Tumors of the Nervous System.* London, Edward Arnold, 1959.)

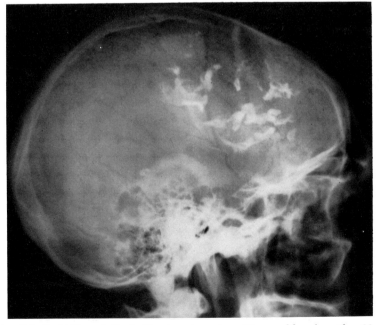

Figure 16–11. Calcified bifrontal Grade II astrocytoma in a 60-year-old male with a 23-year history of seizures. (Courtesy of Dr. James Bull.)

bellum, fills the fourth ventricle, and then invades the brainstem. It also infiltrates the leptomeninges, from which seeding can occur to remote areas of the brain and spinal cord. It is a very cellular tumor; the cytoplasm is scanty and mitoses are abundant. The clinical features are those of a tumor of the fourth ventricle: vomiting, headaches, papilledema, nystagmus, and ataxic gait. In young children, the sutures may spread under the influence of increasing intracranial pressure. Late in the disease, additional symptoms may arise from seeding to the spinal cord or cauda equina. Complete surgical extirpation is impossible, but these tumors are moderately susceptible to x-ray therapy. The whole of the nervous system has to be irradiated because the tumor spreads so widely. For this reason, it is desirable to confirm the diagnosis by biopsy. This is an exception to the general rule that biopsy should never be carried out on a brainstem tumor because it so often precipitates a worsening of the patient's condition. With radiation, survival for as long as five years has been reported, but it is usually considerably less.

Tumors classified as medulloblastomas are sometimes found in the cerebral hemispheres of adults, but there is some doubt as to their true nature. The prognosis in this group is better than in the classical cerebellar variety; five-year survival is not uncommon.

Ependymomas. These tumors account for about 4 per cent of all gliomas. They arise from the ependymal epithelium and are therefore found in the ventricles, especially the fourth ventricle, and in the central canal of the spinal cord. The tumor is usually separate from brain tissue and may be encapsulated. The degree of malignancy varies from a very benign type composed of adult ependymal cells to a relatively malignant form composed of primitive ependymoblasts. Microscopy discloses a cellular growth composed of columnar and polygonal cells with rounded nuclei and a rather granular cytoplasm. The ependymal cilia disappear except in cells on the ventricular surface. Calcification is

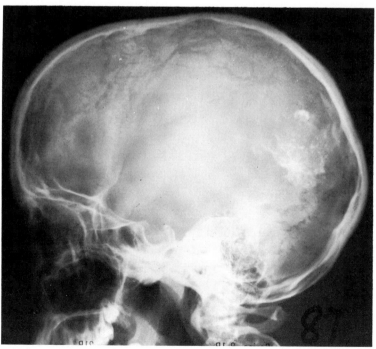

Figure 16–12. Calcified oligodendroglioma. (Courtesy of Dr. R. H. Chamberlain.)

occasionally present. Ependymomas occur predominantly in children and young adults. The symptoms and signs are those of a ventricular or spinal tumor. The treatment of choice is surgical extirpation followed by irradiation, but the rate of recurrence is high.

Oligodendrogliomas. The oligodendroglioma is usually found in the cerebral hemisphere of middle-aged adults.[5] It comprises about 5 per cent of all the gliomas and appears as a firm, pinkish tumor which is not demarcated from the surrounding brain and which is often calcified in its peripheral parts (Fig. 16-12). Such calcification, however, does not necessarily imply that the lesion is wholly benign. Its cells are large and rounded, with a well-formed membrane and relatively clear cytoplasm. Mitoses are rare. Seeding sometimes occurs along the cerebrospinal pathways. Although these tumors are usually benign, their size, deep situation, and invasive characteristics make total removal impossible in most instances. Partial removal sometimes results in an extension of useful survival for several years, but in other cases, surgical intervention seems to accelerate the growth, and this factor has to be taken into account in deciding whether surgery is indicated or not.

GANGLIONEUROMA AND GANGLIOGLIOMA

Tumors are sometimes encountered which contain both mature ganglion cells and glial elements. In some, the ganglion cells are the most conspicuous element, the glial cells being scanty and showing little or no evidence of proliferation. In others, the tumor looks like a glioma but contains ganglionic elements. These tumors usually occur in children and young adults and are most common in the floor of the third ventricle but can also be found in the frontal lobes, the basal ganglia, and the spinal cord. Occasionally, the tumor exhibits malignant changes, notably in the cells of glial

origin. They are variously referred to as neuroblastomas, spongioneuroblastomas, glioneuroblastomas, etc., and are classified by Kernohan as neuroastrocytomas, Grades 2 to 4. Complete surgical removal is impossible and they are but moderately sensitive to radiation therapy.

TUMORS OF THE MENINGES

The meningiomas are by far the most prominent tumor of this group, but the dura may also be invaded by carcinomatous or sarcomatous metastases, while the leptomeninges may be invaded by seedings from intracerebral gliomas and by diffuse metastatic deposits from extracranial growths, such as carcinomas, sarcomas, melanomas, lymphomas, and the leukemias.

Meningiomas. Meningiomas account for about 15 per cent of all primary intracranial tumors, occur mainly in middle life, are more common in women than in men, and are usually supratentorial in location. They can also arise from the spinal dura, especially in middle-aged women.

Pathology. Meningiomas arise from the arachnoid villi and are therefore attached to the dura; an exception is the rare meningioma of the lateral ventricle, which originates in the tela choroidea. They usually compress the underlying structures, without invading them, but sometimes they penetrate the dura to invade the bones of the skull, and they may perforate the falx or the tentorium cerebelli and enlarge on both sides of the septum, giving rise to a dumbbell tumor.

The histological diversity of the meningiomas may be judged from the fact that Cushing and Eisenhardt divided them into nine types, with 20 subvarieties. But, in general, there is so little correlation between histological type and biological behavior that Courville's simpler classification is preferable. He divided the meningiomas into five types: (1) syncytial, arising mainly from endothelial cells, (2) transitional, (3) fibrous, mainly from fibrous tissue elements,

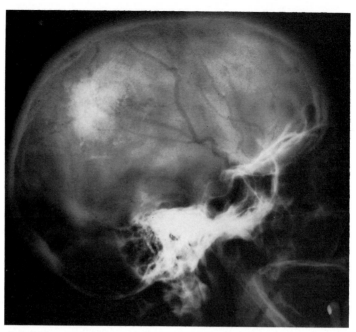

Figure 16–13. Calcified parasagittal meningioma in a 45-year-old woman, showing prominence of the left middle meningeal artery. The foramen spinosum was enlarged. There was a history of slight right-sided jacksonian attacks for 7 years. (Courtesy of Dr. James Bull.)

(4) angioblastic, resembling the capillary angioblastomas, and (5) malignant forms, i.e., sarcomas.

The syncytial type is characterized by poorly defined polygonal cells with large nuclei which are arranged in sheets intersected by vascularized trabeculae. In the transitional type, the cells are arranged in whorls which are separated by spindle-shaped cells; the whorls often contain psammoma bodies—concentric layers of calcium salts deposited in degenerated cells (Fig. 16–13). The fibrous type is composed of interlacing bundles of elongated spindle cells containing fibroglial fibrils; reticulin and collagen fibers are present between the individual cells, and whorls are less conspicuous than in the transitional type. The angioblastic variety is a highly cellular tumor containing many blood spaces lined with capillary endothelium; reticulin fibrils are present between the cells. The malignant meningiomas are characterized by the presence of mitoses, rapid growth, and the capacity to infiltrate surrounding brain and bone.

A circumstance which can give rise to medicolegal embarrassment is the fact that Cushing and Eisenhardt obtained a history of trauma in nearly one-third of their cases, and in some there was a striking correlation between the site of the tumor and the site of the original injury, but since both injuries and neoplasms are common, coincidences are to be expected. In most intracranial meningiomas, there is no history of head injury. Zülch has reviewed some of the literature bearing upon this subject.[102]

Clinical Features. In general, meningiomas grow very slowly and it is not uncommon for symptoms to have been present for several years before the patient is admitted to hospital for treatment. A second feature is their predilection for certain anatomical sites within the brain and spinal cord. Less than 10 per cent of all intracranial meningiomas occur in the posterior fossa; of the remainder, about one-half are situated over the convexity of the hemisphere and one-half at the base. Common situations are parasagittal, frontal, parietal, the floor of the anterior fossa, the sphenoidal ridge, the petrosal ridge, and the suprasellar region. Less commonly, they are found in the cerebellopontine angle, over the convexity of the cerebellum, on either side of the tentorium cerebelli, anterior to the brainstem,[14] at the foramen magnum, or in one of the lateral ventricles.[35]

The presenting features may be focal or generalized seizures, symptoms of raised intracranial pressure, or slowly progressive focal neurological deficit related to the site of the tumor. Occasionally, they present as a visible swelling of the overlying skull in the absence of neurological symptoms and signs. The skull adjacent to the dural attachment of meningiomas may be normal, eroded, or exceptionally dense; local diploic channels are often enlarged.

Parasagittal Meningiomas. The majority of meningiomas are situated in the parasagittal region at the edge of the sagittal sinus (Fig. 16–13). Most of them occur between the coronal suture and the posterior parietal area of the brain, the anterior frontal and occipital regions being relatively immune. The tumor may grow down the side of the falx, or it may spread over the surface of the hemisphere. Many are close to the upper part

of the motor cortex, and this is fortunate because they are apt to betray their presence at an early stage by focal seizures and progressive motor or sensory signs affecting the foot and leg. If the tumor spreads forward between the frontal lobes, grasping and groping reflexes may be encountered. If the tumor is large, mental symptoms may be present. Aphasia, and hemiparesis involving the upper limb as well as the leg, perhaps resulting from interference with the supplementary motor area on the medial side of the hemisphere, may confuse the issue. Bone rarefaction and increased vascular markings are commonly seen in parasagittal meningiomas. In a few cases, the sagittal sinus is invaded and obstructed. These are vascular tumors and removal may be difficult but the results are often excellent, and even when the sagittal sinus has to be resected to prevent recurrence, this does little harm because a compensatory venous circulation has already developed by the time the patient comes to surgery.

Convexity Meningiomas. These are less common than the parasagittal variety, and hyperostosis of the overlying bone is less common. Most of them are situated in the central area along the

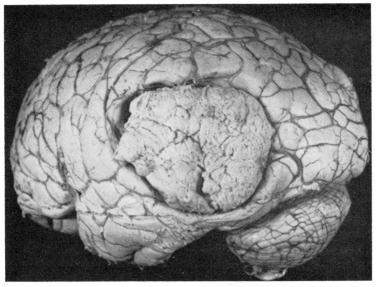

Figure 16–14.   Meningioma. (From Wechsler, I.: *Clinical Neurology.* 9th Ed. W. B. Saunders Co., Philadelphia 1963.)

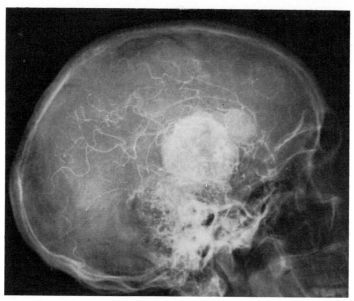

Figure 16–15.   This meningioma, displayed by arteriography, caused a parkinsonian tremor of the right hand for 19 years. Intracranial pressure was normal. Plain x-rays were negative. Slight aphasia was present for a few days following successful removal of the tumor.

coronal suture (Fig. 16–14) or in the mid-parietal region, and they are difficult to distinguish on clinical grounds from gliomas in the same regions; bone changes are helpful in diagnosis and the angiographic appearances are usually characteristic (Fig. 16–15).

Olfactory Groove. These are not uncommon. They are often bilateral and they may grow to a great size before their presence is recognized. They give rise to frontal lobe symptoms and the only signs that suggest their extracerebral situation may be anosmia on one or both sides. The diagnosis has to be confirmed by contrast studies.

Suprasellar Region. These tumors, which arise from the tuberculum sella, are not uncommon. Growing upward, they come to involve the optic nerves and chiasm, and they may compress the third ventricle and produce obstructive hydrocephalus and hypothalamic disturbances. Hyperostosis of the tuberculum sellae is often present. Meningiomas in this situation usually occur in older individuals than is the case with craniopharyngiomas, but the latter occasionally produce symptoms for the first time in late adult life.[82]

Sphenoid Ridge. These occur in two forms. Most of them are rounded tumors which grow from the dura along the ridge, the major mass of the neoplasm being in the anterior fossa. When situated on the inner third of the ridge, they may involve the optic nerve and chiasm and often invade the orbit, producing proptosis and ocular motor paresis. They may also involve the undersurface of the frontal lobe and the tip of the temporal lobe. Those arising from the middle third of the ridge tend to be silent in their development and usually present as cases of raised intracranial pressure with little in the way of localizing signs, but upward pressure on the striatal region may cause extrapyramidal signs. Those on the outer third of the ridge may also grow to a large size without producing gross lateralizing signs, and when signs do appear they usually consist of contralateral weakness of the face and tongue, followed by weakness of the upper limb. As these tumors are situated in the sylvian fissure, an important pathway for cerebrospinal fluid to the convexity of the brain, they cause an increase of intracranial pressure at an early stage.

The second type of sphenoid ridge

meningioma takes the form of a thin growth (meningioma en plaque) which does not raise intracranial pressure or compress the brain but gives rise to sclerosis and enlargement of the sphenoid bone.[11] The lesser wing and orbital roof are chiefly affected and the process may spread to the greater wing. The symptoms and signs are related to the overgrowth of bone and include proptosis, mechanical disturbance of ocular movements, optic atrophy, sclerosis of the optic canal, and a palpable tumor at the pterion. Occasionally, the sclerotic process affects the optic canal only, and rarely, the hyperostosis is associated with a large intradural mass.

Petrosal Meningioma. This tumor lies under the temporal lobe, along the superior petrosal sinus. Most of them are located near the medial end of the ridge and involve the fifth and sixth nerves. They tend to displace the brainstem, pushing it against the contralateral edge of the tentorium, thus producing spastic hemiplegia on the same side as the tumor. Occasionally, these tumors grow from the posterior part of Meckel's cave and, after involving the trigeminal nerve, they expand backwards into the posterior fossa in much the same way as neurofibroma of the trigeminal nerve.

Tentorial Meningioma. Occasionally a meningioma arising on the upper surface of the tentorium will penetrate this structure and invade the posterior fossa. The combination of supratentorial and posterior fossa symptoms and signs will suggest the diagnosis.

Posterior Fossa Meningiomas. These are not uncommon. They can occur in the cerebellopontine angle, over the cerebellar convexity, and anterior to the brainstem along the clivus of the sphenoid.[14] As noted above, the posterior fossa may also be invaded by a tumor originating from the dura over the posterior part of Meckel's cave, or from the upper surface of the tentorium. Meningiomas arising in the region of the foramen magnum are described in the section on spinal tumors.

Meningiomas in the lateral recess are perhaps the most common and are difficult to distinguish from acoustic nerve tumors because impairment of eighth nerve function is the first symptom in many cases, but in general, cranial nerve paralysis is less severe, the characteristic enlargement of the internal auditory meatus is absent, cerebellar dysfunction is more marked, and the protein content of the cerebrospinal fluid is less. *Classical tic douloureux may be the only symptom of such a tumor.*

When the tumor is situated over the cerebellar convexity, the symptoms and signs are those of an intrinsic cerebellar tumor, but an increase of diploic vascularity may be seen on x-rays. A clivus meningioma[14] produces a brainstem syndrome from compression of the midbrain and pons, together with symptoms and signs of raised intracranial pressure; it may spread downwards to the foramen magnum and produce additional symptoms from compression of the medulla and upper cervical cord. Meningiomas arising from the tentorium may spread upwards and downwards, involving the undersurface of the temporal and occipital lobes as well as the cerebellum. Homonymous field defects are an early sign of a meningioma starting in the region of the torcular.

Other Sites of Meningiomas. These tumors can also occur in other situations, including the lateral ventricle, the lateral edge of the velum interpositum, and deep in the sylvian fissure. Multiple meningiomas have been encountered, usually associated with generalized neurofibromatosis.

Laboratory Aids. Spinal tap may or may not disclose a rise in intracranial pressure. The protein content may be normal or slightly raised; high figures are rare and a high protein level in the presence of a cerebellopontine angle tumor usually indicates a neurinoma and not a meningioma. Plain x-rays will sometimes show hyperostosis or erosion of bone in the neighborhood of the tumor. Isotope scanning is useful, but angiography is necessary to show the situation and size of the tumor and will also determine its feeding vessels, so that surgery can be planned so as to secure these at an early stage. Most meningiomas acquire their main blood supply from the external carotid artery, and it is therefore desirable to include this vessel in the arteriographic study when a meningioma is suspected on clinical grounds or is suggested by the results of internal carotid angiography. The blood supply of the rare intraventricular meningioma comes from the posterior cerebral artery, and the posterior circulation has to be visualized in these cases, but they can also be identified by air studies and brain scan.

Treatment. Meningiomas are not sensitive to radiation, and are treated by surgical removal whenever possible. They tend to recur if tumor cells are left behind, but because of their slow growth, the patient often enjoys years of good health.

EXTRADURAL TUMORS

A number of tumors arising in tissues external to the dura may come to invade or compress the brain. Most of these are bone tumors, either primary or metastatic, in which neural involvement is of secondary importance. Chondrosarcoma of the skull base may extend both internally and externally, as may nasopharyngeal carcinoma. Both of these may be impossible to distinguish from chordoma on neurological grounds, but other physical signs and radiological evidence help to distinguish them.

Primary sarcoma of the skull is rare, and in most instances it occurs in cases of Paget's disease of bone. Diploic epidermoids seldom compress the brain, since they tend to decompress themselves by eroding the outer table of the skull. Metastatic carcinoma is a common cause of tumors of the skull, but cerebral involvement is usually due to other metastases in the meninges or brain substance. Osteolytic lesion in the skull may also be caused by multiple myelomata and by the xanthomata of lipoid disease.

Acoustic Neurinoma (Neurofibroma, Perineural Fibroblastoma, Schwannoma)

Pathology. Acoustic neurinomas account for about 5 per cent of all primary intracranial tumors. The tumor usually arises just within the internal auditory meatus, which it usually expands before filling the cerebellopontine recess. The seventh and eighth nerves are either buried within it or stretched over it, and it may spread up to the fifth nerve or down to involve the lower cranial nerves. In time, the tumor will compress the pons and cerebellum. It is supplied by the anterior inferior cerebellar, internal auditory, and pontine arteries; severance of pontine vessels during surgical removal can cause fatal pontine infarction. Acoustic neurinomas are sometimes bilateral.

The tumor is composed of dense interlacing fibrous bands, separated by loose reticulin fibrils. The cells are elongated, with oval nuclei arranged in rows, like a palisade. The degree of vascularity varies widely, and areas of necrosis may be present.

Clinical Features. The tumor grows slowly and may attain a considerable size before the correct diagnosis is suspected, which is usually within three years of the onset of symptoms but may be considerably longer.[74]

The first symptom is progressive unilateral nerve deafness. Tinnitus is common, and episodes of vertigo occur in some cases from involvement of the vestibular component of the eighth nerve.[28, 36] This triad—nerve deafness, tinnitus, and vertigo—is easily mistaken for Meniere's disease. The patient may complain of discomfort behind the ear long before intracranial pressure is raised. Slight facial weakness is common, but it may amount to little more than slowness of movement in the eyelids and the angle of the mouth on the affected side, and the corneal reflex may be sluggish because of this. Later on, the reflex is lost if the tumor involves the sensory root of the trigeminal nerve, and paresthesias and sensory impairment in the face may be present. By the time the tumor has reached the fifth root, it is quite large and will have started to compress the lateral lobe of the cerebellum, giving rise to nystagmus, ataxia of the ipsilateral limbs, and a tendency to deviate to the affected side. Ultimately, pressure on the brainstem can induce unilateral or bilateral pyramidal and sensory signs, and by this time internal hydrocephalus is likely to be present, with consequent generalized headache, papilledema, diplopia, and vomiting. Mental symptoms may be present before or after the tumor is removed. Caudal extension of the tumor may implicate the ninth, tenth, and eleventh nerves. Cutaneous neurofibromas are often present, but full-fledged von Recklinghausen's disease is a rare association.

Laboratory Aids. If the patient can hear at all on the affected side, air conduction will be found to be better than bone conduction, absolute bone conduction is reduced, and loudness recruitment is absent or incomplete; in *cochlear* deafness, sounds which can be heard at all appear louder in the deaf ear than in the normal ear, i.e., recruitment is present, whereas in auditory nerve lesions, relative deafness persists however loud the stimulus. Furthermore, whereas in cochlear deafness, the intelligibility of spoken speech does not improve with loudness, it may do so in nerve deafness. Impairment or loss of the caloric labyrinthine responses is the rule in all but the smallest acoustic neurinomas. These signs are important, because careful otologic investigation of all cases of perceptive deafness or vertigo will sometimes disclose an eighth nerve tumor when it is small and easily removable.[28]

X-rays will *sometimes* show enlargement of the internal auditory meatus on the affected side, and fractional pneumoencephalography discloses a filling defect in the cerebellopontine angle in all but the smallest tumors. When the results are equivocal, a positive contrast medium should be used.

The electroencephalogram remains normal until the intracranial pressure is raised, and then the findings are nonspecific.

The spinal fluid protein is usually in the region of 200 to 300 mg. per cent, *but can be within normal limits in the case of a very small tumor.* The pressure may be either normal or raised, depending mainly on the size of the growth at the time the test is done.

Differential Diagnosis. In early cases, the symptoms and signs may suggest Meniere's syndrome, but audiometry will often disclose the absence of recruitment, which constitutes an imperative indication for further investigation. The distinction between cochlear and nerve deafness can also be helped by Bekesy audiometry (p. 113).

Other tumors in the lateral recess may give a very similar picture, especially the hemangioblastoma and epidermoid cysts, but on the whole, cranial nerve palsies are slighter, and hearing loss is less complete. Moreover, the internal auditory meatus is not expanded. A meningioma in the recess may give a similar picture, although deafness is less severe, the protein in the cerebrospinal fluid is lower and may be normal, and bone erosion when present is not confined to the internal meatus. Gliomas may grow into the angle from the cerebellum or brain stem and occasionally a tumor in the pons itself may mimic an eighth nerve tumor, but in these cases the history is usually shorter and the signs are usually bilateral. Arachnoiditis in the lateral recess has been described as producing similar clinical features. The nature of this process is obscure, and the pressure of an arachnoid cyst in this area—or anywhere else for that matter—should not be presumed to explain the symptoms until careful search has confirmed the absence of an underlying disease; such cysts overlying a small acoustic nerve tumor can be mistaken for the primary pathological process.

Treatment. Radiation therapy has little effect. Complete surgical extirpation is desirable but is sometimes impossible. The best results are obtained in very small tumors which can be peeled off the eighth nerve without inducing facial weakness; their recognition depends largely on the otological methods described above. Operative mortality and postoperative morbidity have been reduced in recent years by approaching the tumor through the temporal bone, and by carrying out the removal with the help of a dissecting microscope.

TRIGEMINAL NEURINOMA

This is a rare lesion.[84] Of a total of 95 verified trigeminal neurinomas described in the literature, 10 have occurred in adolescents. The tumor arises from sheath cells of the nerve and may develop either in the gasserian ganglion or on the root of the nerve. Paresthesias and sensory impairment are followed by weakness of the masticatory muscles. Facial pain is not common. The trigeminal symptoms and signs are followed by paresis of the third, fourth, or sixth nerve, and ipsilateral cerebellar signs may occur. Compression of the brainstem may lead to internal hydrocephalus. In the late stages, there is erosion of the floor of the middle fossa and of the petrous apex. Carotid and vertebral arteriograms dis-

close displacement of vessels, with or without a tumor stain. Involvement of the fifth nerve by metastatic tumor or carcinoma of the nasopharynx has to be considered in the differential diagnosis.

Neurinomas occasionally occur on other cranial nerves, notably the third, ninth, tenth, and eleventh. They are extremely rare and the diagnosis is made by consideration of the symptoms and signs and inspection of the growth at operation.

CRANIOPHARYNGIOMA

These tumors arise from the remnants of Rathke's pouch. They accout for 5 per cent of all primary intracranial tumors and about 15 per cent of all cerebral tumors in children. They usually lie above the sella (Figs. 16–16 and 16–17) and consist of a mass of multilocular cysts containing a turbid fluid. Occasionally they are predominantly solid. Histologically, there are 3 main types: cysts lined with columnar epithelium which secretes mucus, a squamous epithelioma with areas of cystic degeneration, and an adamantinoma consisting of epithelial

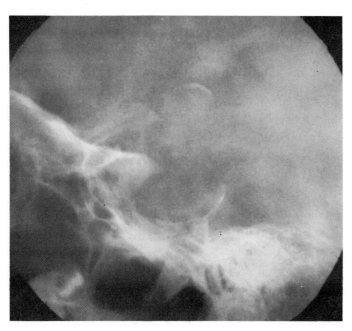

Figure 16–16. Craniopharyngioma in a nine-year-old girl. The sella is grossly enlarged, and there is suprasellar calcification. (Courtesy of Dr. James Bull.)

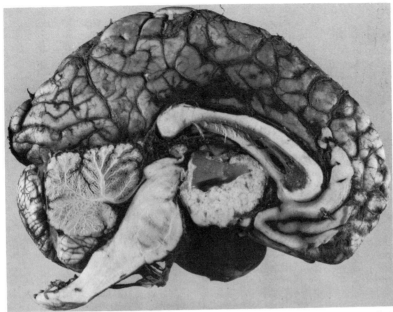

Figure 16–17. Craniopharyngioma. (Courtesy of Ayer Laboratory, Pennsylvania Hospital, Philadelphia.)

cells which form a reticulum resembling the enamel of a developing tooth.[81]

These tumors are congenital in origin and commonly give rise to symptoms in childhood, but they can lie dormant for many years, only to produce symptoms in middle age or advanced age.[82] Sometimes they remain silent throughout life.

Clinical Features. In general, symptoms develop very slowly, but occasionally the onset appears to be rapid or abrupt because of the sudden development of a dramatic symptom, such as headache, visual loss, diabetes insipidus,[23] or (in the elderly) mental disturbances or orthostatic hypotension.[71, 82]

The symptoms and signs may be divided into 4 groups: those due to an expanding mass, those due to hypopituitarism, those caused by involvement of the hypothalamus, and mental disturbances. In children, the presenting symptom may fall under any one of the first three headings, but in adults, visual symptoms usually appear early, endocrine disturbances are inconspicuous, symptoms of raised intracranial pressure appear late or not at all, and mental symptoms are relatively common. Seizures are uncommon at all ages.

Expansion of the tumor gives rise to headache and vomiting; papilledema is rare. Pressure on the optic nerve, chiasm, or optic tract produces appropriate impairment of the visual fields, but unlike what happens in pituitary tumors, the field loss may start in either the upper or lower quadrants, and is apt to fluctuate in degree from time to time. Diplopia is not uncommon. Hemiparesis, a late development, occurred in 18 per cent of Jefferson's series of 57 cases. The clinoid processes are eroded, but the sella is not usually ballooned. Suprasellar calcification has been present in more than 50 per cent of reported cases.

Hypopituitarism is responsible (in children and adolescents) for retardation of growth, genital underdevelopment, hypoadrenocorticism and hypothyroidism. In adults, decreased libido, amenorrhea, and hypothyroidism may be present, and postmenopausal lactation has been described. Episodic arterial hypotension may be the presenting symptom in an adult, presumably from hypoadrenocorticism.

Hypothalamic symptoms (in the young) include obesity, hypogenitalism,[23] somnolence, and diabetes insipidus. The clinical picture may be that of Fröhlich syndrome. Sexual precocity is very rare.

Mental symptoms varying from loss of memory to progressive dementia were present in 50 per cent of Russell and Pennybacker's 24 elderly subjects with craniopharyngioma[82]; they are probably due, in part at any rate, to pressure on the temporal and frontal lobes.

Treatment. Contrast studies are desirable to outline the tumor before operation. Treatment consists of surgical evacuation of the cyst and the removal of as much of the cyst wall as possible. This can be hazardous, because the vessels of the circle of Willis are stretched around the mass, and the hypothalamus is in intimate contact with it. These tumors are generally regarded as being insensitive to x-ray therapy.

CHORDOMA

The chordoma, a rare congenital tumor, arises from notochordal remnants over the dorsum sellae or at the junction of the sphenoid and occipital bones. It is also found in the lumbosacral region of the spinal cord. The tumor is white and smoothly nodular, the cut surface resembling cartilage in appearance. It is highly invasive, spreading along the base of the skull in all directions. Extensive bone destruction occurs, and the tumor may erode into the nasopharynx. Cranial nerves are progressively interrupted, and the brainstem may be compressed. The tumor is to be suspected in the presence of multiple cranial nerve palsies and erosion of the floor of the skull as seen in x-rays. Fortunately, chordomas grow very slowly, and some relief may be obtained from partial removal.

DERMOIDS AND TERATOMATA

These tumors account for 4 per cent of all intracranial tumors, and for about 18 per cent of all spinal tumors in childhood. They may be cystic or solid and contain tissues derived from any of the germinal layers of the embryo. They tend to be located along the central axis—in the region of the third ventricle, the suprasellar space, the pineal recess, the fourth ventricle, and the distal end of the spinal cord. The tumor is present from birth, and symptoms usually develop in the first decade but may be delayed to adult life. The symptoms and signs are appropriate to their situation. Calcification in the tumor mass can sometimes be seen on x-ray pictures, but the diagnosis cannot be made with any certainty before operation.

Treatment is surgical. The results depend on the situation of the tumor and on its degree of malignancy. Of 15 patients reported by Ingraham and Bailey,[47] two were living more than five years after the operation without evidence of recurrence, five were still living less than five years after operation without recurrence, two were living but with evidence of recurrence, and six had died.

EPIDERMOIDS (CHOLESTEATOMAS, PEARLY TUMORS)

These are rare, and occur both in the head[93] and in the spine. The most common sites are the cerebellopontine angle, the suprasellar region, the fourth ventricle, the pineal recess, and the convexity of the hemispheres. The tumors vary in size from small nodules to large masses, are sharply demarcated, and may have a pearly appearance. They consist of layers of large, finely granular cells. Although they are encapsulated and separated from the surrounding tissues, their tendency to fill every available nook and cranny around them makes their removal difficult.

Epidermoids situated within the bones of the skull seldom affect the nervous system, but appear as a lump under the scalp. X-ray reveals wavy erosion of one or both tables of the skull. Occasionally the tumor arises in the petrous bone,[12] in which position it can involve the facial nerve and the cochlea. In this event, there is a slowly progressive paralysis of the face, combined with cochlear deafness and radiological evidence of excavation within the petrous temporal bone.

When situated intracranially, they tend to progress very slowly unless they are so situated as to cause internal hydrocephalus, as for instance in the cerebellopontine angle or fourth ventricle. There are no special features which enable the nature of the tumor to be diagnosed before operation. It should be completely removed, but this may be impossible by reason of its position. Prolonged periods of survival may be achieved by partial removal.

PITUITARY TUMORS

Pituitary tumors account for from 10 to 15 per cent of all intracranial tumors and are most commonly encountered in young and middle-aged adults. They are divided into three types—chromophobe adenomas, acidophilic adenomas, and the rare basophilic adenomas. The tumors are usually benign, but in exceptional cases carcinomatous changes take place. The symptoms and signs are the result of endocrine effects and pressure of the tumor on the sella and neighboring structures.

Chromophobe Adenoma

This is by far the commonest of the pituitary tumors. It is made up of polygonal cells arranged in sheets, with a roughly alveolar pattern; vascular connective tissue lies between the alveoli. The cytoplasm does not ordinarily contain chromophilic granules but, exceptionally, mixed tumors are found which contain a few granules. The tumor is usually solid, but cysts are occasionally present and some of these are due to previous hemorrhage or infarction. The enlarging mass compresses the remainder of the gland, giving rise to hypopituitarism, and expands and erodes the walls of the sella. Finally, it breaks through the dural diaphragm to compress the chiasm, optic nerves, and the base of the third ventricle.[50] Lateral extension into the middle fossa brings the mass into contact with the temporal lobe, and even the cerebral peduncle may be involved. Rarely, the tumor erodes into the sphenoidal sinus or cavernous sinus.

The chromophobe adenoma is usually considered to be entirely nonsecretory, but occasionally the patient exhibits what Bailey and Cushing described as "fugitive acromegaly," a combination of mild acromegaly and anterior pituitary insufficiency. Moreover, thyrotoxicosis, galactorrhea, and Cushing's syndrome have been observed in conjunction with these tumors. At the time of writing, the reason for these associations is not known with any certainty, but it has been suggested that the presence of the chromophobe adenoma alters the secretory rate of eosinophilic and basophilic cells, or that in certain instances the adenoma itself secretes trophic substances.

Clinical Features. A frontal or bitemporal headache is often an early symptom, but this is sometimes preceded by signs of endocrine disorder. The headache is probably due to pressure on the walls of the sella and the dural diaphragm. The adenoma depresses gonadal, thyroid, and adrenocortical functions. In consequence, the patient tends to put on weight and tires easily. In men, there is loss of bodily hair, lack of libido, and impotence, while women complain of irregular menstruation or amenorrhea. If the tumor arises in childhood, which is uncommon, growth is arrested and gonadal development does not occur. In adults, the skin is soft, slightly yellow in color, and there may be an increase of fat around the hips, shoulder girdle, and breast. Decreased thyroid function is manifested by lethargy, intolerance to cold, and sleepiness. The basal metabolic rate may be lowered. Diminution in secretion of adrenocortical hormone reduces water excretion; most patients adapt to this by drinking less, but if fluids are force—as in hospital, for instance—water intoxication can be precipitated. Excretion of urinary 17-ketosteroids following an injection of ACTH is subnormal.

Occasionally, when there is rapid and extensive destruction of the pituitary gland, the syndrome of pituitary cachexia develops, with profound asthenia, hypotension, pallor, emaciation, hypoglycemia, and electrolyte disturbances. Rarely, a chromophobe adenoma produces the features of the Cushing syndrome.

Diabetes insipidus does not occur unless the tumor erupts from the sella and involves the pituitary stalk, and it is uncommon even under these circumstances.

Visual disturbances occur when the tumor grows out of the sella and comes into contact with the optic nerves, chiasm, or optic tracts. This subject has been fully explored by Hughes.[46] The type of visual defect varies widely, according to which structures are involved. Usually, the central portion of the chiasm comes to be affected first, and this results in impairment of vision in the upper temporal fields. Most patients perform well on tests for visual acuity, and it requires examination on the tangent screen to disclose the trouble. Intermediate isopters are usually affected first, but the peripheral field is the first to show complete loss of light perception. Visual loss starts in the upper temporal quadrant and spreads to the lower temporal and lower nasal quadrants, in that order. The upper nasal quadrant may not be affected until very late in the disease. When the chiasm is prefixed, the tumor may involve its posterior part initially with the appearance of bitemporal hemianopic scotomas, which appear first in the paracentral region of the upper temporal quadrant, spread to the lower temporal quadrant, and then break through into the upper temporal peripheral field. When the chiasm is postfixed, the main pressure may fall on one or both optic nerves, causing a paracentral scotoma with quadrantic features. Exceptionally, there is a true central scotoma resembling that of retrobulbar neuritis. Posterior and lateral extension of the growth may bring it into contact with the optic tracts, or even the optic radiation, producing homonymous hemianopia. In all cases, there is considerable disparity between the field defects in the two eyes. The discs will eventually exhibit primary optic atrophy when the chiasm or optic nerve is involved but, however large the tumor, papilledema is uncommon if optic atrophy is already present.

If the tumor extends upwards it will come to involve the floor of the third ventricle and this gives rise to hypersomnolence, diabetes insipidus, and — occasionally — coma. Changes in temperature regulation and in pulse and respiration are uncommon. Upward displacement of the floor of the third ventricle can lead to internal hydrocephalus and a rise of intracranial pressure.

Extension into the temporal lobe causes uncinate seizures. Hemiparesis results from pressure on the cerebral peduncle; sometimes it occurs acutely and mimics a vascular accident. The third cranial nerve may be involved, with consequent diplopia. A nonparetic diplopia is sometimes encountered in the presence of bitemporal hemianopia; the double vision appears to be caused by an intermittent slight divergence of the visual axes.

Rarely, an invasive tumor of the pituitary will involve the cavernous sinus, producing paresthesias and pain in the face and paralysis of the third and fourth cranial nerves on that side. When headache has been present, it sometimes diminishes or disappears when the tumor erupts from the sella through the diaphragm or into the cavernous sinus; the latter mode of extension is very rare.

Hemorrhage into the tumor can give rise to so-called pituitary apoplexy. This is described on page 450.

Laboratory Aids. The x-ray appearances are characteristic. The sella is enlarged, mainly at the expense of the posterior wall and of the posterior part of the floor; the more compact bone in the anterior wall is relatively resistant to pressure. The floor deepens, and this deepening may be more on one side than the other, in which event lateral x-ray pictures give the impression of a double floor. The posterior wall and the

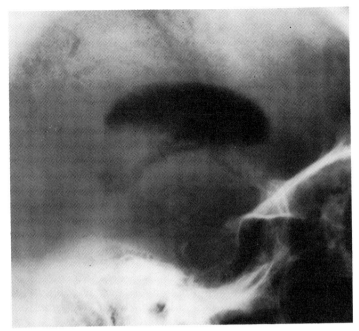

Figure 16–18. Pituitary adenoma in a 72-year-old woman with a six-month history of visual impairment. There is destruction of the floor of the sella and of the posterior clinoid processes. The anterior end of the third ventricle is elevated and crescentic in outline. (Courtesy of Dr. James Bull.)

posterior clinoids are decalcified and eroded (Fig. 16–18). Enlargement of the sella is occasionally brought about by a cystic extension of the subarachnoid space; in this event, pneumoencephalography discloses that the pituitary fossa is empty. An empty sella can also result from infarction of the pituitary tumor.

Examination of the visual fields by both perimetry and the tangent screen is obligatory.[46, 49] Not only does it indicate what the tumor is doing to the visual pathways, but it can also be used to study the progress of the disease.

Differential Diagnosis. The clinical picture of a chromophobe adenoma may be simulated by other tumors in this region. Craniopharyngiomas can involve the chiasm and optic tracts, but they seldom produce the characteristic ballooning of the sella, and stippled calcification is often seen. Gliomas of the optic nerve[16] and chiasm are more common in children, and while they may cause erosion of the clinoid processes, they do not usually enlarge the sella; on the other hand, forward extension of the tumor along the optic nerve will enlarge the optic foramen on the affected side. Meningiomas arising from the dura in the region of the pituitary fossa can produce bitemporal hemianopia and hypothalamic symptoms, but here again they do not usually enlarge the sella itself. Aneurysms sometimes produce visual field changes reminiscent of a pituitary tumor and can also invade the sella turcica. This is a rare event, but the fact that it can happen emphasizes the value of angiography in diagnosis. In order to define the full extent of a pituitary tumor, it is desirable to carry out both pneumoencephalography and bilateral carotid angiography.

Clinical Course. Chromophobe adenomas grow very slowly, and it may take many years before the tumor is large enough to produce blindness or significant damage to the hypothalamus. However, the course of the disease may be interrupted by hemorrhage into the tumor, which constitutes a neurosurgical emergency.

Treatment. This depends on the nature and size of the tumor. If there is no evidence of extrasellar extension, x-ray therapy is the method of choice, though these tumors are less sensitive than the acidophilic and basophilic adenomas. In the presence of a large extrasellar extension, surgery is indicated, but if there is extensive involvement of the hypothalamic region or temporal lobe, the operative prognosis is poor. Otherwise, the results of operation are usually good, so far as recovery of vision is concerned. Even when acuity has fallen to mere light perception, full fields and 20/20 vision may return. However, if light perception has been absent in an eye for more than a few weeks, no return of function is to be expected.

Patients who have undergone bilateral adrenalectomy for Cushing's syndrome occasionally develop a chromophobe adenoma of the pituitary. These are treated by radiation, followed by surgery if the growth of the tumor is not arrested.

Eosinophilic Adenomas

These seldom occur in pure form but are usually associated with a large number of chromophobe cells—a mixed adenoma. The tumor contains large cells with eosinophilic granules in the cytoplasm, and the secretion from these cells is responsible for many of the clinical features of acromegaly and pituitary gigantism. The growth-diabetogenic factor is currently assumed to be one protein molecule with dual properties. When secreted in excess, it gives rise to gigantism or acromegaly, and about one-third of all acromegalics develop diabetes mellitus as a consequence of blockade of insulin action in the tissues and the exhaustion of the beta cells of the pancreas.

Clinical Features. Acromegaly is usually a disease of middle life, but has been known to start in adolescence or even in childhood. Pituitary gigantism usually starts at puberty.

The early symptoms of acromegaly include impotence in the male and amenorrhea in the female. Frontal or bitemporal headache may be present from the start, but sometimes it is long delayed, and even when present it is variable in severity. Deep pain on one or both sides of the face and "rheumatism" in the joints and muscles can cause difficulties in diagnosis when they occur before the characteristic changes in personal appearance. Excessive sweating is often complained of.

The hands, feet, face, and skull gradually enlarge. This process is often accompanied by pain, particularly in the fingers, toes, and face. There is coarsening of the skin and subcutaneous tissues of the face and scalp, and enlargement of the mandible gives rise to prognathism, with separation of the teeth in advanced cases. As time goes on, dorsal kyphosis gradually develops, and the skeletal muscles become weaker and thinner.

There is a general enlargement of the viscera; in particular, the heart enlarges, in the absence of hypertension or valvular disease. As was already stated, about one-third of all acromegalics develop diabetes mellitus. Hypermetabolism is usually present, though without clinical or laboratory evidence of thyrotoxicosis; it is probably due to the metabolic effects of the growth-diabetogenic hormone. Persistent or sporadic galactorrhea may occur. The growth hormone responsible for acromegaly decreases renal excretion of phosphates so that an elevated plasma phosphate concentration, in the absence of renal disease, indicates that the tumor is active.

The neurological effects of an eosinophilic adenoma are similar to those of the chromophobe type, as described above. In addition, however, thickening of the tissues of the wrist can give rise to a unilateral or bilateral median carpal tunnel syndrome at any stage of the disease.

In pituitary gigantism, excessive growth begins at or about puberty; the arms, legs, and trunk are long, and the hands and feet are large and well formed. Later on, acromegalic characteristics appear in some cases, with increase in size of the lower jaw and spacing of the teeth, enlargement of the tongue, and thickening of the subcutaneous tissues of the face, hands, and feet. Sexual development is sometimes precocious, and both libido and potency may be excessive at first, in contrast to the situation in hypogonadal gigantism. Growth may continue up to the age of 25 or 30 years, and there is delayed fusion of the epiphyses. As in acromegaly, insulin-resistant diabetes is apt to develop. Eventually, the muscles become weak and wasted, and scoliosis develops.

Diagnosis. The physical appearance of acromegaly cannot be mimicked by any other condition. Pituitary gigantism must be distinguished from hypogonadal gigantism which occurs as a result of atrophy, disease, or damage to the gonads. When this happens before the epiphyses are united, the result is a characteristic type of long-limbed, eunuchoid gigantism. The patient remains sexually infantile and the voice unbroken; secondary sexual characteristics do not appear. A very rare form of gigantism is the so-called cerebral type,[89] which is characterized by excessive height, large hands and feet, mental retardation, and clumsiness of movement. In a case reported by Appenzeller, there was persistent fever and evidence of a failure of central temperature control, sustaining the notion that these cases are of "cerebral" origin. More than one case can appear in the family.

Treatment. These tumors are relatively radiosensitive and even if visual loss has started, it is better to rely on radiotherapy than to attempt surgery. As in chromophobe adenomas, the surgical prognosis is poor once the tumor has involved the floor of the third ventricle or the temporal lobe.

Basophilic Adenoma

These tumors are rare. They are small and seldom present as a tumor, but the endocrine disturbances to which they give rise are striking. The latter were first described by Cushing in 1932, and the term "Cushing's *disease*" or "pitui-

tary basophilism" should be reserved for hyperadrenocorticism resulting from a functioning pituitary tumor. "Cushing's *syndrome*," on the other hand, is used for symptoms and signs which arise from the presence of excessive 11-oxysteroids in conditions other than basophilic adenoma of the pituitary. At the present time, the most common cause of Cushing's syndrome is the administration of steroids for therapeutic purposes, but it can also arise in the course of adenoma and hyperplasia of the adrenal cortex, malignant tumors of the thymus, pancreas, lung, and other organs, and hypothalamic lesions. It may occur transiently during pregnancy.

Clinical Features. Women are more often affected than men, and the onset is usually in the middle decades of life. Obesity develops in the trunk and proximal portions of the limbs. Purple striae appear in the skin of areas which have increased in size, notably the lower abdomen and the limb girdles. The face becomes rounded and reddish blue in color, and there is often an increase of facial hair in women. The patient complains of fatigue and muscular weakness, and wasting of the muscles may be severe enough to suggest the presence of a myopathy. There is usually amenorrhea or impotence. Hypertension is common, and both hyperglycemia and polycythemia can occur. Generalized osteoporosis is usual; it is attributed to a negative protein balance.

Mental symptoms are common in all forms of Cushing's syndrome. A decline in sexual capacity and chagrin over a deteriorating personal appearance contribute to psychoneurotic disorders, the pattern of which is sometimes related to the previous personality of the patient. In addition, however, there are symptoms that suggest that the metabolic disturbance has a physical effect on the brain. These include difficulty in concentration, poor memory, weakness of attention, and wide and sudden shifts of mood, which appear to be unrelated to current events or antecedent experiences. Similar symptoms are sometimes encountered in patients who have been taking steroids for a long time.

The true basophile adenoma does not expand the pituitary fossa, or spread beyond its confines, but, as noted above, a chromophobe adenoma will sometimes present the features of pituitary basophilism and in this event, the fossa is expanded and the growth may spread to involve the chiasm.

Laboratory Aids. The quantity of free cortisol excreted in the urine is increased. Excretion of 17-ketogenic steroids is depressed by dexamethazone and is increased during the administration of corticotrophin. However, even when the cortisol secretion rate is increased, the problem still remains as to whether this is due to a pituitary tumor or to extracranial disease.

Treatment. A variety of treatments have been employed, including irradiation of the pituitary gland, the implantation of radioactive gold and yttrium, and adrenalectomy. The Italian literature, in particular, emphasizes the value of intrapituitary implants, although these are not free from the risk of producing diabetes insipidus, cerebrospinal rhinorrhea, and bacterial meningitis. The more conventional approach, as recommended by Danowski, is subtotal adrenalectomy, followed by total adrenalectomy if the former proves ineffective. Hypophysectomy, electrocoagulation of the pituitary gland, and sectioning of the pituitary stalk have also been advocated.

Untreated, these cases often show reduced resistance to infections, and death can occur from generalized infection following trivial injuries, such as a pinprick or tooth extraction. Apart from infections, the usual cause of death is cardiac failure, cerebral hemorrhage, or uremia.

Pituitary Apoplexy

Hemorrhage into a pituitary tumor can lead to an abrupt worsening of neurological symptoms.[3] The tumor outgrows its blood supply, and this results in necrosis and secondary hemorrhage, which may appear for no apparent reason, or which may follow head injury or radiation to the pituitary region.

Hemorrhage occurs suddenly, and the consequent enlargement of the tumor leads to compression of the chiasm, optic nerves, and cavernous sinus. Sometimes the blood penetrates the capsule of the gland and appears in the spinal fluid.

The presenting symptom is usually an abrupt impairment of vision, which may take the form of blindness in one eye and less severe visual failure in the other. This is accompanied by headache, and if subarachnoid hemorrhage is present, there will be signs of meningeal irritation. The patient may be drowsy. Other symptoms that have been described include hemiparesis from compression of the middle cerebral artery, facial pain, diplopia from involvement of the third and fourth cranial nerves in the cavernous sinus, and "pituitary coma." If the presence of a pituitary adenoma has not been recognized before the hemorrhage, the symptoms are apt to suggest a primary subarachnoid hemorrhage from an intracranial aneurysm, and a pressure cone can be simulated by the combination of headaches, stiffness of the neck, diplopia, and increasing stupor or coma.

Accurate and prompt diagnosis is desirable because pressure on the optic nerves and the hypothalamus can be relieved only by removal of the blood clot within the bulging capsule of the tumor. Large doses of cortisone should be given before, during, and after operation. Untreated, the condition is likely to be fatal. Spontaneous cure can also occur[98] but should not be relied upon. Infarction and small, nonfatal hemorrhages into a pituitary tumor can sometimes lead to a remission of the endocrine features caused by the tumor. This has been seen in acromegaly and in pituitary basophilism. Amelioration of diabetes mellitus has also been known to occur as the result of pituitary infarction; conversely, diabetes is one of the recognized causes of pituitary infarction.

Hemangioblastoma (Angioblastoma, Angioreticuloma, etc.)

This tumor accounts for about 2 per cent of all primary intracranial neoplasms. It is found at any age, but its peak incidence is in middle life. It can occur on its own, or in association with retinal angiomatosis; in the latter event, it is often familial and may be associated with cysts of the pancreas and kidney, angiomas of the liver and skin, hypernephroma, or adrenal tumors.[81] The association of cerebellar hemangioblastoma and retinal angiomatosis is known as the von Hippel-Lindau disease.

Pathology. These tumors are usually solitary, but more than one tumor may be found in the posterior fossa. The most common site is the cerebellum, but they may be also found in the medulla and in the spinal cord. They are seldom found in the cerebral hemispheres.

Hemangioblastomas are true mesodermal tumors which are presumed to arise from the mesenchymal vascular network. They consist of solid sheets of angioblastic cells with or without vascular spaces of capillary or cavernous type. The tumor may be solid, well encapsulated, and highly vascular, or the mass may be largely cystic, the actual tumor being represented by a small mural nodule, in which event the cyst wall contains no tumor cells but consists of glial tissue. A highly proteinous fluid collects in the cyst or leaks into the spinal fluid, which is often yellowish and has a high protein content. The tumor also elaborates an erythropoietic substance, which causes polycythemia in some cases.

Clinical Features. Hemangioblastomas of the cerebral hemisphere are rare. Like angiomatous malformations, they can be asymptomatic for years, and then seizures appear, or they may give rise to minimal focal signs without evidence of progression. Stippled calcification may be visible radiologically.

In *cerebellar hemangioblastomas* the clinical picture is that of a slowly growing tumor in the cerebellum or cerebellopontine angle. Those lying in the lateral recess can be difficult to differentiate from a meningioma or acoustic neurinoma, but the rise of protein in the cerebrospinal fluid tends to be greater than with a neurinoma, and the internal auditory meatus is not enlarged. Differentiation from an astrocytoma of the cerebellum may be impossible unless there are associated angiomatous malformations elsewhere, such as a retinal hemangioma. This usually appears as a small nodule at the periphery of the lower pole of the retina, fed by a tortuous artery and drained by a dilated vein which often contains pink blood. Eventually, degenerative retinal changes occur, with hemorrhage, exudate, and detachment.

Angiography is the diagnostic method of choice. The raised cerebrospinal fluid protein is suggestive. X-rays will occasionally reveal increased vascularity of the overlying bone, but this can occur in other tumors.

Spinal hemangioblastoma can occur in the cord, amid nerve roots, or in the extradural space, usually in the thoracic region, and gives rise to the features of progressive cord compression.[99] The presence of skin nevi or a retinal angioma is suggestive.

Progress and Treatment. Hemangioblastomas are slowly progressive, and severe incapacity eventually occurs.

Surgical removal is possible in some instances, but the location of the mass and its extreme vascularity make this a hazardous procedure. Fortunately, these tumors are radiosensitive, and radiation is employed to reduce the size and vascularity of the tumor before attempting to remove it.

NASOPHARYNGEAL TUMORS

Neoplasms arising in the nasopharynx often involve the cranial nerves by entering the basal foramina. In adults, these growths are usually carcinomatous, but in children, sarcomas are more likely to be encountered. The Chinese are prone to a peculiar growth, sometimes referred to as a lymphoepithelioma, which is apt to infiltrate widely without producing much in the way of a mass in the nasopharynx; consequently, neither inspection nor palpation may reveal the tumor.

Of 381 patients with nasopharyngeal malignant tumors reported by Thomas and Waltz,[92] 113 were found to have neurological complications, and in many cases, these symptoms were the first to appear. Intractable facial or head pain may be the only symptom for some time. It is commonly unilateral and may superficially resemble tic douloureux. Nocturnal exacerbations of pain are not uncommon. Blockage of the eustachian tube may produce middle-ear deafness and tinnitus, while nerve deafness may result from involvement of the eighth nerve in the temporal bone. Infiltration of the soft palate may immobilize it and give rise to a "nasal" voice. The combination of a nasal intonation and trigeminal pain with or without diplopia should always suggest the need for a careful search of the nasopharynx. Other cranial nerves are often involved, notably the third, fourth, and sixth nerves, and there may also be loss of vision in one eye, loss of smell, facial weakness, dysarthria, hoarseness, and weakness of the sternomastoids. Cranial nerve palsies can occur without pain and *without symptoms related to the nasopharynx.*

Metastatic deposits can occur in the brachial plexus and the spinal cord. Occasionally, a large intracranial mass gives rise to the feature of a primary tumor. Both meningitis and brain abscess may occur from the spread of infection from the nasopharynx along the pathways opened up by the tumor.

In time, x-rays will disclose erosion of the base of the skull and encroachment on the nasopharyngeal air space, but failure to see a tumor does not rule it out. Suspicious lymph nodes in the neck may be removed for examination, and biopsy of a seemingly normal nasopharynx will occasionally prove positive.

These tumors do not lend themselves to surgical extirpation and are best treated by radiation or by a combination of radiation and chemotherapy. Survival time following treatment ranges from a few months to several years.

Tumors of the Glomus Jugulare

The glomus jugulare is part of a chemoreceptor system which includes the carotid and aortic bodies. The system consists of small glomera, one of which is situated on the dome of the jugular bulb; a similar body, the glomus tympanicum, may be situated on the tympanic branch of the glossopharyngeal nerve.[100]

These small, slowly growing, locally invasive tumors may arise from any one of the glomera, or from several simultaneously.[44, 100] The growth is composed of rounded cells arranged in small alveolar clusters separated by fine reticulin fibers and vascular channels, the whole being surrounded by a zone of dense collagen. The tumor spreads into the middle ear and into the posterior fossa. Metastases can occur if the tumor invades the jugular vein. Multiple cases have occurred in a single family.[55]

Clinical Features. Symptoms commonly occur in middle age, and women are more often affected than men. In the great majority of all cases the initial symptoms are aural: tinnitus, middle-ear deafness, otitis, pain, and occasional vertigo. There is often a long history of a discharging ear. Vascular polypi may be seen behind or bulging through the drum. These symptoms continue for many years before the tumor spreads to involve the cranial nerves. About 50 per cent of reported cases have had evidence of intracranial extension, characterized as a rule by the very slow development of paralysis in one or more of the lower cranial nerves on the side of the tumor. There may be diplopia from sixth nerve involvement, facial paralysis, deafness and vertigo from infiltration of the eighth nerve, palatal weakness, and paralysis of one side of the tongue. Nystagmus, cerebellar ataxia, and pyramidal signs are infrequent, and a rise in intracranial pressure is exceptional. A bruit has been present in a few cases. Rarely, the tumor does not invade the middle ear, the symptoms being confined to paralysis of the lower cranial nerves.

Treatment. The tumors are extremely vascular, and surgery is hazardous. Radiotherapy is the method of choice.

Colloid Cysts of the Third Ventricle

These small cysts, filled with colloid material, arise from paraphysial remnants in the anterior part of the third ventricle. The wall is composed of cuboidal and columnar ciliated cells and a layer of connective tissue. Being pedunculated, they can alter their position on movement of the head, and it is thought that this is the reason for the intermittent attacks of internal hydrocephalus which are their most characteristic clinical feature.[77] This also applies, of course, to tumors in the fourth and lateral ventricles as well. The cysts are usually found in adolescents and young adults.

The traditional but by no means the only form of presentation is with repeated attacks of headache and mental confusion, with or without papilledema, lasting a few days. There may be dizziness, vertigo, vomiting, generalized weakness, sudden giving way of the legs, and diplopia in these attacks. The author has seen two patients who were admitted to a mental ward because an acute confusional state dominated the clinical picture. If and when the obstruction is relieved, the symptoms disappear, only to recur at shorter and shorter intervals until obstruction is permanent and complete. Other patients present with chronic hydrocephalus of gradual development, and the prevailing symptoms may be headache, mental dulling, and (as in so many cases of internal hydrocephalus) unsteadiness of gait. Apathy and inaccessibility gradually increase, ending either in akinetic mutism or in coma. Exceptionally, there is increasing dementia without headache or papilledema.[79] A 2 to 3 per second bobbing tremor of the head and trunk has also been described in association with internal hydrocephalus caused by a large cyst of the third ventricle. Hyperglycemia and glycosuria can occur in the acute episodes, but they are more commonly encountered in gliomas which infiltrate the walls of the third ventricle.

The differential diagnosis between a colloid cyst and other tumors in this region cannot be made with any certainty on the basis of the clinical symptoms and signs, but depends on the demonstration of a filling defect in the third ventricle. If air pictures give an equivocal result, an opaque medium should be used.[10]

Treatment is by surgical extirpation; reasonably good results are to be expected in the majority of cases.

Papilloma of the Choroid Plexus

These very rare tumors are usually found in the fourth ventricle but may also occur in the lateral and third ventricles. They appear as red, mulberry-like growths which grow to a large size and may undergo cystic degeneration. The tumor consists of papillae which have a central core of connective tissue covered by cuboidal epithelium. Some are relatively benign, while others are highly malignant; the latter may seed into the subarachnoid space. They are usually encountered in children or young adults and present with the nonspecific picture of a tumor within the ventricular system. As is to be expected, the cerebrospinal fluid protein is increased, and a pleocytosis may be present. The location of the tumor is determined by complete visualization of the entire ventricular system. Complete extirpation is difficult and often impossible, but the tumor is sensitive to deep x-rays and a preliminary course of such treatment may so reduce the size and vascularity of the tumor as to allow safe surgical removal at a later date. The end results are poor because in most instances the tumor recurs.

Tumors of the
Lateral Ventricle

Tumors of the lateral ventricle are rare (Fig. 16–19). In addition to the papilloma of the choroid plexus already described, other tumors found in this situation include ependymomas, meningiomas,[35] angiomas, and teratomas. Most of them occur in infancy or childhood, but no age is exempt. The symptoms are those of raised intracranial pressure, which can give rise to false localizing signs, and localization depends more upon ventriculography than on the clinical features. The operative mortality is in the region of 50 per cent.

PINEAL TUMORS

Pinealocytomas and the more malignant pinealoblastomas are very rare. A tumor in this situation more often turns out to be a teratoma or a glioma, and pineal cysts large enough to cause symptoms are usually due to cystic degeneration within a teratoma. Pineal tumors occur in both sexes, and in both children and adults.

Clinical Features. The symptoms and signs are neurological rather than endocrinological in origin. The hypogonadism and the sexual precocity which sometimes occurs in boys are not due to pineal secretions but to infiltration of the hypothalamus. Recently, a melanocyte-contracting substance (melatonin) and a substance which stimulates adrenocortical aldosterone secretion have been isolated from the gland, but there is no evidence that these substances play any part in the symptoms produced by pineal tumors in man.

The anatomical situation of these tumors is such that they are apt to cause internal hydrocephalus at an early stage (Fig. 16–21). Consequently, headache, papilledema, and vomiting may occur early, and false localizing signs due to brainstem displacement may complicate the picture. In other cases, the first symptoms are due to infiltration of the midbrain. Paralysis of conjugate upward gaze, pupillary inequalities, and loss of the reflexes to light and convergence are more common than diplopia. Tinnitus and partial deafness may be present from infiltration of the medial geniculate

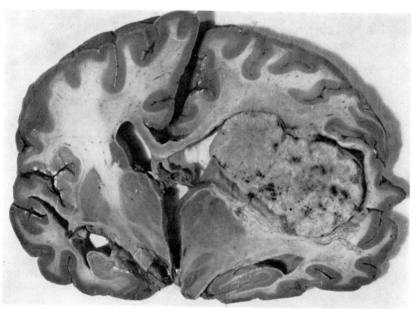

Figure 16–19.   Large intraventricular meningioma. (From Russell, D. S., and Rubenstein, L. J.: *Pathology of Tumors of The Nervous System*. London, Edward Arnold, 1959.)

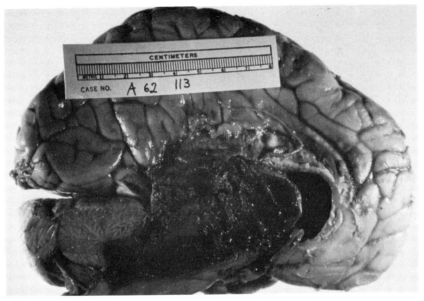

Figure 16–20. Pinealoma. (Courtesy of Children's Hospital of Philadelphia.)

Figure 16–21. Ventriculogram showing dilatation of the lateral ventricles
caused by tumor of the pineal. (Courtesy
of Children's Hospital of Philadelphia.)

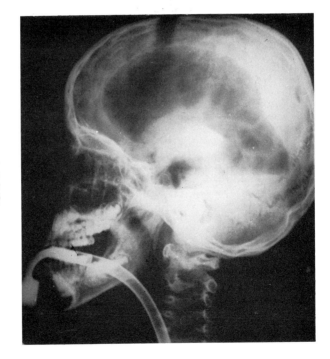

nuclei. Cerebellar ataxia and a tendency to fall backward reflect involvement of the superior cerebellar peduncle. In a series reviewed by Smith,[87] hemiplegia and sensory loss were rare.

Extension of the tumor into the hypothalamus can give rise to diabetes insipidus, the salt-losing syndrome, hypogonadism, and—very rarely—precocious puberty. The latter is usually found in boys.

Diagnosis is aided by the presence of stippled calcification around the pineal, but final diagnosis depends on brain scanning and on air contrast studies which, in the brow-down position, show the outline of a tumor abutting on the posterior part of the third ventricle.

Treatment. Owing to their situation, these tumors are not amenable to surgical extirpation, but fortunately they often respond fairly well to radiation, and survival for five or more years is not uncommon. If internal hydrocephalus has occurred, ventriculocisternostomy has to be carried out before radiation is embarked upon.

Metastatic Tumors

Metastatic tumors account for some 10 to 20 per cent of all intracranial tumors, the lower figure coming from neurological and neurosurgical units and the higher estimate from general hospitals. The precise figure does not matter. What does matter is that metastases are relatively common, and that they can cause symptoms before there is any evidence of the primary tumor. A less common form of invasion of the central nervous system is so-called carcinomatous meningitis. Visceral carcinomas can also give rise to disorders of the central and peripheral nervous system through a variety of metabolic pathways, without actually invading the nervous system. These are listed below.

Metastatic Deposits. The commonest growth to metastasize to the brain is carcinoma of the lung, followed in order of frequency by carcinoma of the breast,

the gastrointestinal tract, and the urinary tract. Intracranial metastases from sarcomatous tumors are rare. Chorioepitheliomas are rare but are apt to metastasize to the brain. Malignant tumors of the eye may spread directly into the brain.

Metastases are not difficult to diagnose when there is collateral evidence of a primary tumor elsewhere. However, it is not uncommon, particularly in the case of bronchial carcinoma, for the cerebral metastases to produce symptoms before the primary tumor can be identified either clinically or radiologically. The difficulty is compounded by the circumstance that in many cases only one major metastasis is present, thus mimicking a primary brain tumor (Fig. 16–22).

The pressure of the spinal fluid may be elevated or normal, depending on the volume of the metastatic deposits and the amount of edema they provoke. The protein content and cell count may be raised if the tumor has spread to the surface of the brain or ventricles. Of the contrast studies which can be carried out in these cases, brain scans are particularly useful in revealing multiple lesions. In a substantial number of cases, however, the pathological nature of the tumor is only revealed by brain biopsy. Exploratory craniotomy is justified when there is doubt as to the diagnosis.

Carcinomatosis of the Meninges. Although diffuse involvement of the leptomeninges is less common than metastatic intracerebral deposits, it is not rare. It may present as a subacute meningitis, with headache, mental symptoms, and paralysis of one or more cranial nerves. The cerebrospinal fluid pressure may be normal or increased, and there is commonly a mononuclear pleocytosis and a decreased sugar content. Tumor cells may be found in the fluid, but the absence of such cells does not invalidate the diagnosis. The course is progressive, with death occurring within a few weeks.

In less acute cases, the meningeal infiltration picks out individual cranial nerves without symptoms of meningeal irritation. Exceptionally, the presenting

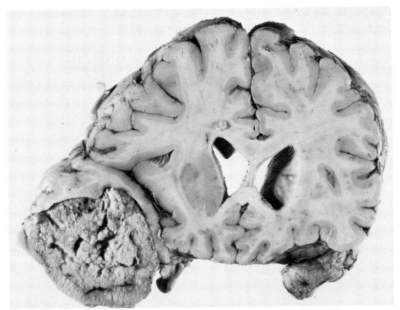

Figure 16–22. Metastatic carcinoma. (Courtesy of Ayer Laboratory, Pennsylvania Hospital, Philadelphia.)

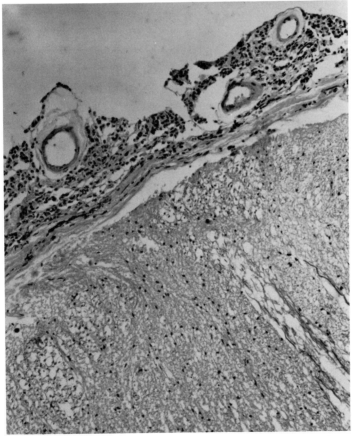

Figure 16–23. Metastatic carcinomatosis of the meninges. (Courtesy of Ayer Laboratory, Pennsylvania Hospital, Philadelphia.)

Table 16–2.   Neurological Complications of Cancer

Invasion by fungi and viruses
Fungal meningitis
Herpes zoster and herpes simplex
Progressive multifocal leukoencephalopathy

Degenerative conditions of the nervous system and muscles

Degenerative encephalopathies	Carcinomatosis myelopathies
Cerebellar degeneration	Carcinomatosis polyneuropathy
Central pontine myelinolysis	Carcinomatosis myopathy

Metabolic Disturbances

Hypoglycemia	Hypercalcemia
Hyponatremia	Cushing's syndrome
Hypokalemia	Porphyria

symptom is that of rapidly advancing dementia which is caused by diffuse infiltration of the meninges, cerebral cortex, and limbic system, a condition which has to be distinguished from other forms of carcinomatous encephalopathy.

Nonmetastatic Neurological Complications of Cancer

Neurological symptoms occurring in the course of visceral cancer of lymphoma are not always or necessarily caused by direct invasion of the nervous system. Malignant disease, including the lymphomas and leukemias, increases the patient's susceptibility to infection by viruses and fungi, and this susceptibility is further enhanced by radiotherapy and the administration of steroids. Secondly, cancer sometimes has metabolic effects on the brain, spinal cord, peripheral nerves and muscles. For convenience, these complications are listed here but are described under appropriate headings elsewhere.

THE LYMPHOMAS AND LEUKEMIAS

Hodgkin's Lymphoma

Hodgkin's lymphoma seldom occurs in the brain but is not uncommon as a source of spinal compression.[88, 97] The difference is probably accounted for by the tendency of the growth to spread into the epidural space from contiguous, paravertebral lymph nodes in the mediastinum and abdomen. Intracranial deposits usually occur in the dura and produce symptoms by infiltrating cranial nerves, raising intracranial pressure, and compressing adjacent brain. Intracerebral, as opposed to extracerebral, deposits are extremely rare. Sohn and his colleagues[88] found only two cases in the literature of Hodgkin's granuloma with discrete macroscopic deposits within the brain, and added a third case in which the granuloma involved the hypothalamus, fornix, septum pellucidum, optic nerves, optic chiasm, certain cranial nerves, medulla, and spinal cord. In rare cases, seizures and focal symptoms of acute onset have occurred in the course of the disease without any autopsy evidence of lymphomatous infiltration of the brain or spinal cord, but with multiple areas of demyelination consistent with a diagnosis of multifocal leukoencephalopathy.

A third neurological complication of Hodgkin's disease is peripheral polyneuropathy, which can take two forms, a symmetrically and predominantly distal polyneuropathy, presumably of metabolic origin, and mononeuritis multiplex caused by random infiltration of nerve roots and peripheral nerves.

Hodgkin's Sarcoma

This condition can occur in the brain without evidence of lymphoma elsewhere in the body. The growth shows a notable predilection for the temporal lobe, but because of its extreme rarity it is likely to be a surprise finding at operation.

Lymphosarcoma of the Brain

Lymphosarcoma of the brain is less uncommon that Hodgkin's sarcoma. It was found in 22 cases of a series of 1773 patients suffering from lymphosarcoma.[97] Because the deposits are usually in the meninges, cranial nerve palsies are common, and the intracranial pressure can be raised by blockage of the subarachnoid space at the base of the brain.

There is a higher incidence of herpes zoster in Hodgkin's disease and lymphosarcoma than can be accounted for by chance, and the same applies to fungal meningitis. Cryptococcal infections can appear as subacute meningitis and can also mimic a rapidly growing tumor of the posterior fossa. A search for evidence of lymphoma should always be carried out in patients with fungal meningitis.

The Leukemias

Symptomless infiltration of the meninges, brain, and spinal cord is common in the leukemias.[97] When symptoms do occur, they may take the form of seizures, raised intracranial pressure, or a frank intracerebral or subarachnoid hemorrhage. Such symptoms are apt to appear late in the disease, when the diagnosis is already established.

Multiple Myeloma

Neurological complications usually occur late in multiple myeloma, but occasionally they are the first to appear as the result of spinal, intracranial, or orbital deposits. Spinal compression is by far the most common neurological complication (see Fig. 16–27).[17, 97]

Intracranial myeloma usually starts in the skull and spreads thence to the dura and so into the brain. There are three main types of presentation: single or multiple cranial nerve palsies, a single intracranial mass, and diplopia and proptosis from orbital deposits. Headache may be severe, mild, or absent. In all cases, the diagnosis is helped by demonstration of radiotranslucent deposits in the ribs and other bones, or by localized osteoporosis. Bence Jones protein is present in the urine in some cases, and serum electrophoresis may disclose hyperglobulinemia.

The treatment of the reticuloses is beyond the scope of this book.

INTRACRANIAL TUMORS IN CHILDREN

Intracranial tumors in children increase in frequency up to the seventh year, after which the incidence declines until a second rise occurs at or around puberty.

Unlike tumors in adults, the majority are subtentorial, and tend to develop in the midline. Consequently, they commonly cause obstructive hydrocephalus at an early stage; an exception is glioma of the pons, which rarely blocks the aqueduct, but causes multiple cranial nerve palsies and vomiting. Of the supratentorial tumors, spongioblastoma of the optic nerve and chiasm[16] occurs mainly in children, and the same applies to craniopharyngiomas and papillomas of the choroid plexus. Gliomas of the cerebral hemispheres account for only about 10 per cent of all brain tumors in children, and meningiomas are uncommon; pinealomas, dermoids, and teratomas commonly give rise to symptoms after age 15. Metastases are far less common than in adults, because visceral carcinoma is not frequent in childhood. Nevertheless, metastases do occur from sarcomas, hypernephromas, and the lymphomas, and gliomas of the retina may extend into the brain.

Clinical Features. In infancy, the onset of raised intracranial pressure may be delayed because the sutures separate and the skull enlarges to accommodate not only the tumor but also (in the case of a subtentorial growth) the expanded lateral ventricles. Whereas in adults the onset of obstructive hydrocephalus is commonly due to a tumor, in infants it is usually caused by atresia of the sylvian aqueduct or meningeal adhesions around the base.

In brainstem gliomas, vomiting is usually early, before a rise of intracranial pressure occurs, and it is only too often ascribed to "cyclic vomiting" or is regarded as a symptom of an upper respiratory infection or gastrointestinal upset. Headache is common; it is apt to be present early in the morning, and may be aggravated by change of posture. Papilledema occurs early in many subtentorial tumors of childhood, but in glioma of the pons, it may be late in appearing. Because most tumors in children occur beneath the tentorium, seizures are less prominent than in adults. Whereas convulsions occurring for the first time in adult life immediately suggest the possibility of a tumor, this is not the case in early childhood, a period in which convulsions are usually due to other causes.

In children under the age of about seven years, an intracranial bruit does not necessarily indicate the presence of an arteriovenous malformation or fistula.

PSEUDOTUMOR CEREBRI (BENIGN INTRACRANIAL HYPERTENSION)

Definition. The term "pseudotumor cerebri" was introduced in 1914 by Nonne for a group of cases displaying increased intracranial pressure, papilledema, and normal cerebrospinal fluid, which followed a benign, self-limited course. It is likely that some of the cases described as serous meningitis by Quincke in 1893 belonged to this group.

Symonds' term "otitic hydrocephalus" applies specifically to high intracranial pressure caused by thrombosis of the dural venous sinuses following otitis media and other infections.[78, 91]

Etiology. The condition is thought to be due to an endocrine or metabolic disturbance because (1) it occurs predominantly in women, between the menarche and the menopause; (2) it is often associated with menstrual irregularity and sometimes with pregnancy; (3) obesity is often present;[41] (4) galactorrhea has occurred in some cases; (5) brain swelling has been known to occur periodically, with each menstrual period; and (6) it can occur in asthmatic children treated with steroids.[24] Nevertheless, many patients with pseudotumor cerebri are conspicuously healthy in all other respects, and apart from obesity and menstrual irregularity in some, they display no overt evidence of endocrinopathy. Excretion of 17-ketosteroids and 17-hydroxycorticosteroids is normal. Oldstone[73] has reported absence of the normal response to metyranone in six patients, but it is not certain whether this evidence of disturbance in the pituitary-corticotrophic-adrenal axis is primary or is secondary to the rise of intracranial pressure.

Clinical Features. The patient usually looks healthy and alert. Headache can be an early symptom, but it is seldom severe or localized, and often it is absent. Amaurosis fugax is common, and persistent impairment of vision from papilledema may follow. Papilledema may occur in the absence of headache or other symptoms. Dizziness and diplopia occasionally occur, but vomiting is rare. The presence of seizures or focal neurological deficits other than diplopia throws doubt on the diagnosis.

Papilledema is usually the sole physical sign. The blind spot is enlarged; reduction of the peripheral fields occurs in advanced cases and is of ill omen, signifying that unless the intracranial pressure is reduced, consecutive optic atrophy is likely to occur. Iron deficiency anemia is present in some cases.

Prognosis. The condition may go on for weeks or months. Spontaneous remission without treatment is not unknown, but it should never be relied upon to occur, because of the danger to sight. Irretrievable blindness is the penalty for carelessness in the treatment of this syndrome.

Differential Diagnosis. Cerebral tumor is by far the most common cause of headache and papilledema, and must be sought for by meticulous visualization not only of the ventricular system but also of the subarachnoid space. Large tumors in the cerebellopontine angle or over the dorsum sellae, for instance, may be clinically silent except for the presence of papilledema; rarely, a large aneurysm may present in similar fashion. Raised intracranial pressure can be caused by metastatic disease of the dural sinuses.[69] A recent history of infection, whether of the ear, nasal sinuses, or elsewhere in the body, is an indication for careful study of the venous phase of the arteriogram. Cisternal arachnoiditis can cause a communicating hydrocephalus, with headache and papilledema.

Brain swelling and papilledema, occasionally encountered in vitamin A intoxication in children and young adults, Addison's disease, hypoparathyroidism, sustained steroid therapy in children, severe pulmonary emphysema, and the pickwickian syndrome, will not cause confusion because each of these conditions produces characteristic satellite symptoms and signs.

Once the diagnosis has been established, oral administration of corticosteroids should be started at once (e.g., 40 mg. Prednisone per day, for a week, followed by 15 mg. daily for as long as required). If this fails to halt the process, a ventricular-atrial shunt is needed. If, by reason of geographical distance or other circumstances, surgery has to be delayed, recourse can be had to the old-fashioned method of removing from 15 to 30 ml. of spinal fluid every day, or every other day, depending on the cerebrospinal fluid pressure. It is vital to employ every available method to reduce intracranial pressure if papilledema is increasing and the peripheral visual fields are diminishing.

SPINAL TUMORS

Incidence. Tumors of the spinal cord are less common than intracranial growths, and are rare in children.[29, 40]

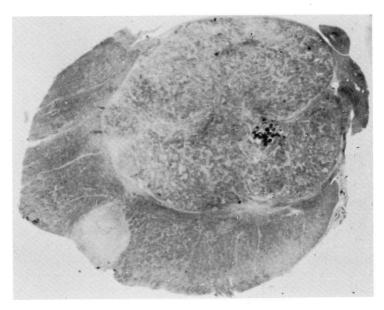

Figure 16–24. Ependymoma of the spinal cord. (Courtesy of Department of Neuropathology, Philadelphia General Hospital.)

The sexes are equally affected except in the case of meningiomas, which are commoner in women. Metastatic tumors are relatively common in adults.

Pathology. Primary intraspinal tumors occur in the same varieties as are found intracranially, but astrocytomas and oligodendrogliomas are uncommon, and the ependymomas account for about half of all neoplasms arising within the substance of the cord.[81, 85, 86] Meningiomas and neurofibromas account for almost two-thirds of all primary spinal tumors; this is fortunate, because they are discrete and extramedullary, and are usually situated on the posterior or posterolateral aspect of the cord, a position which facilitates surgical removal. Uncommon tumors include lipomas, teratomas, and cholesteatomas. Malignant ganglioneuromas usually start in the chest and reach the spinal canal via the intervertebral foramina. Hematogenous spread from carcinoma elsewhere is exceedingly rare in the cord itself, but cord compression from extradural or intradural deposits or from metastases in the vertebrae is common. In Hodgkin's disease and multiple myeloma, symptoms of cord compression usually occur late in the disease,[97] but occasionally they are the first to appear. Compression can occur in leukemia, but acute damage from hemorrhage into or around the cord is more common. Vascular malformations are not rare.[99]

From the pathological point of view, primary intraspinal tumors behave very much like their intracranial equivalents. An exception is the neurofibroma of the cauda equina, which is usually less encapsulated and more malignant than the acoustic neurinoma; the tumor fills the lumbar sac, and may extend outward through the foramina. The cord oligodendroglioma differs from the cerebral type in tending to spread via the subarachnoid space; it often arises from the filum terminale.

Many intramedullary tumors are accompanied by syringomyelia-like cavitation of the cord. They were present in 155 of 186 cases reported by Poser. The reason for this association is not known, but it appears unlikely that the cavitation is always due to secondary necrosis. In addition, the central canal may be dilated for a considerable distance both above and below the tumor (a hydromyelia).

Seeding from an intracranial glioma can produce multiple secondary deposits in the subarachnoid space from the foramen magnum to the lumbar sac. As a rule this is a late development, and the patient does not live long enough for the deposits to grow large enough to produce spinal compression.

The Mechanics of Spinal Compression

The spinal cord is smaller than the canal in which it lies, so at first there is room for a tumor to expand, especially posteriorly.

Extramedullary tumors, which are by far the most common, disturb function by local pressure at the point of contact with the cord, by displacement of the cord against the hard spinal canal, and by interference with the blood supply to the cord, thereby producing lesions within its substance ("compression myelitis"), and by compression of nerve roots.

In time, the mass of the tumor and the edematous cord will block the subarachnoid space.

Clinical Features. In the days before contrast myelography, the localization of spinal tumors and the differentiation between extramedullary and intramedullary types depended solely on a careful weighing of evidence derived from the history and physical examination. Such clinical evaluation can provide the right answer in some cases, but it is often impossible to be sure of the correct level and extent of the tumor, whether it be intramedullary or extramedullary. Myelography provides a more accurate means of identifying the level of the lesion, and may help to distinguish between intramedullary and extramedullary tumors,

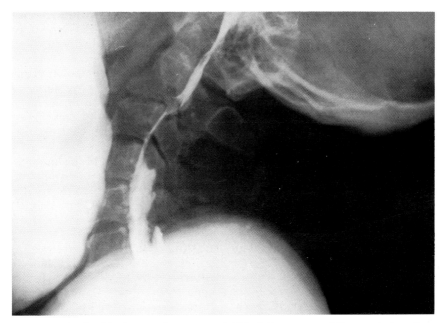

Figure 16–25. Myelogram showing partial block by a tumor of the cervical cord.

but the diagnosis depends, in the final analysis, on inspection of the exposed cord.

ONSET. The mode of onset is usually slow, and the course is steadily or intermittently progressive. The earliest symptom may be pain, paresthesias, weakness, or sphincter symptoms.

Pain is the presenting symptom in more than 50 per cent of all cases of intraspinal tumors, whether intramedullary or extramedullary. In some cases, it is a persistent midline ache which is usually worse at night. More often it takes the form of a root pain, on one or both sides, which is aggravated by coughing and straining, and by jolting the spine. The patient may adopt a bizarre posture to avoid it. Sometimes the pain does not appear to originate in the back at all but is of root distribution, and in this event it may falsely suggest the presence of thoracic or abdominal disease. These early pains may come and go *over a period of many months* before other signs of cord involvement become obvious. Sometimes the pain is replaced by an uncomfortable sense of constriction, as from a tight girdle, situated above, at, or below the level of the tumor. Diffuse pain may be present below the level of the lesion; it is thought to be due to irritation of the spinothalamic tracts. Thus, pain in the lumbar region and legs can be experienced as a result of compression of the cervical or thoracic cord.[25] Local tenderness may be present not only over the spine but also in the area to which the pain is referred and this adds to the risk of mistaking the pain of a spinal tumor for evidence of visceral disease.

Paresthesias in the form of pins and needles, numbness, tightness, coldness, etc., are very common. If they are due to root irritation, they are felt in the periphery of the affected dermatomes. If they result from cord compression, they appear in the feet, buttocks, and hands, and less often in the trunk. In cervical and thoracic tumors, flexion of the neck can produce showers of pins and needles down the spine and into the limbs (Lhermitte's sign). This can also occur in combined system disease, multiple sclerosis, spondylosis, and other diseases of the cervical cord.

SENSORY DISTURBANCES. Objective sensory signs are sometimes absent in the early stage of spinal compression from extramedullary tumors, though subjective paresthesias may be prominent. In the less common intramedullary group, objective sensory impairment occurs earlier, but is often slight and difficult to elicit. With unilateral involvement of posterior roots, there is mild depression of pain and touch sensibility in the periphery of the affected dermatomes, whereas in central lesions there is bilateral or unilateral loss of pain and temperature sensibility in the areas corresponding to the segmental distribution of the tumor. In time, the long sensory tracts will be involved in both types of lesion, with sensory loss below the level of the lesion. With a unilateral tumor, there is usually loss of pain and temperature on one side and impairment of vibration and touch on the other, but this is not always the case; compression from an extramedullary mass, neoplastic or otherwise, will sometimes give a pattern of sensory loss which is more appropriate to an intramedullary lesion. Depression of pain and temperature sensibility on one-half of the body, and pyramidal weakness on the opposite side, constitute the Brown-Séquard syndrome, signifying a lesion confined to one-half of the cord.

In extramedullary tumors, the upper level of sensory loss may be considerably below the level of the lesion, and is denser peripherally than proximally, whereas in intramedullary lesions, sensory impairment is usually maximal at the level of the tumor and less marked peripherally; relative sparing of the sacral segments, especially in the perianal area, is not uncommon in thoracic and cervical tumors.

MOTOR DISTURBANCES. Motor symptoms may occur before or after the onset of sensory disturbances. If they are due to affection of the motor pathways in the cord, the limbs feel heavy and tire easily. A leg may buckle when the patient puts weight on it. If the hand is affected, there is a tendency to drop things before weakness is obvious. In the case of a cervical tumor, weakness first appears in one arm, then in the leg on that side, followed in its turn by the opposite leg and hand, in that order. Sometimes difficulty in walking is greater than it should be, as judged by the degree of weakness, because sensory ataxia is present owing to involvement of the posterior columns. The discrepancy between the patient's incapacity to walk and the presence of reasonable power in the legs may falsely suggest the presence of hysteria.

A second source of muscular weakness is damage to the anterior horn cells, either by direct pressure or by interference with the blood flow in the anterior spinal artery. The latter explanation probably applies to the weakness and wasting of the small muscles of the hand which sometimes occurs in high cervical tumors. Atrophic weakness is sometimes seen in the lower limbs in tumors of the lumbosacral segments of the cord because the motor roots are involved. In such cases, the legs are hypotonic, and the extensor plantar reflex which would ordinarily be expected is abolished by lower motor neuron paralysis of the muscles which dorsiflex the foot and toes. Tumors of the cauda equina will, of course, produce lower motor neuron paralysis in the legs.

Spinal compression causes spasticity below the level of the lesion. There is loss of abdominal reflexes, hyperactive tendon reflexes, extensor plantar responses, and ankle clonus. The degree of spasticity varies widely from case to case; it is often absent in cord compression of sudden onset. Case-to-case variations may perhaps be accounted for by the relative extent to which the corticospinal and reticulospinal pathways are involved. Hypertonicity is a greater source of disability than weakness in some cases. It is more marked in the extensor groups than in the flexors, and sooner or later extensor spasms will occur. With complete physiological transection of the cord, the extensor spasms give place to painful flexor spasms, and the legs are held in an attitude of generalized flexion.

SPHINCTER DISTURBANCES. Sphincter symptoms are common but are very seldom the first to appear. If the compression is above the level of the sacral segments, the bladder becomes irritable and spastic, with consequent frequency and precipitancy of micturition; sometimes there is incontinence. If, however, the sacral segments or the efferent fibers to the bladder are involved, dribbling incontinence results. If tone persists in the sphincters and the detrusor is paralyzed, the patient may be able to overcome retention by manual compression of the lower abdomen when he wishes to void. Bowel function is less disturbed. There is usually constipation and retention of feces, but incontinence will occur if the stools are loose.

OTHER SIGNS. Tumors of the thoracic and cervical cord can disturb sweating below the level of the lesion. At first, sweating may be increased, but as compression increases, it is lost—a useful sign which can be elicited by passing the hand lightly down the trunk: The fingers will pass from moist to dry skin at approximately the level of the lesion.

Impotence can occur with a lesion at any level of the cord, but is prominent and early in affections of the sacral segments and cauda equina.

Papilledema occasionally occurs in tumors of the cervical, thoracic, or lumbar cord, and disappears if the tumor is removed. No satisfactory explanation has been offered for this curious and misleading phenomenon.

Regional Syndromes

The Foramen Magnum. Tumors at the foramen magnum may be half inside and half outside the skull. Consequently, they can involve the eleventh and twelfth cranial nerves, and may produce cerebellar symptoms. Rarely, intermittent attacks of unconsciousness occur, probably as a result of transient internal hydrocephalus. Compression of the posterior columns gives rise to appropriate sensory loss at an early stage. Pain in the distribution of the second occipital root is common, and is often aggravated by movements of the head. Flexion of the head produces paresthesias down the trunk and into the legs in some cases. Motor symptoms develop early, and are usually seen first in the arm on the affected side, spreading thereafter to the ipsilateral leg and contralateral leg and arm, in that order. Cutaneous sensory loss is first discerned in the upper cervical root zones; later on, compression of the cord produces appropriate sensory impairment below the level of the lesion.

Papilledema can occur if the tumor extends into the posterior fossa. Partial or complete block is usually found on lumbar puncture, and myelography will define the lower end of the tumor.

Cervical Region. In addition to the distal motor and sensory disturbances common to spinal compression at all levels, weakness, wasting, and fibrillation are often seen in the muscles of the neck, shoulder girdle, and upper arm; the diaphragm on the affected side may be paralyzed. Lesions of the fifth cervical segment produce weakness of the supinator longus, biceps, deltoid, rhomboids, and spinati. Sensory impairment may be found on the lateral aspect of the arm and forearm; it will occasionally involve the thumb as well. Inversion of the supinator reflex is a reliable sign of a lesion of the fifth cervical segment; the contraction of the supinator and biceps (C5) is lost, but flexion of the fingers (C6–7) is exaggerated. A tumor involving the sixth root or segment may produce pain down the outer side of the arm, paresthesias in the thumb and index finger, slight sensory blunting along the anterolateral border of the arm, forearm, and index finger, weakness of the triceps, and slight weakness of the extensor of the wrist, with consequent partial wrist drop. If the seventh segment or root is involved, pain may be felt down the outer aspect of the arm and forearm, and it may also spread into the pectoral muscles, which are supplied by the sixth and seventh cervical roots. Sensory impairment is maximal in the middle finger, and it may also be found in the posterior aspect of the forearm and arm. There is weakness of the flexors of the wrist and the flexors and extensors of the fingers, and the triceps jerk is lost. Tumors involving the eighth root can produce pain down the inner aspect of the arm and forearm, together with sensory impairment in the ring and little fingers and on the medial side of the forearm. There is weakness and wasting of the small muscles of the hand, and Horner's syndrome may be present.

The Thoracic Region. In tumors of the thoracic cord, the arms are spared. Tumors of the lower six thoracic segments will cause weakness of the lower abdominal muscles, so that when the abdomen is contracted, the umbilicus deviates upward (Beevor's sign). Motor, sensory, and sphincter disturbances conform to the usual pattern, and a girdle sensation is common. Unilateral root pains radiating to the lower part of the chest or abdomen may simulate disease of the lungs, pleura, or abdominal viscera. At this stage, there may *or may not be* other motor and sensory indications of spinal cord compression.

Lumbosacral Segments. A large number of functionally important segments are compressed into this small part of the spinal cord; quite small tumors can therefore produce considerable incapacity. In the early stage, a tumor involving the first and second lumbar segments can give rise to root pain in the groin and testicle, together with impotence and loss of the cremasteric reflexes, but weakness, sensory loss, and bladder symptoms rapidly supervene. Affections of the third and fourth segments will weaken the quadriceps, abolish the knee jerk, accentuate the Achilles reflex, and produce an extensor plantar response. Growths in this situation can produce a rather complicated clinical picture, because they involve the roots of the cauda equina as well as the spinal cord, thus leading to a combination of upper and lower motor neuron lesions.

Pain, either unilateral or bilateral, and of approximately sciatic distribution, is sometimes the presenting symptom of tumors in this region,[67] but it is usually possible to distinguish it from the more common pain of a prolapsed intervertebral disc by the fact that the pain is more diffuse, tends to be bilateral, and is often associated with paresthesias in the distribution of more than one root. A growth in the lumbosacral region, however, can produce sciatic pain with a distribution which is indistinguishable from that of an irritative lesion of the fourth or fifth lumbar root, but as time goes on, other telltale symptoms and signs appear—diffuse paresthesias, sphincter symptoms, or an extensor plantar reflex. In intramedullary lesions of this area, sensory loss may be limited to the perianal area (S3–S5).

The Cauda Equina. Neoplasms of the cauda equina[29, 67, 86] are rare. Meningiomas, small fibromas of the root sheaths, and giant tumors are the least uncommon. Lumbar pain is usually absent in the early stages, but it may occur in association with rigidity later on. Freedom from symptoms in the back may be misleading when the patient complains only of pain in the legs, especially if it is limited to the lower part of the limbs, but when it is influenced by change of posture, by movements of the spine, or by coughing and sneezing, it points to a spinal or intraspinal origin.

The pain may be unilateral or bilateral, distal or proximal. It is commonly of roughly sciatic distribution, whatever the situation of the tumor, but occasionally it may be felt in the front of one thigh or in the region of the adductors. It is a feature of firm, slowly growing neoplasms and is less marked in quickly growing infiltrative masses. Remissions of pain are not uncommon, and in an important minority, pain may precede the development of neurological signs by several months.

Tingling, numbness, or thermal sensations are a common accompaniment and may involve one or more dermatomes. Weakness and wasting are prominent, and fasciculation may be seen in the affected muscle. Eventually, sensory loss is prominent, its distribution depending on the roots affected. It may start in the perianal area (S3–S5). Tumors situated high up in the cauda equina may interfere with all the tendon reflexes, and there may be loss of cremasteric reflex as well; sometimes, though pain is unilateral, reflex changes are found bilaterally. Impotence arising early in the history indicates disease in the neighborhood of the conus, but it may also occur temporarily as the result of long-continued pain. Sphincter disturbances usually appear early.

Differential Diagnosis. The most common cause of cord compression after the age of 40 is spondylosis with a posterior osteophytic ridge or bar. For convenience, however, the list of conditions which can mimic a spinal tumor are dealt with in alphabetical order.

AMYOTROPHIC LATERAL SCLEROSIS. This condition can mimic a tumor when it starts with weakness, atrophy, and fasciculation in one limb, or as slowly progressive spastic weakness of the legs, but it is excluded by the presence of root pains, paresthesias, a girdle sensation, sensory impairment, early sphincter symptoms, and abnormalities in the spinal fluid. The disease is painless except for muscle cramps.

ANGIOMATOUS MALFORMATIONS. Angiomatous malformations may present as a sudden partial or complete transverse lesion of the cord, usually preceded by root pain, or with gradual and often intermittent symptoms of cord dysfunction. Since other tumors sometimes behave thus, the diagnosis depends on demonstrating the characteristic appearance of a malformation by myelography, or selective aortography, but small intramedullary vascular tumors can seldom be identified as such unless they bleed into the cord and subarachnoid space. Rarely, auscultation over the spine will disclose a bruit. Neurofibromatosis is present in some cases.

ARACHNOIDITIS *(Meningitis Serosa Circumscripta, Chronic Spinal Meningitis).* This condition can occur (1) in relationship to active spinal disease, (2) as a result of previous meningitis, injury, spinal anesthesia, or myelography, or (3) without these antecedents. Since operation usually fails to relieve the symptoms, there is often doubt whether arachnoiditis is the cause of the symptoms or whether some other underlying process is responsible. Arachnoiditis commonly gives rise to slowly progressive spastic weakness of the limbs. There is usually complete or incomplete spinal block, and myelography discloses a highly characteristic appearance: Drops and strings of contrast medium are held up at various levels of the cord and cannot be shifted by altering the patient's position.

BASILAR IMPRESSION (PLATYBASIA). This can mimic a very slowly growing tumor at the foramen magnum.[72] The diagnosis depends on radiological demonstration of basilar invagination: In a lateral view, part of the odontoid process will lie above a line drawn from the back of the hard palate to the posterior border of the foramen magnum (Chamberlain's line).

CEREBRAL PARAPLEGIA. This term is applied to spastic weakness of the legs caused by a bilateral parasagittal lesion of the motor cortex. If headache and seizures are absent, the resemblance to a spinal lesion can be close. Papilledema can occur in spinal tumors, further confusing the situation. Pointers to a spinal origin are root pains, a sensory level, and evidence of lower motor nerve involvement at the level of the tumor. Headache, seizures, and electroencephalographic abnormalities suggest a cerebral origin.

DÉJERINE-SOTTAS DISEASE (HYPERTROPHIC POLYNEURITIS). This disease can superficially resemble tumor of the cauda equina in that it gives rise to atrophic weakness and sensory loss in the legs, but its progress is exceedingly slow, sphincter symptoms are absent, the peripheral nerves are thickened, the condition is usually familial, and congenital abnormalities—clubbed feet, kyphoscoliosis, and cerebellar symptoms (nystagmus, dysarthria, intention tremor)—are not uncommon. Occasionally, the thickening of the roots within the spinal canal is sufficient to compress the cauda equina or cord.

EPIDURAL ABSCESS. Epidural abscess is recognized by severe pain in the back or neck, the development of weakness, sphincter disturbances, and sensory loss over a period of hours, and the presence of a focus of infection elsewhere in the body. The evolution of symptoms is far more rapid than is the case in a primary spinal tumor.

FUNGAL INFECTIONS OF THE NERVOUS SYSTEM. Infections by fungi usually produce subacute meningitis or meningoencephalitis; less often, they give rise to a large granuloma (e.g., a toruloma), which may mimic a tumor of the brain or cord. The organism can usually be found in the spinal fluid. Fungal infections are most common in debilitated individuals and in patients suffering from Hodgkin's disease and other lymphomas.

HODGKIN'S DISEASE. The lymphomas usually cause spinal compression late in the disease, and the compression is commonly situated in the thoracic region. Pyrexia, anemia, bone pain, enlargement of the liver, spleen, or lymph glands, and widening of the mediastinal shadows will suggest the correct diagnosis. In rare instances, compression of the spinal cord occurs before other signs are apparent, in which event the diagnosis will be made at operation.

HYDATID CYSTS. Cysts of this type occur in the vertebral column or in the epidural space. The bone is excavated, the radiological appearance resembling that of a myeloma. Spinal compression can occur. The diagnosis is to be thought of in patients who are living, or have lived, in areas where infestation is common. Casoni's cutaneous test may be positive or negative. There may be eosinophilia and clinical or radiological evidence of cysts elsewhere in the body, notably in the lungs, liver, long bones, and pelvic bones. Spinal compression can also be caused by *cysticercosis.*

INTERVERTEBRAL DISC DISEASE. Compression of the cord and cauda equina can occur either as the result of herniation of the nucleus pulposus or from spondylosis. The latter is common, but since some degree of spondylosis is common after the age of 50, the fact that it is present does not necessarily prove

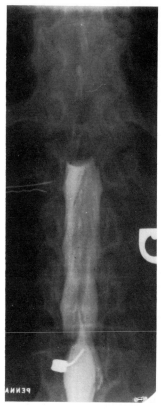

Figure 16–26. Myelogram showing obstruction of the column by a meningioma at L1 and a disc herniation between L3 and L4.

it responsible for the patient's symptoms (Fig. 16–26). There may be an accidental association of multiple sclerosis, subacute combined degeneration of the cord, or spinal tumor.[9]

KYPHOSCOLIOSIS. Advanced congenital kyphoscoliosis is an occasional cause of very slowly developing paraplegia; neurological symptoms occur only when the deformity is extreme. Root pains are usual, and they may be present for years before weakness of the legs becomes apparent. Motor signs are more prominent than sensory signs, and deterioration is very slow. Progression can sometimes be prevented by orthopedic measures to stabilize the spine.

LEUKEMIA. Leukemia usually produces symptoms as a result of extramedullary or intramedullary hemorrhage, and the onset is therefore abrupt, but occasionally leukemic deposits give rise to rapidly evolving spinal compression.

MALIGNANT METASTASES. Such metastases in the extradural space or in the vertebrae are common and give rise to spinal compression. The symptoms develop rapidly and progress faster than is usual in primary tumors of the cord. Sudden cord compression is sometimes caused by collapse of a vertebral body, but more often there is little or no radiological evidence of bone involvement, and the abrupt damage to the cord is presumably due to thrombosis of the spinal vessels. A primary growth may or may not be evident. The sedimentation rate is usually elevated in spinal metastases, whether the primary tumor is obvious or not. Evidences of denervation in the paraspinal muscles may be found by electromyography at an early stage in some cases.

MULTIPLE SCLEROSIS. After the age of 40, this disease sometimes causes slowly progressive pyramidal weakness of the limbs, with or without paresthesias in the fingers and toes or in the feet alone.

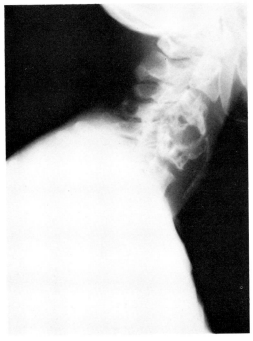

Figure 16–27. Invasion of the bodies of three cervical vertebrae by a myeloma. Despite signs of cervical cord compression, the patient had neither pain nor stiffness of the neck.

In the absence of a history of previous incidents, or of telltale signs of multiple lesions, examination of the spinal fluid and myelography are necessary to exclude a cord tumor. A high gamma globulin level in the cerebrospinal fluid or a paretic Lange curve in the absence of serologic evidence of syphilis is suggestive of multiple sclerosis.

MYELOMA. Myeloma acts like a spinal tumor (Fig. 16–27), and its distinction from other sources of cord compression depends on the demonstration of translucent "holes" in other bones, or (occasionally) of generalized osteoporosis. Bence Jones protein will be present in the urine in about 60 per cent of these patients, and atypical plasma cells can sometimes be found in the circulating blood. There is a significant rise in plasma globulin as determined by electrophoresis.

MYOPATHIES. Myopathies starting in the pelvic girdle and proximal muscles of the legs cause weakness and fatigue of the lower limbs which can mimic a neurological condition, but the reflexes are normal at first, and there is no sensory loss or sphincter difficulty. In myositis, the muscles are sometimes tender and may pit on pressure. Muscle biopsy may or may not be positive in the early stages of this complex group of diseases.

PAGET'S DISEASE. This malady can narrow the vertebral canal and compress the spinal cord.[94] It can also produce neurological symptoms by causing basilar impression (Fig. 16–28). There may or may not be pain in the spine, and neurological evidence of spinal compression comes on very slowly. The diagnosis is made by the radiological appearance of the vertebrae, long bones, skull, and pelvis, and elevation of serum alkaline phosphatase. Metastases from prostatic carcinoma can produce a rather similar radiological appearance in the vertebrae, but the *acid* phosphatase level is elevated.

POTT'S DISEASE. This is a common cause of spinal compression in countries in which bovine tuberculosis is rife. Spinal angulation following collapse of a vertebra can contribute to compres-

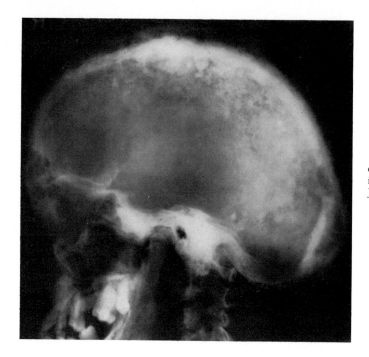

Figure 16–28. Paget's disease of the skull, with marked basilar invagination. (Courtesy of Dr. James Bull.)

sion, but granulation tissue and cold abscess play a more significant role in most cases. Local tenderness over the site of the caries, the characteristic radiological appearance, a high sedimentation rate, and evidence of past or present tuberculosis (lungs, lymph glands, kidney, epididymis, etc.) help to confirm the diagnosis.

SUBACUTE COMBINED DEGENERATION OF THE CORD (COMBINED SYSTEM DISEASE).   In this disease, there is no pain, sphincter symptoms are absent until late, and the combination of peripheral neuropathy, pyramidal signs, macrocytic anemia, and achylia gastrica is distinctive. In a few patients weakness of the legs and paresthesias of the hands and feet precede the blood changes, and the diagnosis can then be established by the Schilling test, or by failure of the patient to absorb radioactive vitamin B_{12}. If a patient with pernicious anemia and neurological symptoms continues to deteriorate despite adequate treatment with vitamin B_{12}, reinvestigation is called for to establish the reason for deterioration.

SUBACUTE NECROTIC MYELITIS.   This rare disease can simulate compression of the lumbosacral segments by giving rise to a mixture of upper and lower motor neuron weakness, sensory loss, sphincter symptoms, and raised cerebrospinal fluid protein (Chap. 15). Myelography is necessary to exclude a tumor or other pathology.

SYPHILIS.   Neither tabes dorsalis nor acute syphilitic transverse myelitis is likely to cause confusion. Gumma of the cord is rare, but it can resemble a rapidly growing spinal neoplasm. In hypertrophic cervical pachymeningitis (which is not always syphilitic), the dura is greatly thickened over several segments, giving rise to root pains and atrophic weakness in the upper limb; ultimately there may be features of spinal cord compression. In Erb's syphilitic paraplegia, a rare disease, there is very slowly progressive spastic weakness of the legs, accompanied by early sphincter symptoms but without sensory loss. The diagnosis of these conditions is helped by positive serology of the blood and spinal fluid, lymphocytic pleocytosis and rise of protein in the spinal fluid in the active phase of the disease and evidence of syphilis elsewhere in the body. Myelography is mandatory if the patient is suffering from spinal compression because a positive serology does not necessarily mean that the symptoms are due to syphilis. If antisyphilitic treatment improves the symptoms, it goes some way to confirm the diagnosis, but failure to improve, as for instance in Erb's syphilitic paralysis, does not exclude a syphilitic origin.

Treatment of Spinal Tumors. Surgical treatment is indicated when there is evidence of compression of the spinal cord or the roots of the cauda equina, but the degree of success will depend partly on the surgical accessibility of the tumor and partly on the degree of incapacity which is already present at the time of operation. With extradural tumors, remarkable restoration of function may occur even when spastic weakness of the legs has been present for a year or more, but little improvement is to be expected when flaccid paraplegia has resulted from extensive damage to the cord. Partial removal followed by x-ray therapy can produce beneficial results. The best results are obtained in meningiomas and neurinomas. Care of the bladder, the prevention of bed sores, and the treatment of reflex muscle spasms and contractures are carried out on the same lines as for the care of paraplegia following spinal injury (p. 514).

Pain can be a problem. It can be treated by bilateral percutaneous cervical cordotomy but if the expectation of life is short, the patient can usually be made comfortable and slightly euphoric by the old-fashioned but reliable Brompton mixture, each dose of which contains ½ grain of morphia and an ounce of gin or whiskey, flavored with honey.

NEUROFIBROMATOSIS (VON RECKLINGHAUSEN'S DISEASE)

Neurofibromatosis is an inherited disease characterized by café-au-lait patches and multiple tumors of nerve roots, peripheral nerves, and cranial nerve roots. It is sometimes associated with other developmental abnormalities, notably syringomyelia, and there is an unusually high incidence of meningiomas and gliomas in affected persons.

Mild forms of the disorder are extremely common, and the question arises as to the criteria needed for diagnosis of the "disease." There should be both café-au-lait spots and one or more neurofibromas. In the course of a comprehensive study, Crowe and his colleagues[21] also emphasized the number of café-au-lait spots; they calculated that the risk of developing neurofibromatosis is one in 50 for people with five or more spots, as against one in 4000 for individuals with only one spot.

Etiology. The disorder appears to be due to a genetically determined abnormality which results in pigmentary changes in the skin and overgrowth of ectodermal and mesodermal elements in the skin, nervous system, and other organs.

Pathology. Tumors in the peripheral nerves are of three types: (1) single cutaneous neurofibromas derived from the connective tissue of small terminal branches of peripheral nerves, (2) neurofibromas arising from the sheath of nerve trunks, and (3) large plexiform neurofibromas with overgrowth of adjacent subcutaneous tissue. Tumors also occur on cranial and spinal nerve roots. Sarcomatous change can occur in neurofibromas of any type, but this is rare.[38]

Abnormalities found outside the nervous system include polycystic disease of the lung and osteitis fibrosa cystica. Local overgrowth of connective tissue may cause hemihypertrophy of the tongue, face, or an extremity.

Clinical Features. Although the lesions may be present in the skin and nerves at birth, they are seldom recognized before puberty. In a full-blown case, the skin is covered by hundreds of small pedunculated or sessile growths which are round, soft, and painless. They are most numerous on the trunk, and vary in size from a pinhead to an orange. Some of them are bluish in color because an angiomatous element is present. Sometimes there is gross overgrowth of the tissues around a plexiform neuroma ("elephantiasis neuromatosis"). Subperiosteal neurofibromas can cause pain, swelling, local rarefaction, and spontaneous fractures. Tumors may occur in the mediastinum and retroperitoneal area and are not uncommon on the eighth and fifth cranial nerves, on the spinal roots, and in the cauda equina.

Whereas intracranial and intraspinal neurofibromas usually interfere with function, the skin tumors seldom give rise to symptoms. Occasionally, they become painful when situated in an area exposed to pressure, and exceptionally they give rise to pain and paresthesias within the distribution of the affected nerve. Motor symptoms are extremely rare.

In most cases, the worst result of neurofibromatosis is cosmetic. Not only may there be multiple neurofibromas and café-au-lait spots, but "port wine" nevi and pedunculated anemic nevi are also often present. The overgrowth of tissue which occurs in association with plexiform neuroma can be extremely disfiguring.

Treatment. There is nothing that can be done for these patients except to remove tumors and hypertrophic folds of skin if they are in the way or are painful or disfiguring. The removal of single tumors is attended by a high rate of recurrence, and it is said that such surgical intervention may lead to an increased rate of growth.

Other Tumors of Peripheral Nerves

Solitary tumors of peripheral nerves are rare. The benign schwannoma is a neoplasm of slow growth which can be encountered on the flexor aspect of the limbs, on the intercostal nerves, and on the brachial plexus. When it arises from an intercostal nerve in the posterior mediastinum, it can grow through the intervertebral foramen into the spinal canal, forming a dumbbell tumor. These growths give rise to pain and paresthesias with or without sensory loss or muscular weakness in the distribution of the affected nerve. The malignant schwannoma[38] is usually found on large nerve trunks, and although it does not infiltrate the surrounding tissues, it can recur after removal and can also metastasize to distant areas, such as the lung. About 50 per cent of published cases have occurred in von Recklinghausen's disease.

Metastatic deposits from carcinomas elsewhere in the body seldom involve the peripheral nerves but may envelop the brachial or lumbar plexus, giving rise to paresthesias, weakness and wasting, and sensory impairment, in that order. Surprisingly, pain may be absent when infiltration is confined to a plexus, but it can be very intense, as in Pancoast's tumor, as a result of infiltration of the adjacent ribs and spine. Pelvic endometriosis can "metastasize" to the sciatic nerve and to the spinal cord.

REFERENCES

1. Andrew, J. S., and Nathan, P.: Lesions of the anterior frontal lobes and disturbances of micturition and defecation. *Brain* 87:233, 1964.
2. Appleby, A., Foster, J. B., and Hudgson, P.: The diagnosis and management of the Arnold-Chiari anomalies in adult life. *Brain* 91:131, 1968.
3. Argires, J. P., and Nelson, J.: Pituitary Apoplexy: A review of the literature and two case reports. *Southern Med. J.* 59:785, 1966.
4. Bailey, P.: *Intracranial Tumors.* 2nd Ed. Charles C Thomas, Springfield, Ill., 1948.
5. Bailey, P., and Bucy, P. C.: Oligodendrogliomas of the brain. *J. Path. Bact.* 32:735, 1929.
6. Bailey, P., and Cushing, H.: *Tumors of the Glioma Group.* J. B. Lippincott Co., Philadelphia, 1926.
7. Bell, D. S.: Speech functions of the thalamus inferred from the effects of thalamotomy. *Brain* 91:619, 1968.
8. Bouchard, J., and Pierce, C. B.: Radiation therapy in the management of neoplasms of the central nervous system, with a special note in regard to children: Twenty years' experience. *Amer. J. Roentgenol.* 84:610, 1960.
9. Brain, W. R., Northfield, D., and Wilkinson, M.: The neurological manifestations of cervical spondylosis. *Brain* 75:187, 1952.
10. Bull, J. W. D., and Sutton, D.: The diagnosis of paraphysial cysts. *Brain* 72:487, 1949.

11. Castellano, F., Guibetti, B., and Olivecrona, H.: Pterional meningiomas "en plaque." *J. Neurosurg.* 9:188, 1952.

12. Cawthorne, T., and Griffith, A.: Primary cholesteatoma of the temporal bone. *Arch. Otolaryngol.* 73:252, 1961.

13. Cheek, W. R., and Taveras, J. M.: Thalamic tumors. *J. Neurosurg.* 24:505, 1966.

14. Cherington, M., and Schneck, S. A.: Clivus meningiomas. *Neurology* 16:86, 1966.

15. Chusid, J. D., and DeGutierrez-Mahoney, C. G.: Glioblastoma of septum pellucidum. *J. Neurosurg.* 11:251, 1954.

16. Chutorian, A. M., Schwartz, J. F., Evans, R. A., and Carter, S.: Optic gliomas in children. *Neurology* 14:83, 1964.

17. Clarke, E.: Cranial and intracranial myelomas. *Brain* 77:61, 1954.

18. Cooper, I. S., Kernohan, J. W., and Craig, W. McK.: Tumors of the medulla oblongata. *Arch. Neurol. Psychiat.* 67:269, 1952.

19. Critchley, M.: *The Parietal Lobes.* Edward Arnold Publishers, Ltd., London, 1953.

20. Critchley, M.: Phenomenon of tactile inattention with special reference to parietal lesions. *Brain* 72:538, 1949.

21. Crowe, F. W., Schull, W. J., and Neel, J. V.: *A Clinical, Pathological, and Genetic Study of Multiple Neurofibromatosis.* Charles C Thomas, Springfield, Ill., 1956.

22. Dandy, W. G.: Congenital cerebral cysts of the cavum septi pellucidi and cavum vergae: *Arch. Neurol. Psychiat.* 25:44, 1931.

23. Danowski, T. S.: Craniopharyngioma with involvement of the hypophysis and hypothalamus. *Clinical Endocrinology*, Vol. I. Williams and Wilkins Co., Baltimore, 1962, Chap. 14

24. Dees, S. C., and McKay, H. W.: Pseudotumor cerebri during treatment of children with asthma by steroids: Report of three cases. *Pediatrics* 23:1143, 1959.

25. Dodge, H. W., Svien, H. J., Camp, J. D., and Craig, W. M.: Tumors of the spinal cord without neurologic manifestations, producing low back pain and sciatica. *Proc. Mayo Clin.* 26:88, 1951.

26. Dow, R. S., and Moruzzi, G.: Frontal ataxia. *Physiology and Pathology of the Cerebellum.* University of Minnesota Press, Minneapolis, 1958, p. 404.

27. Elliott, F. A.: *Handbook of Neurology*, Vol. 2. North Holland Publishing Co., Amsterdam, 1969, Chap. 24.

28. Elliott, F. A., and McKissock, W.: Acoustic neuroma: Early diagnosis. *Lancet* 2:1189, 1954.

29. Elsberg, C. A.: *Surgical Disease of the Spinal Cord, Membranes, and Nerve Roots: Symptoms, Diagnosis, and Treatment.* Paul B. Hoeber Div., Harper and Row, New York, 1941.

30. Foley, S.: Benign forms of intracranial hypertension in "toxic" and "otitic" hydrocephalus. *Brain* 78:1, 1955.

31. Foster, J. B., Hudgson, P., and Pearce, G. W.: The association of syringomyelia and congenital cervico-medullary anomalies: Pathological evidence. *Brain* 92:25, 1969.

32. Frazier, C. H.: Tumor involving the frontal lobe alone. A symptomatic survey of 105 verified cases. *Arch. Neurol. Psychiat.* 35:525, 1936.

33. Gardner, W. J.: Hydrodynamic mechanism of syringomyelia: Its relationship to myelocele. *J. Neurol. Neurosurg. Psychiat.* 28:247, 1965.

34. Gassel, M. M.: False localizing signs. *Arch. Neurol.* 4:526, 1961.

35. Gassel, M. M., and Davies, H.: Meningiomas in the lateral ventricles. *Brain* 84:605, 1961.

36. Givre, A., and Olivecrona, H.: Surgical experiences with acoustic tumors. *J. Neurosurg.* 6:396, 1949.

37. Gordy, P. D.: Neurinomata of the gasserian ganglion. *J. Neurosurg.* 22:90, 1965.

38. Gore, I.: Primary malignant tumors of nerve. *Cancer* (N.Y.) 5:278, 1952.

39. Grant, D. K.: Papilledema and fits in hyperparathyroidism with a report of three cases. *Quart. J. Med.* 22:243, 1953.

40. Grant, F. C., and Austin, G. M.: The diagnosis, treatment, and prognosis of tumors affecting the spinal cord in children. *J. Neurosurg.* 13:535, 1956.

41. Greer, M.: Benign intracranial hypertension. VI: Obesity. *Neurology* 15:382, 1965.

42. Guttmann, L.: Statistical survey of one thousand paraplegics and initial treatment of traumatic paraplegia. *Proc. Roy. Soc. Med.* 47:1099, 1954.

43. Guttmann, L.: The problem of treatment of pressure sores in spinal paralysis. *Brit. J. Plastic Surg.* 7:196, 1955.

44. Henson, R. A., Crawford, J. B., and Cavanagh, J. B.: Tumors of the glomus jugulare. *J. Neurol. Neurosurg. Psychiat.* 16:127, 1953.

45. Howell, D. A.: Upper brain-stem compression and foraminal impaction with intracranial space occupying lesion and brain swelling. *Brain* 82:525, 1959.

46. Hughes, B.: *The Visual Fields.* Blackwell Scientific Publications, London, 1954.

47. Ingram, F. D., and Bailey, O. T.: Cystic teratomas and teratoid tumors of the central nervous system in infancy and childhood. *J. Neurosurg.* 3:511, 1946.

48. Ingraham, F. D., Bailey, O. T., and Barker, W. F.: Medulloblastoma cerebelli. *New Eng. J. Med.* 238:171, 1948.

49. Jane, J. A., and McKissock, W.: The importance of failing vision in early diagnosis of suprasellar tumors. *Brit. Med. J.* 2:5, 1962.

50. Jefferson, G.: Extrasellar extension of pituitary adenomas. *Proc. Roy. Soc. Med.* 33:433, 1940.

51. Jefferson, G.: The differential diagnosis of lesions of the posterior fossa. *Proc. Roy. Soc. Med.* 46:719, 1953.

52. Kearns, T. P., Salassa, R. M., Kernohan, J. W., and MacCarty, C. S.: Ocular manifestations of pituitary tumor in Cushing's syndrome. *Arch. Ophthal.* 62:242, 1959.

53. Kelly, R.: Colloid cysts of the third ventricle. *Brain* 74:23, 1951.

54. Kernohan, J. W., and Sayre, G. P.: Tumors of the central nervous system, atlas of tumor pathology. Armed Forces Institute of Pathology, Washington, D.C., Section X, Fasc. 35, 37, 1952.

55. Ladenheim, J. C., and Sachs, E.: Familial tumors of the glomus jugulare. *Neurology* 11:303, 1961.

56. Langfitt, T. W., Weinstein, J. D., and Kassell, N. F.: Cerebral vascular paralysis produced by intracranial hypertension. *Neurology* 15:622, 1965.

57. Lassman, L. P., and Arjona, V. E.: Pontine gliomas in childhood. *Lancet* 1:913, 1967.

58. Lichtenstein, B. W.: Cervical syringomyelia and syringomyelia-like states associated with Arnold-Chiari malformation and platybasia. *Arch. Neurol. Psychiat.* 49:874, 1943.

59. Lysak, W. R., and Svien, H. J.: Long term follow-up of patients with pseudotumor cerebri. *J. Neurosurg.* 25:284, 1966.

60. McKissock, W., and Paine, K. W.: Primary tumors of the thalamus. *Brain* 81:41, 1958.

61. McLauren, R. L., Bailey, O. T., Schurr, P. H., and Ingraham, F. D.: Myelomalacia and multiple cavitations of spinal cord secondary to adhesive arachnoiditis: An experimental study. *Arch. Path.* 57:138, 1954.

62. McNealy, D. E., and Plum, F.: Brainstem dysfunction with supratentorial mass lesions. *Arch. Neurol.* 7:10, 1962.

63. Malamud, N.: Psychiatric disorders with tumors of the limbic system. *Arch. Neurol.* 17:113, 1967.

64. Matson, D. D., and Crofton, F. D. L.: Papilloma of the choroid plexus in childhood. *J. Neurosurg.* 17:1002, 1960.

65. Meyer, J. S., and Barron, D. W.: Apraxia of gait, a clinico-pathologic study. *Brain* 83:261, 1960.

66. Milansky, A., Cowie, V. A., and Donohue, C.: Cerebral gigantism in childhood. *Pediatrics* 40:395, 1967.

67. Milnes, J. M.: The early diagnosis of tumors of the cauda equina. *J. Neurol. Neurosurg. Psychiat.* 16:158, 1953.

68. Molinatti, G. M., Camanni, F., Massara, F., et al.: Implantation of the sella turcica with 90-yttrium in the treatment of Cushing's syndrome of pituitary origin. *J. Clin. Endoc.* 27:861, 1967.

69. Mones, R. J.: Increased intracranial pressure due to metastatic disease of venous sinuses: A report of 6 cases. *Neurology* 15:1000, 1965.

70. Netsky, M. G.: Syringomyelia. A clinicopathological study. *Arch. Neurol. Psychiat.* 70:741, 1953.

71. Northfield, D. W. C.: Rathke-pouch tumors. *Brain* 80:293, 1957.

72. O'Connell, J. E., and Turner, J. W. A.: Basilar impression of the skull. *Brain* 73:405, 1950.

73. Oldstone, M. B. A.: Endocrinological aspects of benign intracranial hypertension. *Arch. Neurol.* 15:362, 1966.

74. Olsen, A., and Horrax, G.: Symptomatology of acoustic tumors with special reference to atypical features. *J. Neurosurg.* 1:371, 1944.

75. Patterson, R., DePasquale, N., and Mann, S.: Pseudotumor cerebri. *Medicine* 40:85, 1961.

76. Penfield, W., and Roberts, L.: *Speech and Brain Mechanisms.* Princeton University Press, Princeton, N.J., 1959.

77. Poppen, J. L., Reyes, V., and Horrax, G.: Colloid cysts of the third ventricle. Report of 7 cases. *J. Neurosurg.* 10:242, 1953.

78. Ray, B. S., and Dunbar, H. S.: Thrombosis of the dural sinuses as a cause of pseudotumor cerebri. *Ann. Surg.* 134:376, 1951.

79. Riddoch, G.: Progressive dementia without headache or changes in the optic discs due to tumors of the third ventricle. *Brain* 59:225, 1936.

80. Rigolosi, R. S., Schwartz, E., and Glick, S. M.: Growth-hormone deficiency in acromegaly: Results of pituitary apoplexy. *New Eng. J. Med.* 279:362, 1968.

81. Russell, D. S., Rubinstein, L. J., and Lumsden, C. E.: *The Pathology of Tumors of the Nervous System.* Edward Arnold, London, 1959.

82. Russell, R. W. R., and Pennybacker, T. B.: Craniopharyngioma in the elderly. *J. Neurol. Neurosurg. Psychiat.* 24:1, 1961.

83. Scherer, H. J.: The forms of growth in gliomas. *Brain* 63:1, 1940.

84. Schisano, G., and Olivecrona, H.: Neurinoma of the gasserian ganglia and trigeminal root. *J. Neurosurg.* 17:306, 1960.

85. Shenkin, H. A., and Alpers, B. J.: Clinical and pathological features of gliomas of the spinal cord. *Arch. Neurol. Psychiat.* 52:87, 1944.

86. Slooff, J. L., Kernohan, J. W., and MacCarty, C. S.: *Primary Intramedullary Tumors of the Spinal Cord and Filum Terminale.* W. B. Saunders Co., Philadelphia, 1964.

87. Smith, R. A.: Pineal tumors. *Univ. Mich. Med. Bull.* 27:33, 1961.

88. Sohn, D., Valensi, Q., and Miller, S. P.: Neurologic manifestations of Hodgkin's disease. *Arch. Neurol.* 17:429, 1967.

89. Sotos, J. F., Dodge, P. R., Muirhead, D., et al.: Cerebral gigantism in childhood. A syndrome of excessively rapid growth with acromegalic features and a nonprogressive neurological disorder. *New Eng. J. Med.* 271:109, 1964.

90. Sprague, J. M., Chambers, W. W., and Stellar, E.: Attentive, affective, and adaptive behavior in the cat. *Science* 133:165, 1961.

91. Symonds, C. P.: Otitic hydrocephalus. *Neurology* 6:681, 1956.

92. Thomas, J. E., and Waltz, A. G.: Neurological complications of nasopharyngeal tumors. *J.A.M.A.* 192:103, 1965.

93. Toglia, J. U., Netsky, M. G., and Alexander, E.: Epithelial (epidermoid) tumors of the cranium. Their common nature and pathogenesis. *J. Neurosurg.* 23:384, 1965.

94. Turner, J. W. A.: The spinal complications of Paget's disease. *Brain* 63:321, 1940.

95. White, H. H.: Brainstem tumors occurring in adults. *Neurology* 13:292, 1963.

96. White, P., and Ross, A. T.: Inanition syndrome in infants with anterior hypothalamic neoplasms. *Neurology* 13:974, 1963.

97. Williams, H. M., Diamond, H. D., Craver, L. F., and Parsons, H.: *Neurological Complications of Lymphomas and Leukemias.* Charles C Thomas, Springfield, Ill., 1959.

98. Wright, R. L.: Hemorrhage into pituitary adenomas. Report on two cases with spontaneous recovery. *Arch. Neurol.* 12:326, 1965.

99. Wyburn-Mason, R.: *The Vascular Abnormalities and Tumors of the Spinal Cord and Its Membranes.* Henry Kimpton, London, 1943.

100. Zacks, S. I.: Chemodectomas occurring concurrently in the neck (carotid body), temporal bone (glomus jugulare) and retroperitoneum. Report of a case with histochemical observations. *Amer. J. Path.* 34: 293, 1958.

101. Zimmerman, H. M., Netsky, M. G., and Davidoff, L. M.: *Atlas of Tumors of the Nervous System,* Lea and Febiger, Philadelphia, 1956.

102. Zülch, K. J.: *Brain Tumors: Their Biology and Pathology.* 2nd Amer. Ed. Springer Publishing Co., Inc., New York, 1965.

103. Zwetnow, M.: Cerebral blood flow autoregulation to blood pressure and intracranial pressure variations, *Scand. J. Clin. Lab. Invest.,* Suppl. 102, 1968.

CHAPTER SEVENTEEN

Nutritional Disorders

BERIBERI

Beriberi is characterized by peripheral neuropathy and cardiac failure, occurring as a result of inadequate availability of vitamin B_1 in relation to the patient's carbohydrate intake.[26]

Etiology. The disease occurs as a result of long-continued deficiency of vitamin B_1 (thiamine) intake in persons on a relatively high carbohydrate diet. It does not occur in pure starvation, but is seen when the vitamin intake falls below 0.3 mg./1000 nonfat calories. In this event, there is insufficient thiamine present for the complete metabolism of glucose, and pyruvate accumulates in the tissues. Beriberi can also result from inadequate absorption of thiamine from the gastrointestinal tract as a result of chronic dysentery and steatorrhea, and exceptionally a mild form can occur as the result of the prolonged use of relatively insoluble sulfonamides which destroy the colonic bateria that normally synthesize vitamin B_1. The polyneuropathy which sometimes occurs in hyperemesis gravidarum is considered to be due to thiamine deficiency; occasionally it is accompanied by retrobulbar neuropathy and nerve deafness. Chronic alcoholism with its attendant gastritis and hepatic derangement predisposes individuals to beriberi.

Pathology. In the chronic type there is widespread degeneration of the peripheral nerves, ranging from slight degeneration to complete disappearance of the myelin sheaths and axons.[23] There is little, if any, interstitial reaction. Similar changes have been described in the renal and splanchnic plexuses. Chromatolysis may be found in anterior horn cells of the lumbar cord and also in the cells of the posterior root ganglia. In cardiac beriberi, there is dilatation of the heart with chronic venous congestion and generalized edema.

Clinical Features. Subacute and chronic beriberi is usually divided into wet (cardiac) and dry (neuritic) types, but mixed forms are common. In the wet form of the disease, there is edema of the limbs which later spreads to the trunk and is associated with serous effusions in the peritoneal and pleural cavities. The pulse is rapid and weak, and sudden death may occur. The neuritic form starts with tingling and a sense of numbness in the feet, pain in the calves, and weakness in the legs; the latter is most severe peripherally, so that foot drop develops. The weakness is associated with tenderness of the muscles, absent ankle jerks, and peripheral cutaneous sensory impairment. If the disease is allowed to continue, weakness and sensory impairment of peripheral distribution occur in the upper limbs, with loss of tendon reflexes. Aphonia may occur from degeneration of the laryngeal nerves.[11]

Rarely, an acute form is seen. Over the course of one or two days, there is anorexia and vomiting, and a rapidly progressing paralysis of the legs, arms, and trunk, together with the features of congestive heart failure. Death may occur within as little as two days.

Laboratory Aids. The protein content of the spinal fluid is normal. The plasma pyruvate level is raised above the normal upper limit of 1.2 mg./100 ml. of blood when the patient has been fasting for four hours. Some of the toxic neuropathies resemble vitamin deficiency neuropathy clinically, and in doubtful cases help can be derived from the pyruvate tolerance test. Two doses of 50 gm. of glucose are given by mouth at 30 minute intervals. The blood pyruvate is estimated 30, 60, and 90 minutes after the first dose. In normal persons it does not rise above 1.4 mg. per cent, but in patients with thiamine deficiency values over 2.0 gm. are usually obtained. After two weeks of intensive parenteral vitamin B_1 treatment, pyruvate tolerance returns to normal in vitamin B_1 deficient subjects. Tolerance is also abnormal in intoxications with substances which interfere with SH groups (e.g., heavy metals), which are essential to the normal functioning of the enzyme systems responsible for pyruvate oxidation, *but it does not return to normal after vitamin B_1 administration.*

Prognosis. The cardiac manifestations clear up rapidly on treatment, but the neuritic symptoms may take months to disappear if degenerative changes have already occurred in the peripheral nerves.

Treatment. For the first week, 100 mg. of thiamine should be given intravenously every day; thereafter, the patient should receive 10 mg. daily by mouth. It is usual to supplement this treatment with the whole vitamin B complex. The patient should be given a mixed diet. In some prisoners of war who had been on a totally inadequate diet for several years, the neuritic symptoms at first became worse when the diet was increased. Congestive heart failure re-quires absolute bed rest. When thiamine deficiency is secondary to disease of the gastrointestinal tract or liver, appropriate treatment must be given to prevent the condition from occurring again.

THIAMINE DEFICIENCY IN INFANTS

This condition occurs in breast-fed infants and is due to maternal nutritional deficiency. There are gastrointestinal, cerebral, neurological, and cardiac symptoms. The infant fails to thrive, loses weight, and is fretful. Vomiting and diarrhea are almost always present. Cardiac weakness appears, with tachycardia, cyanosis, and peripheral edema. The cerebral manifestations are those of Wernicke's encephalopathy—ptosis, ocular palsies, nystagmus, and ataxia. Choreiform movements and weakness of the laryngeal nerves may also be present. Untreated, the patient rapidly lapses into coma. Prompt intravenous administration of thiamine can save life unless the patient is already moribund.

Lesions resembling those of Wernicke's encephalopathy are also found in *subacute necrotizing encephalomyelopathy,* a rare disease of childhood, which is often familial. It appears in the first year of life and progresses to a fatal termination within 12 months. Brain biopsy from one patient showed a gross deficiency of thiamine triphosphate,[9] although thiamine and its other phosphate esters were present in normal concentrations. It has been suggested that in this disease some factor or factors inhibit the formation of thiamine triphosphate.

PELLAGRA

The disease is characterized by cutaneous eruptions, gastrointestinal disturbances, and mental symptoms, coupled in a minority of cases with the symptoms of peripheral neuropathy and signs of pyramidal degeneration.

Etiology. The cutaneous eruption is due to deficiency of nicotinic acid.

The associated angular stomatitis results from riboflavin deficiency, and the peripheral neuropathy is probably due to lack of thiamine. The degenerative changes in the pyramidal tracts, when present, are attributed to deficiency of vitamin B_{12}. The disease occurs in ill-nourished people. Pellagra can occur in the midst of plenty, as for instance in patients who refuse to eat, in chronic alcoholics, and in individuals with chronic gastrointestinal disorders which prevent the absorption of vitamins.

Pathology. In severe cases, there is chromatolysis, poor staining of cell nuclei, and increase of pigment in the cells of the cerebral cortex and basal ganglia.[15, 19] Degeneration has been found in the dorsal columns of the spinal cord, the pyramidal and spinocerebellar tracts, and the peripheral nerves, but these spinal features are probably due to associated thiamine and vitamin B_{12} deficiency.

Clinical Features. The skin eruption occurs chiefly on the exposed parts of the face, neck, forearms, and legs.[26] Starting as an erythema which may resemble sunburn, it progresses to a reddish-brown roughening of the skin. Angular stomatitis and dermatitis of the scrotum are frequently encountered. The tongue is painful, fiery red, and fissured, and in severe cases the epithelium may be shed, leaving a smooth surface. There is usually nausea, anorexia, abdominal cramps, and recurrent diarrhea. Achlorhydria is common.

Mental disturbances are prominent.[24] The patient is irritable, cannot sleep, and suffers from memory impairment and slowness of cerebration. In severe cases, psychotic episodes can occur; these may take the form of an acute confusional state, maniacal outbursts, or hallucinatory episodes. Signs of peripheral neuropathy and spinal cord degeneration are less prominent than the dermatitis and mental disturbances, and they may be absent. The peripheral neuropathy is akin to what is found in neuritic beriberi. There may also be spastic ataxia with impairment of proprioception in the legs,

increased knee jerks, and extensor plantar responses.

Untreated, the disease runs a protracted course lasting many years. Commonly, the first attack and subsequent exacerbations of the disease occur in the spring and early summer.

When the skin lesions are not prominent, and the factor of malnutrition is not obvious, the condition may be mistaken for subacute combined degeneration of the cord, but careful scrutiny of the tongue and skin, and the history of recurrent gastrointestinal upsets, will indicate the true state of affairs.

Treatment. The diet should be well balanced, with a high caloric content. Nicotinic acid should be given in doses of 100 mg. five times a day by mouth, or 10 to 20 mg. may be injected in saline four times a day. If severe encephalopathy is present, 100 mg. of nicotinamide should be given intravenously and a similar amount intramuscularly every day, together with 100 mg. five times a day by mouth. A high caloric diet, including a quart of milk per day, is desirable. If the spinal cord or peripheral nerves are involved, it is wise to administer 1000 μg. vitamin B_{12} and 100 mg. thiamine by intramuscular injection twice a week.

LATHYRISM

Outbreaks of spastic weakness of the legs have frequently occurred in India during times of famine if the lathyrus pea has been included in the diet in large quantities; when pea flour is included in a *normal* diet, the disease is unlikely to develop. It has been suggested that the condition may result from the destruction of some essential factor in the food by the lathyrus pea rather than from a direct toxic action on the spinal cord.[11]

Pathology. Degenerative changes have been found in the pyramidal tracts and in the dorsal columns.

Clinical Features. The onset is usually sudden, with pain in the back and weakness and stiffness of the legs. There are no symptoms referable to the cranial nerves. Paraplegia develops rapidly, with increased tendon reflexes and extensor plantar responses. Paresthesias occur, but objective sensory loss is not described. Even if ingestion of the lathyrus pea is stopped, spastic weakness of the legs may be permanent. There is no known treatment.

STARVATION NEUROPATHIES

Under conditions of prolonged protein and vitamin deficiency, coupled with a relatively high carbohydrate intake, nutritional neuropathies are not limited to beriberi, pellagra, or Wernicke's encephalopathy, but include retrobulbar neuropathy, nerve deafness, laryngeal palsy, spinal ataxia, the "burning feet" syndrome, spastic paraplegia, and a myasthenic type of bulbar paralysis. These may be present singly or in varying combinations.[11] They occur almost exclusively in tropical and subtropical regions; they were not seen, for instance, in prisoner-of-war camps or concentration camps in Germany during World War II. In Jamaica, Nigeria,[31] and Senegal, a similar spectrum of disorders is found in individuals who cannot be described as starving or even grossly undernourished, but whose diet is poor.[25] Optic atrophy, nerve deafness, pyramidal signs, polyneuropathy, and sensory ataxia occur in varying combinations, with or without other evidence of vitamin deficiency. It has been suggested that in this group of cases, the disorder may be due to a combination of vitamin deficiency and the ingestion of cassava (manioc tapioca), which contains cyanide. Demyelination can be produced in animals by giving repeated small doses of cyanide, and in man, cyanides possibly play a role in the demyelination found in Leber's optic atrophy and in tobacco amblyopia.

Retrobulbar Neuropathy. Retrobulbar neuropathy was seen in those who took part in the siege of Madrid in the Spanish Civil War and in prisoners of war in Japanese prison camps during World War II.[11, 16, 26] It has also been recorded in the civilian populations of Nigeria and Jamaica. The neuropathy occurs either on its own or in association with other nutritional disorders, and is probably due to vitamin B deficiency. Impairment of vision is bilateral, and usually comes on insidiously over a period of weeks; exceptionally, severe visual loss occurs in a matter of a few days.[16] There is loss of central vision in the form of centrocecal scotomas, the peripheral fields being unaffected at first. There is temporal pallor of the discs. In contrast to the night blindness of vitamin A deficiency, vision is worse during the day. Normal vision can be restored if treatment is started early by the administration of vitamin B_{12}, but once optic atrophy has appeared, no improvement can be expected.

Bilateral Nerve Deafness. Bilateral nerve deafness of gradual onset and progressive course is usually associated with retrobulbar neuropathy or other features of vitamin B deficiency in prisoners of war, but it is rare in beriberi.[11, 26] Evidence of labyrinthine disorder in the form of vertigo was common among prisoners in Batavia in World War II and was associated with deafness in a minority of cases.

Laryngeal Palsy. Laryngeal palsy is sometimes associated with pharyngeal weakness, and it occurs in association with other evidence of nutritional neuropathy, including classic beriberi.[11] There is weakness of adduction and abduction of the vocal cords, and the voice is weak and hoarse.

The "Painful Feet" Syndrome. Unpleasant burning paresthesias of the feet are sometimes seen in alcoholic neuropathy and in peripheral vascular disease; in the latter, paresthesias can occur without the usual signs of peripheral neuropathy. The condition was described as "acrodynia" in the siege of Paris during the Franco-Prussian War and as the "paresthetic-causalgia syndrome" in the siege of Madrid. It was common among prisoners of war in Japanese prison camps.[11] It is probably due to a deficiency of pantothenic acid, which is necessary for the complete oxidation of pyruvate, because normal volunteers deprived of pantothenic acid have developed burning paresthesias.[4] The condition starts with tingling in the feet, which soon gives place to intense burning sensations and shooting pains; discomfort is worse at night, preventing sleep, and in severe cases the patient experiences exquisite discomfort on putting the foot to the ground. It is said to be relieved by daily injections of 40 mg. of calcium pantothenate; in prisoners of war, it was helped by a diet rich in vitamin B complex. When the "burning feet" syndrome is the result of alcoholic neuropathy or peripheral vascular disease, it is more resistant to treatment.

Ataxia. Ataxia, due to impairment of position sense in the legs, is prominent in some cases of prolonged malnutrition.[31] It is usually accompanied by loss of vibration sense in the toes, peripheral sensory impairment, tenderness of the calf muscles, and absence of ankle jerks. The arms are unaffected, and there are no signs of cerebellar disease. Generally speaking, the clinical picture is that of peripheral neuropathy with an unusually severe impact on proprioceptive nerve fibers, but in a few cases the tendon reflexes remain brisk and the plantar responses are extensor, indicating that the spinal cord is also involved. Treatment is by the administration of the entire vitamin B complex, together with re-educational exercises for the control of ataxia.

Spastic Paraplegia. An outbreak of spastic paraplegia occurred in the Changi Camp in Singapore in 1942 and 1943. Mental disturbances and spastic weakness of the legs came on rapidly; sometimes the arms were affected as well. A few patients died, and survivors either recovered completely or were left with residual evidence of pyramidal disorder. The condition was reminiscent of lathyrism, but the lathyrus pea was not part of the diet in this group of cases, and the precise cause of the condition remains unknown.[11]

Bulbar Paralysis. In 1944, there was an outbreak of a myasthenia gravis-like syndrome among American prisoners of war in Cabanatuan.[18] The symptoms were induced by fatigue and were improved by rest and administration of potassium chloride and neostigmine. There was blurring of vision, diplopia, ptosis, and weakness of the muscles of the face and neck, together with dysphagia and dysarthria. Sporadic outbreaks of a somewhat similar condition occurred in Switzerland in 1886 and in Japan in 1896.

SUBACUTE COMBINED DEGENERATION OF THE CORD (COMBINED SYSTEM DISEASE, FUNICULAR MYELOSIS)

Subacute combined degeneration of the cord is usually associated with pernicious anemia and is characterized pathologically by degeneration of the peripheral nerves and posterior and lateral columns of the spinal cord, and clinically by a combination of spasticity, ataxia, and peripheral neuropathy. It is seen in all races, but it is most common in persons of North European stock. It is very rare in children and usually affects people over 40 years of age.

Etiology. The neurological damage is due not to anemia but to defective absorption of vitamin B_{12} which is necessary as a coenzyme for nucleoprotein synthesis. The absorption of vitamin B_{12} requires the presence of a gastric intrinsic factor which is absent in addisonian pernicious anemia. The associated achylia gastrica is not responsible, for occasionally subacute combined degeneration of the cord occurs in patients with free acid. It occurs on rare occasions in diabetes and in elderly subjects with hypochromic anemia, and also in association with megaloblastic anemia caused by the fish tapeworm (*Diphyllobothrium latum*),[6] fatty diarrheas, partial or total gastrectomy, and in patients with a blind loop of intestine following anastomosis or with a dilated loop of intestine proximal to a stricture. In the

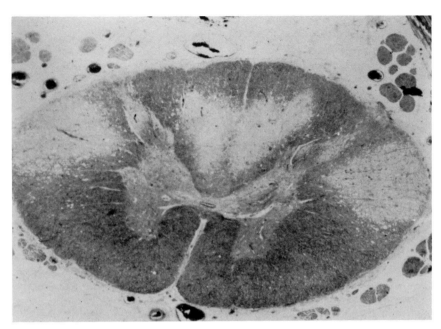

Figure 17–1. Subacute combined degeneration of the cord (posterolateral sclerosis). (Courtesy of Department of Neuropathology, Philadelphia General Hospital.)

last two instances, the defective absorption of vitamin B_{12} may be related to bacterial growth because normal absorption of the vitamin can be restored by treatment with antibiotics. It is thought that the bacteria use the vitamin B_{12} content of the food.

Pathology. Degeneration occurs in the peripheral nerves, spinal cord, and, to a lesser extent, the cerebral hemispheres.[23] In the cord, it is most marked in the posterior columns (causing sensory ataxia), and in the corticospinal tracts. The myelin sheaths swell and break up, after which the axons degenerate, and the debris is absorbed by macrophages. This process is at first patchy in distribution and imparts a spongy appearance to cross sections of the spinal cord (status spongiosus). There is fragmentation of the myelin and degeneration of the axons of the peripheral nerves, with minor secondary changes in the anterior horn cells. Small foci of demyelination may occur in the brain. The bone marrow is hyperplastic, with megaloblasts predominating. The peripheral blood shows hyperchromic macrocytic anemia; nucleated red cells may

be present, and there is leukopenia with relative lymphocytosis; myelocytes are present in severe cases.

Clinical Features. The disease starts insidiously, with paresthesias in the toes, feet, and fingertips. These gradually become more obtrusive, and soon the patient begins to find that his legs are becoming weak and unsteady. The hands become clumsy, so that the patient has difficulty in doing up buttons. There may be complaints of shooting pains in the feet and legs, or of a tight girdle sensation around the chest or abdomen, and the patient may experience showers of pins and needles down the back and into the limbs when he flexes his neck (Lhermitte's sign); the latter is also seen in other diseases of the spinal cord.

The neurological symptoms are usually accompanied by the pallor, lassitude, dyspepsia, and sore tongue of pernicious anemia, *but in some instances, the neurological symptoms precede the anemia.*

The nature of the physical signs depends on the relative impact of the disease on the peripheral nerves, the posterior columns, and the pyramidal tracts.

If peripheral nerve degeneration predominates, there is weakness, hypotonia, slight wasting, and impairment of the peripheral tendon reflexes. The plantar response is physiological in the early stages, but sooner or later extensor responses will be present. There is an early loss of vibratile and joint sensibility in the toes, spreading later to the ankle joints, the knees, and the hands; the loss of vibration is more widespread than can be explained by the peripheral neuropathy alone, and may involve the sacrum early in the disease because of posterior column degeneration. There is slight peripheral impairment of touch, pain, and temperature in the legs, and the same changes appear later in the hands. Tenderness of the calf muscles is an important sign, indicating the presence of peripheral neuropathy.

When degeneration of the posterior and lateral columns dominates the clinical picture, the legs become spastic, weak, and ataxic. The tendon reflexes are increased, the abdominal reflexes are impaired, and the plantar responses are extensor, but even in this variety of the disease, there is often evidence of polyneuropathy in the form of tender calf muscles and slight cutaneous sensory impairment of peripheral distribution. Ataxia is due mainly to the loss of proprioception caused by posterior column degeneration.

Sphincter symptoms are usually late in appearing, but in untreated cases there is ultimately paraplegia in flexion, gross weakness of the upper limbs, and incontinence of urine and feces.

The cranial nerves are spared, with the exception of the optic nerve.[27] Bilateral central scotomas have been reported; these may occur early or late in the disease and may also be present in pernicious anemia without any evidence of subacute combined degeneration of the cord.

Mental symptoms are seldom seen nowadays, but they were common and sometimes severe prior to the discovery of the value of liver extract and vitamin B$_{12}$.[12] Irritability, confusion, amnesia, depression, paranoid trends, and severe psychotic reactions have been recorded. The mental symptoms are seen in patients without severe anemia, and also in patients whose anemia has been brought under control, and are therefore regarded as secondary to the degeneration of the cerebral white matter which occurs in the disease. This conclusion is sustained by the presence of generalized slow waves in the electroencephalogram of severely affected individuals.

Laboratory Aids. The spinal fluid is normal. There is usually a histamine-fast achlorhydria, and the blood count and bone marrow will eventually provide evidence of macrocytic hyperchromic anemia, although this may be absent in the early stages. The icteric index may be elevated. The Schilling test will disclose defective absorption of vitamin B$_{12}$. The plasma vitamin B$_{12}$ level is usually below 100 $\mu\mu$g./ml. The appearance of marked reticulocytosis 10 days after an injection of vitamin B$_{12}$ or crude liver extract helps to confirm the diagnosis.

Clinical Course. Whereas spontaneous remissions are not infrequent in pernicious anemia, the neurological symptoms are slowly progressive and lead to death if untreated. Neurological improvement usually starts within two months of the commencement of treatment, and the first aspect to improve is the peripheral neuropathy. If incapacity is still present at the end of six months of thorough treatment, further improvement is unlikely.

Treatment. Progress of the disease can be arrested by intramuscular administration of vitamin B$_{12}$. Two hundred micrograms of the vitamin should be given every day for two weeks, and weekly for the next two months. Thereafter, a maintenance dose of 50 μg. every three or four weeks will usually suffice to keep the blood count in the neighborhood of 5,000,000 red cells/mm.^{3} Two milliliters of the crude liver extract can be used in place of the vitamin. Iron should also be given for the first two months, while the blood count is rising. Folic acid is contraindicated; it aggravates the neurological condition. It is essential to warn the patient with addisonian pernicious anemia that the treatment will have to be continued indefinitely. Physiotherapy and re-educational exercises are indicated for patients severely incapacitated by weakness and ataxia.

NUTRITIONAL DISORDERS OF ALCOHOLISM

The nutritional disorders of alcoholism include polyneuropathy, Wernicke's syndrome, Korsakoff's syndrome, cerebellar degeneration,[13] and retrobulbar neuropathy.[28] Central pontine myelinolysis and Marchiafava's disease may also be nutritional in origin. The cause of alcoholic myopathy is not known at present.

Alcoholic Polyneuropathy

The commonest neurological manifestation of alcoholism is a distal, symmetrical polyneuropathy. Pathologically, it is characterized by wallerian degeneration, and there may also be segments of nerves in which the myelin is lost but the axis cylinders remain. As in all nutritional types of generalized forms of polyneuropathy, degeneration is most intense in the longest nerves and in their most distal portions.

Etiology. This condition is often equated with neuritic beriberi and is, therefore, attributed to a specific deficiency of thiamine, but it must be emphasized that the nutritional factors involved in alcoholic polyneuropathy are not fully defined. Deficiency of pyridoxine and pantothenic acid can also cause degeneration of peripheral nerves, as can lack of vitamin B_{12}. It will be recalled that, during treatment of tuberculosis with isoniazid, a conditioned deficiency of vitamin B_6 is produced, with neuropathy as an important manifestation. The rarity of wet beriberi in communities in which alcoholic polyneuropathy is rife implies that the re-

lationship of vitamin B deficiency to the latter is not fully understood. It must be allowed, however, that patients who continue to drink excessive quantities of alcohol seem to be protected from polyneuropathy if they are on a well-balanced diet containing an adequate amount of the entire vitamin B complex.

Clinical Features. In the mild type, there is asymptomatic wasting of the leg muscles with depression of the knee jerks and absence of the ankle jerks. The calf muscles are tender, and there is often patchy impairment of pain and touch sensation over the toes and feet. The situation may deteriorate rapidly, so that in a few days the patient is severely incapacitated; this is reminiscent of the acute deterioration which is sometimes seen in tropical beriberi.

In severe cases, there is a slowly progressive development of paresthesias in the toes, feet, and distal portions of the legs. Paresthesias may take the form of numbness and tingling, or there may be bitter complaints of "burning feet." This may be so severe that the patient does not dare put the foot to the ground, and dislikes having his feet touched. There may also be complaints of dull pain with lancinating exacerbations similar to the lightning pains of tabes. Peripheral wasting, weakness, sensory impairment, and loss of peripheral stretch reflexes are the rule. Some degree of foot drop is usual; wrist drop is rare. The triceps, biceps, and supinator jerks are usually intact, but if there is peripheral weakness, the finger jerk is reduced or lost. In early cases, especially when neuropathy is predominantly sensory in type, the reflexes may be brisker than normal.

The protein content of the spinal fluid is usually normal, but it may be slightly elevated in severe cases. Even with the best treatment, recovery is a slow process, taking a year or more, and the patient may be left with persistent weakness of the distal musculature. The cornerstone of treatment is the daily administration of thiamine, parenterally in the first instance, and later by mouth. Physiotherapy may help, but it is badly tolerated by patients with severe pain, paresthesias, and tenderness. If foot drop is permanent, an appliance is necessary to correct it.

Wernicke's Encephalopathy

This condition was first described by Wernicke in 1881. It is usually due to acute thiamine deficiency in chronic alcoholics but also occurs in diseases of the gastrointestinal tract and occasionally in hyperemesis gravidarum.[7] Typical cases occurred in Changi Camp, Singapore, during World War II as a result of vitamin deficiency and a predominantly carbohydrate diet; most of the patients also developed neuritic beriberi.

Pathology. There is patchy necrosis of nerve cells in the hypothalamus, the mamillary bodies, the periaqueductal region, and the vestibular nuclei.[2, 28] Punctate hemorrhages are present in only about 50 per cent of cases (Fig. 17–2). They are not an essential feature of this disease and probably reflect a bleeding diathesis caused by hepatic or renal disease.

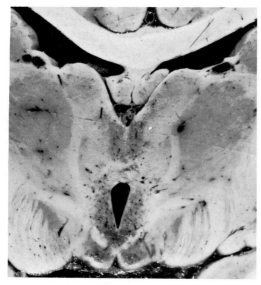

Figure 17–2. Wernicke's encephalopathy. The wall of the third ventricle is discolored and there are many small hemorrhages. (From Robbins, S.: *A Textbook of Pathology.* 2nd Ed. W. B. Saunders Co., Philadelphia, 1962.)

Histopathological changes similar to those occurring in Wernicke's disease are found in subacute necrotizing encephalomyelopathy in infants. This is not a nutritional disease, but it is pertinent to the present theme in that brain biopsy has shown an absence of thiamine triphosphate, which is present in the normal brain.

Clinical Features. The onset is rapid, with diplopia, mental changes, and ataxia. Diplopia is usually due to weakness of the external recti, together with some paresis of conjugate movement. Nystagmus is common. In advanced cases, the pupils may be small and nonreacting. Ataxia affects the legs most, so that standing and walking may be impossible, or the condition may be limited to slight unsteadiness of gait and inability to perform heel-to-toe walking. The labyrinthine responses to caloric stimulation may be reduced or absent,[14] unilaterally or bilaterally, and this probably contributes to the instability of stance and gait. Polyneuropathy is often present. Mental changes of varying degree are found in the great majority of cases; usually the patient is apathetic, disoriented, and forgetful. A smaller number are agitated, confused, and hallucinated; these may show all the features of delirium tremens. Yet other patients display the features of Korsakoff's psychosis. The body temperature may be subnormal.

Untreated, Wernicke's encephalopathy is likely to be fatal, but cases of moderate severity clear up rapidly with proper treatment; in severe cases, the mental state clears very slowly, and the patient may be left with a Korsakoff's psychosis for many months. The ataxia and ocular symptoms are due solely to thiamine deficiency, but some other factor may be responsible for the mental changes.

Treatment. The patient should be given 100 mg. of thiamine by injection daily for a week, followed by 50 mg. daily by mouth for as long as is necessary. It is desirable to give the other components of the vitamin B complex as well, notably nicotinamide.

Korsakoff's Syndrome

This syndrome is variously defined, but as described by Korsakoff in 1887, it consisted of confusion, defective memory for recent events, a tendency to confabulate, and polyneuritis. However, the amnesia-confabulatory aspect of the syndrome can occur in nonalcoholic patients with subarachnoid hemorrhage, head injuries, cerebral tumors, meningitis, and toxemia of pregnancy. In alcoholics, mental symptoms may be present in the absence of polyneuropathy, but they are often associated with the features of Wernicke's encephalopathy.[21, 28]

The patient's memory for recent events is poor. He may not remember things which happened a few minutes previously; familiar faces and surroundings are forgotten, so that he readily becomes disoriented as to place and time, and this causes confusion and apprehension. The memory blanks are filled in with detailed but fictitious accounts of his activities, and these may be so convincing and circumstantial that the examiner accepts them in good faith. Some of this confabulation probably represents a reliving of long-past events, so that they are not so much fictitious as dislocated in time. In some cases, confabulation is not apparent, or it is so only to a very slight extent.

It is not only the capacity to form and retain memories which is disturbed; there is also impairment of perception and of concept formation, and the result is gross disturbance of mind, mood, and behavior in the more severe cases. The patient may be either quiet or noisy, or one phase may succeed the other. Complete recovery occurs in only a small proportion of patients, most patients continuing to show some defect of memory after the acute phase has passed. The treatment is the same as for Wernicke's encephalopathy.

Retrobulbar Neuropathy

Retrobulbar neuropathy is described on pages 87 and 479.

Cerebellar Degeneration

This condition occurs predominantly in middle-aged males who have been hard drinkers for a considerable time and who have been chronically undernourished.[13, 29] It is regarded as a nutritional disease. Pathologically,[22] there is more or less circumscribed degeneration of the vermis and the anterior and superior aspects of the hemispheres. The outstanding symptom is cerebellar ataxia of gait, which comes on very slowly over weeks or months and may then stabilize; sometimes there is rapid worsening of ataxia following an alcoholic spree. Incoordination of the hands, intention tremor, cerebellar dysarthria, nystagmus, and truncal instability are mild in comparison with the difficulty in gait. The condition can coexist with polyneuropathy and Wernicke's disease.

Central Pontine Myelinolysis

In 1959, Adams and his colleagues[1] described a hitherto unrecognized entity characterized by a symmetrical area of demyelination in the base of the pons, in three patients with chronic alcoholism and in one with scleroderma with nutritional deficiency. Most of the cases published since then have been in alcoholics, and the disease has been observed in association with Wernicke's disease, pellagra, and alcoholic cerebellar degeneration,[3] but it also occurs in nonalcoholics.[8]

The lesion takes the form of a single symmetrical focus of demyelination of variable size, in the center of the basis pontis. There is extensive demyelination and reduction in the number of oligodendrocytes, but the axis cylinders, nerve cells, and blood vessels are relatively preserved. There is also pathological evidence of a peripheral neuropathy in some cases.

The disease presents as a rapidly developing quadriplegia with pseudobulbar palsy, but in many instances the lesion is too small to cause symptoms and is only discovered at autopsy. When symptoms do appear, death commonly follows in from three to four weeks. There is as yet no effective treatment.

Alcoholic myopathy is described on page 548.

MARCHIAFAVA-BIGNAMI'S DISEASE

First described in 1898 by Carducci, a pupil of Marchiafava, this disorder is found in association with chronic alcoholism or malnutrition or both, predominantly but not exclusively in Italians. It is thought to be a form of alcoholic encephalopathy.

Pathologically, the disease is characterized by sharply demarcated areas of demyelination of the central fibers of the corpus callosum and (in some cases) of the anterior commissure, cortical subarcuate fibers, the centrum ovale, the optic chiasm, and the cerebellar peduncles (Fig. 17–3). There is demyelination in the affected areas, with persistence of axons but no inflammatory changes.[17, 23]

The clinical picture is so unspecific that antemortem diagnosis is seldom possible. Following a period of gradual intellectual decline, usually but not always in an alcoholic, there is a rapid onset of symptoms, which may appear so abruptly as to suggest a vascular lesion. In other cases, there is a premonitory period of apathy and akinesia. There may be agitation, severe memory loss, delirium tremens, hallucinations, seizures, and dysarthria or aphasia. Dementia increases, and pyramidal signs appear in the limbs. The symptoms and signs are so like those of some cases of a rapidly advancing tumor of the corpus callosum that the differential diagnosis should not depend on a history of alcoholism or malnutrition alone: Contrast studies are necessary in order to exclude the possibility of a neoplasm. Syphilis of the nervous system and presenile dementia have also to be excluded by appropriate studies. The disease is slowly progressive and results in death in three to six years. There is no treatment.

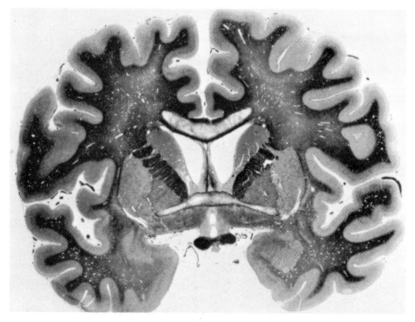

Figure 17–3. Marchiafava-Bignami disease, showing degeneration of the anterior commissure and the cortical portion of the corpus callosum. (From Baker, A. B.: *Clinical Neurology*. Paul B. Hoeber Div., Harper and Row, New York, 1955.)

REFERENCES

1. Adams, R. D., Victor, M., and Mancall, E. L.: Central pontine myelinolysis. *Arch. Neurol. Psychiat.* 81:154, 1959.
2. Bailey, F. W.: Histopathology of polioencephalitis hemorrhagica superior (Wernicke's disease). *Arch. Neurol. Psychiat.* 56:609, 1946.
3. Bailey, O. T., Bruno, M. S., and Ober, W. B.: Central pontine myelinolysis. *Amer. J. Med.* 29:902, 1960.
4. Bean, W. B., and Hodges, R. E.: Pantothenic acid deficiency induced in human subjects. *Proc. Soc. Exp. Biol. Med.* 96:693, 1954.
5. Bethell, F. H., Castle, W. B., Conley, C. L., and London, I. M.: Present status of treatment of pernicious anemia. *J.A.M.A.* 171:2092, 1959.
6. Bjorkenheim, G.: Neurological changes in pernicious tapeworm anemia. *Acta Med. Scand.*, Suppl. 260, 140:1, 1951.
7. Campbell, A. C. P., and Biggart, J. H.: Wernicke's encephalopathy (polioencephalitis haemorrhagica superior): Its alcoholic and nonalcoholic incidence. *J. Path. Bact.* 48: 245, 1939.
8. Chason, J. L., Landers, J. W., and Gonsalez, J. E.: Central pontine myelolysis. *J. Neurol. Neurosurg. Psychiat.* 27:317, 1964.
9. Cooper, J. R., Itokawa, Y., and Pincus, J. H.: Thiamine triphosphate deficiency in subacute necrotizing encephalopathy. *Science* 164:79, 1969.
10. Cravioto, H., Korein, J., and Silberman, J.: Wernicke's encephalopathy. *Arch. Neurol.* 4:510, 1961.
11. Denny-Brown, D.: Neurological conditions resulting from prolonged and severe dietary restriction. *Medicine* 26:41, 1947.
12. Ferraro, A., Arieti, S., and English, W. H.: Cerebral changes in the course of pernicious anemia and their relationship to psychic symptoms. *J. Neuropath. Exp. Neurol.* 4: 217, 1945.
13. Furmanski, A. R.: The deficiency state cerebellar syndrome. *J. Nerv. Ment. Dis.* 114: 519, 1951.
14. Ghez, C.: Vestibular paresis: A clinical feature of Wernicke's disease. *J. Neurol. Neurosurg. Psychiat.* 32:2, 1969.
15. Greenfield, J. G., and Holmes, J. M.: A case of pellagra; the pathological changes in the spinal cord. *Brit. Med. J.* 1:815, 1939.
16. Hobbs, H. E., and Forbes, F. A.: Visual defects in prisoners of war from Far East. *Lancet 2:* 149, 1946.
17. Ironside, R., Bosanquet, F. D., and McMenemey, W.: Cerebral demyelination of the corpus callosum (Marchiafava-Bignami's disease). *Brain* 84:212, 1961.
18. Katz, C. J.: Neuropathologic manifestations found in a Japanese prison camp. *J. Nerv. Ment. Dis.* 103:456, 1946.
19. Langworthy, O. R.: Lesion of the central nervous system characteristic of pellagra. *Brain* 54:291, 1931.
20. Leikin, S. L.: Pernicious anemia in childhood. *Pediatrics* 25:91, 1960.
21. Malamud, N., and Skillikorn, S. A.: Relationship between Wernicke and Korsakoff syndrome. *Arch. Neurol. Psychiat.* 76:585, 1956.
22. Mancall, E. L., and McEntee, W. J.: Alterations of the cerebellar cortex in nutritional encephalopathy. *Neurology* 15:303, 1965.
23. Meyer, A.: Anoxias, intoxications, and metabolic diseases. *Neuropathology.* Edited by Greenfield, J. G., Edward Arnold Publishers, Ltd., London, 1958, Chap. 4.
24. Spies, T. D., Aring, C. D., Gelperin, J., and Bean, W. B.: The mental symptoms of pellagra: Their relief with nicotinic acid. *Amer. J. Med. Sci.* 196:461, 1938.
25. Spillane, J. D.: Tropical neurology. *Proc. Roy. Soc. Med.* 62:403, 1969.
26. Spillane, J. D.: *Nutritional Disorders of the Nervous System.* E. & S. Livingstone, Edinburgh, 1967.
27. Turner, J. W. A.: Optic atrophy associated with pernicious anemia. *Brain* 63:225, 1940.
28. Victor, M., and Adams, R. D.: Effect of alcohol on the nervous system. *Res. Pub. Ass. Res. Nerv. Ment. Dis.* 32:526, 1953.
29. Victor, M., Adams, R. D., and Mancall, E. L.: A restricted form of cerebellar cortical degeneration occurring in alcoholic patients. *Arch. Neurol.* 1:579, 1959.
30. Victor, M., and Dreyfus, P. M.: Nutritional diseases of the nervous system. *World Neurol.* 2:862, 1961.
31. Williams, A. O., and Osuntokun, B. O.: Peripheral neuropathy in tropical (nutritional) ataxia in Nigeria. *Arch. Neurol.* 21:475, 1969.

CHAPTER EIGHTEEN

Trauma

Head injuries are commonly divided into two categories, closed and open. The latter group includes injuries in which there is a compound fracture of the skull, with or without penetration of the dura mater and brain; these are surgical problems, in the first instance at any rate, and will not be discussed in any detail. This section is mainly concerned with damage to the brain and cranial nerves resulting from closed inuuries.

Physical Mechanisms and Pathology of Closed Injuries. When the unsupported head is hit by a large, blunt instrument, the skull may or may not fracture, but the brain and its blood vessels are liable to damage brought about by a sudden movement in space — an acceleration injury.

Similarly, sudden arrest of the moving head causes a deceleration injury to the brain and the blood vessels. The damage caused by acceleration and deceleration injuries is essentially the same, so they will be considered together.

In both, the effects depend on the momentum and on the direction of the force. If it is sufficient to cause indentation of the skull at the point of impact, it brings about a momentary high-pressure wave which passes towards the foramen magnum, and the shearing stress produced in this way[12, 15, 21] can rupture nerve fibers[50] and small blood vessels in the cerebral hemispheres and brainstem.

Second, if the direction of the blow is tangential, it imparts a rotary twist to the head, which can be equally damaging to nerve fibers and blood vessels. Holbourn[21] investigated the effects of blows administered to human skulls containing a gelatin model of the brain and concluded that sudden rotation of the skull about any axis sets up shearing stresses sufficient to disrupt tissue. If high-speed cinematography is used, swirling movements of the brain can be observed to result from blows to the head in monkeys whose skulls have been replaced by transparent plastic material. Shearing stresses are also set up between the skull and the brain because at the moment of impact the skull is accelerated or decelerated more abruptly than the brain within it; this leads to rupture of veins passing from the brain to their points of attachment to the dural sinuses.

Deformation of the cranium may also cause contusion of the brain underlying the point of impact, whether a fracture has occurred or not. Linear stresses resulting from the blow can also rupture nerve fibers and blood vessels along the line of force, and can cause contusion of the brain at the opposite side of the skull. The latter accounts for "contre coup" lesions. Sudden movements of the brain in the skull, linear or rotary, also result in contusion in areas in which the brain is insecurely anchored to its

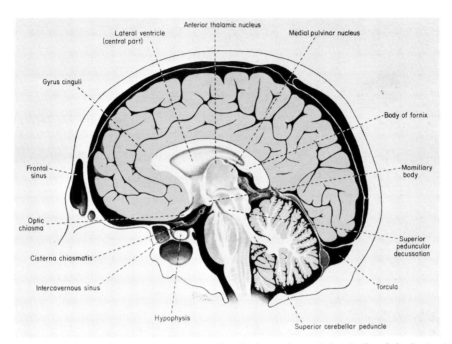

Figure 18–1. The brain, showing gross topographical relationships of the skull and the brain. (Adapted from Delmas, A., and Pertuiset, B.: *Craniocerebral Topometry in Man.* Charles C Thomas, Springfield, Ill., 1959.)

coverings or in which the inner surface of the skull is irregular. Thus, the anterior and basal aspects of the frontal and temporal lobes are frequently found to be bruised in fatal closed head injuries (Fig. 18–2).

Fracture of the skull is not entirely a measure of the force of the impact. Thin skulls fracture more easily than thick ones, and elderly skulls are more brittle than those of young adults. A linear fracture crossing the course of the middle meningeal artery may rupture it or its accompanying veins, causing extradural hemorrhage, and fractures of the vault can tear the dural sinuses and their tributaries, with consequent subdural hemorrhage or thrombosis. Linear fractures of the base may stretch or tear any of the cranial nerves, the olfactory being the most vulnerable; anosmia may follow an occipital or frontal injury which is insufficient to cause unconsciousness. Fractures running into the middle ear or nasal air sinuses are important because if the mucous membrane and dura are torn, cerebrospinal rhinorrhea follows, and air can be forced into the brain by a

sneeze or by blowing the nose, thus causing a pneumoencephalocele; this can rupture into the lateral ventricle. A greater danger is meningitis stemming from the passage of microorganisms into the subarachnoid space. If the gap in the dura underlying the fracture is not repaired, there is a risk of recurrent attacks of meningitis in the years ahead. Facial injuries can fracture the posterior wall of the frontal sinuses, with similar results.

Damage to the brain varies with the severity of the blow. In very mild injuries, there may be neither macroscopic nor microscopic evidence of damage,[6] and it has been suggested that if as the result of shearing stresses nerve fibers are stretched rather than torn, the functional effects may be reversible, thus accounting for what is usually called concussion, i.e., immediate loss of consciousness with flaccid paralysis, followed shortly by complete recovery.

When the injury has been more severe, the brain may appear normal to the naked eye, but microscopy reveals alterations in the Nissl substance of the ganglion

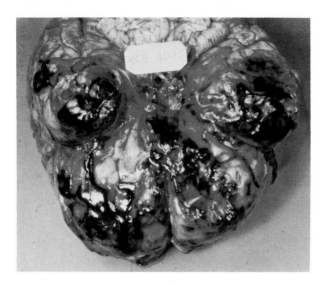

Figure 18–2. Hemorrhagic contusions of the inferior surface of the frontal and temporal lobes. (Courtesy of Department of Neuropathology, Philadelphia General Hospital.)

cells in the cortex, basal ganglia, and brainstem.[39] Moreover, tearing of fibers and slight surface contusions are sometimes seen even when, to judge by the length of the post-traumatic amnesia, the blow was not severe.

Generally speaking, however, widespread rupture of nerve fibers resulting from shearing stresses is encountered only in severe injuries. In these cases, silver impregnation shows numerous retraction balls—a blob of axoplasm at the point of rupture[50]—and diffuse demyelination (Fig. 18–3). These changes are particularly well marked in the white matter of the hemispheres and brainstem in patients who have remained in coma for a prolonged period, but are more marked in the hemisphere than in the brainstem in cases of traumatic dementia. Ultimately, there is dilatation of the ventricles.

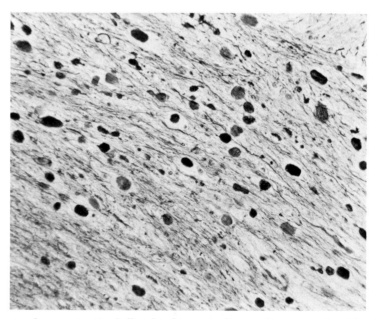

Figure 18–3. Axoplasmic retraction balls related to severed axons after severe closed head injury. (Silver impregnation.) (Courtesy of Dr. Sabina Strich.)

Damage to small blood vessels within the brain gives rise to multiple cystic cavities and discrete scars in the white matter, basal ganglia, and brainstem.

Small foci of necrosis are often found in the pituitary, and occasionally there is ischemic infarction of the entire anterior lobe.[3] It is likely that some of the metabolic disturbances which may follow a head injury are related to these lesions. Diabetes insipidus, on the other hand, is caused by damage to the pituitary stalk or the adjacent portion of the hypothalamus.

Severe brain injury frequently causes local or diffuse cerebral edema. As in other parts of the body, focal contusion produces local edema but in the case of the brain, impairment of vascular autoregulation is an additional hazard.[47] Under normal circumstances, the cerebral vessels adapt to changes of blood pressure and bodily posture and thus maintain a more or less constant blood flow through the brain, but the capacity for autoregulation can break down as the result of head injury, and when this occurs the intracranial vessels dilate under the influence of the systemic blood pressure. This can cause acute brain swelling, and it may be the cause of the rapidly fatal swelling which sometimes occurs in infants and young children after comparatively minor head injuries.[29] Brain swelling is further increased by intracranial vasodilatation if the pCO_2 is allowed to rise as the result of an inadequate airway or defective pulmonary ventilation.

During recovery, the products of hemorrhage and necrosis are removed by the phagocytic action of microglia, and the injured areas are replaced by glial scar tissue derived from the astrocytes. A superficial injury associated with laceration of the meninges frequently results in a meningocerebral cicatrix, which is a potential cause of epilepsy. Glial scar tissue in or near the cortex results in shrinkage, with traction on surrounding blood vessels, and it is thought that this too may be epileptogenic. If the scar is extensive, it may cause traction on the walls of the lateral ventricle, which are distorted. A large area of hemorrhage or necrosis may eventually result in the formation of a cyst, which may communicate with one of the lateral ventricles — traumatic porencephaly. Leptomeningeal adhesions at the base can cause communicating hydrocephalus.

Whiplash injuries[38] are discussed on page 511, but it is desirable to point out that many head injuries are necessarily accompanied by sudden flexion, extension, or rotation of the neck. These movements can produce hemorrhages on the surface of the brain and cervical cord.

The pathological findings following a head injury can also be modified by traumatic thrombosis of the middle cerebral or internal carotid artery, and by massive intracerebral hemorrhage occurring at the time of the injury.[16] Hemorrhage and thrombosis can also occur days or weeks after the accident. When the head injury has been accompanied by fractures of long bones, multiple petechial hemorrhages from fat embolism[46] may be present in the brain (p. 374).

Clinical Manifestations of Brain Injury

Concussion and Contusion. It is doubtful whether a clinical distinction can be made between concussion and contusion.[51] The traditional distinction between the two is based upon the assumption that the symptoms of the former are due to diffuse functional effects of the injury, and the latter to structural damage. According to this doctrine, the symptoms of concussion are completely reversible, and any residual symptoms are assumed to be due to contusion. Another distinction which is often made is that the duration of unconsciousness in uncomplicated concussion is brief, lasting not more than a minute or two, more persistent unconsciousness being attributed to contusion. This can no longer be regarded as a valid distinction. In the first place, rupture of nerve fibers in the white matter has been found in patients who suffered brief unconsciousness, but who died from other causes. Secondly, recovery from unconsciousness can be delayed for hours or days, and yet the patient may make a complete recovery. Moreover, contusion may occur without unconsciousness, as in crushing injuries where the head undergoes neither deceleration nor acceleration. Again, there are many cases in which a bullet has passed right through the skull without causing loss of consciousness. For these reasons, many prefer to use the term "post-traumatic syndrome" for all symptoms following head injury.

When the blow is of moderate severity, there is immediate loss of consciousness and generalized flaccid paralysis, so that the subject collapses or falls. Recovery of consciousness and motility may occur within a minute or two, after which there may be no further symptoms. Occasionally, this is followed by a period of automatism, during which the patient seems to act more or less normally—as for instance in the football player who is knocked out but who gets up after a few seconds and continues the game. However, when this happens off the football field, it is often possible to observe minor aberrations of conduct or thought during this period. In other cases, recovery from the initial stage of unconsciousness is followed by vomiting and headache, the latter continuing for some hours.

In more severe injuries, recovery of consciousness in the sense of clear and continuous awareness of and memory for current happenings may be delayed for hours, days or weeks. The return of consciousness passes through phases of coma, semicoma, confusion (often with delirium), and automatic behavior. The plantar responses may be extensor in the early stages, and there is often incontinence or retention of urine. It is important that the level of consciousness be estimated as soon as possible after the injury and at regular intervals thereafter, until it is clear that satisfactory progress is being made. Sustained deterioration should always arouse the suspicion of increased intracranial pressure from meningeal or intracerebral hemorrhage or from brain swelling. When the head injury has been accompanied by fractures of long bones and other injuries, fat embolism[9, 46] in the brain may complicate the picture (p. 374).

Rough but adequate measures of the depth of unconsciousness can be made as follows: At the deepest level—coma—the patient shows no response to external stimuli or to inner needs. At the next level, there is some evidence of integrated behavior—for example, a distended bladder provokes restless bodily movements, and a painful stimulus causes a change of facial expression or purposeful attempts at avoidance. With further improvement, the patient still is largely inaccessible, but occasionally he will show adequate responses to simple commands, forcibly given and if necessary reinforced by appropriate gestures, e.g., "put out your tongue," "take my hand," etc. At a still higher level, the patient may give relevant answers to simple questions, such as, "What work do you do?", "How old are you?", "What is your name?" Finally, the patient arrives at the stage in which, although he is confused and disoriented, he is capable of conversation and of appropriate behavior, but even when he seems to have regained full consciousness he will often be unable to recall this period, or will remember only certain highlights. Events with emotional associations, such as a visit from a relative, may be recalled, and at this stage the patient may respond naturally to his surroundings and answers questions intelligently. It is important to distinguish between the period of unconsciousness as verified by nurses and relatives, and the period of complete or patchy amnesia, as reported by the patient following recovery. The period of amnesia (between the time of the accident and the full recovery of continuous memory) is a better yardstick to the severity of brain damage than is the period of apparent unconsciousness.

There is often amnesia for the events

immediately preceding the injury. In cases of slight concussion, the retrograde amnesia extends for no longer than a few seconds, but in more severe injuries, it may include periods up to several hours, or even several days. The longer periods of retrograde amnesia usually decrease with the passage of time after recovery, but the post-traumatic amnesia remains constant.[1]

In severe injuries, areas of contusion are likely to be present, but the symptoms and signs of such damage may be difficult to detect in a stuporous patient. They are of the kind to be expected as the result of focal damage—dysphasia, hemianopia, hemiparesis with appropriate reflex changes, unilateral sensory impairment, and so on. Contusion of the brainstem will result in dysarthria, pupillary changes, ocular palsies, nystagmus, diminution of corneal reflexes, ataxia, and signs of pyramidal disease on one or both sides.[28] Isolated cerebellar contusion is rarely seen. The effects of frontal and temporal lobe contusion injuries cannot be detected until the patient recovers consciousness. Frontal lobe injuries can give rise to facile and inappropriate behavior, while damage to the temporal lobe is apt to cause defective memory, especially for recent events. Rarely, the patient loses all sense of personal identity and cannot recall events over a period of several years. It is thought to be caused by bilateral damage to the hippocampal gyri.[37]

The presence of blood in the spinal fluid is a helpful sign of severe injury. This may be of practical value when it comes to the assessment of residual symptoms at a later date, but it must be emphasized that lumbar puncture can be a lethal procedure in the presence of increased intracranial pressure from extradural, subdural, or intracerebral hemorrhage and should not be performed in the presence of signs of a pressure cone (p. 424).

Metabolic Disturbances. Injuries to the brain may be followed by disturbances of water balance, serum electrolytes, and renal function, and neurogenic

hyperventilation can cause respiratory alkalosis. Damage to the hypothalamus and pituitary stalk can cause diabetes insipidus; this is easily detected in conscious individuals, but the unconscious patient cannot draw attention to his fluid needs and unless they are met, dehydration and hypernatremia will result. Even in the absence of diabetes insipidus, dehydration and hypernatremia with consequent increase of osmolarity can occur from failure to administer sufficient fluids, and it should be noted that liquid requirements are increased by hot weather, fever, and hyperventilation. On the other hand, water intoxication can result from the administration of excessive amounts of dextrose solution without an adequate intake of salt. The cerebral salt-losing syndrome can also occur following head injuries. Both dehydration and water intoxication can produce symptoms in their own right, thereby complicating the clinical picture (p. 585). Potassium retention is seldom encountered, but it is more dangerous than sodium retention because it can lead to paralysis of the limbs and sudden cardiac arrest. The latter can occur without clinical warning, but the danger can be avoided by watching for the high T waves and widening of the QRS complex, which betoken hyperkalemia. These EKG changes are easily distinguished from the inverted T waves which are so often found following severe head injuries and subarachnoid hemorrhage (Chap. 21).

There is often a moderate rise of blood urea following head injury, but it is uncertain whether this is due to increased metabolism or to the effects of the head injury on renal excretion. Respiratory alkalosis from overbreathing is not uncommon. Hyperglycemia, with consequent glycosuria, can occur from injuries to the base of the brain; it reacts briskly to modest doses of insulin.

POST-TRAUMATIC CEREBRAL SYNDROMES

The most common of these is the so-called *postconcussional syndrome*,[51] characterized by headache, dizziness, difficulty in concentration, abnormal liability to mental fatigue, anxiety, and depression. Second, diffuse cerebral demyelination and focal contusions can give rise to *traumatic dementia*,[1, 43, 55] sometimes called "chronic traumatic psychosis"; fortunately, this is far less common than postconcussional syndrome. Third, specific *neurological deficits*[1, 28] may arise as a result of focal damage to the brain or cranial nerves. These are not necessarily associated with a significant degree of traumatic dementia. Fourth, *traumatic epilepsy*,[23, 24, 42, 55] is not uncommon, particularly after penetrating injuries. Whereas the postconcussional syndrome is usually unassociated with dementia, focal disabilities, or seizures, these three are apt to occur together in varying combinations, but it is convenient to describe them separately.

The Postconcussional Syndrome. Although, for the reasons stated on page 491, this term lacks pathological specificity, the symptoms are clear-cut. They appear with monotonous regularity following mild and moderate head injuries, regardless of age, sex, or race. They are sometimes regarded as psychogenic, but the consistency with which the same symptoms appear after injuries to the head in thousands of patients bears witness to a physical basis. This is not to deny the possibility of psychological factors in some cases; it is obvious that they sometimes play an important part in the aggravation and perpetuation of the symptoms. It may be, as Symonds has put it, that the effect of brain injury is to make the patient slightly "less of a man and more of a child" and, as a result, his reactions to external and internal stresses may prove to be inadequate or neurotic. Should the patient have shown any evidence of neurosis before the accident, the liability to neurotic patterns of behavior is increased. Nevertheless, the postconcussional syndrome occurs in tough-minded persons whose injuries have been sustained in sporting activities, when there is no question of com-

pensation and when other circumstances are such that there is no cause for anxiety, apart from the patient's concern with his own symptoms.

Although there are striking exceptions, the incidence of the postconcussional syndrome increases with the length of the post-traumatic amnesia. With post-traumatic amnesia of one hour or less, the average period of incapacity is about four weeks, while with post-traumatic amnesia lasting between one and seven days, the severe symptoms may last for eight or nine weeks or even longer. They may be minimal or even absent, however, following very severe head injuries which have given rise to prolonged unconsciousness, marked focal disabilities, or dementia.

The headache is variable in situation, is sometimes associated with tenderness of the scalp at the site of the blow, and is variously described as throbbing, dull, or stabbing. It is relieved by rest and quiet and is aggravated by noise, heat, emotional strain, physical exertion, stooping, and mental effort.

The dizziness usually consists of a sense of instability or lightheadedness induced by sudden changes of posture, and it is sometimes associated with momentary blacking-out of vision. Sometimes the patient complains of dizziness on extreme lateral gaze. Occasionally, true vertigo is complained of, either on movements of the head, or on assuming a particular posture, and in these cases, nystagmus can be induced by the movement or posture that produces the patient's symptoms. In the more common "dizziness" of the postconcussional syndrome, however, nystagmus is rarely observed, a circumstance which may lead the unwary to conclude that the patient's symptoms are functional. In most cases, however, caloric and rotational tests will reveal disturbance of labyrinthine function, and the more discriminating the test, the greater will be the number of positive results. Thus, the bithermal test of Fitzgerald and Hallpike produces a greater yield than a crude ice-water test. Similarly, abnormalities not demonstrable by simple methods can sometimes be identified if rotational and caloric stimulation are carried out in the dark, or with the eyes closed, to abolish fixation. This has to be done with the aid of the nystagmograph. Nevertheless, even the most elaborate methods sometimes fail to disclose labyrinthine dysfunction in patients who continue to complain of posttraumatic dizziness; conversely, Toglia found impaired labyrinthine responses in some patients whose symptoms had ceased.[55]

Audiometry will sometimes provide collateral evidence of damage to the internal ear. The most common finding is high-frequency sensory-neural impairment, accompanied by loudness recruitment and difficulty in auditory discrimination. Occasionally, there is conduction deafness due to dysarticulation of the ossicles. Severe permanent deafness is rare. Tinnitus is frequently present; it is usually described as a ringing or hissing sound in cases of sensory-neural deafness; a roaring sound suggests damage to the middle ear.

There are often complaints of irritability, dislike of noise, mental and physical fatigability, sweating, palpitations, and insomnia. Tolerance for alcohol is reduced. There is difficulty in concentrating, and the patient is apt to be forgetful. Conventional psychometric tests may show little amiss except difficulty in concentration and slight impairment of immediate memory. Anxiety is usually conspicuous. Discomfort related to the head, as with pain in the region of the heart, is very frightening to the uninformed, and fears of mental incapacity are aggravated when the patient finds that he cannot concentrate as well as before. The situation is further complicated by worry over financial and domestic problems and by concern over the issues of compensation and litigation.

Chronic Traumatic Psychosis. Very rarely, the confusional state following a severe head injury fails to improve beyond a certain point, and the patient remains incapable either of managing his own affairs or of making normal social adjustments. In most of these patients, there has been clinical evidence, in the earliest stages, of focal brain injury— aphasia, apraxia, hemiplegia, diplegia, etc. The focal symptoms tend to improve over the years.

Exceptionally, bilateral damage to the hippocampal region causes retrograde amnesia extending back for months or even for years.[37] Although the patient retains the knowledge and the skills acquired before the accident and is able to think clearly and behave normally in a social sense, he has no memory whatever for the events of his life covered by the period of the amnesia. Associated with this is a gross defect of memory for recent events, and dislocation of the personal time sense. The patient will not remember whether his last meal was breakfast or dinner and is unable to recall events from hour to hour or from day to day. Since oblivion for the past can be convenient under certain circumstances, care must be taken before ascribing a lengthy retrograde amnesia to organic damage. Careful psychometric tests will remove doubt in such cases.

Lesser degrees of residual mental disorder are not uncommon after severe injuries. These defects can take two forms, which are sometimes found in combination. There is impairment of attention, memory, arithmetical ability, and judgment, which are revealed by the patient's inadequacy in his daily tasks and which can be measured by psychometric tests.

There may also be disorder of personality. The formerly considerate and well-behaved man becomes quarrelsome, liable to sudden rages, untrustworthy, sexually promiscuous, and neglectful of domestic and professional duties; alternatively, he may show unwonted apathy, lack of initiative, and loss of interest in his surroundings and future. The combination of personality change and intellectual impairment is often accompanied by a lack of insight. The patient may insist on returning to work and may claim that his performance is as good as before the injury, although his employers find him unreliable and ineffective.

In children, behavior disorders may be

the outstanding residual symptoms of a severe head injury. In contrast with his pretraumatic disposition, the child becomes quarrelsome, aggressive, disobedient, and untruthful, and these unwelcome traits may persist in some cases so that with advancing years, delinquency becomes a problem. This situation bears a striking resemblance to the behavioral disorders following encephalitis lethargica in children.

Progressive deterioration occurring years after head injury indicates the presence of some other disease. Occasionally, the symptoms of general paresis make their appearance following a head injury. The presenile dementias of Pick and of Alzheimer are not traumatic in origin, but they are among the conditions which have to be excluded by appropriate investigation when progressive mental deterioration appears in the years following a head injury. The same applies to the syndrome of normal pressure hydrocephalus with dementia and ataxia of gait (p. 209).

Traumatic Epilepsy. The term "traumatic epilepsy"[23, 24, 42] refers to seizures arising months or even years after trauma to the head in patients who have not had seizures in the past; it does not properly apply to seizures occurring solely within the first few days after injury, although the risk of epilepsy at a later date is enhanced in patients who have had early seizures. Convulsions are particularly common in young children and may occur after minor injury.

The incidence of late epilepsy after closed head injuries of a severity to require admission to hospital has been variously estimated at between 3 and 6 per cent. In the majority of these cases, the first seizures occur within two years of the injury; if no attacks have occurred in these two years, there is no more than a 10 per cent risk of attacks occurring at a later date. In closed head injuries, the risk of late epilepsy is increased when the post-traumatic amnesia is longer than 24 hours and when there has been a depressed fracture and focal contusion.

The risk of seizures is far greater after penetrating injuries, especially in those

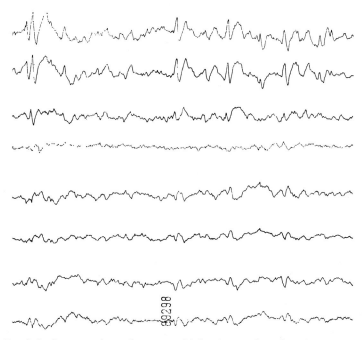

Figure 18–4. Focal discharge in the right temporal lobe (upper three lines) in a patient suffering from generalized epileptiform seizures dating back to a blow on the temple from a baseball.

involving the sensory-motor cortex. In general, the chance of developing epilepsy is in the neighborhood of 40 per cent if the cortex has been penetrated by bone splinters or a foreign body, and about 10 per cent after severe focal contusion without penetration. Fortunately, these cases show a marked tendency to improve; with advancing years, the attacks are apt to become less frequent and less severe.

Traumatic epileptic seizures may be focal or generalized (Fig. 18–4). Occasionally, they take the form of psychomotor attacks. Under anticonvulsant treatment, the attacks become infrequent and may cease. Electroencephalography may reveal a *localized* epileptogenic focus,[20] and in this event surgical excision of the lesion will reduce or abolish the seizures in about 50 per cent of the cases so treated.

Traumatic Encephalopathy. Pugilists who have taken a lot of punishment over a number of years sometimes show signs of mental and physical deterioration, to which the popular term "punch drunk" is given.[49] This condition is characterized by impairment of memory and concentration, mild confusion, lack of insight, emotional instability, and a slowing of reaction time, which impairs efficiency and therefore leads to further knockouts if the patient continues in pugilism. There is tremor of the head, intention tremor of the hands, defective convergence, and slurring of speech. Gait becomes slow and unsteady, and there is clumsiness of movement in the upper limbs. The picture resembles that of a person in a permanent state of moderate alcoholic intoxication. Seizures are not uncommon.

When the symptoms have appeared, they progress slowly for a year or two, and then come to a halt, provided that further head injuries are avoided. The patient, lacking insight, is willing to fight all comers, and can hardly be restrained from doing so. As in the case of any severe traumatic psychosis, pneumoencephalography usually discloses some degree of ventricular dilatation and cortical atrophy, and may also reveal disappearance of the septum pellucidum.[49] Needless to say, not all neurological or psychological disturbances in former boxers are necessarily traumatic in origin.

Traumatic Neurosis. Neurotic patterns of behavior are common after any form of accident, whether the head is injured or not, but they are particularly frequent after head injuries, not only because a blow to the head is more significant to the patient than an injury elsewhere in the body, but also because brain damage can reduce the patient's capacity to deal with life's problems.

Traumatic neuroses usually arise in persons with a previous history of emotional instability as judged by the work record, domestic life, or previous breakdowns, but such evidence may be lacking in persons who have had the good fortune to escape excessive stress. In some cases, the accident is simply the culminating point in a series of stresses, as for instance in the case of a soldier who has stood up to battle strain for many months and then suddenly breaks down after a trivial blow to the head. Analogous cases are not rare in civilian life, although the nature of the stresses is different. Psychological trauma as the result of a terrifying experience at the time of the injury can produce psychoneurotic reactions, particularly in mild injuries, which are unaccompanied by a merciful oblivion. Neurotic patterns of behavior usually result from circumstances arising out of the accident—the possibility of prosecution or litigation, hopes of compensation, inability to pursue a former occupation, and fear of permanent incapacity.

The symptoms of traumatic neurosis vary from case to case; anxiety, depression, hysterical conversion, hysterical amnesia complicating post-traumatic amnesia, and hypochondriacal obsessions are common. Infantile regression may occur. It is often difficult to decide which symptoms are organic and which are functional. Each case must be judged on its merits, without prejudice, on the basis of a careful history, a complete neurological and psychiatric examination, and special studies.

Prognosis of Closed Head Injuries. It has already been stated that complete recovery is usual in patients suffering from the so-called postconcussional syndrome and that the duration of the incapacity is roughly proportional to the post-traumatic amnesia in emotionally stable persons.

The mortality rate in cases of severe head injury has been dramatically reduced in recent years. In the 1930's the mortality rate for all cases of head injuries admitted to hospital was in the region of 20 per cent. This has been reduced to about 3 to 4 per cent in institutions in which expert care is available. A striking example of this improvement is provided by Lewin: Of 150 patients who remained in continuous coma for more than a month, 95 survived, and 33 per cent of these returned to their normal work; 25 per cent remained severely disabled. Increased survival rates have been achieved largely by preventing unconscious patients from dying of respiratory obstruction, infections, brain swelling, dehydration, and untreated intracranial hematomas. On the other hand, it is probable that intensive treatment of severe head injuries has increased the number of severely disabled survivors, who would have died under less favorable conditions.[4]

The outlook for complete recovery from the effects of moderate and severe head injuries is vitiated by advancing age and *by previous head injuries.* Patients with personality disorders and intellectual impairment which persist for more than two years seldom show further improvement. In children and young adults, there may be slow but progressive recovery from focal disabilities.

Treatment of Closed Head Injuries. In discussing the management of head injuries, no attempt will be made to deal with the surgical aspects of the problem or with the treatment of infections or other complications, but attention will be directed to the principles underlying the treatment of the unconscious patient and to the management of convalescence.

Head Injury Without Unconsciousness. In these cases, it is important to be aware that occasionally contusion of the brain occurs without unconsciousness. In any case of severe local injury to the scalp, an x-ray of the skull is mandatory. It is wise to keep the patient under observation for at least 24 hours, bearing in mind the possibility of epidural or subdural hemorrhage after trivial injuries. It is also desirable to remember that a patient can walk into hospital with a bullet in his brain and that if the entry wound is in the hairy scalp, it may be difficult to find.

Head Injury with Loss of Consciousness. Following transient unconsciousness, bed rest and observation for 48 hours is indicated, notwithstanding the fact that ill effects seldom follow neglect of this precaution in healthy young adults. It is impossible to foretell the effect of such injury: Many persons will have no symptoms at all; others will develop the postconcussional syndrome. A very small minority will develop an extradural or subdural hematoma, the latter being more common in persons over the age of 40 and in alcoholics of all ages. If headache or other symptoms persist, the period of bed rest must be extended, but it is important to reassure the patient and his family as to eventual recovery and to avoid undue solemnity, because it is only too easy to promote neurotic attitudes by excessive therapeutic zeal. The tempo of convalescence will have to be adjusted in accordance with the patient's symptoms. It may be possible to allow a return to work within a few days, or return may have to be deferred for weeks. Good judgment has to be exercised in this matter because premature resumption of full activities may provoke or aggravate headaches, dizziness, and irritability, while too protracted a convalescence can foster neurosis. An early explanation of the nature of the injury and reassurance as to the future will do much to prevent unhealthy attitudes in the patient and in well-meaning but overanxious relatives. A minor head injury can be the occasion, rather than the cause, of a neurotic illness.

Severe Head Injury with Prolonged Unconsciousness. When the patient is first seen, there is no reliable way of knowing whether unconsciousness is going to be prolonged or not, but in general, the more severely injured patients are likely to be in deep coma and in shock. Before doing anything else, a good airway must be ensured; this is easier to maintain with the patient in the lateral position, but if there is any doubt about the efficacy of ventilation, an endotracheal tube should be inserted or a tracheostomy performed. The only accurate way of ascertaining whether ventilation is adequate is through routine analysis of arterial blood samples for pO_2, pCO_2, and pH. Hypercapnea increases brain swelling by dilating the cerebral circulation, and if prolonged, it leads to respiratory depression and also to an outpouring of endogenous catecholamines, which in their turn produce peripheral vasoconstriction and therefore elevate the blood pressure. The latter can be dangerous if the autoregulatory capacity of the cerebral vessels is impaired. Humidified oxygen can be delivered through the catheter or the tracheostomy, but it must be remembered that the use of excessive concentrations of oxygen can mask the existence of hypoventilation.

Shock is treated by giving blood, plasma, or plasma expanders. The patient should receive 2500 ml. of 5 per cent glucose solution daily, of which 500 ml. should be in sodium chloride solution. The amount of fluid required can be altered according to the volume and specific gravity of the urine.

An indwelling catheter should be inserted *at once* to prevent bladder distention and to allow accurate measurement of urinary output.

The patient's skin must be washed daily, dried carefully, and powdered on flexor and interdigital surfaces. Soiling should be cared for immediately. Oral hygiene should be attended to and the lips should be prevented from drying and cracking by the application of an appropriate ointment.

The patient should be moved hourly to prevent pressure sores.

Accumulations of mucus must be removed by suction; this should be carried out as gently as possible so as not to provoke excessive coughing, which temporarily raises the intracranial pressure.

Plasma electrolyte levels should be estimated daily until it is certain that they have not been disturbed. Checks should be made for hypochloremia, hyponatremia, hypernatremia, and hyperkalemia; the last is the most dangerous because it can cause paralysis and sudden cardiac standstill.

Attempts to reduce cerebral swelling by administration of intravenous urea or mannitol are often effective for a short time, but they may be followed by a reactive increase of brain swelling and should in general be avoided except in cases of extreme emergency. Adrenocorticoids are more effective.

Hyperthermia should be treated by the use of a cooling blanket or an ice pack. In addition, there is evidence that lowering the body temperature to between 86° and 88°F. (30° to 31°C.) for several days after the injury may improve the prognosis.

Restlessness can be very troublesome, exhausting the patient and nurses alike. Morphine is contraindicated because even very small doses will sometimes induce respiratory depression. Intramuscular paraldehyde in doses of 5 ml. or more is safe but is not always effective. Ten to 40 mg. of triflupromazine can be effective when given by slow intravenous injection, but other tranquilizers of the phenothiazine series can be used in its place, and barbiturates given by intramuscular injection are sometimes effective.

A wide-spectrum antibiotic should be given in full doses from the start, in order to prevent pulmonary and urinary infection. They are doubly important in the presence of fractures leading into the ear and accessory nasal sinuses and in compound fractures of the vault.

Seizures during the immediate post-traumatic period can be treated by the intramuscular injection of 200 mg. Dilantin twice a day in an adult. Status epilepticus is most easily controlled by intravenous Valium (p. 140) followed by full doses of Dilantin.

During the recovery phase, headache can be severe and may require effective doses of codeine phosphate or Demerol (pethedine).

The question of spinal tap is beset by difficulties. The withdrawal of 10 to 15 ml. of fluid sometimes relieves headache, but the procedure carries the risk of precipitating or aggravating a tentorial pressure cone, and in this connection it must be remembered that normal or low pressures, as measured by spinal manometry, do not necessarily reflect the intracranial pressure, since uncal herniation associated with a hematoma or brain swelling will prevent the transmission of pressure to the spinal arachnoid space. Therefore, lumbar puncture should never be carried out if the patient displays diencephalic or midbrain symptoms.

Convalescence

There can be no hard or fast rules as to how long the patient should be kept in bed or how long a time should be devoted to convalescence, because individual reactions vary so widely. However, most patients with moderate head injury should start getting out of bed within two weeks. There is no evidence that prolonged bed rest has any special virtue, and in elderly patients it has many disadvantages. Whether the patient is up and about or in bed, he should be protected from mental effort, worry, noise, and fatigue. Ideally, mental and physical activity should be increased in graduated fashion, pausing at each step until the patient is free of symptoms, but although this is often possible, there are many patients in whom progress is

so slow that the range of activity has to be widened despite the persistence of symptoms, and this applies particularly to overanxious and introspective persons who are apt to develop neurotic reactions.

Occupational therapy is useful, but it must be remembered that after severe injuries the patient is easily fatigued, both mentally and physically, and that if he is overtaxed, symptoms will be aggravated, thus leading to discouragement and to an increased liability to neurosis. Any patient showing evidence of neurosis should receive psychiatric help, and in this connection it is necessary to emphasize the need for a gentle, firm, and uncensorious attitude on the part of the doctor, nurse, or relatives. Those showing severe intellectual loss or change of personality and those with traumatic epilepsy may find it necessary to change their occupation and manner of life. The assistance of social workers is invaluable in this situation, and a little effort expended on finding the correct niche for the individual will save trouble later on.

THE SCALP AND CRANIUM

Any severe injury to the head will bruise, lacerate, or perforate the scalp. It may be difficult to detect small wounds in the hairy scalp, even in cases in which the skull has been fractured and the brain penetrated, as for instance by a bomb splinter or a small caliber bullet. In adults, pericranial hematomas absorb well, but in infants they form easily, disperse poorly, and may eventually calcify, with the production of an unsightly lump; this can be prevented by evacuating the hematoma.

Although damage to the skull is not as important as injury to its contents, the detection of fractures is important for two reasons. A fracture indicates that an injury has been sustained—a matter of both medical and medicolegal importance, although it must be remembered that the brain can be severely injured in the absence of a fracture. Second, the situation and nature of a fracture have a bearing on immediate treatment and future developments. Thus, fractures through the middle meningeal groove or across dural sinuses carry a risk of extradural hemorrhage, while fractures which communicate with the accessory air sinuses or with the ear provide a pathway for the inward spread of infection, and the same is true of compound fractures of the vault. Depressed fractures and, in particular, those in which fragments of bone have penetrated the brain, constitute an indication for surgical intervention. In compound fractures, effective debridement is essential for the prevention of infection. Bone fragments and foreign bodies must be removed if possible, not only to reduce the chances of infection, but also to reduce subsequent liability to seizures. Dural tears associated with fractures of the frontal sinuses and rhinorrhea should be repaired to prevent meningitis. The only evidence of a tear may be escape of cerebrospinal fluid from the nose or ear, and careful inquiry should always be made on this point, since many patients assume that a dribble of fluid from the nose or a postnasal drip is merely evidence of nasal congestion.

Cerebrospinal Rhinorrhea

Fractures involving the air sinuses and ear are often but not always marked by an escape of the cerebrospinal fluid, especially when the head hangs down. Moreover, air can be driven into the brain, producing a pneumocele, as a result of blowing the nose or sneezing. In many cases, the rhinorrhea ceases spontaneously, but when it persists for more than a week or two, surgical repair is required in order to reduce the chances of ascending infection into the meninges and brain at a later date.

Nontraumatic cerebrospinal fluid rhinorrhea[26] is more uncommon. It can occur when the base of the skull is eroded by a tumor or by osteomyelitis. It has been seen in both obstructive and communicating hydrocephalus. Congenital defects of the cribriform plate can be associated with a pulsating subarachnoid cyst, which can rupture and thus cause rhinorrhea. Sometimes the subarachnoid space sends a downward extension into the sella, and this provides the anatomical basis for an escape of the cerebrospinal fluid through a persistent craniopharyngeal canal; pneumoencephalography will disclose air within the sella.

The disorder presents as a drip or flow of clear fluid from one nostril, which may be increased or decreased by changing the position of the head or straining. The liquid can be identified as cerebrospinal fluid by identifying its glucose content, which is easily done by the use of glucose-oxidase impregnated Testix, as used by diabetics for urine testing. It is more difficult to localize the site of the fistula. Plain x-rays of the skull seldom help. If a radioactive isotope is injected into the cisterna magna, a scanning technique can be employed to demonstrate whether or not some of it passes into the nose, but the precise tract can seldom be identified by this means. Occasionally, the rhinorrhea will cease following a spinal tap, but if it persists, efforts must be made to identify and close the fistula in order to protect the patient from the risk of meningitis.

Injuries to the Cranial Nerves

Any cranial nerve can be injured by bruising against the bone, disruption of its blood supply, fractures of the canal or foramen through which it leaves the skull, sudden stretching of the nerve by displacement of the brain at the moment of impact, local pressure by hemorrhage or edema, or penetrating injuries.[1] The olfactory nerve is more often injured than any other, followed in order of frequency by the facial, the eighth, the second, and the nerves of the extrinsic muscles of the eye.

The olfactory nerve is often damaged by frontal blows which fracture the ethmoid, and by shearing stresses in occipital and parietal injuries. Recovery from complete anosmia is unlikely if it is still present three months after the injury. Surprisingly, not all patients with complete anosmia complain of deficient taste. The patient with permanent anosmia should be warned that he will be unable to smell poisonous fumes, a matter of importance to chemists, gas workers, and miners.

The optic nerve may be torn by penetrating wounds, but is more commonly injured indirectly by closed fractures involving the frontotemporal region.[54] In some cases, the trauma is comparatively slight; the injury probably results from torsion or stretching of the nerve with consequent damage to its blood supply. The lesion is usually situated in the region of the optic canal. Loss of vision may be complete or partial, and is usually unilateral. In partial lesions, the defect varies from a small scotoma to a large irregular sector defect.[54] In severe cases the direct pupillary reaction to light is lost, but the consensual reaction is preserved. Even in complete lesions the optic discs look normal for the first two or three weeks, after which pallor becomes apparent. Some degree of recovery is to be expected in about half the cases; this takes place during the first four weeks, after which no further improvement is to be expected. Attacks of partial or complete amaurosis lasting seconds or minutes occur occasionally during recovery from severe head injury. They pass off in time, and there is no known explanation for them.

Chiasmal lesions are rare, and usually occur with frontal trauma. They are marked by bitemporal field defects, which may be complete or incomplete. In some instances, the optic nerve on one side is involved as well. Polyuria, polydipsia, and obesity may develop if the nearby hypothalamus has been injured. Rarely, arachnoiditis develops around the chiasm with gradual and intermittent deterioration of vision. Surgical attempts to free the chiasm from adhesions may lead to further deterioration of sight.

A penetrating injury or contusion of the occipital lobe can cause homonymous hemianopic field defects. When the tip of the lobe is damaged, the defects are central, homonymous, congruous, and scotomatous.

The third, fourth, and sixth cranial nerves are involved in about 3 per cent of cases of head injury. The abducens is more often involved than the other two; in some cases it is affected in fractures of the petrous temporal bone with or without damage to the facial and auditory nerves; damage to the nerve may also result from a hematoma of the orbit. Comparatively trivial injuries to the orbit may cause fourth nerve paralysis. Partial or complete third nerve palsies are usually due to a hematoma in the orbit. Diplopia from nerve injury must be distinguished from that which occurs as a result of displacement of the eye by fracture of the maxilla. Dilatation and paralysis of one pupil is sometimes seen as a result of a blow to the eye; the condition usually recovers after a few days. It can be mistaken for dilatation of the pupil occurring as a result of a tentorial pressure cone in the presence of an extradural or subdural hematoma. Increased intracranial pressure with coning may also lead to a variety of ocular motor palsies, which are apt to vary from hour to hour (p. 428).

The trigeminal nerve: Sensory loss in the distribution of the frontal and maxillary branches is not uncommon as a result of injury to the face; damage to the mandibular divisions from basal fractures is much less common. Injury to the supraorbital and infraorbital branches, followed by partial regeneration, may lead to unpleasant paresthesias in the area of skin affected, and a few patients subsequently develop pain resembling that of tic douloureux, which is not always relieved by sectioning of the trigeminal sensory root.

The facial nerve may be involved in fractures of the petrous temporal bone, leading to immediate and usually complete facial paralysis on the affected side, together with bleeding from the ear and some degree of deafness. Less often, paralysis appears two to 10 days after the injury. The prognosis is good in the delayed type, recovery taking place in a few weeks, but it is adversely affected by coincident otitis media. Treatment is as for Bell's palsy, with the added necessity of vigorously combating any infection there may be in the middle ear. Some assistance in prognosis is furnished by electromyography, for if paralysis is still complete by the third week and there is evidence of complete denervation of the facial muscles, improvement is likely to be slow and may be incomplete.

Damage to the eighth nerve in association with fracture of the middle fossa can cause deafness in one or both ears, and the loss of hearing is usually of the middle ear type. This type of deafness usually improves, but when the nerve has been damaged, full recovery cannot be expected. Tinnitus may be troublesome and persistent, particularly in introspective subjects. True vertigo of great intensity is an occasional sequel to labyrinthine damage, but it usually passes off quickly, leaving the patient somewhat unsteady on his feet and with a sense of dizziness on quick movements of the head. It is probably due to concussion of, or hemorrhage into, the labyrinth. Minor degrees of labyrinthine damage are more common and are usually accompanied by changes in labyrinthine responses.[55] Positional vertigo (page 101) is seen occasionally.

The ninth, tenth, eleventh, and twelfth cranial nerves occasionally are involved by fractures of the base or by penetrating injuries, and they may be associated with paralysis of the cervical sympathetic.

Extradural Hematoma

Although extradural hematoma is an uncommon condition, occurring in less than 1 per cent of all head injuries,[16] it is important because unless treated promptly it always leads to death. The hematoma usually results from rupture of the middle meningeal artery, less often from injury to the dural sinuses. Additional hemorrhage from diploic vessels helps to swell the size of the collection. Extradural hemorrhage usually takes place in the middle fossa, but occasional examples are encountered in relation to the superior sagittal sinus and in the posterior fossa from the transverse sinus.[32] The injury is often slight, but if it has been severe, the clinical picture will be complicated by the presence of cerebral concussion and contusion. In most cases, there is a linear fracture across the line of the middle meningeal artery. Middle meningeal hemorrhage has also been recorded in penetrating wounds. Occasionally it occurs without a fracture.

Clinical Features. The condition is commonly encountered in young adults but it can occur in infants and children. In most cases, bleeding is rapid and symptoms develop within a few hours of injury; rarely the clot grows slowly and in this form two or three weeks may elapse before the diagnosis becomes evident.

The presence of extradural hemorrhage following a head injury is suggested by three events: depression of the level of consciousness after a lucid interval, the symptoms and signs of cerebral compression, and the delayed appearance of focal neurological signs after injury.

Deterioration in the level of consciousness is usual. The classic story is an initial short period of unconsciousness followed by a lucid interval and then a return of unconsciousness. However, the lucid interval may be obscured by coma due to brain injury or alcoholic intoxication. Occasionally there is no immediate loss of consciousness following the blow but unconsciousness appears minutes, hours, or days later. Very rarely there is no unconsciousness at any time, and the patient merely complains of headaches, drowsiness, and increasing hemiparesis. Another rare form shows alternating periods of confusion and semiconsciousness over a period of days, a condition more suggestive of a subdural hematoma. A lucid interval is certainly not pathognomonic of extradural hemorrhage, for its occurs occasionally in young children who become unconscious as a result of post-traumatic cerebral swelling,[29] and it is also a prominent feature of subdural hematoma. There may also be a lucid interval between the time of a head injury and the subsequent development of intracerebral hemorrhage or infarction. Again, there is often no recovery of consciousness when the brain injury is severe, and the advent of an extradural hematoma is marked by a deepening of unconsciousness, slowing of pulse, and a rise of blood pressure, although this sequence does not necessarily mean the presence of bleeding, for it may occur as a result of widespread cerebral edema. A lucid interval occurred in only 25 of 56 cases of verified extradural hematomas reported by Gurdjian and Webster.[16]

In the conscious patient, headache may develop, the pulse rate drops, and respiration becomes slower. In some cases there is an early rise of blood pressure, but this is insignificant if intracranial pressure rises slowly. Generalized or jacksonian seizures may occur. Papilledema is usually absent because of the rapidity with which the condition develops, but it may occur in the rare subacute and chronic cases. When the clot is situated low in the middle fossa, as is usually the case, the symptoms and signs of a tentorial pressure cone develop rapidly (page 424); there is stiffness of the neck, ipsilateral and sometimes bilateral third nerve palsy with pupillary dilatation, disturbance of ocular movement, and sometimes ptosis. Occasionally a constricted pupil is found on the side of the hemorrhage, and in some instances the pupils are unaffected. Compression of the brain may produce contralateral hemiparesis, but sometimes ipsilateral hemiplegia occurs from pressure of the cerebral peduncle against the edge of the tentorium on the opposite side. Decerebrate rigidity, caused by uncal herniation with consequent midbrain compression, is a dangerous development.

The cerebrospinal fluid pressure is high, and the fluid may be clear or bloodstained. Spinal tap should be avoided if the signs suggest the presence of a pressure cone. X-rays will often reveal a fracture of the skull, and if the pineal is calcified, it may be shifted away from the affected side. The echoencephalogram may show a shift of midline structures, but time should not be wasted on laboratory procedures in the face of rapidly advancing clinical symptoms and signs.

Diagnosis depends more upon the evolution of the condition, as judged by the changing pattern of symptoms and signs, than upon the clinical picture at any given time. Suggestive features are a progressively increasing degree of unconsciousness, unilateral pupillary dilatation, ophthalmoplegia, the appearance of new signs or the aggravation of those already present, and the presence of a fracture across the middle meningeal groove. In some cases, exploration will show some other condition; occasionally, an acute subdural hematoma simulates an extradural clot while in other cases there is insufficient extradural or subdural blood to account for the symptoms, and opening of the dura discloses a tense and edematous temporal lobe containing multiple small hemorrhages. The surgical removal of this mass of damaged brain can save life.

Difficulty may also arise in severe injuries when, after an initial period of improvement, the level of unconsciousness starts to fall, pulmonary edema develops, and the general condition deteriorates rapidly. Local signs are absent, and there is no evidence of a pressure cone. This can be due to cerebral swelling from generalized contusion, and no benefit can be expected from decompression.

An abrupt worsening of the patient's condition after head injury, often with the development of hemiplegia, is sometimes due to intracerebral hemorrhage or carotid thrombosis. Prompt recognition of this situation, followed by emergency surgery, may save life. Deterioration in the level of consciousness can also result from water intoxication caused by the excessive administration of fluids containing insufficient salt. Hypernatremia can itself cause irritability, disorientation, disturbance of memory, seizures, and impairment of consciousness. Hyperkalemia can also occur following severe contusion of the brain and brainstem. Elevation of blood urea and hyperglycemia are occasionally found, but there is no evidence that they affect the level of consciousness. Increased drowsiness with a rise of temperature and a lowering of cerebral spinal fluid pressure can occur in the first few days following head injury, as a result of dehydration. This can be recognized clinically by dryness of the skin and tongue and concentration of the urine, and it can be relieved by the administration of saline. Finally, slowly progressive deterioration in the level of consciousness may follow head injuries in elderly people, in whom the most careful examination fails to reveal any of the above causes. Infection of the lungs or urinary tract may precede final dissolution.

Treatment. In most cases, the condition develops rapidly and surgical intervention is urgently needed; delay of an hour or even less may prejudice the patient's chances of survival. The site of exploration is determined by the focal signs, the presence of bruising or edema of the scalp, and the situation of the fracture as determined by x-ray. In the most urgent cases, it is necessary to make burr holes without waiting for x-rays to be done.

Subdural Hematoma

Subdural hemorrhage may be acute, subacute, or chronic.[16, 31] The *acute form* includes cases in which symptoms develop within hours of injury, and this type requires surgical intervention within three days. The injury may be major or minor; this form of hematoma can occur as a result of severe vomiting or a bout of coughing. The *subacute form* is seen in patients whose recovery from a head injury is interrupted within two or three weeks, while the *chronic* hematoma becomes clinically apparent three weeks or more after the injury. The acute and subacute forms increase in frequency to a peak at about 70 years of age, whereas the chronic type has a maximum incidence in the 60's, although it is not rare in children and adolescents.[2] The total incidence is difficult to estimate with accuracy, but it may be as high as 20 per cent if both survivors and fatal cases are included. The chronic variety has a better surgical prognosis than the acute and subacute forms, and it is more common in males than females. Hemorrhagic states predispose to all types of subdural hematoma, including those produced by anticoagulants and cirrhosis of the liver.

ACUTE SUBDURAL HEMORRHAGE

This condition, which may be unilateral or bilateral, usually results from tearing of bridging veins from the brain to the dural sinuses, but it can also occur from a contusion of the brain, with tearing of small vessels and rupture of the overlying membranes, so that a clot collects in the subdural space. It can result from penetrating wounds and from birth injuries. The clot is usually situated in the frontal or temporal region, but no area is immune. Since the injury causing the acute form of subdural hemorrhage is commonly severe, it is apt to be associated with contusion and laceration of the brain; skull fracture may or may not be present. Rarely, an acute hematoma occurs as a result of bleeding from an aneurysm, arteriovenous malformation, hemorrhagic blood dyscrasia, or brain tumor.

The clinical signs are caused by a rapid rise of intracranial pressure, followed by localized compression of the brain, and the development of a tentorial pressure cone with uncal herniation. This occurs over a period of hours or a day or two. There may or may not be a lucid interval, depending upon the severity of brain damage. The spinal fluid is usually bloodstained. Diagnosis is confirmed by arteriography and echoencephalography. Electroencephalography is seldom helpful because it often fails to lateralize the lesion and because bilateral dysrhythmia is usually present as a result of the brain injury.

The liquid clot is aspirated through burr holes; in the few cases in which it is semisolid, an osteoplastic flap may have to be turned.

The prognosis in this type of case is worse than in the chronic variety of subdural hematoma. The mortality is over 50 per cent, and survivors have a prolonged convalescence with considerable liability to subsequent convulsive seizures. Both acute and chronic psychotic manifestations and personality defects may be present for a long time after the accident. The prognosis for ultimate recovery is better in children and young adolescents than it is in older persons.

SUBACUTE SUBDURAL HEMATOMA

This comes on within two or three weeks after injury, and the symptoms and signs develop less rapidly than in the acute form. It is commonly regarded as an early form of chronic subdural hematoma, as described below.

CHRONIC SUBDURAL HEMATOMA

Etiology. Chronic subdural hematoma usually occurs following a blow to the head, but can be caused by a fall on the buttocks, a whiplash injury, a bout of coughing or vomiting, hyponatremia in infants, pneumoencephalography, and operations on the cauda equina entailing a loss of spinal fluid. Sometimes there is no history of injury or other provocative factor; this can be the case in children. Chronic alcoholism and the use of anticoagulants predispose subjects to subdural bleeding, as does any condition causing cerebral atrophy.

Pathology. The hematoma is usually situated over the hemispheres, but it can occur under the temporal lobe, around the chiasm, at the occipital pole, or in the posterior fossa (Fig. 18–5). It is often bilateral. There is a collection of bloody fluid in a cavity lined with laminated blood clot and bounded externally by a layer of connective tissue 1 to 4 mm. thick, which adheres to the dura and contains many new capillaries and lake-

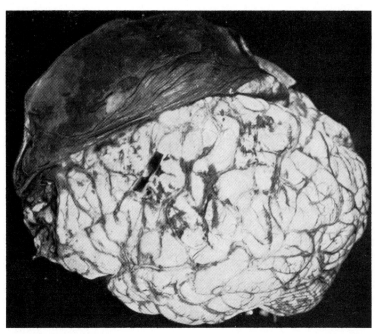

Figure 18–5. Chronic subdural hematoma. (From Wechsler, I.: *Clinical Neurology.* 9th Ed. W. B. Saunders Co., Philadelphia, 1963.)

like spaces filled with normal blood. On the inner surface, there is a thin layer of connective tissue covered with a single layer of mesothelial cells, which lies against the arachnoid. The inner and outer layers unite at the periphery of the hematoma. The appearance of the internal membranes suggests that it is the inner portion of the dura which has been stripped off by the hematoma. The clot may undergo intermittent variations in size, which are reflected in the fluctuating symptoms and in the changing pressures of the cerebrospinal fluid. It is thought that the pressure changes are due to recurrent hemorrhage from the vascular external layer. The hematoma usually increases in size and the subjacent brain is compressed and displaced. This process causes a shift of midline structures, with pressure on the diencephalon, and—ultimately—a tentorial pressure cone. In some cases, the hematoma stops enlarging and becomes organized, resulting in a spontaneous "cure." Calcification may occur (Fig. 18–6).

Symptoms. Of all intracranial space-occupying lesions, the subdural hematoma is the most deceptive because its manner of presentation is so variable.[16, 31] It may mimic a vascular accident, a cerebral tumor, or a psychosis, or it may simply cause a severe headache. The most common presentation is headache followed by fluctuating drowsiness or stupor and the features of a tentorial pressure cone. Local compression of the subjacent brain may or may not produce appropriate symptoms and signs (e.g., hemiplegia); usually it does not.

Headache may be severe, slight, or absent, and it may be over the site of the hematoma or generalized. The patient may be alert, drowsy, or stuporous, and rapid changes in the level of consciousness may occur. Ultimately, when the brainstem is compressed by a pressure cone, coma results from pressure on the ascending reticular formation.

Signs of local pressure are variable. When the clot is situated over one hemisphere, weakness of the contralateral limbs may or may not be present. Rarely,

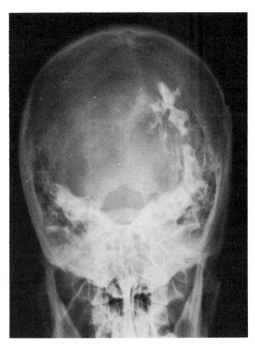

Figure 18–6. Calcified subdural hematoma. (Courtesy of Dr. R. H. Chamberlain.)

infarction of the brain under the hematoma will bring on an abrupt hemiplegia, aphasia, or other localized defect which can be mistaken for a primary vascular accident. With the onset of a pressure cone, ipsilateral motor signs may appear because the crus is pushed against the edge of the opposite tentorium. Sometimes there is a generalized paratonia or Gegenhalten before pyramidal signs develop.

When a tentorial pressure cone occurs, the pupil on the affected side becomes dilated and fixed, and ultimately a complete third nerve palsy develops. Sometimes the posterior cerebral artery is nipped, giving rise to contralateral homonymous hemianopia. As the pressure cone develops, the neck becomes stiff, and decerebrate rigidity appears on one or both sides.

Seizures are uncommon. Disturbances of mind, mood, or behavior may be early features (especially in elderly subjects), presenting before the level of consciousness is significantly depressed. The mental symptoms may vary greatly from hour to hour.

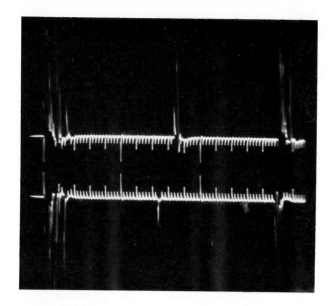

Figure 18–7. Echoencephalogram in a case of left-sided subdural hematoma, showing deviation of midline structures to the right.

Slight edema of the disc and a few retinal hemorrhages may appear, but frank papilledema is uncommon.

The pulse is often slowed, and the blood pressure may be moderately elevated. Cheyne-Stokes respiration may be encountered, but this gives place to rapid, stertorous respiration as pressure on the midbrain develops (p. 425). Needless to say, it is undesirable to let a subdural hematoma develop thus far without surgical intervention.

Laboratory Aids. Spinal tap is to be avoided. Echoencephalography is a simple, rapid, and nontraumatic procedure for detecting a shift of the midline structures, such as occurs in large unilateral hematomas over the convexity of one hemisphere (Fig. 18–3), but there is no shift if bilateral hematomas of equal size are present.

Skull x-rays may or may not show a fracture. The pineal is often displaced to the opposite side, or downward in the case of bilateral parasagittal collections, but it can remain in its normal position despite the presence of a subdural hematoma large enough to produce symptoms.

Arteriography shows displacement of the middle cerebral vessels away from the inner table of the skull. Both sides should be examined because bilateral hematomas are not uncommon.

Electroencephalography[20] may show depression of activity over the hematoma, but the tracing can be completely normal in the presence of a considerable clot, for which reason this form of investigation is unreliable. A brain scan can disclose a subdural hematoma, but care must be taken not to be misled by a hematoma of the scalp.

If the condition of the patient is worsening rapidly, it is wiser to do burr holes than to waste time on academic speculation and complex diagnostic procedures. This applies with particular force to the patient in whom there is reason to suspect that a tentorial pressure cone is imminent.

Treatment. Treatment is surgical. Burr holes are made not only at the suspected site but also on the opposite side. The dura is opened and the fluid contents of the hematoma are washed out with saline. When the collection is large, it is advisable to make counter openings elsewhere. If the hematoma is solid, or largely so, or if there is massive brain swelling, a bone flap must be turned which adequately exposes the lesion and permits its complete removal.

Following the operation, the brain may not expand immediately, for which reason it is necessary to drain the subdural space. Fresh bleeding may occur,

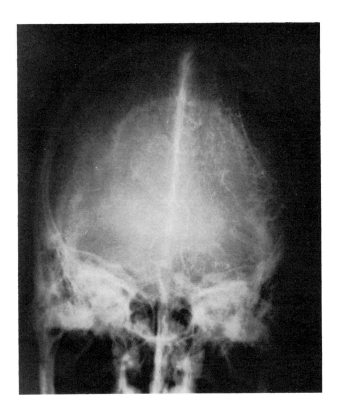

Figure 18–8. Venous phase of the arteriogram, showing left parietal subdural hematoma.

especially in the elderly and in alcoholics with liver damage.

SUBDURAL HEMATOMA IN INFANTS

The condition differs from the adult variety in several respects.[22, 61] It usually arises as a result of excessive moulding of the head during childbirth with consequent rupture of bridging veins, or from postnatal injury; the tendency to bleed can be increased by the presence of subclinical scurvy. It can occur as a result of vomiting and diarrhea, with consequent hypernatremia. Extravasation usually spreads widely on either side of the superior sagittal sinus. The infant is a poor feeder, irritable, apt to vomit, and liable to seizures. Enlargement of the head is noticed at about the fourth month, and may mimic hydrocephalus, but percussion yields a dull note. The sutures separate, and the anterior fontanelle may bulge. Neurological signs are inconspicuous, sixth nerve palsy being the most common. X-ray reveals enlargement of the skull, and there may be a notable increase in the size of the middle fossa on one side. Transillumination may disclose a shadow. Diagnosis is confirmed by puncturing the subdural space lateral to the margin of the anterior fontanelle with a large-bore needle; the fluid should not be aspirated, but should be allowed to drip out; sudden removal of large bilateral hematomas may be followed by profound shock, so not more than 15 ml. should be removed from each side at one time. The procedure is repeated daily for one to two weeks. When, as a result of this and of supportive measures, the patient is deemed fit for craniotomy, bilateral burr holes are made to evacuate the remaining fluid and to see whether a solid membrane is present; if it is, it should be removed because an organized clot can restrict the growth of the brain beneath it.

Subdural Hygroma

Subdural hygroma is an uncommon condition in which symptoms resembling those of a chronic subdural hematoma are produced by an encysted collection of clear fluid in the subdural space.[60] It is usually caused by a head injury with tearing of the arachnoid and the passage of cerebrospinal fluid into the subdural space. It is assumed that the rise of pressure encountered in these collections is caused by a ball valve action at the site of the vent in the arachnoid. Occasionally a subdural effusion occurs secondary to meningitis, especially in children. Rarely, a hygroma has resulted from rupture of the arachnoid in cases of communicating hydrocephalus.

The clinical features of hygroma are the same as those of chronic subdural hematoma, and the diagnosis can be made only by angiography and exploration. The prognosis for recovery is good following drainage.

Intracerebral Hemorrhage Following Head Injury

Intracerebral hematoma is less common than the subdural variety but more frequent than epidural hemorrhage. Gurdjian and Webster found it in 36 of 950 cases of head injury.[16] These hemorrhages are the result of acute contusion of blood vessels deep in the brain. They are usually found in the frontal and temporal regions, and occasionally in the cerebellum. They follow severe head injuries and therefore a skull fracture is commonly present, and the cerebrospinal fluid is usually bloody. As is to be expected from the deep location of the hematoma, contralateral hemiplegia is usual.

The diagnosis is confirmed by angiography, and the treatment is prompt surgical evacuation. The same diagnostic and therapeutic procedures are called for in people who suffer an abrupt intracerebral hemorrhage weeks after head injury. This condition is sometimes referred to as *late traumatic apoplexy*, and it is not always clear whether the original trauma should be regarded as coincidental or responsible. Sudden hemiplegia after head injury is occasionally due not to cerebral hemorrhage but to thrombosis of the middle cerebral or internal carotid artery. This will be disclosed by arteriography. Injuries to the neck alone may also cause thrombosis of the internal carotid artery, with consequent hemiplegia.

The Electroencephalogram in Head Injuries

In animals, the EEG record immediately after the impact of a concussive blow is either isoelectric or flat.[20] This is succeeded by diffuse slow waves which, in the case of very mild injury, give place to a normal alpha rhythm within a few minutes, but which may persist for weeks or months in more severe trauma. The widespread slow activity ranges from 1 to 7 c./sec., and may be interrupted by bouts of high-voltage, 2 to 3 c./sec. waves. Generally speaking, the deeper the coma, the slower the waves, and in this sense the severity of trauma and the amount of generalized EEG abnormality run parallel, but the immature brain of infants and children sometimes show disproportionately severe EEG disturbances, either focal or generalized, after trivial injuries.

The return to normal may be rapid or slow, complete or incomplete, according to the severity and nature of the injury.[20, 55, 59] When the dura has been penetrated, focal abnormalities are apt to persist for months or years after the injury. Sometimes the generalized disturbances pass off, but a focal abnormality slowly develops at or near the site of a cortical scar. Owing to the contrecoup effect, this focus may be situated at a point remote from the site of the blow — in the opposite hemisphere, for instance. In such cases, seizures usually appear sooner or later, whereas the persistence of diffuse dysrhythmia carries with it less likelihood of seizures.

Care must be exercised in the interpretation of electroencephalograms in patients who complain of postconcussional "blackouts"; such symptoms should not be regarded as epileptic unless they are associated with paroxysmal seizure patterns, and even then the relationship may be coincidental because, since idiopathic epilepsy and head injuries are both common, seizures and paroxysmal EEG discharges found after a head injury are not necessarily due to trauma. The best way to establish a causal connection between brain injury and dysrhythmia is to carry out serial recordings at intervals; if there is no improvement in the record as time goes on, it may be due to some additional condition.

The findings in subdural hematoma are variable, and from a diagnostic point of view, they are unreliable. Depression of electrical activity over the site of the hematoma does occur, but it is by no means the rule; a slow wave focus may be found, or there may be generalized slowing as a result of increased intracranial pressure, coincidental brain injury, or both.

The electroencephalogram provides little help in the assessment of the headaches, fatigability, and memory weakness of the postconcussional state.[59] These symptoms may persist after the EEG has returned to normal, but this does not necessarily mean that the symptoms of which the patient complains are unreal. There is, in fact, no objective method of determining whether postconcussional symptoms are wholly organic or are being prolonged as a neurosis.

Whiplash Injury

This type of injury commonly occurs to passengers sitting in a stationary car when it is hit from behind by another vehicle.[13] The sudden forward acceleration of the body causes violent hyperextension and subsequent flexion of the neck, leading to overstretching of the muscles and ligaments of the neck. The upper cervical cord is probably stretched as well, but clinical evidence of damage to the cord is unusual unless the situation is complicated by the presence of backward-protruding spondylitic ridges which narrow the cervical canal.

Little is known about the pathological effects of whiplash injury on the central nervous system of man, but in experimental animals, whiplash injuries which are unaccompanied by a head injury have been found to produce chromatolysis in cells of the brainstem, damage to nerve fibers in the cervical cord, and hemorrhage over the surface of the brain —notably in the parietal and parasagittal areas, the tips of the frontal and temporal lobes, the infero-orbital and temporooccipital areas, the brainstem, and the upper cervical cord.[38] These hemorrhages are consistent with the shearing stresses caused by sudden rotational movements of the skull.

Clinical Features. In the absence of a coincident head injury, unconsciousness rarely occurs as a result of a whiplash injury. A characteristic feature of the condition is that the symptoms do not usually appear until several hours after the accident. The patient is apt to consider himself uninjured and to refuse medical help. Later that day, or the next morning, there is pain in the neck and head, stiffness in the occipital region and across the shoulders, and a general sense of malaise. The patient also complains of lightheadedness, dizziness, irritability, fatigability, and difficulty in concentration—symptoms that are indistinguishable from those of the postconcussional syndrome. Torres and Shapiro[52] report that the EEG changes following pure whiplash injuries are similar to those seen after concussion from a head injury. It would seem, however, that the EEG eventually reverts to normal, because in the author's experience it is usually within normal limits by the time the patient is referred for a neurological consultation on account of the undue persistence of symptoms.

As in the postconcussional syndrome, there is a vexatious lack of objective clinical signs, but Toglia found abnormal caloric responses in 50 of 80 cases, and an abnormal threshold to rotary tests in 9 of 16 patients.

In most cases, the symptoms gradually abate over a period of several weeks, but as in the postconcussional syndrome, they are apt to persist for many months in emotionally unstable individuals, in cases in which compensation or litigation lies ahead, and in individuals who are under personal or domestic stress.

Treatment. In the acute phase, the wearing of an adjustable plastic collar is the conventional treatment, but the time comes when the patient has to be weaned from this device. There are no set guidelines on this point, but on the evidence available at present, it seems reasonable to dispense with the collar in 3 to 4 weeks after the injury, unless there is clear evidence of damage to the cervical spine or the intervertebral discs.

Birth Injuries

Injuries sustained by infants during parturition are usually the result of difficult labor, but too rapid moulding of the head during precipitate labor can also be harmful. Results include fractures of the skull, subdural hematoma, contusion of the brain, and traction injuries to the brainstem, spinal cord, and brachial plexus.

Fractures of the vault are of little consequence if the blood vessels and brain escape injury. Fractures of the base can sever the optic or facial nerves, but survival is rare because of the severity of the associated brain injuries in such cases.

Contusion of the brain can result from a depressed fracture. In other cases, excessive traction on the legs in breech presentations pulls the medulla and cerebellar tonsils into the foramen magnum, thus causing widespread hemorrhagic contusion. Liability to this type of injury is increased in the presence of malformation of the foramen magnum and upper vertebrae.

It is probable that excessive molding of the skull thrusts the inframedial border of the temporal lobe through the tentorial hiatus, and contusion sustained in this way may be one cause of the incisural sclerosis which is found in some cases of temporal lobe epilepsy. Other results of focal contusion include monoplegia, hemiplegia, hemianopia, and (rarely) diplegia. The most common of these is infantile hemiplegia.

SPINAL CORD INJURIES

Etiology. Road accidents and falls from heights account for most spinal cord injuries in civilian life. Injuries from accidental electrocution or as a result of being struck by lightning can cause disruption of the cord, and additional damage may be sustained if the victim is flung violently to the ground by the shock. Angulation of the neck can cause massive herniation of an already protruding disc and can also damage the vertebral arteries.[44] Cord injuries may also be sustained in infants during delivery.

Pathology. Spinal concussion is a convenient clinical term for transient spinal paralysis which passes off completely within a few hours. For obvious reasons, the pathology of this recoverable condition is unknown. In more severe injuries, there is contusion of the cord. In its mildest form this is accompanied by swelling of the cord within the tough and inelastic pia, with partial or complete interruption of conduction; edema tends to increase for 48 hours and then declines over a period of about a week.[1] In yet more severe injuries, there may be tearing of meninges and nerve roots, epidural, subdural, and subarachnoid hemorrhages, and cavitation of the cord. Cavities may be found extending longitudinally several segments above and below the point of maximum injury. Hemorrhage into the cord is less common, but it too may spread upward and downward; it usually remains confined to the central gray matter. Rarely, *hematomyelia* occurs hours or even a day or two after the injury, causing a rapid increase in the physical signs. It may also occur, with devastating effect, after comparatively slight trauma and after strains such as lifting a heavy weight, laughing, or a bout of coughing. It is probable that in such instances the strain has caused rupture of a minute angiomatous malformation within the cord. The author has seen this happen in two cases of hereditary telangiectasia.

Fracture dislocations are commonest in the lower cervical and lumbar areas, but because the cord is smaller than the vertebral canal, considerable degrees of bone displacement are possible without cord compression. Hemorrhage into the canal is present in such cases, but since the blood can spread upward and downward, cord compression from this factor is unusual.

The most severe of all injuries, and one from which no recovery can be expected, is transection of the cord; it occurs infrequently as a result of fracture dislocation and is usually due to penetrating wounds.

The process of recovery is marked by rapid reduction of edema, absorption of hemorrhage, fibrosis of the meninges, and gliosis of the injured part of the cord.

Clinical Features. At the onset, all neurological function is usually lost below the level of the lesion. There is complete flaccid paralysis, total sensory loss, loss of sweating below the level of the lesion, and paralysis of the bowel and bladder—a condition of so-called spinal shock. What happens next depends on how severely the cord is injured. In the mildest cases, sometimes referred to as spinal concussion, there is a rapid return of function, and the patient may appear virtually normal within a matter of hours. This happy outcome is most often seen in children. In more severe injuries, flaccid paralysis lasts for days or even a week or two; then tendon reflexes return and eventually become hyperactive, extensor plantar responses are apparent, and sensation starts to return. In the initial phase of spinal shock, there is paralysis of both the sphincter and the

detrusor of the bladder, but when reflex activity returns, retention of urine is almost the rule; if incontinence occurs, it is usually the result of overdistention. The legs show a varying degree of spasticity which is mainly in the extensor groups, and the tendon reflexes are hyperactive.

In still more severe cases, paraplegia (or tetraplegia) persists. In paraplegia-in-extension, there is persistent hypertonicity of the adductors of the thighs, the quadriceps, and the extensors of the ankle. The knee and ankle jerks are exaggerated, clonus is common, and tapping the patellar tendon on one side may cause contraction of the adductors on both sides. The plantar reflexes are extensor. Withdrawal of one leg in response to a noxious stimulus to the foot may be accompanied by increased extension of the contralateral leg—the crossed extensor reflex. Paraplegia-in-extension is thought to be due to involvement of the corticospinal (pyramidal) tracts, with relative sparing of the reticulospinal tracts. Paraplegia-in-flexion, on the other hand, implies damage to both the corticospinal and reticulospinal pathways. The thighs and knees are flexed, the tendon reflexes are reduced, ankle clonus is seldom obtainable, and the plantar responses are extensor.

Involuntary muscle spasm may be present.[25] It may be either flexor or extensor in distribution. Flexor spasms are usually encountered in cases of paraplegia-in-flexion, and may be accompanied by sweating and evacuation of the bladder—a mass reflex. This can occur with both complete and incomplete lesions of the cord, and is found in over 50 per cent of all patients with severe lesions. The spasms are aggravated by overdistention of the bladder, bed sores, and other sources of irritation. They have usually been attributed to the removal of inhibitory influences from above, but there is evidence that the proximal end of the isolated portion of cord is hyperexcitable to mechanical and electrical stimuli, and that mass reflexes can be reduced or abolished by cutting the dorsal columns below the level of the lesion.[45] This suggests that factors associated with scarring at the point of injury are partly responsible for the increased reflex excitability of the isolated segments of the cord.

Flaccid paraplegia with rapid wasting and permanent loss of the knee and ankle reflexes occurs with severe lesions involving the anterior horns of the lumbar segments and the cauda equina. In such cases there are no involuntary spasms of the leg muscles, but contractures are liable to occur and must be guarded against by appropriate physiotherapy and splints.

Involvement of the autonomic system below the level of the lesion is common. At first, sweating is abolished distal to the level of the injury, a fact which is of practical value when looking for evidence of a spinal cord lesion in a patient who is unconscious as a result of a coincident head injury. Later, with return of reflex functions in the distal segment of the cord, sweating may be increased. As mentioned, the bladder is always affected. At first, both the detrusor and the sphincter are paralyzed, and if the lumbosacral segments of the cord are pulped, paralysis will be permanent. With lesions higher up, retention of urine is the rule because the sphincter recovers before the detrusor, and if incontinence occurs, it is usually due to overflow. Involuntary micturition will often accompany involuntary muscle spasms, especially in paraplegia-in-flexion. Priapism is frequent. Peristalsis is inhibited by severe transverse lesions of the upper thoracic region, and paralytic ileus may therefore develop. When the lesion is complete and is above the sixth thoracic segment, diseases of the abdominal viscera which would normally cause pain may no longer do so.

Pain is common after incomplete spinal injuries. Sometimes it is due to irritation of nerve roots at the level of the injury. A second type is characterized by intense burning and tingling sensations involving the entire body below the level of the lesion; the patient may also complain of an exaggerated awareness of visceral sensations.

Laboratory Findings. The spinal fluid is usually bloodstained in the early stages of a severe spinal injury, and manometric evidence of block is often present. The latter can be due to several factors, alone or in combination: fracture dislocation, protrusion of an intervertebral disc, edema of the cord, and extradural, subdural, or intramedullary hemorrhage. After about a week, edema will usually subside. If there is no block at the beginning and it becomes apparent later on, it can be due to the formation of dense adhesions around the area of injury, or (rarely) to abscess formation.

X-rays are essential. Sometimes a fracture will be seen at some distance from the level of cord injury, as determined by clinical signs.

Prognosis. It is impossible to give a prognosis within the first day or two. The outlook depends on the patient's age and general health, the presence or absence of other injuries, success or failure in the avoidance of renal infection and pressure sores, and, above all, the degree of damage to the cord. In cases with open wounds, it is usually possible to determine the precise state of affairs at the time of debridement. If the cord is not actually transected, there is always hope for some degree of recovery, although it may be several months before the first clinical evidence thereof appears. It is unlikely that there will be any significant improvement after a period of three years, though skillful rehabilitation will enable the patient to make increasingly better use of the functions that remain.

Treatment. Fractures, dislocations, and penetrating injuries should be treated in accordance with modern surgical and orthopedic principles.[44] Early attention to the bladder and to the skin over pressure points will save trouble later on. An indwelling catheter should be introduced at once, to avoid the overdistention which does so much to promote infection of the bladder and kidneys.[33] Subsequently, tidal drainage can be introduced. Avoidance of bed sores in bedridden patients is helped by frequent change of position, rubbing the skin over pressure points, and the application of spirit, powder, or a silicone spray. In certain fracture dislocations, the use of a Stryker frame is desirable, because the patient can be changed from the face-up to the face-down position without being handled. Thus, it is possible to change the weight-bearing areas of the skin at frequent intervals with little effort and minimum risk. When bed sores are present there is often a fall of plasma protein and secondary anemia; blood transfusion is indicated in these circumstances.

Laminectomy for the relief of pressure on the cord from edema or hemorrhage is of doubtful value; it can lead to a catastrophic herniation of the edematous cord when the dura is opened. Most authors therefore advise against surgical decompression, unless there is progression of the neurological signs, and rely on steroids to reduce edema. Manometric block found soon after spinal trauma is not by itself an indication for laminectomy.

It is usual to administer antibiotics over the first week or two to forestall infection of the lungs, urinary tract, and—in compound fractures—of the spinal canal itself.

Abdominal distention must be guarded against. A Miller-Abbott tube into the duodenum, and rectal tubes, will afford relief. Pitressin (1 ml.) or neostigmine (5 mg.) can be given intramuscularly. Hot packs to the abdominal wall can be effective.

Physiotherapy should be initiated as soon as possible to keep the limbs and joints in good condition. However, in patients liable to the mass reflex, excessively vigorous physiotherapy can increase the spasms. The intramuscular injection of from 5 to 15 mg. of Valium will often relieve spasms. In cases of total transection of the cord, or when there is reason to believe, after a long convalescence, that no further recovery can be expected, spasms limited to a muscle or muscle group are dealt with

by division of peripheral nerves, by anterior rhizotomy, or by the injection of boiling saline into the cord below the level of the lesion. When there is doubt as to whether further improvement can occur or not, it is probably wiser to interrupt the dorsal columns below the level of the lesion.[45] Medical rhizotomy induced by subarachnoid injection of 20 per cent phenol in Pantopaque has also proved effective.[36]

Rehabilitation. Much can be done to help a paraplegic person over his psychological and physical handicaps. That many severely incapacitated individuals are eventually able to earn a living and to take part in social life should be emphasized from the start, because effective rehabilitation depends as much on the patient's will and enthusiasm as on the efforts of others. There is a place for physical therapy, the intelligent use of supportive apparatus, orthopedic surgery, and vocational training. Wherever possible, the patient should be referred to a rehabilitation center, and the referral should be early rather than late. When no such center is available, both physician and patient can derive much benefit from perusal of the considerable literature on the subject.[18, 25, 30, 36, 41]

Birth Injuries to the Spinal Cord and Brainstem

Excessive longitudinal traction on the trunk during breech delivery, or on the head during cephalic delivery, is more likely to damage the cord and brainstem than the spine itself because the latter is slightly elastic and the former are not. Such injuries can lead to sudden death during or shortly after labor, and to diplegia or quadriplegia in those who survive the first few hours. Complete transection of the cord is rare.

On the basis of postmortem examination of the brain and spinal cord of a large number of infants, Towbin[53] has estimated that these injuries may be responsible for as much as 10 per cent of all neonatal deaths in the United States.

Lower estimates are usually forthcoming from institutions which do not include routine examination of the spinal cord in autopsies of the newborn. The most common finding is profuse epidural hemorrhage extending over the cervical and upper thoracic regions of the spinal cord. This may be accompanied by tears of the dura, subdural hematoma, subarachnoid hemorrhage, edema and congestion of the cord, diffuse neuronal damage, and focal softening and hemorrhage into the substance of the cord. More important as a cause of neonatal mortality are hemorrhages into the brainstem and hemorrhagic contusion of the inferior surface of the cerebellum resulting from acute herniation of the cerebellar tonsils during spinal traction. Malformations of the foramen magnum and upper cervical vertebrae may facilitate such injuries, and damage to the vertebral arteries can compound the situation by causing infarction in the brainstem and inferior surface of the temporal lobes.

Clinical Features. There is difficulty in getting the baby to breathe. When it starts to do so, respiration is shallow and irregular and punctuated by periods of apnea. These symptoms signify medullary distress and are accompanied by profound shock; death usually occurs within a few hours. In less severe cases, it is noted within a day or two that the legs are flaccid and immobile and that there is retention of urine and feces. The abdominal musculature and intercostal muscles are paralyzed, and the cry is weak. In those who survive the first few weeks, reflex activity returns to isolated portions of the cord; the legs are flexed at the hip and knee, the tendon reflexes are brisk, and from time to time a mass reflex appears. If the spinal lesion is incomplete, as is usually the case, the legs are spastic but not completely paralyzed, and they are held in extension. Retention of urine with overflow incontinence is present whether transection is complete or not.

Avulsion of motor roots of the mid-cervical segments can give rise to lower motor neuron paralysis of one or both arms; the nature of this paralysis can be identified by electromyography.

The prognosis is usually poor, early death being the rule in cases of total or subtotal transection. Life may be prolonged for a time by scrupulous attention to the skin and control of urinary infection.

The diagnosis is obvious in the most severe cases. In others, the initial hypotonia of the legs may suggest amyotonia congenita, but this syndrome is excluded by the presence of bladder symptoms and sensory loss, and by the limitation of atonia to the lower half of the body. In mild cases, the spastic condition of the legs may mimic cerebral diplegia, but the history of breech delivery and the presence of a sensory level consistent with a spinal cord lesion will indicate the correct diagnosis.

PERIPHERAL NERVE INJURIES

The term "injury," as used in this section, includes penetrating wounds, acute and chronic pressure lesions, and tearing of nerves or plexuses by stretching.

Etiology and Pathology

PENETRATING WOUNDS.[40, 48] These are the most common source of *acute* nerve injury. The nerve may be severed completely or incompletely, it may be bruised by the passage of a high-velocity bullet through adjacent tissues, or it may be disrupted by the inadvertent injection into it of an irritant substance. The peripheral portion of the nerve undergoes degeneration: A few days after injury, the myelin sheaths become swollen and stain less intensely with hematoxylin, the cells of the sheath of Schwann multiply, and the axons swell and break up into small pieces. The Schwann cells become actively phagocytic and engulf the myelin, and the peripheral segment of the nerve ultimately consists of Schwann cells and connective tissue which act as a guideline for regenerating axons. The portion of nerve proximal to the injury undergoes a less marked change: degeneration occurs for a short distance proximal to the injury and the parent cell becomes rounded and swollen, while its nucleus travels to the periphery and the Nissl substance undergoes chromatolysis. The muscles supplied by the affected nerve show an increase of sarcolemmal nuclei and a loss of staining properties; the fibers split, their nuclei degenerate, and they are replaced by fibrous tissue if regeneration does not occur.

Regeneration of myelinated fibers may start as early as the second day, and of nonmyelinated fibers by the fourteenth day. The axons of the stump sprout out in disorderly fashion, forming terminal bulbs and spheres, and seek to penetrate the peripheral segment but make no attempt to invade the surrounding tissue; growing nerve fibers avoid mesoderm, and if they encounter it in the form of fascia or muscle between the severed ends of the nerve, they recoil upon themselves and form a tangled skein of interlacing fibers—a neuroma. If there is no such obstruction, the axons grow at the rate of about 1.5 mm./day in healthy young adults. Myelination is slower, starting 15 to 30 days later and spreading peripherally from the point of injury. Under optimal conditions, motor fibers make their way to muscle and sensory fibers to sensory endings; we do not know the explanation of this remarkable phenomenon, but it determines the degree of functional recovery. Some fibers do in fact take the wrong turning: An axon which formerly supplied the skin over the tip of the thumb may eventually arrive at its base, so that a stimulus applied at the base will feel as if it comes from the tip; a touch fiber may connect with a temperature receptor giving rise to perversion of sensation. Bearing in mind the complexity of the motor and sensory pathways, it is remarkable that functional recovery is as good as it so often is.

After crush injuries of the nerves, several motor filaments may go down the original endoneural tube, but only one connects with the old motor end-plate. After nerve sectioning, recovery is slower; nerve fibers do not occupy all the available endoneural tubes, and those that fail to find an old end-plate establish connections with muscle fibers by means of new, simplified end-plates.[62] Misdirection of nerve fibers sometimes occurs; thus, a fiber destined for muscle *a* arrives at muscle *b*, but the disorganization of function which occurs as a result of this misdirection can be overcome by training and re-educational exercises.

PRESSURE LESIONS. These occur as a result of acute or chonic compression of a segment of nerve. The acute variety is seen when a nerve is compressed by a tourniquet or when a superficial nerve (e.g., radial, peroneal) is nipped between the bone and a hard surface during sleep or anesthesia. It occurs from pressure upon the axillary nerves in unreduced dislocation of the shoulder joint, and from compression of the lumbosacral cord between the fetal head and the pelvic brim. The chronic type occurs when peripheral nerves are exposed to long-continued mild pressure. Thus a nerve may be slowly strangled by callus formation or by a tumor arising from an adjacent bone; the median nerve may be compressed in the carpal tunnel; the ulnar nerve is exposed to recurrent pressure where it lies behind the medial epicondyle and also as it enters the hypothenar eminence.

The clinical and pathological effects of pressure are largely due to interruption of the blood supply to the affected segment of nerve. This causes an initial impairment of conductivity, followed by structural damage.[5, 10] It has been shown that the application of pressure to a segment of nerve for periods up to two hours results in a recoverable loss of conduction without histological change; more prolonged exposure gives rise to longer-lasting but still recoverable paralysis, together with demyelination of the affected segment, and if the pressure persists still longer, there is a complete anatomical lesion with subsequent degeneration in the whole of the distal segment and a corresponding delay in recovery. In cases of slight or intermediate severity, motor fibers are more affected than sensory ones, and it is not uncommon to find a considerable degree of weakness without any sensory loss at all after the first few days; in some cases, cutaneous sensation is normal while deep sensibility is impaired. Sympathetic fibers are the least vulnerable of all.

In chronic cases, in which the pressure has been present for some time, the nerve is narrowed in the area of constriction, with a firm bulbous enlargement—a neuroma—immediately proximal to it. The peripheral portion of the nerve shows the usual histological picture of degeneration, partial or complete.

TEARING OF ROOTS, PLEXUSES, AND PERIPHERAL NERVES BY OVERSTRETCHING. This type of injury to the brachial plexus occurs as the result of falls on the tip of the shoulder, forceful elevation of the shoulder, and traction on the fetal arm during labor. Violent falls on the shoulder are not uncommon in motorcyclists, and the upper roots of the plexus are damaged. Tearing of the lower roots occurs when an individual who is falling from a height tries to save himself by holding onto a support. Traction on the arm during labor can cause either an upper plexus lesion (Erb's paralysis) or a lower plexus lesion (Klumpke's paralysis), depending on which way the fetus is descending. The peroneal and radial nerves can be injured by violent movements of the limbs.

In severe traction injuries, the root sheath is torn and there is wide separation of the ends. Even when there is no complete rupture of continuity, the internal damage may be considerable, extending as much as 15 cm. along the nerve. Fibrosis follows, and generally speaking, the prognosis is poor with or without surgical intervention.

Clinical Features of Nerve Injuries

Complete severance of a mixed peripheral nerve gives rise to (1) flaccid paralysis, followed by atrophy and changes in electrical excitability; (2) sensory loss, both superficial and deep; (3) loss of sweating within its cutaneous distribution; (4) loss of stretch reflexes; (5) loss of pilomotor reflexes; (6) eventual trophic disturbances in the skin, nails, bones, and joints.

Motor Signs. To determine the extent and degree of paralysis, each muscle must be tested separately and the results recorded, so that subsequent progress can be assessed with accuracy. The numerical index system is a convenient method: The figure 5 is used for the ability to contract a muscle against powerful resistance, 4 for contraction against gravity and slight resistance, 3 for contraction against gravity alone, 2 for movement obtained only when gravity is eliminated, 1 for a visible flicker of contraction, and 0 for complete paralysis. Having mapped out the motor loss, one can usually decide the site of the lesion and whether it is complete or not, but in some cases the problem is complicated by other factors. Of these, anomalies of innervation are important, inasmuch as persistence of movement in a muscle within the paralyzed group may be due either to incompleteness of the lesion or to an anomalous supply from an adjacent motor nerve. The best way of deciding this is to block the collateral nerves with procaine and then repeat the examination.[19] A further difficulty is introduced by trick movements whereby an ingenious patient learns to circumvent some of his incapacity by using nonparalyzed muscles to carry out the work of those which are affected. For instance, abduction of the fingers can be achieved despite paralysis of the interossei by contraction of the long extensors while the fingers are slightly flexed at the metacarpophalangeal joints. Or gravity may be used to assist paralyzed muscles, e.g., wrist drop can be masked by supinating the forearm and thus allowing the wrist to dorsiflex under its own weight. For other examples of trick movements, the reader should consult Pollock and Davis.[40]

A further source of confusion is the

presence of injuries to tendons and muscles themselves, which add to the paralysis. Ultimately, adhesions around joints and in tendon sheaths aggravate the incapacity and thus help to obscure the amount of neurogenic paralysis. Trauma to arteries may also confuse the picture by inducing ischemic paralysis of peripheral nerves other than those injured by direct violence, and by causing changes in the muscles themselves; the latter become weak or paralyzed, and manifest any degree of pathological change, from cloudy swelling to a patchy fibrosis which gives the muscle a hard, wooden consistency. Muscle biopsy is useful in deciding whether paralysis of a muscle is due to nerve injury, ischemia, or both.

Aggravation of organically determined weakness by hysteria or malingering is a common event. There is usually an underlying profit motive, whether in the realm of compensation, avoidance of professional or domestic responsibilities, or resolution of a personal conflict.

Sensory Signs and Symptoms. Sectioning of a pure sensory nerve does not cause subsequent pain, but discomfort may be felt as a result of injuries to blood vessels and other tissues. On the other hand, incomplete lesions of mixed nerves —notably the median and the sciatic— will occasionally be followed by the excruciating burning pain of causalgia or by a dull ache in the distribution of the nerve (p. 531). Paresthesias within the area of sensory denervation are common during the recovery period; they may be elicited by stimulating the skin or by percussing the nerve itself. The latter is sometimes employed to estimate the degree of recovery, in the belief that the most peripheral point along the nerve at which tapping can elicit paresthesias is the point to which new fibers have grown (Tinel's sign), but the method is unreliable.

When a sensory nerve is injured, sensory loss is confined to the skin; sensibility from joints and muscles is conveyed in motor nerves and is therefore lost in lesions of motor or mixed nerves.

Cutaneous loss is most easily determined by light touch and pinprick; thermal loss usually follows the latter so closely that its separate assessment has no practical value. During recovery, the quality of the response, the patient's ability to locate the stimulus, and his capacity for two-point discrimination provide additional information as to the progress of recovery.

Sensory findings following nerve injury are liable to misinterpretation in the presence of anomalous innervation, arterial injuries, and hysteria or malingering.

Immediately after nerve section, cutaneous loss to light touch, pain, and temperature is found over the whole area supplied by the nerve; there is an inner core of complete loss, surrounded by a marginal zone in which some sensation remains owing to overlap from adjacent nerves. In this hypoesthetic zone, the threshold is high, the response excessive, and localization poor. These are features of partial denervation. Within six weeks, the area of pain loss often shrinks around its periphery, not because of regeneration of the severed nerve but because the marginal area of skin is invaded by pain fibers from adjacent uninjured nerves.[57]

The cutaneous distribution of individual nerves varies somewhat from case to case, as does the degree of overlap between adjacent nerves. When there is doubt whether a sensory nerve is completely severed or not, or whether more than one nerve is involved, the method of nerve block analysis is useful.[19] Additional information can be obtained from sweating tests. The sudomotor fibers of the sympathetic nerves reach the skin via the sensory nerves, and sweating ceases when the latter are cut. The method devised by Guttmann is accurate.[17] The skin of the limb is dusted with a powder containing iodine and starch, and the patient is made to sweat by placing him under a heat cradle. Perspiration takes place over the normal skin, turning the powder blue, whereas no color change is observed over the affected area. This technique can also demonstrate the scattered pinpoints of sweating which herald regeneration. Alternatively, the area of anhidrosis may be mapped out by measuring the electrical resistance of the skin; dry skin has a higher resistance than moist skin. It is easier but less accurate than Guttmann's method, and does not disclose the pinpoint sweating referred to above.

When the nerve injury is accompanied by damage to a major artery of the limb, the area of peripheral sensory loss is often increased by the effect of ischemia on other peripheral nerves. The muscles are tender, in contrast to the loss of muscle pain which occurs after sectioning a mixed nerve, and the signs of arterial occlusion will usually be obvious. Discrepancies in sensory findings may also be due to hysteria or malingering, and in such cases sweat tests are useful in mapping out the area of organically determined impairment.

Trophic Disturbances. When there is loss of superficial sensibility to painful and thermal stimuli, the patient is apt to injure the skin without knowing it. Denervated tissues do not heal readily. The skin is smooth and dry, the hair falls out, and the nails become brittle. The combination of repeated trauma and lack of reparative power can give rise to painless ulcers. Arthropathies similar to the Charcot joint of tabes and syringomyelia occasionally occur in denervated joints, and the bones become brittle. Superficial trophic lesions recover fairly rapidly when sensation starts to return.

SIGNS OF REGENERATION

Generally speaking, the order of recovery is as follows: (1) sensory symptoms—tingling, formication, dull pain—accompanied by the return of crude pain sensibility and punctate sweating; (2) the halt of muscle atrophy, with a return of tone and the presence of action potentials as determined by electromyography (p. 23); (3) gradual return of motion; (4) increasing capacity for sensory discrimination. Curiously enough, tendon reflexes which have been lost seldom return even in the presence of good motor and sensory function.

Sensation. Many patients report a "different feeling" in the area of sensory loss as the first symptom of recovery. It may be associated with a dull aching pain, which is not to be confused with causalgia. The first objective sign is the reappearance of sensibility to crude pain (e.g., pinching the skin) in the area of isolated supply: Early sensory improvement in the marginal areas is not necessarily a sign of regeneration (p. 519). Crude pressure, pain, and thermal sensibility return together, in a patchy manner; the threshold is high, the stimulus cannot be localized accurately, and the sensation evoked is diffuse and may be unpleasant in character. As regeneration proceeds, there is a return of intermediate degrees of temperature, pain, and touch; localization improves, and two-point discrimination ultimately becomes possible.

Motor Recovery. Proximal muscles usually recover before distal ones, and many nerves exhibit a definite order of recovery after suture. Return of function should be looked for first in the extensors of the wrist after a radial nerve lesion, in the peronei and extensor digitorum longus in sciatic palsy, and in the pronator teres and flexor carpi radialis in median lesions. Indications of regeneration can be obtained by electromyography (p. 23) before they are apparent clinically. As power returns, there is at first a lack of precision in the movements; the muscle will not always do what the patient wants it to, partly because of proprioceptive impairment and partly because some regenerating fibers may have gone to the wrong muscle. Much can be done to expedite functional recovery by re-educative exercises.

Recovery can be delayed for many reasons. Regeneration of the nerve fibers may be prevented by imperfect apposition of the cut ends or by ischemia from coincident arterial injury, or it may be slowed by general ill health or old age. Even if regeneration is satisfactory, it avails little if the muscles have been allowed to undergo contracture and the joints have stiffened. The word "allowed" is used advisedly because these complications are usually avoidable. The return of lymph and venous blood from a limb depends partly on muscular activity; when the latter is absent, edema occurs, followed by fibrosis and the deposit of a network of collagen fibers through the soft tissues and around the joints. Under these circumstances, the joints become stiff, the tendons adhere to their synovial sheaths, and the denervated muscles undergo progressive interstitial fibrosis and contracture. A second form of muscle shortening, occurring in unparalyzed antagonists, is a physiological response which can usually be prevented by exercises and splinting.

TREATMENT

Nonoperative Treatment. Care of the muscles and joints of the limb should start as soon as the diagnosis of a nerve injury has been made, whether operative intervention is intended or not, since the maintenance of mobility is as important as nerve regeneration. Each joint of the affected limb should be put through a complete range of movements several times a day; the patient can do much of this himself if skilled supervision is lacking. Splinting is desirable to prevent the overstretching of paralyzed muscles by gravity or by nonparalyzed antagonists and to prevent shortening in active muscles, but splints should be easily removable so as not to interfere with exercises. Daily galvanic stimulation may retard muscle atrophy. Re-education during recovery is exceedingly valuable, because regenerating axons do not always reach the correct muscle or portion of muscle, and this gives rise to incoordination of movement which can be overcome only by intensive re-education, starting with the performance of simple movements and going on to more complex tasks. The entire motor-sensory complex has to be trained anew.

Surgical Treatment. Repair of a severed nerve may be done immediately, or it may be deferred. The arguments for and against primary suture lead to the conclusion that in the great majority of cases, it is better to do a planned operation soon after the initial wound has healed than to attempt immediate primary suture.[48] Little is lost by the delay, and much may be gained. At the time when debridement is carried out, it is desirable to bring the ends of the nerve together by two stitches, so placed as to prevent rotation of the cut ends, and to leave it at that until the wound has healed.

Lesions of Individual Peripheral Nerves

The Great Occipital Nerve (C2). This nerve provides unimportant motor filaments to the neck muscles and supplies sensation to the posterior half of the scalp. Its main clinical interest lies in the frequent occurrence of pain, sometimes associated with paresthesias and slight hypalgesia within its distribution, in elderly persons with spondylosis of the upper cervical spine. There is no intervertebral disc between the atlas and the axis, so that these symptoms cannot be attributed to a herniation, but they are probably caused by inflammatory involvement of the root where it lies in contact with the joint of Luschka, between the opposing rims of the bodies of the atlas and the axis. The pain is sometimes referred to the temple. Treatment is by physiotherapy, supplemented if necessary by injecting 1 per cent procaine into the tender spots which are usually to be found in the muscles on the affected side of the neck. Wearing a cervical collar can help, but traction is not consistently effective. Tumors in the region of the foramen magnum may cause similar occipital sensory symptoms, but there will usually be evidence of spinal compression as well.

The Great Auricular Nerve (C2-3). The nerve winds around the posterior border of the sternomastoid and ascends

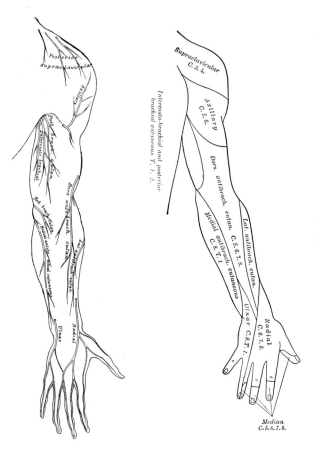

Figure 18–9. Cutaneous innervation of the right upper extremity, anterior view. (From Goss, C. M., Ed.: *Gray's Anatomy of the Human Body.* 27th Ed. Lea & Febiger, Philadelphia, 1959.)

on its surface beneath the platysma in company with the external jugular vein to supply the skin over the angle of the jaw, the back of the auricle, and the lower half of the concha. It is often visibly enlarged in leprosy, and may be involved by herpes zoster.

The Third and Fourth Cervical Nerves. The nerves supply the skin of the neck and infraclavicular region, and provide important motor fibers to the sternomastoid and trapezius. The spinal portion of the eleventh cranial nerve is composed of rootlets from the first to the sixth cervical segments which enter the skull through the foramen magnum and blend with the bulbar root. The nerve thus formed leaves the skull through the jugular foramen, within the same dural sheath as the vagus, and supplies the trapezius and sternomastoid. There are differences of opinion as to which part

of the former muscle is innervated by the accessory and which by the third and fourth cervical nerves, but in practice it is usually possible to localize the lesion by a study of satellite symptoms and signs, in particular by the demonstration of sensory loss over the neck and clavicle (C3–4).

The Phrenic Nerve (C3-5). The nerve supplies the central portion of the diaphragm. It can be paralyzed by: (1) disease of the cervical cord—poliomyelitis, syringomyelia, spondylosis, tumor, caries and fracture dislocations of the cervical vertebrae, and pachymeningitis; (2) affections of the roots, notably neuralgic amyotrophy of the shoulder girdle; (3) disease in the neck and mediastinum—penetrating wounds, tumors, aneurysm of the aorta. Cases of uncomplicated unilateral paralysis of the diaphragm are occasionally seen, without any obvious cause either in the history or on clinical examination. Some are due to congenital absence of muscle fibers in the diaphragm; this is said to occur on the left side only. In others, however, the patient is able to date its onset by the occurrence of dyspnea on effort. Such cases of idiopathic phrenic paralysis must always be examined at frequent intervals to exclude a mediastinal or cervical cord lesion. The diagnosis of diaphragmatic paralysis is suggested by recession of the hypochondrium on the affected side during inspiration, and is confirmed by x-ray screening.

The Circumflex (Axillary Nerve) (C5-6). The nerve winds around the neck of the humerus to enter the deltoid from beneath. It supplies the deltoid and teres minor, and innervates the skin over the former. Deltoid paralysis is common in poliomyelitis, serum neuritis, neuralgic amyotrophy, fracture dislocation of the shoulder and syringomyelia. It can occur from pressure by an unpadded crutch, from tears of the upper roots of the plexus by falls upon the tip of the shoulder, and from downward traction on the arm in breech deliveries. In complete paralysis, the arm can be abducted a short way by the supraspinatus, and some people can actually abduct fully but weakly despite complete paralysis of the deltoid. In incomplete lesions, the movement obtained depends on which portion of the muscle is spared; the posterior fibers retract the arm, the anterior fibers draw it forward, and the large intermediate mass of the muscle abducts it. In the treatment of deltoid paralysis it is important to prevent the formation of adhesions in and around the shoulder joint by putting the joint through a complete range of movement thrice daily. In the early stages, an abduction splint should be applied.

The Long Thoracic Nerve (C5-6-7). This nerve supplies the serratus magnus, which holds the scapula to the chest wall during movements of the upper limb, and rotates the inferior angle upward and laterally when the arm is held out in front of the body. In serratus palsy, the patient has difficulty in using the arm because the scapula is no longer fixed, its medial border standing out like a wing when the patient is asked to push the hand forward against resistance. It is often difficult to assign a cause for isolated paralysis of the long thoracic nerve. It can occur as a result of a blow to the neck, or from carrying a heavy weight on the shoulder. Poliomyelitis, neuralgic amyotrophy, and serum neuritis are occasionally responsible. Sometimes it complicates the cervical rib syndrome, the nerve being involved at the point where it crosses the uppermost rib.

The Suprascapular Nerve (C5-6). The supraspinatus and infraspinatus muscles are supplied by this nerve. As it passes backward and downward from the plexus to the scapula, it is liable to injury from carrying of heavy weights on the shoulder; it is often involved in neuralgic amyotrophy.

The Musculocutaneous Nerve (C5-6). This nerve supplies the brachialis, biceps, and coracobrachialis, and continues below the elbow as the lateral cutaneous nerve of the forearm to the base of the thenar eminence. Paralysis is usually due to direct injury; flexion of the elbow and supination of the forearm are weak, but sensory loss is usually slight, owing to overlap from contiguous nerves. The biceps reflex is lost.

The Radial (Musculospiral Nerve (C5-8). The nerve winds round the radial groove of the humerus to supply the triceps, supinator longus, and the extensors of wrist, fingers, and thumb. It supplies the skin over the lower third of the radius, and a variable area over the dorsum of the wrist, first interosseous space, back of the thumb, and back of the proximal two phalanges of the index and middle fingers. Sensory loss is often limited to the space between the first two metacarpals. The cardinal sign of paralysis is wrist drop (Fig. 18–10).

The radial nerve is very vulnerable to fractures of the shaft of the humerus, callus formation and bony tumors in the region of the radial groove, sustained

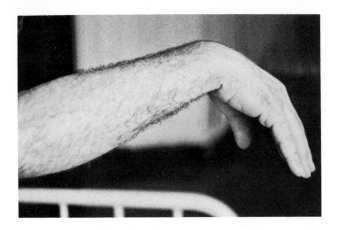

Figure 18–10. Wrist drop from radial nerve compression. (Courtesy of Dr. A. M. Ornsteen.)

pressure, as for instance from going to sleep with the arm over the back of a chair or using an unpadded crutch, gunshot wounds, imperfectly placed intramuscular injections, and tourniquet paralysis. Paralysis of radial distribution is seen in some forms of polyneuritis (notably lead, alcohol, diphtheria), in polyarteritis nodosa, in diseases of the spinal cord such as poliomyelitis and neurosyphilis, and occasionally in neuralgic amyotrophy, but there is usually additional evidence of disease in other peripheral nerves.

In complete palsy, e.g., with a lesion in the axilla, there is failure to extend the elbow, wrist, fingers, and thumb, and weakness of supination owing to involvement of the supinator brevis. The grip is weak because inability to extend the wrist puts the long flexors at a mechanical disadvantage. When the arms are held out, the wrist flexes under the weight of the hand and the fingers are slightly bent. The affected muscles undergo atrophy, and electromyography will show evidence of denervation. *There may be normal reactions to electrical stimulation in the early stages of paralysis produced by pressure.* The prognosis of radial palsy depends on the type and severity of the causal lesion. Mild cases of compression recover soon, and open wounds have a more favorable outlook than is the case in ulnar or median lesions. Trophic disturbances, other than wasting, are exceptional, and causalgia is almost unknown. Treatment depends

on the cause, but it is necessary to emphasize that wearing a cock-up splint to keep the wrist and fingers in partial extension can be harmful because it leads to stiffening of the joints. Such splints can be worn with advantage during occupational therapy, since they increase the efficiency of the flexors of wrist and fingers and so enable the patient to do work that would otherwise be impossible, but they should be discarded for at least 12 of every 24 hours.

The Posterior Interosseous Nerve. In the antecubital fossa, the radial nerve divides into a superficial sensory branch and the posterior interosseous nerve; the latter passes through the supinator brevis, winds around the neck of the radius, and then passes distally along the interosseous membrane. It supplies the supinator, the extensors of the wrist and fingers, and the abductor and extensor of the thumb (Fig. 18–11). It has no cutaneous sensory functions. Paralysis of the muscles supplied by this nerve may be sudden or slow in onset. In nontraumatic cases submitted to exploration, the findings have included enlargement of the bicipital bursa, lipomas, fibromas, and entrapment neuromas.[58] The natural prognosis of this condition is poor, but improvement can follow surgical exploration and the correction of whatever situation is present.

The Median Nerve (C6-7-8, D1). This nerve is derived from the outer and inner cords of the brachial plexus, and supplies the long flexors of the forearm (with the

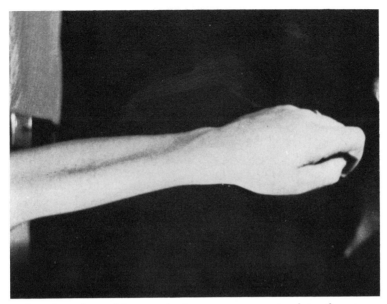

Figure 18–11. Partial paralysis of the posterior interosseous nerve involving the extensors of the fingers. The extensors of the wrist have been spared. (Courtesy of Dr. A. M. Ornsteen.)

exception of the flexor carpi ulnaris and the medial half of the flexor digitorum profundus), the pronators, the lateral two lumbricales, abductor pollicis, opponens pollicis, and half the flexor pollicis brevis. The cutaneous fibers of the median nerve are derived from the outer head (C6-7), and supply the palmar aspect of the thumb, index, middle and lateral side of the ring fingers, the back of the terminal phalanges of the same fingers, and the lateral half of the palm. Median paralysis is a crippling disaster because it paralyzes the grip and weakens pronation, two of the most important movements of the body. It usually results from penetrating injuries, and when the nerve is incompletely severed, there is a small but definite risk of subsequent causalgia. Maladroit intravenous injections into the cubital veins may enter the medial nerve. Compression of the nerve in the carpal tunnel (p. 530) may lead to motor and sensory loss in the hand. Paralysis of muscles within the median territory, but without sensory loss, occurs in poliomyelitis, amyotrophic lateral sclerosis, and lead poisoning; wasting of the thenar eminence may be the first sign of syringomyelia and leprosy. The median nerve sometimes supplies the flexor carpi ulnaris and all the deep flexors of the fingers, and may even supply the adductor of the thumb. Conversely, the ulnar nerve may encroach on median territory.

The Ulnar Nerve (C8, D1). The ulnar nerve arises from the medial cord of the brachial plexus and runs downward through the axilla on the medial side of the axillary artery, between it and the axillary vein, continuing downward on the medial side of the brachial artery as far as the middle of the arm. Here it pierces the medial intermuscular septum and descends in front of the medial head of the triceps to the interval between the medial epicondyle and the olecranon where it lies in a groove on the back of the epicondyle, and is liable to compression between the bone and any hard surface upon which the elbow may be leaning. This is especially apt to occur in the presence of cubitus valgus. The nerve then dips down between the two heads of the flexor carpi ulnaris, at which point it can be injured by repeated forceful contraction of the muscle in heavily muscled individuals. This gives rise to ulnar palsy which is similar to that produced by lesions behind the elbow, but local tenderness is found about an inch distal to the medial epicondyle, and at operation a traumatic neuroma may be found as the nerve dips between the two heads of the muscle. It is important to distinguish between these two forms of ulnar palsy, because whereas transposition of the nerve to the front of the elbow may be required when it has been injured behind the elbow, the operation of choice in the more distal variety of entrapment is to provide more room for the nerve at the site of constriction.

The ulnar nerve supplies the flexor carpi ulnaris, the medial half of the flexor digitorum profundus, the hypothenar muscles and interossei, the medial two lumbricals, the adductor pollicis, and (usually) the medial part of the flexor pollicis brevis. It supplies sensation to the back of the wrist on the medial side, the ulnar border of the hand, the hypothenar eminence, the little finger, and the medial half of the ring finger. The skin over the medial border of the forearm is supplied by the median cutaneous nerve (C8, D1) which arises from the medial cord of the plexus. Consequently, if signs of ulnar palsy are present in the hand, and there is also sensory loss in the proximal forearm, the lesion must be in the upper arm, brachial plexus, roots, or spinal cord. A complete lesion at the elbow causes weakness of the flexor carpi ulnaris and the ulnar intrinsic muscles of the hand, and sensory loss and anhidrosis of ulnar distribution. The resultant deformity, the *main en griffe,* is characterized by flattening of the hypothenar eminence, hollows between the medial flexor tendons in the palm owing to wasting of the lumbricals and interossei, overextension of the metacarpophalangeal joints of the medial two fingers, and flexion of their distal joints. It is important to keep the fingers extended in line with the hand while testing the interossei, in order to obviate trick movements carried out by the long flexors and extensors of the fingers.

Ulnar paralysis can be caused by: penetrating wounds at any level; occupations involving pressure on the nerve at the base of the hypothenar eminence, as in racing cyclists and users of vibrating tools such as pneumatic drills; repeated pressure on the nerve behind the elbow, which is especially likely to occur in the presence of cubitus valgus in persons whose occupation entails leaning the elbows on a hard surface for much of the working day, or in patients confined to bed who are in the habit of raising themselves on their elbows; compression of the nerve behind the two heads of flexor carpi ulnaris as described; fracture dislocation of the elbow; and leprosy, chronic lead poisoning, polyarteritis nodosa, and hypertrophic polyneuritis.

Ulnar paralysis must be distinguished from the effects of lesions involving the brachial plexus, the eighth cervical root, and the spinal cord. A cervical rib can cause weakness and atrophy of the muscles supplied by the ulnar in the hand. Damage to the eighth cervical root will paralyze *all* the intrinsic muscles of the hand, but sensory loss will be confined to the medial half of the palm, the little finger, and the whole of the ring finger. It is often associated with Horner's syndrome on the same side. The cause is usually obvious—penetrating wounds, cervical spondylosis, traction injuries, and birth injury—but upward extension of carcinoma of the lung from the superior pulmonary sulcus is an occasional cause which is easy to miss if the chest is not x-rayed. Diseases affecting the cervical cord include poliomyelitis, amyotrophic lateral sclerosis, neoplasm, and syringomyelia. Tumors situated in the *upper* part of the cervical cord occasionally give rise to wasting of the small muscles of the hand in addition to signs of pressure on the long tracts; this is probably due to pressure on the anterior spinal artery with consequent ischemia of the lower cervical segments. Wasting of the hand occasionally precedes atrophy of the feet and leg muscles in peroneal muscular atrophy. It may also occur in lesions of the contralateral parietal lobe; the reason for this is not known.

The Anterior Crural Nerve (L2-3-4). The nerve enters the thigh underneath Poupart's ligament, lateral to the femoral artery. It supplies the quadriceps, sartorius, and pectineus; the hip and knee joints; the skin over the front and inner aspects of the thigh; and, via the long saphenous nerve, the inner aspect of the leg between the knee and ankle. The nerve is seldom injured except by penetrating wounds. Extension of the knee is impossible, and flexion of the hip is weak, so the disability is greatest when the patient attempts to walk up stairs. Direct injuries apart, most of the disturbances within the territory of this nerve are due to diseases affecting the lumbar roots, the cauda equina, and the lumbar segments of the cord. Femoral neuritis, in the sense of interstitial neuritis of rheumatic origin, is rare, if indeed it occurs at all. Anterior femoral

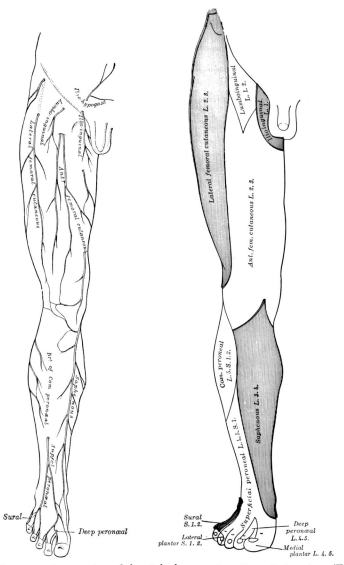

Figure 18–12. Cutaneous innervation of the right lower extremity, anterior view. (From Goss, C. M., Ed.: *Gray's Anatomy of the Human Body.* 27th Ed. Lea & Febiger, Philadelphia, 1959.)

pain is usually due to a prolapse of the third or fourth lumbar disc, or spondylosis of the lumbar spine with root involvement. The quadriceps in common with the muscles of the pelvic girdle is often involved bilaterally in the muscular dystrophies and myopathies.

Lateral Cutaneous Nerve of the Thigh. (See page 531.)

The Obturator Nerve (L2-3-4). The nerve supplies the abductor longus, brevis, and gracilis muscles, and the skin of the upper part of the inner aspect of the thigh. It may be injured by dislocations of the hip joint and in parturition. There is weakness of adduction and external rotation of the femur. Pain in the obturator distribution is usually due either to a prolapsed disc involving one of its roots of origin, a pelvic mass, or an obturator hernia.

The Sciatic Nerve (L4-5, S1-2-3). Fibers from the fourth and fifth lumbar roots pass downward, as the lumbosacral

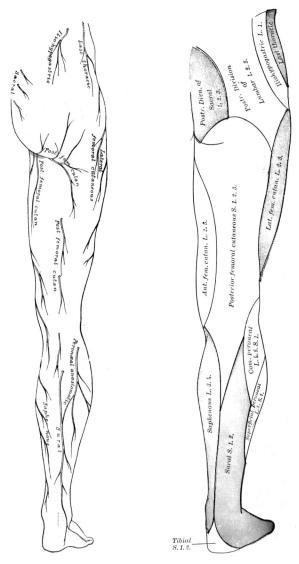

Figure 18–13. Cutaneous innervation of the right lower extremity, posterior view. (From Goss, C. M., Ed.: *Gray's Anatomy of the Human Body.* 27th Ed. Lea & Febiger, Philadelphia, 1959.)

cord, over the brim of the pelvis, crossing the sacroiliac joint as they do so. They are liable to compression by the fetal head during labor and are occasionally involved by the spread of disease, notably tuberculosis, from the sacroiliac joint. Within the pelvis, they unite with the upper three sacral roots to form the sciatic nerve, which is sometimes invaded or pressed upon by pelvic neoplasms. Rarely, it is invaded by endometriosis. The nerve emerges through the greater sciatic notch, at which point it may be injured by fractures of the ischium or by improperly placed intramuscular injections. The division into medial and lateral popliteal takes place at any point between the pelvis and the lower third of the thigh. Branches given off in the thigh supply the glutei, the hip joint, the hamstrings, and part of the abductor femoris. The skin over the back of the thigh and the upper part of the calf is supplied by the posterior cutaneous nerve; some of its branches curve upward to the buttock, and others pass to the scrotum or labium. This nerve, though not a branch of the sciatic, is often involved along with the sciatic in lesions of the pelvis.

The medial popliteal (tibial) nerve supplies the muscles of the calf and sole of the foot, the joints of the ankle and foot, and the skin of the distal half of the back of the calf, the heel, and the plantar aspect of the foot and toes. *The lateral popliteal (common peroneal)* winds around the neck of the fibula, where it is exposed to the danger of pressure and fractures, and divides into anterior tibial and musculocutaneous nerves; sometimes the latter comes off in the popliteal fossa, so that it may be spared in injuries to the neck of the fibula. The anterior tibial supplies all the muscles of the anterior compartment and the extensor digitorum brevis, together with a small triangle of skin at the base of the great and second toes. The musculocutaneous branch supplies the peronei, the lateral surface of the lower third of the leg, and most of the dorsum of the foot. A branch of the lateral popliteal supplies the skin over the upper half of the lateral aspect of the leg. The sciatic nerve thus conveys sensation from the leg below the knee with the exception of a strip on the medial border which is supplied by the long saphenous branch of the femoral nerve (mainly derived from L4).

Sciatic palsy may have its origin at several distinct and easily recognizable levels. In the cauda equina, the descending fibers may be involved by tumors, large herniations of the lumbar discs, arachnoiditis, and hydatid cysts. The roots may be affected by posterolateral disc herniations, spondylosis, fracture dislocations, spondylolisthesis, tumor, and Pott's disease. The lumbosacral cord and the sacral plexus are exposed to the pressure of the fetal head, which can cause complete and sometimes permanent sciatic paralysis as a result of prolonged dystocia, and it may be involved by pelvic neoplasms. Fractures through the ischium can cause serious injury to the nerve.

In the thigh, the nerve is liable to penetrating injuries such as stab wounds, gunshot wounds, and misplaced intramuscular injections. Partial palsy is not uncommon as the result of sitting overlong on a chair with a hard edge, and this is especially liable to occur in patients who, as a result of dieting, have recently lost their protective padding of subcutaneous fat. Foot drop or sciatic palsy can also result from using unpadded supports to support the back of the thighs during surgical operations which require the patient to be in the lithotomy position. Primary interstitial neuritis, once considered to be the usual cause of sciatica, is rare, if it exists at all. Ischemic paralysis of the sciatic nerve may occur from the application of a tourniquet, and is also seen in thrombosis or embolism of the femoral artery.

Complete division of the sciatic nerve causes paralysis of the hamstrings and all the muscles below the knee. If the lesion is at or above the greater sciatic foramen, the glutei are also involved, with the result that the pelvis tilts forward. This is compensated for by a lordosis. Sensory loss involves the leg below the knee excepting only the medial aspect of the leg, ankle, and foot, which are served by the saphenous nerve. The ankle jerk and the plantar responses are lost. Sweating is deficient on the foot except for its medial aspect; the hair falls out and the leg is slightly edematous, especially if it is allowed to hang down. Perforating ulcers may develop on the sole of the foot.

Injury to the external popliteal (peroneal) nerve is usually caused by pressure between the fibula and a hard object, but it can also be brought about by fractures in this area and by squatting for half an hour or so. Rarely, it results from a sudden awkward movement of the leg involving forceful plantar flexion of the foot. There is paralysis with wasting of the peronei and of the anterior tibial group. The foot and toes cannot be dorsiflexed, and eversion is lost. Some degree of inversion is possible in association with plantar flexion. If the nerve is divided above the origin of the lateral cutaneous branch, sensation is impaired over the dorsum of the foot including the first phalanges of the toes, and over the anterior and external aspect of the leg in its lower half; when the lesion is below the origin of the lateral cutaneous nerve, sensation is impaired over the dorsum of the foot only. The ankle jerk is retained, but the distal components of the plantar reflex are lost. However, a noxious stimulus to the sole of the foot will cause contraction of the quadriceps if the pyramidal system is intact, whereas in pyramidal disease such stimulation may lead to a visible contraction of the hamstrings, thus affording evidence of an upper motor neuron lesion even if movements of the foot are paralyzed by a lesion of the peripheral nerves.

The internal popliteal nerve is seldom injured alone, but if injury occurs, the calf muscles and the intrinsic muscles of the foot are paralyzed, and the foot assumes the position of talipes calcaneovalgus. There is anesthesia and analgesia over the sole of the foot. The ankle jerk is lost, and the flexor plantar response is abolished.

Entrapment Neuropathies

The term "entrapment neuropathy"[27] refers to local injury and inflammation caused by mechanical irritation of a peripheral nerve in its course through a fibrous or osseofibrous tunnel or at a point where it abruptly changes its course through the deep fascia or over a fibrous or muscular band. It does not include neuropathies resulting from external pressure on superficial nerves, such as the ulnar at the elbow, the peroneal as it winds around the neck of the fibula, or the interdigital nerves of the foot (Morton's neuroma).

At the point of entrapment, there is an inflammatory response characterized by swelling, degeneration of nerve fibers, and replacement fibrosis. The latter may anchor the nerve to surrounding structures and thereby rob it of its freedom to move during movements of the limb.

The symptoms of these neuropathies include pain, paresthesias, and—in the case of mixed nerves—weakness and wasting of muscles. The pain and paresthesias are usually present at rest as well as during activity, and are often worst at night. The pain, but not the paresthesias, often spreads proximally from the point of entrapment; thus pain from compression of the median nerve in the carpal tunnel may shoot up the arm, and an interdigital neuroma of the foot can cause pain that radiates up the back of the leg. This contrasts with the distal projection of pain which occurs with irritative lesions of nerve roots and plexuses.

The Median Carpal Tunnel Syndrome. This common condition is caused by compression of the median nerve as it runs in its tunnel under the transverse carpal ligament. It is most commonly seen in middle-aged women who have recently engaged in vigorous, manual work, especially if they are unused to such work, but it can occur in persons of either sex from adolescence onwards. It is sometimes seen in pregnancy and is a common complication of arthritis or tenosynovitis at the wrist. It has been seen in association with acromegaly and sometimes complicates the thoracic outlet syndrome.

The patient complains of paresthesias on the volar aspect of the thumb, index, and middle finger. Sometimes there is pain in the palm, and in rare cases, pain may shoot up the front of the forearm. An unpleasant numbness rather than true pain is the most frequent symptom. It is aggravated by using the hands but is also prone to occur at night or on waking.

In moderate cases, there is slight blunting to pinprick over the median distribution in the hand. Some complain of weakness of the thumb and in long-standing cases there is pronounced weakness and atrophy of the opponens pollicis and the adductor pollicis brevis, the lateral two lumbricals, and the outer head of the flexor pollicis brevis. Sometimes the first dorsal interosseous muscle is involved as well. Although this situation usually takes months to develop, cases are occasionally encountered in which severe sensory and motor signs develop over a matter of two or three days.

In mild cases, the symptoms sometimes disappear spontaneously if the patient desists from manual tasks. In those with arthritis, 5 mg. of prednisone three times a day for three or four weeks can be effective. Local injections of hydrocortisone can help. When these measures fail, the nerve should be decompressed.

Meralgia Paresthetica. This common condition is caused by entrapment of the lateral femoral cutaneous nerve as it pierces the deep fascia to enter the thigh in the region of the ilio-inguinal ligament.[35] It is characterized by the presence of unpleasant numbness and tingling on the anterolateral aspect of the thigh. There is usually a mild degree of sensory impairment over the affected area, but there is no weakness, and the patellar reflex is unaffected. Rarely, the paresthesias are accompanied by pain.

It can occur in the second half of pregnancy and may also appear following a sudden gain in weight. Sometimes it follows an injury to either limb which involves a change in posture.

In most cases, the condition is mild and the patient is able to ignore the situation when informed that the symptoms have no serious implications. If a pelvic tilt is present, a heel lift on the contralateral shoe should be tried. If the severity of the symptoms justifies more active measures, the entrapment should be relieved by surgical neurolysis.

The Tarsal Tunnel Syndrome. This involves entrapment of the posterior tibial nerve or of the plantar nerves between the medial malleolus and the laciniate ligament (the tarsal tunnel). The posterior tibial nerve splits into medial plantar, lateral plantar, and calcanean branches. After leaving the tunnel, the plantar nerves pass through two openings in the origin of the abductor hallucis. Symptoms can arise from entrapment at this point, or in the tunnel itself. There is pain, often of a burning quality, on the plantar aspect of the foot and toes, tenderness at the point of entrapment, and sensory impairment in the distribution of the medial or lateral plantar nerves or both. In long-standing cases, there is weakness of the short flexors of the toes and a greater than normal difficulty in abducting and adducting the toes. The condition can be treated by injection of hydrocortisone and the correction of abnormal postures of the foot, but if these measures fail, surgical neurolysis is needed.

Entrapment neuropathy can also involve other nerves, notably the posterior interosseous nerve of the forearm (p. 524), the ilio-inguinal nerve, and the obturator nerve.

Causalgia

Penetrating wounds which injure mixed peripheral nerves or major plexuses are sometimes followed by intense burning pain in the distal sensory distribution of the affected nerve fibers. It usually occurs following partial interruption of a nerve but can follow total transection.[56] True causalgia occurs in about 3 per cent of all cases of peripheral nerve injuries. It can start at the moment of injury, but more usually it appears within the first week. It is most commonly encountered following injuries to the sciatic and median nerves but can also follow injuries to the brachial plexus and the ulnar, radial, and posterior tibial nerves.

The pain—which is necessarily accompanied by the motor and sensory signs appropriate to the nerve injury—varies from moderate to intense, and has a burning quality. It is aggravated by heat, dryness, physical stimuli, and emotional disturbances. The patient carefully protects the affected part from contact with surrounding objects, and partial relief is sometimes obtained by keeping it covered with cool, moist dressings. When severe, the pain banishes sleep and speedily reduces the patient to a condition of abject misery.

The hand or foot, as the case may be, may display either vasodilatation or vasoconstriction; vasodilatation predominates in the early stages. The area is pinker and warmer than normal and tends to be dry. In the presence of vasoconstriction, the part is colder than on the opposite side, and it is mottled or pale and usually moist. The presence or absence of sweating is determined to some degree by the extent of the injury to the nerve. The skin tends to become glossy, and trophic changes occur in the nails and bones of the affected part. The hand or foot is kept immobile because pain is often induced by movement, and in consequence the joints become stiff.

Though there is no completely satisfactory explanation of causalgia, Doupe and his associates[8] advanced the attractive hypothesis that the pain is due to short-circuiting of efferent autonomic impulses at the site of injury; that is to say, normal efferent impulses traveling in sympathetic fibers in response to thermoregulatory and vasomotor needs, stimulate afferent sensory fibers. This suggestion is supported by the observation that impulses in one fiber can initiate impulses in adjacent sensory fibers at any spot at which the nerve is partially damaged.[14] The theory explains the abrupt disappearance of causalgia when the sympathetic chain is interrupted, either physiologically, by an injection of procaine, or anatomically, by sympathectomy.

Causalgia is not the only type of pain which can follow a nerve injury. Some patients complain of pricking, cutting, tingling, piercing, or throbbing pain, while others suffer from severe "pins and needles." These varieties of discomfort, which lack a burning quality, do not respond to sympathectomy. They often disappear spontaneously after a month or two, but occasionally they persist longer and give rise to emotional disorders. The sharp, radiating pain induced by pressure on a neuroma at the site of injury is easily distinguished from the foregoing.

Sometimes the sole of the foot becomes extremely tender to deep pressure after incomplete interruption of the tibial or sciatic nerve. There is no spontaneous pain, and cutaneous stimuli do not cause discomfort, but pain is experienced in standing or walking, so that the patient has to walk on his heel or on the outer side of the sole. The condition may persist unabated for many months. It has been claimed that the discomfort can be removed by injecting alcohol into the lumbar sympathetic chain.

REFERENCES

1. Brock, S.: *Injuries of the Brain and Spinal Cord, and Their Coverings.* 4th Ed. Springer Publishing Co., New York, 1960.
2. Bull, J. W. D.: The diagnosis of chronic subdural hematoma in children and adolescents. *Brit. J. Radiol.* 22:68, 1949.
3. Ceballos, R.: Pituitary changes in head trauma (analysis of 102 consecutive cases of head injury). *Alabama J. Med. Sci.* 3:186, 1966.
4. Crompton, M. R., Teare, R. D., and Bowan, D. A. L.: Prolonged coma after head injury. *Lancet* 2:938, 1966.
5. Denny-Brown, D., and Brenner, C.: Paralysis of nerve induced by direct pressure and by tourniquet. *Arch. Neurol. Psychiat.* 51:1, 1944.
6. Denny-Brown, D., and Russell, W. R.: Experimental cerebral concussion. *Brain* 64:93, 1941.
7. Dodge, P. R., and Meirowsky, A. M.: Tangential

wounds of scalp and skull. *J. Neurosurg.* 9: 472, 1952.

8. Doupe, J., Cullen, C. H., and Chance, G. Q.: Posttraumatic pain and the causalgic syndrome. *J. Neurol. Neurosurg. Psychiat.* 7: 33, 1944.

9. Evarts, C. M.: Diagnosis and treatment of fat embolism. *J.A.M.A.* 194:899, 1965.

10. Feindel, W., and Stratford, J.: The role of the cubital tunnel in tardy ulnar palsy. *Canad. J. Surg.* 1:287, 1958.

11. Ford, R., and Ambrose, J.: Echoencephalography. The measurement of the position of midline structures in the skull with high frequency pulsed ultrasound. *Brain* 86:189, 1963.

12. Friede, R. L.: Experimental concussion acceleration: Pathology and mechanics. *Arch. Neurol.* 4:449, 1961.

13. Gay, J. R., and Abbott, K. H.: Common whiplash injuries of the neck. *J.A.M.A.* 152:1698, 1953.

14. Granit, R., Leksell, L., and Skoglund, C. R.: Fibre interaction in injured or compressed region of nerve. *Brain* 67:125, 1944.

15. Gurdjian, E. S., and Lissner, H. R.: Photoelastic confirmation of the presence of shear strains at the craniospinal junction in closed head injury. *J. Neurosurg.* 15:58, 1961.

16. Gurdjian, E. S., and Webster, J. E.: Traumatic intracranial hemorrhage. *Injuries of the Brain and Spinal Cord, and Their Coverings.* 4th Ed. Edited by Brock, S., Springer Publishing Co., New York, 1960.

17. Guttmann, L.: Disturbances of sweat secretion after complete lesions of peripheral nerves. *J. Neurol. Psychiat.* 3:197, 1940.

18. Guttmann, L.: Rehabilitation after injuries to the spinal cord and cauda equina. *Brit. J. Phys. Med. Int. Hyg.* 9:130, 1946.

19. Highet, W. B.: Procaine nerve block in the investigation of peripheral nerve injuries. *J. Neurol. Neurosurg.* 5:101, 1942.

20. Hoefer, P. F. A.: The electroencephalogram in cases of head injury. *Injuries of the Brain and Spinal Cord, and Their Coverings.* 4th Ed. Edited by Brock, S., Springer Publishing Co., New York, 1960.

21. Holbourn, A. H. S.: Mechanics of head injuries. *Lancet* 2:438, 1943.

22. Ingraham, F. D., and Matson, D. D.: Subdural hematoma in infancy. *J. Pediat.* 24:1, 1944.

23. Jennett, W. B.: Early traumatic epilepsy: Definition and identity. *Lancet* 1:1033, 1969.

24. Jennett, W. B., and Lewin, W.: Traumatic epilepsy after closed head injuries. *J. Neurol. Neurosurg. Psychiat.* 23:295, 1960.

25. Kaplan, L. I., Grynbaum, B. B., Lloyd, K. E., and Rusk, H. A.: Pain and spasticity in patients with spinal cord dysfunction. *J.A.M.A.* 182:120, 1962.

26. Kaufman, H. H.: Non-traumatic cerebrospinal fluid rhinorrhea. *Arch. Neurol.* 21:59, 1969.

27. Kopell, H. P., and Thompson, W. A. L.: *Peripheral Entrapment Neuropathies.* Williams and Wilkins Co., Baltimore, 1963.

28. Kremer, M., Russell, W. R., and Smyth, G. E.: A midbrain syndrome following head injury. *J. Neurol. Neurosurg. Psychiat.* 10:49, 1947.

29. Lindenberg, R., Fisher, R. S., and Durlacher, S. M.: The pathology of the brain in blunt head injuries of infants and children. Proceedings Second International Congress Neuropathology, 1955, p. 477.

30. Lowman, E. W.: Rehabilitation of the paraplegic patient. *Arch. Neurol. Psychiat.* 58: 610, 1947.

31. McKissock, W., Richardson, A., and Bloom, W. H.: Subdural hematoma. A review of 359 cases. *Lancet* 1:1365, 1960.

32. McKissock, W., Taylor, J. C., Bloom, W. H., and Till, K.: Extradural hematoma. *Lancet* 2:167, 1960.

33. Morales, P. A., and Hotchkiss, R. S.: The management of the bladder in traumatic paraplegia. *Arch. Phys. Med. Rehab.* 40:141, 1959.

34. Munro, D.: Rehabilitation of patients totally paralyzed below the waist. *New Eng. J. Med.* 233:731, 1948; 236:223, 1947; 250:4, 1954.

35. Nathan, H.: Gangliform enlargement on the lateral cutaneous nerve of the thigh. Its significance in the understanding of the etiology of meralgia paraesthetica. *J. Neurosurg.* 17:843, 1960.

36. Nathan, P. W.: Intrathecal phenol to relieve spasticity in paraplegia. *Lancet* 2:1099, 1959.

37. Nielsen, J. M.: Amnesia for life experiences. *Bull. Los Angeles Neurol. Soc.* 23:143, 1958.

38. Ommaya, A. K., Faas, F., and Yarnell, P.: Whiplash injury and brain damage. *J.A.M.A.* 204: 285, 1968.

39. Oppenheimer, D. R.: Microscopic lesions in the brain following head injury. *J. Neurol. Neurosurg. Psychiat.* 31:229, 1968.

40. Pollock, L. J., and Davis, L.: *Peripheral Nerve Injuries.* Paul B. Hoeber Div., Harper and Row, New York, 1933.

41. Rusk, H. A.: *Rehabilitation Medicine.* C. V. Mosby Co., St. Louis, 1958, pp. 446–476.

42. Russell, W. R., and Whitty, C. W. M.: Studies in traumatic epilepsy. *J. Neurol. Neurosurg. Psychiat.* 15:93, 1952.

43. Sahy, T. J., Irving, M., and Millac, P.: Severe head injuries: A six year follow-up. *J. Neurol. Neurosurg. Psychiat.* 31:299, 1968.

44. Scarff, J. E.: Injuries of the vertebral column and spinal cord. *Injuries of the Brain and Spinal Cord, and Their Coverings.* 4th Ed. Edited by Brock, S., Springer Publishing Co., New York, 1960.

45. Scarff, J. E., and Pool, J. L.: Factors causing massive spasm following transection of the cord in man. *J. Neurosurg.* 3:285, 1946.

46. Schneider, R. C.: Fat embolism: A problem in the differential diagnosis of craniocerebral trauma. *J. Neurosurg.* 9:1, 1952.

47. Schutta, H. S., Kassell, N. F., and Langfitt, T. W.: Brain swelling produced by injury and aggravated by arterial hypertension. *Brain* 91:281, 1968.

48. Seddon, H. J.: War injuries of peripheral nerves. *Brit. J. Surg.*, Suppl. 2, 1948.
49. Spillane, J. D.: Five boxers. *Brit. Med. J.* 2: 1205, 1962.
50. Strich, S. J.: Shearing of nerve fibers as a cause of brain damage due to head injury. *Lancet* 2:443, 1961.
51. Symonds, C. P.: Concussion and its sequelae. *Lancet* 1:1, 1962.
52. Torres, F., and Shapiro, S. K.: Electroencephalograms in whiplash injury. *Arch. Neurol.* 5:28, 1961.
53. Towbin, A.: Spinal cord and brainstem injury at birth. *Arch. Path.* 77:620, 1964.
54. Turner, J. W. A.: Indirect injuries of the optic nerve. *Brain* 66:140, 1943.
55. Walker, A. E., and Caveness, W. F. (ed.): *Late Effects of Head Injury.* Charles C Thomas, Springfield, Ill., 1970.
56. Webb, E. M., and Davis, E. W.: Causalgia: A review. *Calif. Med.* 69:412, 1948.
57. Weddell, G., Guttmann, L., and Gutmann, E.: The local extension of nerve fibers into denervated areas of skin. *J. Neurol. Psychiat.* 4:206, 1941.
58. Whiteley, W. H., and Alpers, B. J.: Posterior interosseous nerve palsy with spontaneous neuroma formation. *Arch. Neurol.* 1:226, 1959.
59. Williams, D.: The electroencephalogram in chronic posttraumatic states. *J. Neurol. Neurosurg. Psychiat.* 4:131, 1941.
60. Wycis, H. T.: Subdural hygroma: A report of seven cases. *J. Neurosurg.* 2:340, 1945.
61. Yashon, D., Jane, J. A., White, R. J., and Sugar, O.: Traumatic subdural hematoma of infancy. *Arch. Neurol.* 18:370, 1968.
62. Zacks, S. I.: *The Motor Endplate.* W. B. Saunders Co., Philadelphia, 1964.

CHAPTER NINETEEN

Diseases of Muscle

This chapter is devoted to disorders of muscle that are not secondary to disease of the central or peripheral nervous system. They fall into five groups: (1) the genetically determined muscular dystrophies, which are characterized by an extremely slow course and a selective impact on certain muscle groups; (2) various forms of myositis that are not hereditary, come on rapidly, and are generalized rather than selective in their impact; (3) slowly progressive myopathies associated with endocrine disturbances; (4) metabolic disorders characterized by intermittent attacks of weakness or paralysis that is almost global in extent; (5) myasthenia gravis, which is due to a biochemical disorder at the myoneural junction and which is characterized by intermittent weakness of localized groups of muscles induced by their use and relieved by the administration of anticholinesterase drugs.

THE MUSCULAR DYSTROPHIES

The classification of the muscular dystrophies is unsatisfactory because clinical categories overlap and because there is often a lack of correlation between genetic and clinical data. Consequently, the nomenclature is in a state of flux at the present time; the reader is referred to Pearson,[15] Pratt[19] and Walton and Gardner-Medwin[34] for further information.

Progressive Muscular Dystrophy

This disease is genetically determined. It appears in a number of forms, which are distinguished largely by the age of onset and the identity of the muscles which are involved first.[15, 19, 34] The onset is insidious. In all forms, the muscles are picked out in a selective manner, some muscles being involved and others spared. Thus, in the lower limbs, the quadriceps and anterior tibial groups may be weak, while the calf muscles are spared. In the upper limbs, the deltoid and triceps may be relatively spared, while the biceps, brachioradialis, serrati, and pectoral muscles are involved early. Such selectivity, occurring more or less symmetrically on the two sides of the body, is a diagnostic clue that is particularly valuable in the early stages of the disease, or when a family history is lacking, since there is no other disease in which slowly developing atrophy and weakness assume this pattern. Hypertrophy or pseudohypertrophy of the calf muscles and some of the muscles of the shoulder girdle is another valuable clue, but often it is absent. The tendon

535

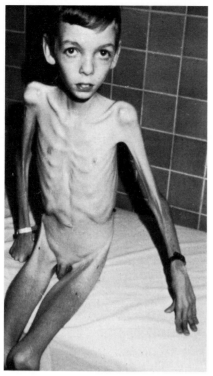

Figure 19–1. Progressive muscular dystrophy. (Courtesy of Children's Hospital of Philadelphia.)

Laboratory Aids. There is an excessive output of creatine and diminished cretininuria, but this happens in other myopathies. Serum aldolase levels are increased by a factor of 10 in the early stages of the disease. Creatine kinase activity may be increased three hundred fold in early cases, and it may be elevated before clinical signs appear. Female carriers of the gene can be detected in the Duchenne type by the presence of an elevated serum creatine kinase.

Electromyography shows a decrease in mean action potential amplitude and duration, and a reduced territory of single motor units. There is a moderate increase in polyphasic potentials. Nerve conduction is normal.

Differential Diagnosis. The diagnosis is suggested by the insidious onset and slow course of weakness in proximal muscles and by the absence of fasciculation and other signs of neurological disease. A positive family history helps, but any patient under review may be the first in his family to exhibit the disease, and sporadic cases occur. Myotonic muscular dystrophy appears first in adult life, tends to involve the peripheral as well as the proximal muscles, and shows the characteristic myotonia; cataracts, early baldness, and gonadal atrophy may or may not be present. Amyotrophic lateral sclerosis begins later and is distinguished by rapid progress, asymmetrical and often distal atrophy, fasciculation, and hyperactive tendon reflexes. Peroneal muscular atrophy can be confused with the rare distal myopathy, but the former shows slight peripheral sensory impairment, which is never present in the dystrophies, and, in the absence of this useful sign, electromyography discloses evidence of denervation. Polymyositis can cause diagnostic difficulty both in children and in adults. However, it is not heredofamilial, progress is as a rule more rapid, and remissions are common; muscular involvement is global rather than selective, the neck muscles are often affected, the muscles are usually tender, dysphagia may occur, atrophy is less severe in proportion to weakness, and the tendon reflexes tend to be spared

reflexes are usually depressed or lost in the affected parts, but in the early stages they are normal elsewhere. Sensation is unaffected. Contractures are common in the later stages, especially in the more severe types; if the calf muscles retain their power and the anterior tibial group are weak, there is bilateral foot drop with flexion of the toes and inversion of the foot. Children thus affected tend to walk on their toes.

Pathology. Common to muscular dystrophies of all types are marked variations in muscle fiber size, fiber splitting, central migration of sarcolemmal nuclei, enlargement of these nuclei, basophilia of the sarcoplasm, fiber atrophy, areas of necrosis and phagocytosis, and infiltration of fat cells.[34] Somewhat similar changes are sometimes seen in polymyositis, but in the latter inflammatory activity is more severe and more widespread and there is often perivascular or interstitial infiltration of lymphocytes and plasma cells.

for a longer period. Dermatitis may or may not be present. In acute cases, the level of serum creatine kinase and other enzymes is increased, as it is in the early stages of rapidly advancing muscular dystrophy, but the sedimentation rate is often high.

"Muscular dystrophy" starting after the age of 50 often proves to be a mild myositis, but biopsy of a muscle undergoing degeneration seldom will settle the question.[24] In *hypertrophia musculorum vera*, true enlargement of the muscles begins in childhood or early adult life, and may be generalized or limited to a limb or to one-half of the body, or even to a group of muscles. In contrast to progressive muscular dystrophy, the muscles are not weak. There is no enlargement of other tissues. The muscle fibers are big but otherwise normal. The tendon reflexes and the electrical responses are normal. The enlargement eventually comes to a halt, and it is not a source of incapacity.

Menopausal "dystrophy," which sometimes responds to corticosteroids, is usually a myositis of varied origins, occurring at the menopause.

Treatment. No specific treatment is available for any of the progressive muscular dystrophies. Regular physical exercise probably delays the onset of contractures, and passive stretching of muscles, carried out several times a day by companions or relatives who have been instructed by a physiotherapist, are useful. Once the child is chair-borne, the provision of a spinal support will delay the onset of kyphoscoliosis. When contracture of the Achilles tendons interferes with walking, surgical lengthening of the tendons, followed by immediate mobilization in a walking cast, is thought to be helpful. It is necessary to utilize the resources of the entire household to prevent premature immobilization.

THE DUCHENNE TYPE. This is the most common and most severe type. In the past, it has been referred to as "pseudohypertrophic muscular dystrophy," but this term should be avoided because hypertrophy is not invariably present and it does occur in other forms. The tongue is often enlarged. The disease is inherited as a sex-linked recessive, occurs almost exclusively in males, and usually becomes apparent toward the end of the third year of life.[19] The muscles of the pelvic girdle are affected first, followed shortly thereafter by involvement of the shoulders. The parents usually report that there is difficulty in walking and in climbing stairs, with frequent falls. Weakness can be discerned in the iliopsoas, quadriceps, gluteus maximus, and sacrospinalis. Enlargement of the calf muscles, and sometimes of the quadriceps, deltoids, or other muscles, occurs in about 90 per cent of all cases at some stage, but the enlargement disappears as the disease advances. The child has a waddling gait and he is unable to rise from the floor without using his hands to "climb up himself" (Gower's sign). Later on, the anterior tibial group and peronei are involved, while the calf muscles, adductors, and hamstrings are relatively spared.

The majority of these children are unable to walk by the time they are 10 years old, and once they are confined to a wheelchair, muscular contractures and skeletal distortion accelerate. Some waste and others become excessively obese.

The central nervous system is normal, apart from the fact that the intelligence quotient is slightly lower than normal.[21] As the disease progresses, there is persistent tachycardia, and the electrocardiogram shows tall R waves in the right precordial leads and deep Q waves in the left precordial leads and limb leads. Death usually results from inanition or respiratory infection in the second decade. There is as yet no treatment for this distressing malady.

THE BENIGN (BECKER) TYPE. This benign variety of progressive muscular dystrophy starts between the fifth and the twenty-fifth year and can be transmitted by affected males through carrier daughters to their grandsons.[34] Weakness and wasting start in the pelvic muscles and later on affect the pectoral muscles. Cardiac involvement is absent, contractures occur late, if at all, and despite considerable disability, the patient may survive for many years.

FACIOSCAPULOHUMERAL TYPE. First described by Landouzy and Déjerine in 1884, this form occurs in both sexes and usually begins in the second or third decade. Occasionally, it has appeared in middle life. It is usually transmitted as an autosomal dominant trait.

The onset is insidious. The lips are everted and weak, so that the patient cannot whistle. Weakness of the zygomatic muscles converts an attempt to smile into a sneer. At the same time, weakness develops in the spinati, rhomboids, pectoralis major, deltoid, biceps, and triceps—the scapulohumeral muscles. The biceps and brachioradialis are sometimes involved first. After a few years, closing the eyes and wrinkling the brow become difficult. In a few cases, the lower extremities are involved (e.g., bilateral foot drop), and in some rapidly advancing cases, there is an exaggeration of the lumbar lordosis. Muscular hypertrophy or pseudohypertrophy is uncommon.

The condition is usually benign, running a prolonged course, with periods of apparent arrest. Complete incapacity is unusual and life expectation is not greatly curtailed.

LIMB GIRDLE MUSCULAR DYSTROPHY. In these cases, atrophy and weakness occur in the limb girdles without involving the face. The disease affects both sexes and usually begins in the second or third decade. In most families, it is transmitted as an autosomal recessive trait, but sporadic cases are not uncommon. Muscle weakness can start in the pelvic or shoulder girdle, and if it starts in the former, it may not appear in the latter for 10 or more years. Enlargement of the calf muscles is not uncommon. In some cases, periods of temporary arrest seem to occur, but in general the degree of disability is severe within 20 years of the onset and the expectation of life is somewhat shortened. As with other forms

of the disease, the later the onset, the longer the period of useful survival.

Rarer Forms of Muscular Dystrophy

Congenital Muscular Dystrophy. In this rare condition, severe hypotonia is present from birth, and it has therefore to be considered among the causes of the "floppy baby" syndrome. Muscular weakness supervenes and may progress slowly or rapidly. Widespread contractures may develop, suggesting arthrogryposis multiplex congenita. Diagnosis depends on the demonstration of histological changes typical of muscular dystrophy which, together with serum enzyme studies and electromyography serve to distinguish the condition from spinal muscular atrophy in infants.

Childhood Muscular Dystrophy. This rare form can exist in both sexes. It comes on in infancy or childhood, and the pattern of weakness resembles that of the Duchenne type, but progression is slower than in the latter, so that the patient may still be able to walk 15 to 20 years after the onset.

The Distal (Gower's) Form of Muscular Dystrophy. This condition appears to be more common in Sweden than elsewhere; it is rare in the United States and Britain. In Welander's study of 250 cases, it was found to be inherited as an autosomal dominant character which appeared in both sexes and usually started after the age of 40. Weakness begins in the small muscles of the hands and in the legs below the knee, and spreads proximally. Progression is usually slow, but in sporadic cases, the course may be comparatively rapid.

Ocular Muscular Dystrophy. This condition, formerly referred to as "progressive nuclear ophthalmoplegia," was identified as a myopathy by Kiloh and Nevin in 1951. The myopathy affects the external ocular muscles. Bilateral ptosis is followed by bilateral external ophthalmoplegia. In most cases, slight weakness of the upper face, neck, and shoulder girdle[11] develops years later.

Oculopharyngeal Muscular Dystrophy.
In this condition, there is dysphagia in addition to ocular myopathy.[34] Inheritance in familial cases is dominant. Symptoms usually arise in the fifth decade or later.

Central Core Disease (Congenital Nonprogressive Myopathy). This rare form of muscular dystrophy is transmitted as an autosomal dominant trait. It gets its name from the fact that the majority of muscle fibers, which are large, display one or sometimes two cores of deeply staining material that is devoid of oxidative enzymes and phosphorylase activity.[25] Mitochondria and endoplasmic reticulum are absent in these areas. The children are hypotonic at birth, and their motor development is delayed. They seldom walk until the age of 4 or 5 years, but although they continue to display weakness of proximal muscles, atrophy does not occur, the reflexes remain normal, and there is no myotonia.

Nemaline Myopathy. This is another nonprogressive form of congenital myopathy. The infant is hypotonic, and motor development is retarded. Weakness persists for some time, but tends to improve. In addition to the diffuse myopathy, which may involve the face, there is usually a high-arched palate, prognathism, and arachnodactyly. The affected muscles show rodlike structures below the sarcolemmal membrane and external to the myofibrils. The rods appear to result from a swelling and degeneration of the Z-bands.

Mitochondrial Myopathies. Shy and Gonatas described what they called "megaconial myopathy," in which muscle fibers contained greatly enlarged mitochondria in the subsarcolemmal region, as well as throughout the fiber. In another type, there was an increase in the number of mitochondria in the muscle fibers—pleoconial myopathy.[34] In both instances, the infant presents as a "floppy baby," and at the age of about 3 or 4 years, a slowly progressive myopathy develops, involving the muscles of the shoulder and pelvic girdles.

Familial Centronuclear Myopathy. In 1966, Spiro, Shy and Gonatas[28] described a congenital myopathy that caused external ophthalmoplegia, ptosis, and weakness of the face and all skeletal muscles. Most of the muscle fibers were smaller than usual, and their nuclei were located centrally. The symptoms were first noted at the end of the first year. The authors suggested that the pathological findings represented the persistence of fetal myotubes. Since then, other cases have been described, which showed a later age of onset, a different mode of inheritance, and different histochemical characteristics, and it appears possible that several forms of disease are being grouped under this name.[1]

MYOTONIA

Myotonia is characterized by delayed relaxation of skeletal muscles after voluntary effort. It can also be induced by percussion and by electrical stimulation, but it is not evident on passive movement. The electromyogram shows runs of high frequency oscillations after voluntary effort has ceased. Myotonia is aggravated by cold and is usually reduced or temporarily abolished by repeated use of the affected muscles. It persists after spinal anesthesia, nerve block, sectioning of the motor nerves, and administration of curare and atropine. It is thought that the defect lies in the membrane of the muscle fiber.

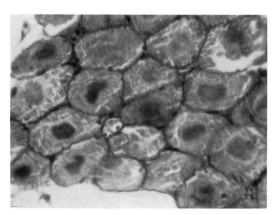

Figure 19–2. Central core disease. (Courtesy of Dr. G. Milton Shy.)

Myotonia Congenita
(Thomsen's Disease)

Myotonia is present from birth and persists throughout life in this heredo-familial disease. The musculature is unusually well developed, and the muscle fibers are larger than normal, with poorly marked cross striation.[34]

There is slowness of relaxation, especially in cold weather. Chewing may be difficult at the commencement of a meal. In some cases, sudden attempts to change position induce myotonia, which freezes the patient in one posture, with the result that he may fall down helpless and remain so for some seconds. After he sneezes, his eyes may remain closed, and his smile may be unnaturally prolonged. When an object is grasped firmly, the patient finds it difficult to let it go. Atrophy does not occur, and sensation and reflexes are unaffected. Mechanical percussion of muscles causes a local dimple, which persists for several seconds, and repeated electrical stimulation induces myotonic contraction; however, a single shock does not do so.

Diagnosis. Dystrophia myotonica is distinguished from myotonia congenita by the onset of symptoms in adult life and the presence of muscular atrophy; cataracts, frontal baldness, and gonadal atrophy may also be present, either in the patient or in other members of his family.

Treatment. Quinine sulfate in doses of 300 mg. three times per day reduces myotonia. Procaine amide has the same effect in doses of 2 to 4 gm. a day, but it can cause nausea, insomnia, and agranulocytosis. Cortisone and ACTH reduce myotonia, but they are not suitable for treating a condition that lasts throughout life. Dilantin in doses of 100 mg. three times per day is said to be helpful.

Dystrophia Myotonica

This condition is transmitted by an autosomal dominant gene and is charac-terized by myotonia, muscular atrophy, cataracts, frontal baldness in the male, gonadal atrophy and other mild endocrine anomalies, impaired pulmonary ventilation, cardiomyopathy, varying degrees of mental defect, and abnormalities of the serum immunoglobulins. The symptoms usually occur for the first time in adult life, but they show a tendency to develop earlier and more severely in successive generations. Affected families show diminished fertility.

Pathology. There is enlargement of scattered fibers, which exhibit less cross striation than normal and contain long rows of centrally placed nuclei. Other fibers show severe degenerative changes similar to those seen in other types of myopathy; ring fibrils, which circle or penetrate muscle fibers at right angles to the normal fibrils, are prominent. Degenerated fibers are replaced by connective tissue and fat. Atrophy of the gonads is the most constant finding, apart from the changes in muscle. The heart muscle has not been affected in the few instances in which it has been examined, despite abnormalities in the electrocardiogram.

Clinical Features. Symptoms usually occur for the first time between the ages of 20 and 50, in persons of either sex.

Myotonia commonly affects the hands, forearms, quadriceps, and tongue, and is usually worse in cold weather. It may be present on voluntary movement or may be found by percussion only. Myotonia and wasting do not necessarily appear in the same muscles.

Muscular wasting and weakness show a predilection for the facial muscles, the sternomastoids, the muscles below the elbows, and the anterior tibial group. The limb girdles are usually spared. Wasting of the sternomastoid makes the neck look excessively thin and long, and the patient ultimately has difficulty in lifting the head from the pillow. Sensation and reflexes are unaffected. A mild degree of mental impairment may develop, and many patients seem to fail to notice their disability until it becomes extreme.

Cataracts are common both in the patient and in unaffected members of the family; the opacities are situated in the cortex of the lens. Frontal baldness may occur early, testicular and ovarian atrophy is frequent, and there is often increased thickness of the vault of the skull and a small sella. Electrocardiographic abnormalities have been found in a significant number of cases; there appears to be a lengthening of the period of isotonic cardiac contraction. Vital capacity and expiratory pressure are often impaired. There is excessive catabolism of immunoglobulin-G.

The disease progresses very slowly. Death from intercurrent maladies usually occurs before the age of 60, but mild cases may remain stationary, and the patient may reach old age.

Diagnosis. The combination of muscular atrophy and myotonia occurs in no other disease. If myotonia is poorly marked, the distinction from other types of muscular dystrophy is made by the characteristic distribution of the wasting, with sparing of the shoulder and pelvic muscles, and by the presence of the systemic features of the disease.

Treatment. The myotonia can be relieved by quinine or procaine amide, as in myotonia congenita, but weakness and atrophy are uninfluenced by these drugs, and there is no known way of arresting the process. Sudden death from cardiac failure is not unknown, and the risk is particularly great during surgical operations. Local anesthesia should be used when possible, and thiopental sodium and muscle relaxants should be avoided.

Paramyotonia Congenita

This condition, first described by Eulenburg in 1886, is a rare familial disorder characterized by the onset in early life of attacks of myotonia of the tongue, face, and extremities, which are precipitated by cold or by cold plus exertion.[19] Without exposure to cold, myotonia can be demonstrated in the tongue only. Some of these patients also suffer from attacks of generalized muscular weakness akin to hyperkalemic periodic paralysis (adynamia episodica hereditaria), while others experience attacks of hypokalemic periodic paralysis.

The treatment is the same as for myotonia congenita together with appropriate treatment for hypokalemia or hyperkalemia in patients who suffer from episodes of paralysis.

INFLAMMATORY DISEASES OF MUSCLE

Myositis

Myositis is occasionally seen as a result of bacterial, parasitic, and fungal invasion of muscles, and the Coxsackie virus causes some cases of epidemic myalgia.

Normal striated muscle is usually resistant to bacterial invasion, but suppurative myositis occasionally occurs secondary to septicemia. The most frequent type of bacterial myositis is the clostridial form, gas gangrene. Muscle fiber degeneration, the most prominent being Zenker's necrosis, occurs in many infectious diseases. The most common parasitic infection is trichinosis. Toxoplasmosis can involve muscles, but this is overshadowed by the other features of the disease. In trypanosomiasis and cysticercosis, the muscles are often invaded, but this does not appear to produce clinical symptoms.

In interpreting the pathology of muscular biopsy material, it must be remembered that previous infections, trauma, electromyography needles, and vascular disease are common sources of histological abnormalities and that not all departures from normal are necessarily relevant in cases of suspected myositis or dystrophy.

The clinical syndromes known as polymyositis and dermatomyositis differ from the foregoing in that they are the central feature of the disease. Pathologically, there is both degeneration and inflammation of skeletal muscle. Phagocytosis

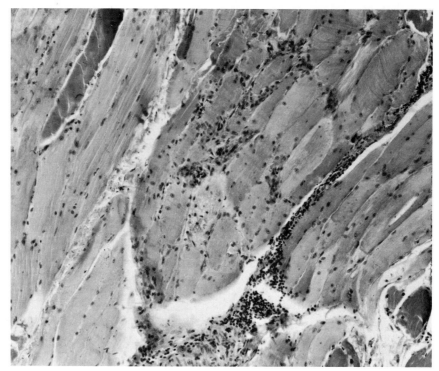

Figure 19–3. Myositis in a case of dermatomyositis. (Courtesy of Ayer Laboratory, Pennsylvania Hospital.)

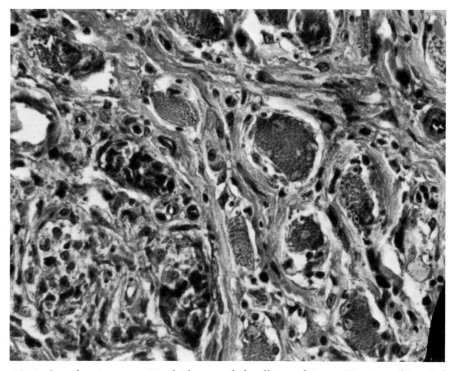

Figure 19–4. Granulomatous myositis which responded well to prednisone. (Courtesy of Ayer Laboratory, Pennsylvania Hospital.)

of degenerating fibers and perivascular inflammatory infiltrations occur. Chou and Gutmann [2] found intracytoplasmic crystalline arrays in muscles of two patients who died from acute dermatomyositis, and they considered that the intracytoplasmic bodies probably indicate infection by a Coxsackie virus. There are acute, subacute, and chronic forms, and the current view is that they are collagen diseases. Polymyositis may exist on its own or in association with dermatitis, rheumatoid arthritis, systemic lupus erythematosus, polyarteritis, scleroderma, or Sjögren's syndrome. Dermatomyositis in persons over the age of 40 is often associated with visceral malignant disease.

Acute polymyositis usually occurs in adults, but it is seen at all ages, including in childhood. There is generalized pain and weakness of the muscles, with or without an erythematous rash. Proximal muscles are more severely affected than distal ones, and the respiratory muscles may be involved. The patient is obviously ill and usually febrile, and the affected muscles are tender and pit on pressure. *Subacute polymyositis* is more common. Constitutional upset is usually absent, and muscle pain is not as prominent as in the acute form. Indeed, the presenting features may be progressive fatigability, weakness, and atrophy of the muscles of the shoulder and pelvic girdles, resembling muscular dystrophy. However, in polymyositis, unlike the dystrophies, the neck muscles are often weak, and dysphagia may also occur. Muscular weakness is greater than the degree of atrophy would appear to justify, and all the muscles within a given group are affected. They are sometimes tender and may pit on pressure. The tendon reflexes are reduced or absent in the affected areas. The skin may show typical scleroderma or lesions similar to those of lupus erythematosus, and even in the absence of a rash, it may be histologically abnormal. Subcutaneous and intramuscular calcification may occur late in the disease.

The sedimentation rate is raised in all acute cases and in about 50 per cent of the subacute ones, and the serum transaminase, aldolase, and creatine kinase are elevated, but diagnosis depends on biopsy and on the presence of creatine in the urine. Electromyography shows a decrease in the size of motor unit action potentials, with an increased percentage of low amplitude polyphasic discharges on voluntary contractions; fibrillation potentials occasionally are seen at rest, presumably because the terminal portions of the motor fibers are involved.

Prognosis. The course of the illness is variable. In the worst cases, death may occur within a month or two; in the best, spontaneous arrest occurs without therapy. Without the use of steroids, the mortality rate is in the region of 50 per cent. Treatment with steroids leads to rapid improvement and a reduction in the previous elevated levels of serum enzymes, but if the steroids are withdrawn, relapse is likely to occur. Treatment may have to be continued for three or more years. Complete recovery is usual in children and young adults treated thus, but in middle-aged patients, the disease is apt to be refractory, and when polymyositis develops over the age of 50, life is often cut short by malignant disease.

Treatment. Prednisone should be given in a daily dose of 60 mg. for a week, thereafter reducing the dose to 40 mg. Subsequent dosage depends on the clinical response and on the level of serum creatinine kinase activity; the objective is to use the smallest effective dose. In refractory patients, a daily dose of 80 units of ACTH can be tried. If respiration is depressed as a result of involvement of thoracic muscles, intermittent positive pressure respiration is needed.

Polymyalgia Rheumatica

Polymyalgia rheumatica, a fairly common condition sometimes called "anarthritic rheumatoid disease," is more common in women than in men and appears chiefly in the fourth and fifth decades. The pathological basis of the condition is unknown (muscle biopsies are negative), and the symptoms and signs constitute a syndrome for which more than one cause may ultimately be discovered. Some patients so designated turn out to be suffering from rheumatoid arthritis, others run a fluctuating but self-limited course, without developing weakness or obvious pathological changes in the affected muscles, and yet others develop temporal arteritis.

The onset may be sudden or gradual. Pain and stiffness appear in the shoulder girdle, pelvic girdle, and thighs, with the distal muscles being spared. Tenderness is slight and may be absent, and true muscular weakness is usually absent, although this is difficult to judge because muscular effort may be inhibited by pain. The patient tires easily. Periarticular pain may be prominent, but actual swelling of the joints is very rare. In the more acute cases there may be constitutional symptoms in the form of sweating, anorexia, slight headache, malaise, and depression. In these, the sedimentation rate is raised, and there may be marked sludging in the conjunctival vessels, as seen by biomicroscopy. The affected muscles may pit slightly on pressure. Striking relief is achieved by the administration of adrenocortical steroids: Prednisone in doses of 5 mg. thrice daily will often suffice, although larger doses are necessary in intractable cases.

Sarcoidosis of Muscle

When muscular weakness and atrophy appear in sarcoidosis, they are usually the result of polyneuropathy, but a few cases have been described in which the sarcoidal infiltration of the muscles has been so widespread as to constitute polymyositis.[26] Sensory changes do not occur, and the stretch reflexes are preserved for longer than would be the case in polyneuropathy of comparable severity. Even in the absence of outspoken

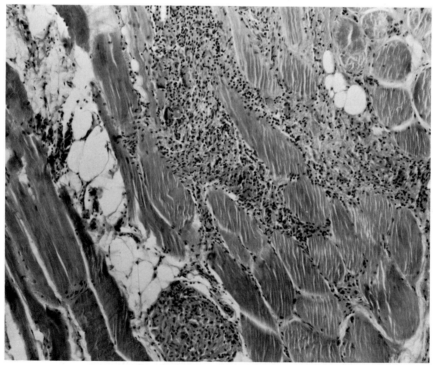

Figure 19–5.   Sarcoidosis of muscle. (Courtesy of Ayer Laboratory, Pennsylvania Hospital.)

weakness and atrophy, random muscle biopsies from people affected by the disease yield a surprisingly high percentage of positive results (Fig. 19–5). Other neurological features of sarcoidosis are described on page 345.

METABOLIC AND ENDOCRINE MYOPATHIES

Disease of the Thyroid Gland

Generalized asthenia and wasting are common in thyrotoxicosis, but in some cases of both hyper- and hypothyroidism, the muscles are affected in a more specific way.[8]

Myasthenia gravis is associated with hyperthyroidism in some 5 per cent of cases, which is more than could be expected to occur by chance. In most cases, the clinical features of the myasthenia are in no way unusual, and thyroidectomy does not influence it. In the condition referred to as *acute thyrotoxic myopathy* or *acute thyrotoxic bulbar palsy*, myasthenia develops rapidly in ocular, bulbar, respiratory, and limb muscles. This can be fatal, but it responds both to neostigmine and to thyroidectomy. Myasthenia has occurred for the first time after thyroidectomy and has also been reported in cases of myxedema. *Hypokalemic periodic paralysis* is more common in thyrotoxicosis than can be explained by chance, and it can be controlled by treating the hyperthyroidism.

Chronic thyrotoxic myopathy is rare. Weakness and wasting are marked, especially in proximal muscles. The muscles of the mouth and pharynx may also be involved, and coarse fasciculation is common. The reflexes related to affected muscles are diminished or lost, and in some cases, the electromyogram shows changes similar to those found in muscular dystrophy. The response to neostigmine may be positive, but often it is negative, and there is no response to Tensilon. The clinical evidence of thyrotoxicosis is often slight, but treatment of the thyroid condition controls the myopathy.

Exophthalmic ophthalmoplegia (malignant exophthalmos; thyrotropic exophthalmos) is a comparatively common condition which occurs in thyrotoxic, euthyroid, or myxedematous adults. It may be accentuated by thyroidectomy. It attacks both sexes. There is edema and lymphocytic infiltration of the orbital tissues; the extraocular muscles are greatly enlarged, and there is an increase of fat in the orbit. The condition usually starts as frank exophthalmos in one or both eyes, but sometimes diplopia is the first sign. The eyes look unduly moist owing to edema of the conjunctiva, which may ultimately become so severe that it bulges over the lower lid. Ptosis may occur, but it is more usual to find widening of the palpebral fissure. The lids may be unable to close over the protruding eyes, and this predisposes to corneal ulceration. The degree of ophthalmoplegia varies. The pupillary reflexes are unaffected. When exophthalmos is severe, papilledema may occur, endangering sight. Rarely, myasthenia gravis is associated with exophthalmic ophthalmoplegia. In most cases, the condition progresses for a few months and then remains stationary. Spontaneous fluctuations are common, making it difficult to interpret the results of therapy.

There is no satisfactory method of treatment. In acute cases, with severe proptosis and papilledema, decompression of the orbit is necessary to save sight. Improvement has been reported from time to time following the use of iodine, thyroid extract, ACTH, cortisone, and x-radiation of the pituitary and orbits, but the results are inconsistent. If acute thyrotoxicosis is present and threatens life, thyroidectomy or treatment by thiouracil is necessary; this can increase the proptosis, but the danger can be reduced by administration of small doses of thyroid during the postoperative period.

In *hypothyroidism* and *sporadic cretinism*, there is sometimes enlargement of the muscles, with moderate weakness and slowness of both contraction and relaxation. The slowness in relaxation is particularly well marked in the quadriceps after tapping the patellar tendon. It has been reported that weakness of the muscles of the shoulders and pelvic girdle can also result from myxedema and that it is improved by treatment with thyroid extract.

OTHER ENDOCRINE MYOPATHIES

In *Addison's disease,* there is generalized muscular weakness coupled with pigmentation of the skin and mucous membranes, hypotension, and a low blood sodium level. The symptoms improve with appropriate treatment, but in untreated patients there may be stiffness of the legs and flexion contractures of the elbows and knees in the late stages.

In *hyperparathyroidism,* there is a considerable sense of muscular fatigue and weakness, together with gastrointestinal disturbances and polyuria. The osteomalacia gives rise to pain in the bones, and there may also be proximal muscle wasting and weakness, with hypotonia.[5] In *hypoparathyroidism,* on the other hand, the muscles are not affected but there may be carpopedal spasms, isolated muscle twitches, generalized seizures, tingling of the extremities and lips, thickening of the nails, loss of hair, cataracts, defects in the enamel of the teeth, hoarseness of the voice, slowness of mind, and a rise of intracranial pressure.

Many patients with *acromegaly*[12] and *pituitary gigantism* complain of generalized muscular weakness and fatigue, but neither the wasting nor the weakness is conspicuous enough to warrant the term "myopathy." The wasting may be the result of a raised metabolic rate.

In *hypopituitarism,* muscular asthenia is profound. There may be considerable wasting of the muscles, but this is apt to be masked by subcutaneous fat. Fatigue

may be so severe as to suggest myasthenia gravis, but the neostigmine test is negative. Limb girdle weakness and wasting is seen in some cases of *Cushing's syndrome* and may occur as the result of prolonged treatment with steroids.

MYOPATHY FOLLOWING MALIGNANT HYPERPYREXIA

Hyperpyrexia is a rare complication of general anesthesia, which may arise during anesthetization or up to 24 hours after receiving the anesthetic.[29] The condition is heralded by tightening of the jaws and stiffness of the respiratory muscles. Spasm and stiffness develop in the limbs as the temperature rises. Respiratory embarrassment leads to cyanosis, tachycardia, and a fall in blood pressure. Convulsions are frequent. Hypokalemia and myoglobinuria have been observed in survivors.

A predisposition to malignant hyperpyrexia appears to be transmitted as an autosomal dominant gene. The serum creatine phosphokinase rises sharply during the acute illness and elevated levels of this enzyme have been found in unaffected relatives. It therefore appears that there is an underlying abnormality of muscle which is "activated" by general anesthesia, irrespective of what anesthetic is given. A hypertrophic myopathy was present in two of the relatives of one patient, who died of malignant hyperpyrexia.[29]

McARDLE'S DISEASE

In 1951, McArdle described the case of a young man in whom physical exercise was limited by weakness, aching, and stiffness.[8, 9] Symptoms developed in any muscle which had been used for a short time, and immediately after exercise, the affected muscles were firm to the touch and remained in a shortened state; thus, the fingers remained partly flexed. Localized painful swellings occur in the affected muscles and, generally speaking, all the symptoms disappear after periods of rest, but in some severely affected individuals, a persistent myopathy eventually develops. Myoglobinuria occurs after exercise in some cases.

Etiology and Pathology. Inheritance is through an autosomal recessive gene. Examination of the muscles reveals an absence of phosphorylase, a high glycogen content, and collections of glycogen underneath the sarcolemmal membrane. Owing to the lack of phosphorylase, the lactic acid content of venous blood does not rise with exercise. Thus, if the circulation to the arm is occluded by a cuff and the patient is asked to open and close the hand rhythmically, blood taken from a vein distal to the cuff fails to show the normal rise of lactate.

Diagnosis. The diagnosis is suggested by the occurrence of painful cramps and weakness following exercise and is confirmed by the absence of a normal lactate response to exercise, and by biopsy. A myopathy resembling McArdle's disease but resulting from a deficiency of phosphofructokinase has been described by Tarui. Other causes of myoglobinuria are discussed on page 548.

POMPE'S DISEASE

In this disorder, glycogen is deposited in muscle, the myocardium, and motor neurons as a result of a lack of amylo-1, 4-glucosidase. The disease is transmitted as an autosomal recessive trait and occurs in two forms. The first of these gives rise to enlargement of the heart and congestive heart failure, with death in the first year. The second type is characterized by marked hypotonia and progressive limb-girdle myopathy. Death usually occurs by the tenth year, but some patients survive until middle life.[6] Unlike some other glycogen storage diseases, hypoglycemic attacks do not occur in this condition.

CARCINOMATOUS MYOPATHY

The remote effects of carcinoma on the nervous system and muscles are listed on page 458. The most common by far is a *neuromyopathy* that may antedate the symptoms of malignancy by months, or even years. Weakness is felt in the lower limbs, and the patient complains of difficulty in rising from a chair and in climbing stairs because proximal muscles are involved first. Eventually, there is difficulty in standing and walking. The upper limbs are less affected, and the bulbar muscles rarely so. Fasciculation is often present in the affected muscles and the tendon reflexes related to these muscles are depressed or absent. Electromyography may show the characteristics of both a myopathy and a neuropathy.

Polymyositis and *dermatomyositis* are more often associated with visceral carcinoma than could occur by chance.

One of the rare manifestations of malignancy is a myasthenia-like fatigability of muscles (*the Eaton-Lambert syndrome*).[7, 10, 20] This is usually associated with oat-cell carcinoma of the bronchus. There is weakness and wasting of the muscles of the limb girdles and of the trunk; occasionally, the bulbar and external ocular muscles are affected, too. The striking thing about these cases is the degree to which their muscles tire after exertion, although in some of them, muscle power increases after *brief* exercise. They can therefore exhibit either a myasthenic or a reversed myasthenic effect. Unlike myasthenia gravis, the tendon reflexes are depressed or absent, and if a motor nerve is stimulated at frequencies of from 10 to 30 per second, there is a progressive increase in the amplitude of response. The weakness is only slightly improved by treatment with neostigmine, and the response to intravenous Tensilon is incomplete.

Both the weakness and the fatigability may be greatly improved by the administration of guanidine in doses of 250 mg. 4 or more times per day. It is believed to facilitate the release of acetylcholine from the presynaptic vesicles. Atrial fibrillation and hypotension have been reported during the course of guanidine therapy; the administration of calcium and atropine is said to reduce the severity of the intoxication.[13]

ALCOHOLIC MYOPATHY

An acute and reversible myopathy can occur in chronic alcoholics following a drinking spree.[16, 17] This type is characterized by generalized weakness and tenderness of muscles, and painful cramps. Serum creatine phosphokinase is elevated, the urine contains myoglobin, and there is a decrease in the lactic acid response to exercise carried out under conditions of ischemia.

Chronic alcoholics sometimes develop increasing weakness and wasting of the limb girdle muscles, which is independent of the peripheral neuropathy that may also be present.[16, 17] The amounts of serum creatine phosphokinase and other enzymes are increased, and biopsy shows scattered areas of necrosis with phagocytosis. Improvement can occur if alcohol is avoided.

PAROXYSMAL MYOGLOBINURIA

Myoglobin appears in the urine as a result of acute damage to muscles. Thus, it may follow muscular ischemia resulting from obstruction of the main artery to the limb and also following crush injuries and damage to muscles following high voltage shock. An episode of myoglobinuria can follow severe exercise in normal persons who are not accustomed to exercise; this is akin to the "paralytic myoglobinuria" which may occur in horses that are subjected to strenuous exercise after prolonged periods of inactivity and good feeding. Myoglobinuria can occur in McArdle's syndrome, acute polymyositis, acute alcoholic myopathy, and as a result of poisoning by barbiturates, carbon monoxide, and sea snake venom. It can occur as a complication of hypokalemia.

Idiopathic Myoglobinuria.[22] This term will probably be found to embrace several conditions, some of which are familial. One type is found predominantly in males in late adolescence or early adult life, and the symptoms are usually provoked by exercise. In the second group, which includes both sexes, the disorder starts in childhood, is not related to exertion, and is sometimes precipitated by infections. As time goes on, the attacks become less severe and less frequent, and ultimately they disappear.

Whatever their origin, the attacks are characterized by muscle weakness, pain and tenderness, and the passage of dark urine. In severe cases, oliguria or even renal shutdown can occur as a result of stoppage of the renal tubules by myoglobin crystals, as in the crush syndrome.

PERIODIC PARALYSIS

Familial Hypokalemic Periodic Paralysis

This is a rare familial disease of unknown etiology characterized by repeated attacks of weakness or paralysis of skeletal muscles, accompanied by loss of tendon reflexes and failure of the muscles to respond to electrical stimulation. During the attack, the plasma potassium falls to less than 3 mEq per liter, and the potassium content of the urine is diminished.

Pathology. The central and peripheral nervous system is normal, but the muscle fibers may show cleft formation and vacuolation. Although plasma potassium falls during the attack, and although the attack itself can be terminated by administering potassium chloride, hypokalemia cannot be the entire explanation for the paralysis, because in normal subjects, serum potassium can be reduced to much lower levels without producing paralysis, and when hypokalemia arises in the course of other diseases, potassium depletion must be severe before paralysis occurs.

Symptoms. The attacks may start in early life but are more common after puberty. They usually occur when the patient wakens in the morning and can sometimes be provoked by a large, high-carbohydrate meal or heavy and violent exertion followed by a period of rest.

The symptoms vary from a transient sense of weakness for a few minutes to a condition of complete immobility of trunk and limbs, which can last for several hours. The bulbar and respiratory muscles are usually spared. Occasionally, the paralysis is localized to a group of muscles or is more marked on one side of the body than on the other. When the worst of the paralysis has passed off, the patient is left with a sense of clumsiness and weakness of the arms and legs, which may persist for as long as one or two days. Some children are left with permanent myopathic weakness.[4] Although smooth muscle is not affected, micturition and defecation may be compromised by the weakness of the skeletal muscles. Sensation is unaffected. The electrocardiogram shows the changes characteristic of hypokalemia (p. 588).

Course and Prognosis. In general, the attacks tend to become less severe and less common as the patient grows older. Death can occur during an attack, but this is very rare.

Differential Diagnosis. Episodes of muscular weakness can occur in the course of primary aldosteronism caused by tumors of the adrenal[3] and in potassium-losing nephritis, renal tubular acidosis, and—very rarely—in thyrotoxicosis. There is no difficulty in establishing the diagnosis in familial cases of periodic paralysis, but a first attack in a sporadic case can pose difficulties. Hysteria is eliminated if there is loss of the tendon reflexes and if the muscles fail to respond to electrical stimulation.

Treatment. The administration of 25 mg. of spironolactone four times daily will reduce the frequency and severity of the attacks,[18] and it is usually thought wise to restrict the consumption of carbohydrates. During the individual attack, potassium salts should be given orally but there is some doubt whether this treatment actually cuts short the duration of the attack.

Hyperkalemic Periodic Paralysis (Adynamia Episodica Hereditaria)

This condition shows a dominant mode of inheritance. In contrast to the hypokalemic form, the onset appears within the first decade, the attacks are milder and briefer (30 to 60 minutes), the serum potassium level rises slightly, and the condition is made worse by the administration of potassium chloride. Occasionally it is associated with myotonia.[31,32]

The attacks can be cut short by the intravenous administration of calcium gluconate, and can be prevented by the administration of 250 mg. of acetazolamide, three times daily, or by 25 mg. of hydrochlorothiazide twice daily.

Normokalemic Periodic Paralysis

This rare form of periodic paralysis differs from the foregoing in several ways. The attacks often develop at night, and they last for days or even weeks. The serum potassium level is within normal limits, but the degree of weakness is increased by the administration of potassium. It is improved by giving large doses of sodium chloride, and it has been reported that the attacks can be prevented by the daily administration of 0.1 mg. of 9-α-fluorohydrocortisone, combined with 250 mg. of acetazolamide two or three times daily.

Benign Congenital Hypotonia (Amyotonia Congenita)

This rare condition is present at birth. The head lolls about in a helpless way, and the range of passive movements permitted is in excess of normal. The movements are feeble, and there is a striking sense of flabbiness when the child is held in the arms, comparable to the experience of handling an anesthetized baby. There is no paralysis, and the tendon reflexes are either normal or somewhat depressed. The electrical responses are physiological, and muscle biopsy shows no pathological changes other than smallness of the muscle fibers.[30, 33]

It is important to identify this condition—no easy task—because, unlike other examples of the "floppy baby" syndrome, the condition usually improves, and a considerable degree of recovery may occur. Some patients continue to have small, weak, and hypotonic muscles throughout life.

The "Floppy Baby" Syndrome

In babies, extreme hypotonia and a considerable degree of motor helplessness are the presenting signs in a number of diseases of the muscles, peripheral nerves, and central nervous system.[33] Diagnosis is usually difficult and, in many cases, only with the passage of time is the cause revealed with certainty.[14]

Disorders of *muscle* include: (1) benign congenital hypotonia, a variety of amyotonia congenita, (2) muscular dystrophy of early onset, (3) metabolic myopathies—e.g., Pompe's disease, cretinism. Extreme hypotonia results from diseases of *the peripheral nerves* in Werdnig-Hoffmann disease (p. 566). Some infants born to myasthenic mothers exhibit hypotonia and weakness of muscles, which pass off in due course.

Marked hypotonia may also be secondary to disease of the *central nervous system*, as in flaccid cerebral diplegia and severe mental deficiency.

Congenital laxity of the ligaments, a nonprogressive and often familial condition, permits affected individuals to become contortionists later in life.

MYASTHENIA GRAVIS

In myasthenia gravis,[32a, 34] weakness and paralysis are induced by continuous use of muscles, with recovery after rest or following the administration of cholinesterase inhibitors. The onset is commonly in the third or fourth decade, but it may begin in childhood or old age. Transient myasthenia can occur in infants born to myasthenic mothers. The prevalence rate in the United States and Britain is in the neighborhood of 3 in 100,000, with a predominance of females in cases starting before the age of 40. Heredity plays no part in the disease, though occasionally more than one case occurs in a family.

Etiology. The etiology is unknown, but the symptoms result from defective transmission of nerve impulses at the myoneural junction; the temporary improvement which follows administration of anticholinesterases, such as physostigmine, neostigmine, Tensilon, and diisopropylfluorophosphate, suggests a disturbance of acetylcholine metabolism at the myoneural junction.

The thymus is thought to be implicated because it exhibits abnormalities in some 50 per cent of all cases, and because thymectomy ameliorates the symptoms in some instances.

Pathology. There are no histopathologic changes in the central nervous system or peripheral nerves, but electron microscopic studies have demonstrated degeneration of the motor end-plates.[35] Lymphorrhages are sometimes found in both affected and unaffected muscles, and there is a significant incidence of myocarditis. Muscle-binding, complement-fixing antibodies are found in the serum of about 60 per cent of patients with this disease, suggesting that an autoimmune process is involved.[27] Tumors of the thymus are found in 15 to 30 per cent of all cases, and germinal center hyperplasia occurs in the majority of nonneoplastic thymus glands from myasthenic patients. Of all patients with a thymoma, 33 to 75 per cent have myasthenia. The nature of the relationship between the thymus and myasthenia is not known.

Symptoms.[32a] The onset is usually insidious but can be abrupt, and the disease usually pursues a fluctuating and irregular course over a period of many years. At first, weakness occurs only when muscles have been used, with recovery after rest, but with the passage of time, muscle weakness may be present to some extent throughout the day. The paresis induced by use usually appears for the first time in the ocular muscles, giving rise to ptosis or diplopia; it may be bilateral or unilateral, and the symptoms are aggravated by using the eyes and are therefore usually either absent or slight in the morning. The condition may remain confined to the eyes, never spreading to the rest of the musculature.

In other cases, the facial or bulbar muscles are first affected. The orbicularis oculi and the retractors of the angles of the mouth are commonly involved. With prolonged talking, the voice becomes weak and the words slurred. Chewing and swallowing become difficult toward the end of a meal. Weakness of the palate gives the voice a nasal character, and nasal regurgitation of fluid may occur during swallowing. Ultimately, the mouth hangs open and has to be supported by the hand. Weakness of the limbs and trunk can be the first symptom, but this usually occurs after the other features have been present for some time. The patient notes that the arms feel heavy and tired when shaving or doing the hair; dressing takes more time than usual, and writing or sewing requires frequent rests. The legs are unduly fatigued by walking. The tendon reflexes usually remain brisk.

Weakness of the muscles of respiration can lead to attacks of dyspnea after exertion or even at rest; this can be fatal. There is often a generalized loss of weight in patients who cannot swallow, but atrophy of weakened muscles is uncommon. Sphincter functions remain normal.

The spinal fluid is normal. Rarely, there is moderate creatinuria, a slight reduction of creatine tolerance, and a decrease of creatine excretion. A thymoma may be visible on radiological examination, but a negative picture does not exclude the presence of a small tumor.

Diagnosis. The weakness of affected muscles is increased by using them and is either abolished or very much benefited by rest and by an injection of neostigmine. Neurosis is a common cause of undue fatigability, especially in the limbs, but it does not lead to diplopia or ptosis; moreover, it is almost always most obtrusive in the early part of the day, improving toward the evening, and there will usually be other indications of emotional disorder. Muscles weakened by disease of the motor pathways or by a myopathy also fatigue more easily than normal but do not fully recover after rest or the administration of neostigmine.

Electromyography shows no evidence of denervation, but there is a characteristic falling off in the amplitude of the motor unit potentials with prolonged use. Quinine in doses of 0.3 to 0.6 gm. increases the symptoms, and the response to curare is excessive and can be dangerous.

In the neostigmine test, 1.0 to 1.5 mg. of the drug is injected intramuscularly, together with 0.6 mg. of atropine. Objective improvement occurs in 20 to 60 minutes in true myasthenia. Tensilon given intravenously in a dose of 2.0 mg. followed in 30 seconds by a further 8.0 mg. has an immediate effect, which lasts a few minutes. Both tests sometimes fail in advanced cases of myasthenia confined to the ocular muscles. Slight improvement following the use of neostigmine is seen from time to time in thyrotoxicosis, polymyositis, and carcinomatous myopathy, but the degree of response is less complete than in myasthenia.

Course and Prognosis. Formerly, untreated patients died within months or a few years from the onset, but the course of the disease was often punctuated by remissions. It is not uncommon for a patient with symptoms confined to the ocular muscles to live 20 or 30 years without any spread of the disease to the rest of the musculature. The prognosis is worst in patients with bulbar symptoms and weakness of the respiratory muscles, but even in these, remissions can occur and may last for years. Among those who have survived for 10 years, death from the myasthenia itself is rare. Rarely, the disease proves fatal in a few weeks. Death usually results from pneumonia or from a myasthenic crisis involving the respiratory muscles, but sudden death (apparently from cardiac failure) is not uncommon. Pregnancy has no consistent effect on the disease.

Modern medication has lengthened life and decreased incapacity during the course of the disease. Thymectomy induces a complete remission in 17 to 25 per cent of all cases, brings considerable improvement to an additional 29 per cent, and produces no response at all in the remainder.

Treatment. The patient must live within the limits imposed by the disease. Complete rest is important during exacerbations. Anesthetics and narcotics should be avoided whenever possible. When there is difficulty with chewing or swallowing, semisolid food is required.

Thymectomy is necessary if medical treatment fails. It is especially beneficial in young female patients who have responded poorly to medical therapy and who have had the disease for less than five years. Myasthenic patients with thymomas do poorly regardless of whether the tumor is removed or not. Irradiation of the thymus may appear to be beneficial, but the fluctuating course of the untreated disease makes this difficult to evaluate. Similar doubts must be entertained as to the value of steroid therapy, since the symptoms sometimes become more severe during treatment.

Myasthenia gravis is treated by the administration of short-acting anticholinesterase compounds — neostigmine (Prostigmine), pyridostigmine (Mestinon), and ambenonium hydrochloride (Mytelase). Longer-acting drugs, such as tetraethylpyrophosphate and octamethylpyrophosphoramide, are effective but are no longer used because of their toxicity. In mild cases, the oral administration of one to six tablets of neostigmine (15 mg.) three times per day is often sufficient to keep symptoms within bounds; the effect may be improved by giving potassium chloride in doses of 500 mg. five times a day. Ephedrine in doses of 25 mg. three times per day can help, but the evening dose should be omitted if it keeps the patient awake. In patients who do not respond to oral administration of neostigmine, the drug should be given by injection in doses of 1 mg. three times or more daily. When there is difficulty in chewing and swallowing, medication is best given 30 minutes before meals. Mestinon has much the same effect as neostigmine, but the effects of a single dose last longer, and it produces fewer muscarinic side effects. Mytelase has an action similar to that of neostigmine, and it is usually given in doses of 10 to 25 mg. every three or four hours. Whatever drug is used, it is necessary to remind the patient that spontaneous remissions are likely to occur and that from time to time he may be able to reduce the dose or to eliminate medication entirely.

In a myasthenic crisis, the patient is in imminent danger of death because of weakness of the respiratory muscles, compounded by inability to keep the airway free from secretions. This situation can occur as a result of either a sudden increase in the severity of the disease (myasthenic crisis) or excessive doses of anticholinesterase drugs to which the patient has become resistant (cholinergic crisis). To differentiate between these, the patient is given an intravenous dose of Tensilon chloride (10 mg.), which will induce brief improvement in a myasthenic crisis, but which will not do so when the patient has become insensitive to anticholinesterase agents. As soon as respiration becomes at all labored, tracheostomy should be carried out, and the patient should be connected with a positive pressure respirator. If the condition proves refractory to drugs, they are withdrawn for 72 hours, and adequate doses of atropine sulfate are given, but care must be taken not to dry up the secretions unduly. By the end of that time, the patient will again start to respond favorably to anticholinesterase drugs, though the amount required will often be less than was necessary for the alleviation of symptoms before the crisis. Round-the-clock nursing care is essential.

REFERENCES

1. Bradley, W. G., Price, D. C., and Watanabe, C. K.: Familial centronuclear myopathy. *J. Neurol. Neurosurg. Psychiat.* 33:687, 1970.
2. Chou, S. M., and Gutmann, L.: Picornavirus-like crystals in subacute polymyositis. *Neurology* 20:205, 1970.
3. Conn, J. W.: Primary aldosteronism, a new clinical syndrome. *J. Lab. Clin. Med.* 45:661, 1955.
4. Dyken, M., Zeman, W., and Rusche, T.: Hypokalemic periodic paralysis. Children with permanent myopathic weakness. *Neurology* 19:691, 1969.
5. Frame, B., Heinze, E. G., Black, M., and Manson, G. A.: Myopathy in primary hyperparathyroidism. *Ann. Int. Med.* 68:5, 1968.
6. Hudgson, P., Gardiner-Medwin, D., Wooford, M., Pennington, R. J., and Walton, J. M.: Adult myopathy in glycogen storage disease due to acid maltase deficiency. *Brain* 91:435, 1968.
7. Lambert, E. H.: Defects of neuromuscular transmission in syndromes other than myasthenia gravis. *Ann. N. Y. Acad. Sci.* 135:367, 1966.
8. McArdle, B.: Metabolic and endocrine myopathies. *Disorders of Voluntary Muscle.* 2nd Ed. Edited by Walton, J. M., Williams and Wilkins, Baltimore, 1969.
9. McArdle, B.: Myopathy due to a defect in muscle glycogen breakdown. *Clin. Sci.* 10:3, 1951.
10. McQuillen, M., and Jonas, R. J.: The nature of the defect in the Eaton-Lambert syndrome. *Neurology* 17:527, 1966.
11. Magora, A., and Zauberman, H.: Ocular myopathy. *Arch. Neurol.* 20:1, 1969.
12. Mastalgia, F. L., Barwich, D. D., and Hall, R.: Myopathy in acromegaly. *Lancet* 2:907, 1970.
13. Nakano, K. K., and Tyler, H. R.: Cardiovascular complications of guanidine therapy in the myasthenic syndrome. *Neurology* 20:408, 1970.
14. Paine, R. S.: The future of the "floppy infant." *Develop. Med. Child. Neurol.* 5:115, 1963.
15. Pearson, C. M.: Muscular dystrophy. Review and recent observations. *Amer. J. Med.* 35:632, 1963.
16. Perkoff, G. T., Dioso, M. M., Bleisch, V., and Klinkerfuss, G.: A spectrum of myopathy associated with alcoholism. I. Clinical and laboratory features. *Ann. Int. Med.* 67:481, 1967.
17. Perkoff, G. T., Hardy, P., and Velez-Garcia, E.: Reversible acute muscular syndrome in chronic alcoholism. *New Eng. J. Med.* 274:1277, 1966.
18. Poskamzer, D. C., and Kerr, D. M. S.: Periodic paralysis with response to spironolactone. *Lancet* 2:511, 1961.
19. Pratt, R. T. C.: *The Genetics of Neurological Diseases.* Oxford University Press, London, 1967.
20. Rooke, E. D., Eaton, L. M., Lambert, E. H., and Hodgson, C. H.: Myasthenia and malignant intrathoracic tumor. *Med. Clin. N. Amer.* 44:977, 1960.
21. Rosman, N. P.: The cerebral defect in Duchenne muscular dystrophy: A comparative clinicopathological study. *Neurology* 20:329, 1970.
22. Rowland, L. P., Fahn, S., Hirschberg, E., and Harter, D. H.: Myoglobinuria. *Arch. Neurol.* 10:537, 1969.
23. Rowland, L. P., Hoefer, P. F. A., and Aranow, H.: Myasthenic syndromes. *Res. Pub. Assn. Res. Nerv. Ment. Dis.* 38:548, 1960.
24. Shy, G. M.: The late onset myopathy. *World Neurol.* 3:149, 1962.
25. Shy, G. M., and Magee, K. R.: A new congenital non-progressive myopathy. *Brain* 79:610, 1956.
26. Silverstein, A., and Sitzbach, L. E.: Muscle involvement in sarcoidosis. *Arch. Neurol.* 21:235, 1969.
27. Simpson, J. A.: Myasthenia gravis: A new hypothesis. *Scot. Med. J.* 5:419, 1960.
28. Spiro, A. J., Shy, G. M., and Gonatas, N. K.: Myotubular myopathy. *Arch. Neurol.* 14:1, 1966.
29. Steers, A. J. W., Tallack, J. A., and Thompson, D. E. A.: Fulminating hyperpyrexia during anaesthesia in a member of a myopathic family. *Brit. Med. J.* 2:341, 1970.
30. Turner, J. W. A.: On amyotonia congenita. *Brain* 72:25, 1949.
31. van der Meulen, J. P., Gilbert, G. J., and Kane, C. A.: Familial hyperkalemic paralysis with myotonia. *New Eng. J. Med.* 264:1, 1961.
32. Van't Hoff, W.: Familial myotonic periodic paralysis. *Quart. J. Med.* 31:385, 1962.
32a. Viets, H. R.: *Myasthenia gravis.* Charles C Thomas, Springfield, Ill., 1961.
33. Walton, J. M.: The limp child. *J. Neurol. Psychiat.* 20:144, 1957.
34. Walton, J. M., and Gardner-Medwin, D.: *Disorders of Voluntary Muscle.* 2nd Ed. Edited by Walton, J. M., Williams and Wilkins, Baltimore, 1969.
35. Zacks, S. I., Bauer, W. C., and Blumberg, J. M.: The fine structure of the myasthenic neuromuscular junction. *J. Neuropath. Exp. Neurol.* 21:335, 1962.

CHAPTER TWENTY

Diseases of the Peripheral Nerves

TERMINOLOGY

The term "neuritis," which means, literally, an inflammation of the nerve, is much misused. Not only is it applied to noninflammatory conditions of the peripheral nerves (for example, diabetic neuritis), but it is also used for disorders in which the peripheral nerves are completely normal, as for instance in sciatic "neuritis," a syndrome usually due to an irritative root lesion. It is doubtful whether there is any such thing as primary interstitial neuritis, which used to be considered responsible for sciatica; true interstitial neuritis with an inflammatory reaction of the supporting elements and secondary parenchymatous involvement is found in herpes zoster, in nerves within an area of sepsis, in Buerger's disease, in leprosy, and as a localized response to mechanical irritation (for example, by a cervical rib).

The terms "polyneuritis," "polyneuropathy," and "peripheral neuritis" signify an affection of multiple peripheral nerves, and comprise two large groups. In one, there is a symmetrical affection of the peripheral nerves; the longest neurons are affected first, so that symptoms appear in the legs before they do in the arms, and the face usually escapes. There is a strong family resemblance between most members of this group, whatever the etiology. In the second and smaller group, the peripheral nerves are involved in an asymmetrical and patchy manner, and the periphery is not necessarily affected more than the proximal parts of the limbs. This syndrome is sometimes known as mononeuritis multiplex.

Pathology. The polyneuropathies show segmental demyelination and axonal degeneration in various combinations.[17] The former, a patchy affair which first appears at the nodes of Ranvier, appears to be the primary event in diabetes, diphtheria, Guillain-Barré syndrome, carcinomatous neuropathy, metachromatic leukodystrophy, and chronic lead poisoning, whereas in the neuropathies due to alcohol, porphyria, triorthocresyl phosphate, isoniazid, and thalidomide, axonal degeneration seems to be primary. This distinction has practical importance in that motor conduction velocities are far more depressed by segmental demyelination than they are by axonal damage; indeed, Gilliatt's experience has led him to conclude that a reduction of 40 per cent or more in motor velocity indicates the presence of segmental demyelination.[17] It must be emphasized, however, that it is rare to find segmental demyelination without loss of continuity of axons in some fibers. Thus, in beriberi and alcoholism, axonal degeneration and segmental demyelination have been described, but conduction velocities are rarely reduced by more than 30 per cent, implying that the axonal degeneration is less significant than the loss of myelin. The greatest reduction of conduction velocities is seen in the hereditary neuropathies, in which the axons are thin and are either demyelinated or poorly myelinated.

Clinical Features. The disorder may be acute, subacute, or chronic. Both motor and sensory fibers are usually involved, but sensory symptoms and signs often dominate certain disorders, such as the neuropathy of diabetes.

Sensory involvement gives rise to distal paresthesias (tingling, numbness, pins and needles, sensations of burning or cold, etc.), and eventually there is impairment of sensation which is greatest in the periphery and shades gradually to normal sensibility proximally. Sensory loss may be limited to the skin but usually affects joint sense and vibration as well; sometimes deep sensibility is more affected than skin sensation. Painful stimuli which reach threshold may be abnormally painful, and the muscles are tender to pressure. Sweating is usually reduced peripherally if sensory involvement is present. In severe cases, orthostatic hypotension may occur from involvement of the sympathetic nervous system.[2]

Motor involvement gives rise to distal weakness or paralysis with hypotonia, and atrophy supervenes after a few weeks. If proprioceptor fibers are affected, motor disability will be increased by sensory ataxia. There is electrical evidence of partial denervation: Slow conduction time, fibrillation action potentials, and small potentials on voluntary effort.

The stretch reflexes of the affected muscles are reduced or lost; the ankle jerks disappear before the knee jerks; the latter may be exaggerated in the early stages of polyneuropathy.

In the presence of *long-standing* severe sensory loss, trophic changes occur. The skin of the feet and hands becomes thin, shiny, and pale; the nails are brittle, and the hair falls out within the area

of sensory impairment. Trophic ulcers may appear.

In addition to the general features of polyneuropathy, certain noxae have their own trademark, e.g., desquamation of the skin of the palms and soles in arsenical poisoning, weakness of convergence in diphtheritic neuropathy, and the telltale features of alcoholism and diabetes. Such signs are useful because in the subacute and chronic forms, one case of polyneuropathy looks very much like another as regards the neurological signs. It is necessary to search into the patient's habits, working conditions, and general health in order to arrive at a correct diagnosis. In a small proportion of cases, exhaustive investigation fails to reveal any cause for the neuropathy.

NEUROPATHY FOLLOWING SERA AND VACCINES

The injection of foreign protein is sometimes followed in one to 12 days by the appearance of an itchy rash, edema of the skin, joint pains, pyrexia, eosinophilia, and enlargement of lymph glands. In a small minority of these cases, the constitutional symptoms are followed or accompanied by an acute neuropathy. Of 100 cases of serum sickness with neurological complications reviewed by Miller and Stanton,[32] there were 74 cases of radiculitis, 10 of polyneuropathy, 10 with cerebral and meningeal complications, four with transverse myelitis, and two with what was described as Landry's paralysis. These complications followed the administration of antisera for tetanus, diphtheria, scarlet fever, gas gangrene, staphylococci, streptococci, pneumococci, or the injection of horse serum, milk, or convalescent poliomyelitis sera. Polyneuropathy may follow bee stings.

Vaccines can give rise to similar symptoms. These have been described following typhoid-paratyphoid vaccination, usually from two to 14 days after the injection. Tetanus toxoid seldom causes neurological trouble, but the administration of antitoxin has been known to

Table 20–1.   Etiology of Peripheral Nerve Disease

"Allergic" Neuropathies	Guillain-Barré syndrome, neuralgic amyotrophy, serum neuropathy.
Collagen Diseases	Disseminated lupus, polyarteritis nodosa, rheumatoid arthritis, Wegener's granulomatosis.
Heredo-familial Diseases	Amyloidosis (primary), Basson-Kornzweig disease, Déjerine-Sottas disease, familial recurrent neuropathy, hereditary sensory radiculoneuropathy, peroneal muscular atrophy, recurrent pressure palsies, Refsum's disease, Werdnig-Hoffman disease, Wolfart-Kugelberg-Welander disease.
Infections (Chap. 14)	Brucellosis, diphtheria, herpes zoster, infectious hepatitis, infectious mononucleosis, leprosy, mumps, typhoid, etc.
Intoxications (Endogenous)	Diabetes mellitus, hypoglycemia, hepatic failure, macroglobulinemia, myxedema, porphyria, uremia.
Intoxications (Exogenous—Chap. 21)	Antimony (emetine), arsenic, benzene derivatives, carbon bisulfide, carbon monoxide, carbon tetrachloride, Dilantin, dinitrophenol, Doriden, Furadantin, Isoniazid, lead, phosphorus compounds (e.g., triorthocresyl phosphate), tick paralysis, trichlorethylene, thallium, Thalidomide, stilbamidine, sulfonamides, vincristine sulfate, etc.
Nutritional Deficiencies (Chap. 17)	Alcoholism, combined system disease, beriberi, hyperemesis gravidarum, Jamaican polyneuropathy, malabsorption syndromes (including Whipple's disease), pellagra, vitamin B_{12} deficiency.
Unclassified	Pink disease, sarcoidosis, polyneuropathy in carcinoma and lymphoma.
Mononeuritis Multiplex	Collagen diseases, embolism, hemorrhage into nerves (anticoagulants, hemophilia), thrombosis (diabetes, Buerger's disease).

cause acute polyneuritis. Pertussis inoculation in infants can lead to convulsions, coma, and hemiplegia from one to 72 hours after the injection. This is a serious condition, and survivors often have permanent residua in the form of mental deficiency, hemiparesis, blindness, or seizures; the effects are cerebral rather than spinal or peripheral in origin.

Inoculation against diphtheria sometimes produces neuralgic amyotrophy, commonly in the arm injected, and a few cases of encephalitis and encephalomyelitis have been reported. The effects of inoculation against rabies are described in Chapter 14; the picture may be one of polyneuropathy, transverse myelitis, or encephalitis.

The explanation for these occasional responses to the administration of foreign protein is not as yet understood. There is ample experimental evidence

to show that, in animals, injection of extracts of nervous tissue combined with adjuvants can produce perivascular demyelinating lesions in the brain and spinal cord, and peripheral neuropathy, but although they are attributed to allergy or delayed hypersensitivity these reactions do not conform to the usual picture of allergic responses.

NEURALGIC AMYOTROPHY (PARALYTIC BRACHIAL NEURITIS)

Definition. Neuralgic amyotrophy[33] is characterized by pain in the region of one or both shoulders, lower motor neuron paralysis of some of the shoulder girdle muscles, and minimal sensory loss. It occurs occasionally in the lower limb.

Etiology. This disease came into prominence during World War II and in nearly 50 per cent of patients, it occurred during convalescence from pneumonia, tonsillitis, or malaria, or after a minor operation. In other patients, an inoculation had been given in the preceding three weeks. Sometimes neuralgic amyotrophy occurs without any such antecedents. It usually occurs in adults.

Clinical Symptoms. The pain starts acutely and may be severe; usually it is felt in the region of the scapula or deltoid, and may radiate down the outer side of the arm as far as the elbow. It usually lasts from 48 hours to a week and then improves, but as it passes off, paralysis appears; rarely, pain continues for some weeks after paralysis has developed. There are no constitutional disturbances. In many cases, the muscles supplied by only one peripheral nerve are affected, the commonest being the serratus magnus (the long thoracic nerve), the spinati (the suprascapular nerve), and the deltoid (the axillary nerve). In others, the muscles supplied by two or more nerves are involved, the usual combination being the spinati and deltoid. The diaphragm may be paralyzed on the affected side. In yet other cases, it is difficult to explain the distribution of paralysis in terms of peripheral nerve or root involvement, and it is possible that the anterior horns are affected. Slight and transient sensory impairment may occur within the territory of the affected roots or nerves. In a few cases, the condition is bilateral, and in some of these, there is an interval of several weeks between the involvement of the two sides. The spinal fluid is normal.

Prognosis and Treatment. As with other peripheral nerve or root lesions, the electrical reactions after three weeks are of considerable value in assessing the prognosis. If there is no reaction of degeneration at this stage, full functional recovery is probable in six to 12 weeks. If there is a reaction of degeneration, it may be many months before improvement in muscle power occurs, and full recovery may be delayed for one or two years. In a very small number of cases, little improvement takes place.

Prednisone in daily doses of 60 mg.

should be given for 10 days, followed by 30 mg. daily for 10 days; the dosage may then be slowly reduced. The shoulder joint should be put through a complete range of movement three times daily in the acute phase, and electrical stimulation of the weakened muscles should be given when pain has subsided.

COLLAGEN DISEASES

Collagen diseases can give rise to peripheral symmetrical sensory-motor polyneuropathy or to involvement of multiple nerves (mononeuritis multiplex).[25] It is common in *polyarteritis*,[31] not unusual in *disseminated lupus* and *advanced rheumatoid arthritis*,[20, 45] and rare in *dermatomyositis* and *scleroderma*. It can occur in *Wegener's granulomatosis*. Some (but not all) of these cases have arteritis of the vasa nervorum. The condition occurs with and without steroid therapy, and may suddenly appear following the withdrawal of steroids. No effective treatment is known for the peripheral neurological complications of collagen diseases.

Polyarteritis Nodosa. Polyarteritis nodosa is an uncommon collagen disease characterized pathologically by necrotizing arteritis of the smaller vessels, leading to thrombosis, aneurysm formation, or rupture. The clinical features are protean and depend on the situation of the lesions, which may involve the kidney, coronary vessels, gastrointestinal tract, peripheral nerves, central nervous system, or subcutaneous vessels. It occurs at any age, but is predominantly a disease of children and young adults.

The neurological features of the disease[31] — which are not present in every case — include headache, vertigo, convulsions, hemiplegia, cranial nerve palsies, cerebellar ataxia, aphasia, mental changes, and polyneuropathy. They may be encountered singly or in various combinations. Vision may be disturbed by thrombosis of the central retinal artery, retinal detachment, hypertensive retinopathy, hemianopia, or paresis of ocular muscles. Peripheral neuropathy may occur in one of two forms: mononeuritis multiplex, or a generalized and symmetrical condition. Other non-neurological features which may occur, either with polyneuropathy or in separate attacks, are loss of weight, anemia, eosinophilia, cutaneous eruptions, and small, tender, pealike aneurysms along the course of superficial arteries. The condition is usually treated, with indifferent success, by the administration of steroids. The prognosis is determined by the effect of the disease on the body as a whole; it is usually poor.

ACUTE FEBRILE POLYNEURITIS (LANDRY-GUILLAIN-BARRÉ SYNDROME)

This disease[21, 53] is characterized by the acute and *usually* febrile onset of rapidly spreading polyneuritis, with or without implication of the cranial nerves and spinal cord; there is usually a considerable increase in the protein content of the cerebrospinal fluid, without pleocytosis. It is not related to the mild polyneuropathy which occasionally develops in the course of prolonged infections, such as typhoid, dysentery, and advancing tuberculosis, which is either wholly or partly nutritional in origin.

In 1859, Landry described the case of a man who developed paresthesias in the feet, followed by flaccid paralysis of the legs, weakness of the upper limbs, and bulbar palsy; he died on the eighth day. There was some objective impairment of tactile sensibility in the feet. This clinical picture can be produced by acute febrile polyneuritis, severe diphtheritic polyneuritis, porphyria, some cases of rabies, and the neuropathy which sometimes follows antirabies inoculation. If the sensory features are excluded from the criteria, acute poliomyelitis, potassium intoxication, and tick paralysis have to be considered. The condition that was described by Guillain, Barré, and Strohl during World War I appears to be identical with Landry's case, and if the term "Guillain-Barré syndrome" is to be used at all, it applies to acute febrile poly-

neuritis, in which disorder the spinal fluid protein is raised, but the cell count remains normal. However, a similar dissociation between cell count and protein content is encountered in many other types of severe polyneuropathy and is not specific for any one disease.

Etiology and Pathology. Acute febrile polyneuritis is most common in adolescents and young adults. The cause is unknown. There is segmental demyelination of the ventral and dorsal roots, with chromatolysis in the sensory ganglia and ventral horn cells. Slight inflammatory changes have been seen in the pia-arachnoid and brainstem.

Clinical Features. The disease often starts with a mild, influenza-like illness or sore throat, the neurological symptoms coming on from three to 12 days thereafter. Weakness, progressing to paralysis, starts in the periphery and sweeps rapidly up the legs, arms, and trunk; it involves the cranial nerves in some cases. Proprioceptive sensory loss may cause ataxia. The paralysis is flaccid, with loss of reflexes. There is usually a slight degree of peripheral sensory impairment; in some cases, paresthesias are complained of, although no sensory loss can be detected. In others, peripheral sensory impairment is obvious. The presence of sensory symptoms and signs is useful in differentiating this condition from poliomyelitis. Facial paralysis, bulbar paralysis, and weakness of the extraocular muscles are quite common. Papilledema is occasionally seen, but its etiology in this context remains obscure. Rarely, proximal muscles of the limbs are more affected than peripheral groups, the paralysis having a more or less segmental distribution. The deep tendon reflexes are lost, and the plantar responses are usually flexor, if the foot can move at all. An extensor response is encountered from time to time, implying spread to the spinal cord or brain. Sphincter symptoms occur in severe cases. Encephalitis may occur, with disturbance of consciousness. In some cases, the features are those of encephaloneuromyelitis.

Orthostatic hypotension is not uncommon. Water intoxication from inappropriate secretion of antidiuretic hormone may complicate the picture.

Diagnosis. The protein content of the spinal fluid is often normal for the first few days, but may ultimately reach a figure of 1000 mg. per cent or more; exceptionally, there is a slight increase of lymphocytes. The cerebrospinal fluid pressure is elevated in severe cases. It must be emphasized that a modest increase of protein with a normal cell count may be found in other conditions, notably in severe diabetic and diphtheritic polyneuropathy, acute encephalomyelitis, and (after the second week) acute anterior poliomyelitis.

The presence of paresthesias and sensory changes helps to exclude poliomyelitis. The neuritis of acute porphyria is distinguished by abdominal pain, a rise of blood pressure, mental symptoms, convulsions, and the presence of porphyrinuria. Diphtheritic polyneuritis is usually preceded by evidence of the local lesions in the nose, throat, or skin, and before the onset of polyneuropathy there is usually blurring of vision due to weakness of accommodation. Other causes of rapidly ascending paralysis are rabies, antirabies inoculation, tick paralysis, and potassium intoxication.

Prognosis. Prognosis is variable; death may occur from bulbar palsy and respiratory paralysis within 48 hours, but the interval between the onset of the disease and the development of respiratory failure may be as long as 20 days. With assisted ventilation, which may have to be maintained for many weeks, complete recovery is possible; there is one report of a case in which complete ventilatory support was required for 266 days, following which the patient recovered.

In a series reported by Hewer and his colleagues, 72 per cent made a full functional recovery, 10 per cent had some residual symptoms, and 17 per cent had fairly severe disability, but only one patient was totally unable to walk.

The disease can recur and there are reports of chronic relapsing cases.[14, 49] Despite their prolonged time course, the clinical and pathological features of these cases suggest that they are variants of the acute disease.

Treatment. From 40 to 60 mg. of Prednisone should be given daily for a week, gradually tapering off to a maintenance dose of 15 mg. per day for three weeks or longer. An artificial respirator is necessary when the respiratory muscles are involved. Tracheostomy should be carried out at the earliest sign of respiratory embarrassment.

THE DIABETIC NEUROPATHIES

Classification. The commonest type of diabetic neuropathy takes the form of a chronic, symmetrical sensory polyneuropathy, which appears first in the lower limbs and seldom involves the arms.[42] The autonomic nervous system is sometimes implicated.[2] Second, there is an uncommon, acute form, marked by severe pain, rapid weakness and wasting of both proximal and distal muscles, peripheral sensory impairment, and loss of the tendon reflexes.[16] Third, two or more peripheral nerves may be involved by mononeuritis multiplex, the pathological basis of which is thrombosis of small radicals of the vasa nervorum.[37] Uremic polyneuropathy may also complicate the late stages of diabetes with renal failure. Diabetic amyotrophy,[16, 26] a myopathy of proximal muscles, is a rare condition which can exist on its own or in combination with polyneuropathy.

Diabetic Polyneuropathy. There is segmental demyelination of the peripheral nerves, predominantly in the lower limbs.[15] The vasa nervorum are diseased; the lumen of the arterioles is narrowed, and the capillary walls are thickened by deposits of PAS-positive material in the basement membrane, but there is no anatomical correlation between the vascular change and the sites of demyelination.[15] In some cases, there is degeneration of the posterior roots and the posterior columns in the lumbar and thoracic segments. The muscles show the changes of neurogenic atrophy and they, too, display prominent thickening of the capillary basement membranes.

This form of diabetic neuropathy is usually mild and is characterized by paresthesias in the toes and feet, with or without shooting pains in the limbs, and cramps. There is tenderness of the calf muscles, depression of the ankle jerks, and depression or loss of vibration sense at the ankles. Sweating may be reduced or lost in the periphery of the legs. Peripheral nerve conduction rates are reduced, even in the absence of clinical signs of neuropathy. Rarely, an extensor plantar response may be found,[16] but this should not be attributed to diabetes until all other possibilities have been excluded. For instance, coincident compression of the cervical cord by spondylosis can confuse the picture. Also, there is a higher incidence of pernicious anemia and subacute combined degeneration of the cord in diabetics than in the general population; Khan[24] found 87 patients with neuropathy in 402 diabetics, and 7 of these exhibited lowered serum vitamin B_{12}. It is probable that vitamin B_{12} deficiency may also account for the progressive optic atrophy which is sometimes seen in diabetes in the absence of diabetic retinopathy.

Cranial nerve palsies, notably of the third or sixth nerve, are not uncommon but are usually transient. In some cases, the abrupt onset suggests that a vascular lesion is responsible.

The symptoms and signs of diabetic neuropathy commonly improve with treatment, although they may sometimes worsen transiently when treatment is first started. In cases of mononeuritis multiplex, however, recovery is usually incomplete.

Peripheral neuropathy is often accompanied by involvement of the autonomic nervous system. Peripheral loss of sweating, referred to above, is the most common but least important symptom. Orthostatic hypotension, retention of urine, nocturnal diarrhea, weakness of the rectal sphincter, and impotence may occur early or late in the disease. The pupils are sometimes small in size and sluggish in their reaction to light, but true Argyll Robertson pupils should not be ascribed to diabetes.

Diabetic Amyotrophy. Diabetic amyotrophy[16, 26] is characterized by the rapid onset of weakness and wasting of proximal muscle groups in patients with poorly controlled diabetes. Pain may be present or absent. There may be coincident evidence of diabetic polyneuropathy, or the amyotrophy may exist on its own. The weakness is often more marked on one side than on the other. Electromyography discloses normal conduction times, and the motor units of the affected muscles are polyphasic and markedly decreased in number. The condition improves when the diabetes is brought under control.

Pathologically, there is moderate variation in size of the muscle fibers and there is increase in the number of sarcolemmal nuclei. Atrophic muscle fibers are interspersed among normal fibers. Electron microscopy reveals electron-dense granules within mitochondria, increased glycogen-containing interfibrillar spaces, and sporadic shrinkage of myofibrils.[19] The capillaries show increased thickness of the basement membrane.

PORPHYRIA

Porphyrinuria[18, 29, 41] is a condition of disordered porphyrin metabolism characterized by the intermittent excretion of photosensitive porphyrins, which turns the urine a dark burgundy color on exposure to light. It is encountered in three forms. *Congenital porphyria* is an extremely rare disease, transmitted as a mendelian recessive and characterized by photosensitivity of the skin (which causes bullous eruptions) and a reddish-brown discoloration of the teeth, excessive growth of bodily hair, and the excretion of large quantities of uroporphyrin I and coproporphyrin I in the urine and feces. Hemolytic anemia may be present, but there are no neurological symptoms. A second form, *porphyria cutanea tarda* is marked by the appearance in adult life of photosensitivity and the development of vesicles following skin trauma or exposure to sunlight. In addition, the patients suffer from abdominal and neurological symptoms similar to those of acute intermittent porphyria, and they may show evidence of liver dysfunction. There are large amounts of uroporphyrin I and III, coproporphyrin I and III, and protoporphyrin IX in the urine and feces. *Acute intermittent porphyria*, which is often familial and which is believed to be transmitted as an autosomal mendelian dominant, is usually seen in adolescents and young adults. There is a heavy excretion of porphobilinogen, porphobilin, and uroporphyrin III in the urine, together with the excretion of increased amounts of coproporphyrin II.

Pathology. The structural changes have been variously described.[13] Sometimes no abnormality has been seen, but many authors have reported patchy demyelination of the peripheral nerves without damage to the axons. The histological picture varies with the duration of the paralysis, its severity and extent, and whether there have been earlier attacks of the disease. Furthermore, the position in the course of the nerve from which the sample is taken has a bearing on the abnormalities found. It seems likely that axons and myelin sheaths are equally affected, the degeneration being of the wallerian type. The more proximal the level at which the nerve is sectioned, the less evidence of damage, so that at the level of the spinal roots little or no change is to be found. Examination of teased preparations of nerve fibers has failed to reveal evidence of segmental demyelination, according to Cavanagh. In the central nervous system, on the other hand, lesions which appear to be ischemic in origin have been found in the cerebral cortex, basal ganglia, and the white matter of the hemispheres. Chromatolysis has been found in the medullary nuclei, especially in the dorsal vagal nucleus, and the vagus and the sympathetic chain may show acute, patchy demyelination and slight axon changes.

Clinical Features. Attacks may occur for no obvious reason, but they sometimes appear to be triggered by alcohol, barbiturates, or sulfonamides. The clinical picture is one of malaise, abdominal colic, a moderate rise of blood pressure, porphyrinuria, and a rapidly advancing polyneuropathy.[39, 41] The latter is usually severe and chiefly motor, producing flaccid paralysis with loss of tendon reflexes. The proximal muscles are often more affected than the distal muscles, and the upper limbs may be more affected than the lower. The cranial nerves, trunk muscles, and sphincters are frequently involved. Sensory disturbances may or may not be present and they may be either of a glove and stocking distribution or may affect the proximal parts of the limbs and trunk in a "bathing trunks" distribution. A striking feature of the neuropathy is the variability in the pattern of muscle involvement which can occur in the same patient in successive attacks. Wasting is rapid, but a remarkable degree of recovery can occur even after widespread and severe paralysis; it may take months for full recovery to occur.

In children, convulsions may occur, and delirium may precede or complicate the neuropathy at all ages. In some cases, the picture is dominated by recurrent mental symptoms in the form of confusion, delirium, disturbance of memory, and disorientation.

Diagnosis. The diagnosis is suggested by the concurrence of abdominal cramps, intermittent hypertension, polyneuropathy, and mental symptoms. The urine may or may not turn burgundy-colored when exposed to light. The diagnosis is confirmed if the urine turns red on the addition of Ehrlich's aldehyde reagent. However, since porphyrinuria is intermittent, repeated spectroscopic tests are desirable, or the glycine loading test[40] may be performed: The patient is given a low-protein breakfast, followed by 25 gm. of glycine at 10:00 A.M. and at 2:00 P.M. The urine is collected hourly and examined for porphobilinogen and its precursor, delta amino levulinic acid, which appears in increased amounts.

Treatment. On theoretical grounds, the administration of vasodilators such as nitrites and papaverine is indicated to relieve spasm of smooth muscles. Peters and his associates[35] have reported that the administration of chelating agents (BAL, EDTA) is effective. Symptomatic relief may be achieved by use of the phenothiazines, e.g., 25 mg. of Thorazine, together with 15 mg. of neostigmine every six hours. Barbiturates are to be avoided.

AMYLOID DISEASE

Three types of amyloidosis exist:[1, 23] (1) a form resulting from chronic suppuration and other diseases associated with extensive tissue destruction, (2) a form associated with multiple myeloma, and (3) a primary form[1, 36, 46] which may be genetically determined. It is this primary form which gives rise to polyneuropathy—a chronic, peripheral, symmetrical sensory-motor disturbance affecting the legs before the arms. It is more common in men than in women, and the onset of symptoms is often delayed until the fifth decade, in which event a median carpal tunnel syndrome may be the first sign of the disease. Amyloid collects in the heart, skeletal muscles, diaphragm, tongue, skin, and viscera. Infiltration of the larynx can cause hoarseness, and enlargement of the tongue may cause dysarthria and dysphagia.[1] In some familial cases, waxy opacities have been found in the vitreous. The serum lipoproteins may be elevated.

PINK DISEASE
(ACRODYNIA, SWIFT'S DISEASE, ERYTHREDEMA)

Acrodynia is a disease of early life characterized by a febrile onset, an irritating rash, and polyneuropathy.

Pathology. Degenerative changes are found in the peripheral parts of the nerves, with considerable degeneration of myelin in the finer nerve bundles. There is widespread chromatolysis of anterior horn cells and proliferation of Schwann cells in the ventral roots. An unexplained feature, present in most cases, is a striking infiltration of the meninges and the spinal cord by small round cells, presumably lymphocytes.

For some time it has been suspected that pink disease might be due to mercury intoxication, since concentrations of more than 50 μg. per liter of mercury are found in the urine of some patients, but this is not a constant finding and the role of mercury in this disorder is uncertain.

Clinical Features. The disease is most prevalent between the ages of four months and four years, but it may occur later. It starts with general malaise, anorexia, irritability, and mild pyrexia. These symptoms may follow an upper respiratory or gastrointestinal infection. After a week or two of ill-defined misery, the rash appears. At first it is a generalized erythema which soon fades from the rest of the body but grows worse in the hands and feet, which become swollen, dusky red, and intolerably itchy. The cheeks, nose, and ears may also suffer. Desquamation occurs, and scratching may lead to secondary infection. There is photophobia, stomatitis, salivation, profuse sweating, and loss of hair. The neurological features may be slight or marked. They appear by the time the rash is well established and take the form of a peripheral sensory-motor polyneuropathy, although it is difficult to estimate the sensory changes with any degree of accuracy in children of this age. Irritability may give place to delirium, but meningism is absent, and the spinal fluid is normal. Leukocytosis is present in the blood. Mild cases recover in four to six weeks, but symptoms can persist for many months; the mortality is 10 per cent or less.

Treatment. Treatment is symptomatic. The child should be given sedatives for insomnia and pain, and it is desirable to tie the hands to prevent scratching or to put them in cotton gloves.

Calamine lotion may be used to relieve the itching. A nutritious, vitamin-supplemented diet should be given. Excessive sweating causes loss of sodium as well as of water, and care must be taken to replace both.

Considerable symptomatic improvement has been reported following the administration of ganglion-blocking agents such as hexamethonium bromide, in doses of 10 to 15 mg. by subcutaneous injection, every six hours.

POLYNEUROPATHY ASSOCIATED WITH CARCINOMA AND OTHER NEOPLASMS

The commonest cause of a *local* neuropathy in visceral carcinoma is metastatic infiltration of nerve roots, plexuses, or peripheral nerves, giving rise to weakness, atrophy, paresthesias, and sensory impairment within the distribution of the affected nerve or nerves. Pain may be absent and sensory loss is seldom as marked as motor dysfunction. Similarly, individual nerves and nerve roots may be involved by Hodgkin's disease, lymphosarcoma, myeloma, and leukemia. These manifestations usually occur in advanced disease, so that the diagnosis is relatively easy. A curious feature of Hodgkin's disease is that when it gives rise to pain, the pain is much aggravated by the ingestion of alcohol.

In carcinoma[6] and the lymphomas,[5] polyneuropathy of slow onset and progressive course can occur in the absence of infiltration of the peripheral or central nervous system. Myelinated fibers show segmental demyelination and axonal degeneration. Symptoms may appear before there is any evidence of a primary tumor. The most common cause is carcinoma of the lung, but it also occurs in carcinoma of the ovary, breast, cervix and uterus, and rectum. The incidence of neuropathy in carcinoma of the lung and breast is not related to the age of the patient, the duration of the primary disease, the amount of weight loss, or the patient's blood group.

Clinical Features.[6, 50, 52] From the clinical point of view, these cases fall into three groups. The least common is a sensory polyneuropathy caused by degeneration of the sensory root ganglia and the posterior columns.[5] It gives rise to a gradually spreading sensory loss which may involve the entire body. All forms of sensibility are affected, and the loss of proprioception gives rise to sensory ataxia. The eighth nerve may also be involved, with consequent deafness.

A mixed sensory-motor neuropathy due to peripheral nerve degeneration is more common. Motor weakness may predominate, but there is usually some degree of peripheral sensory impairment as well.

The third type, termed neuromyopathy,[6, 9] is characterized by weakness and wasting of proximal muscles, with absolute or relative sparing of the distal muscles. The main impact of the disease is on the lower limbs, and the patellar reflexes are lost before the Achilles reflex. It is not always easy to distinguish the respective roles of myopathy and neuropathy in these cases.

Neuropathies caused by visceral carcinoma are gradual in onset and evolution. They are therefore easy to distinguish from the rapidly progressive ascending segmental sensory motor deficit caused by *necrotizing myelopathy*[27] in association with visceral carcinoma. In this condition, there is a patchy and nonsystematized but roughly symmetrical process of subtotal and total tissue necrosis involving both gray and white matter. It gives rise to a flaccid areflexic paraplegia, a rapidly ascending level of segmental sensory loss, and sphincter paralysis. The condition is most marked in the thoracic segments of the cord but may reach the cervical enlargment. There is widespread vascular necrosis and adventitial fibrosis, but these are probably part of the reaction to the necrotizing process rather than the cause thereof.

CHRONIC PROGRESSIVE MOTOR NEURONITIS

This is a rare and perplexing entity characterized by slowly progressive paresis and atrophy of muscles, sensory loss being minimal or absent. It may involve the arms alone, may spread to the legs, or may start in the latter. It commences peripherally and spreads proximally. Paralysis is seldom complete, and atrophy is moderate. Fasciculation may be present. It lasts many months, but it may clear up entirely in a year or more. Occasionally, it progresses steadily over a number of years. It is not a diagnosis to be made lightly; hypertrophic polyneuritis, leprosy, amyotrophic lateral sclerosis, and chronic lead poisoning have to be excluded.

PERIPHERAL NEUROPATHY IN HEPATIC AND RENAL FAILURE

Patients with cirrhosis, a portal systemic shunt, or hepatic necrosis sometimes exhibit mild sensory impairment in the feet and loss of the ankle and knee jerks. Examination of isolated, teased nerve fibers has shown segmental demyelination,[11] a point of some interest in view of the fact that chronic hepatic disease can also give rise to demyelination in the spinal cord.

Chronic renal insufficiency can lead to peripheral neuropathy.[4, 48] It starts insidiously as a predominantly sensory polyneuropathy affecting the feet, with complaints of tingling, burning sensations, numbness, and pins and needles. At this stage, vibration sense is impaired or lost in the feet, and the Achilles reflex is either depressed or absent. If the condition progresses, a modest degree of weakness appears distally.

In severe uremia, the polyneuropathy may start explosively shortly after dialysis is begun. There is severe weakness of the legs and arms, but as dialysis continues, clinical improvement eventually occurs. The cause of this neuropathy is not understood; many factors associated with both uremia and its treatment may play a part—anemia, starvation, infections and the antibiotics used to control them, hypothetical toxins, etc. Massive

doses of thiamine have no effect on the neuropathy.

Peripheral neuropathy has also been described in children suffering from hereditary interstitial nephritis,[28] which is sometimes associated with nerve deafness (Alport's syndrome).

VASCULAR NEUROPATHIES

Atheroma of small vessels can so narrow the lumen as to cause ischemia, and this can be aggravated by thrombosis within the affected vessel. Should this process affect the vasa nervorum of a single nerve, it alone will be involved, but as a rule, the atheroma is generalized and several nerves are affected in the periphery of the limb or limbs. This gives rise to paresthesias, claudication, cramps, and burning pain in the feet; the last is especially liable to arise in bed and when the leg is warm, as, for instance, in bed at night. Moderate sensory loss and muscular weakness accompany these symptoms. In elderly diabetics it is sometimes difficult to determine how much of the neuritis is due to diabetes and how much to atheroma, and whether the sensory changes result from ischemia of the skin or from anoxia of the sensory nerves themselves. Similar difficulties apply to the sensory and motor signs seen in Buerger's disease, in which there is both arterial occlusion and periarterial fibrosis involving adjacent nerves. Careful examination of the vascular responses is important in any adult complaining of pain and paresthesias in the limbs.

Embolism can cause acute paralysis of one or more peripheral nerves in subacute bacterial endocarditis; the prognosis for recovery is usually good.

Hemorrhage into peripheral nerves[34, 43] (usually the sciatic) may occur in hemophilia and in patients on anticoagulant therapy. In the author's experience, complete recovery is to be expected, but it may take months.

Thrombosis of vasa vasorum can cause mononeuritis multiplex in diabetes mellitus and is presumed to be responsible for the mononeuritis multiplex which sometimes occurs in polyarteritis nodosa.

HEREDITARY ATAXIC POLYNEURITIS (REFSUM'S DISEASE)

This is a heredofamilial disorder of the nervous system which usually appears in the first or second decade and is characterized by a slowly progressive, symmetrical peripheral polyneuropathy, with patchy enlargement of the peripheral nerves,[8] cerebellar ataxia, atypical retinitis pigmentosa, and—in some cases—anosmia, nerve deafness, ichthyosis, epiphyseal dysplasia, and electrocardiographic changes suggestive of coronary insufficiency.[8, 38] In some cases, the polyneuropathy has shown distinct remissions. Sudden death due to heart block or acute myocardial infarction has been recorded.

The condition is due to an inborn error of lipid metabolism which leads to the accumulation of large amounts of phytanic acid in serum and tissues.

The cerebrospinal fluid protein is increased and there is an increase in the total serum lipids due to an excess of phytanic acid.

It has been reported that a butter-free, vegetable-free diet causes a marked fall in serum phytanic acid levels, indicating that its accumulation in Refsum's disease is primarily of exogenous origin.

FAMILIAL RECURRENT NEUROPATHY

A rare condition, familial recurrent neuropathy is characterized by the occurrence of intermittent attacks of mononeuritis multiplex in several members of a family, over two or more generations. In some cases, the episodes have been related to pregnancy or to some intercurrent disease. Clinically, the attacks are virtually indistinguishable from those of neuralgic amyotrophy; they show a particular predilection for the shoulder girdle but may also affect the distal portions of the arm or leg. The disorder is localized to a single group of muscles in an individual attack. The onset is with severe pain followed within a day or two by weakness and minimal sensory impairment in the same region. Recovery of function takes several months, as a rule, and may be incomplete. In one family described by Taylor,[47] some of the affected individuals also had episodes of dysphagia and hoarseness, suggesting that the tenth nerve was also involved.

The above condition must be distinguished from a *hereditary liability to pressure palsy*. The episodes consist of painless paresis involving single perceptual nerves. In a family studied by the author and reported by Davies,[10] the father had eight attacks over a period of 35 years, including peroneal palsy and wrist-drop; on one occasion, there was sensory loss in the forehead as a result of resting the brow on the edge of a table for a few minutes. Earle and his colleagues have described four families with this affliction.

HEREDITARY SENSORY RADICULAR NEUROPATHY

Hicks and Denny-Brown[12] have reported a disease which affected 11 individuals of a family of 36 members, in three generations, and which was characterized by a progressive peripheral sensory loss that affected temperature most extensively, then pain, then touch. Vibration and position sense were least affected. Because of the loss of pain and temperature sensibility, indolent trophic ulcers were common in the feet. Progressive deafness can occur, owing to atrophy of the cochlear ganglia.

The pathological basis of the condition is a primary degeneration of dorsal root ganglia together with evidence of degeneration of the olivary nuclei, optic nerves, and cerebellum. The degree of disability is largely determined by the severity of the trophic ulcers in the extremities.

HYPERTROPHIC POLYNEUROPATHY (DÉJERINE-SOTTAS DISEASE)

This is a rare condition, usually but not exclusively heredofamilial in incidence and characterized by thickening of peripheral nerves and slowly progressive peripheral denervation. The thickening is due to excessive cellular connective tissue and collagen around each nerve fiber, which on cross section presents an onion-like appearance of concentric laminated sheaths. The axons degenerate and disappear. There is also thickening of the anterior spinal roots.

Clinical Features. Symptoms appear in childhood or in early adult life. There is a progressive symmetrical involvement of the peripheral nerves, starting distally and spreading proximally, with wasting, weakness, contractures, superficial and deep sensory loss, sensory ataxia, and disappearance of tendon reflexes. Trophic ulcers may appear on the feet. There is palpable thickening of the superficial nerve in the affected parts of the body. Spinal compression can be caused by gross thickening of the spinal roots within the vertebral canal. The trunk and cranial nerves usually escape, but—as is often the case in heredofamilial disease—the picture can be complicated by other abnormalities such as kyphoscoliosis, clubfoot, nystagmus, intention tremor, dysarthria, etc.

The disease usually progresses slowly and intermittently over a number of years.

Diagnosis. The correct diagnosis is suggested by the association of a slowly progressive polyneuropathy and palpable thickening of peripheral nerves. It is confirmed by microscopic examination of one of the minor branches of a peripheral nerve. Adams and his colleagues have described an intermittent but slowly progressive asymmetrical polyneuropathy associated with painful enlargement of nerves. The affected nerves are invested with concentric laminations of dense connective tissue, and there are diffuse and focal collections of inflammatory cells in the perineural and epineural sheaths. The authors reported that clinical improvement followed the administration of steroids.

PROGRESSIVE SPINAL MUSCULAR ATROPHY IN INFANTS (WERDNIG-HOFFMANN DISEASE)

Progressive spinal muscular atrophy of infants is a rare familial disease, usually affecting two or more siblings, in which muscular weakness and atrophy appear as a result of degeneration of the anterior horn cells of the spinal cord. The symptoms are usually noticed for the first time when the infant is about six months old but the disease can start in fetal life, in which event it is evident at birth.

Pathology. There is a conspicuous loss of anterior horn cells, with degeneration of the motor fibers of the peripheral nerves and secondary neurogenic atrophy of the muscle. There is also degeneration of the cells of the nuclei of the motor cranial nerves, notably the twelfth, and slight gliosis is present in the long tracts of the spinal cord.

Clinical Features. When the disease starts in fetal life, the infant shows marked hypotonia and poverty of movement, and is unable to roll over or hold up the head. Movements of the limbs lose their vigor, and ultimately there is complete paralysis, which includes the bulbar muscles. The musculature is hypotonic and atrophied, but wasting may at first be obscured by subcutaneous fat. In this early group, death may occur at any time from one to four months after birth.

When the onset is between two and 12 months, weakness is less severe and the progression less striking; some learn to sit up and crawl or stand. Fasciculation may be noticed both in the periphery and in the tongue, and the tendon reflexes disappear. Cutaneous sensibility and sphincter actions are unaffected. Children in this group may live for six or seven years.

Diagnosis. Familial incidence, the onset of weakness and hypotonia at about six months, and a progressively downhill course form a suggestive triad, but the diagnosis is difficult in the early stages of the disease, especially when the patient is the first in the family to be affected. In these cases, the distinction from other types of the amyotonia congenita syndrome is assisted by electromyography and muscle biopsy. In benign congenital hypotonia, the child is floppy and immobile but has good muscle power, and the tendon reflexes are usually present. (Other causes of the floppy baby syndrome are listed on page 550.)

THE WOHLFART-KUGELBERG-WELANDER DISEASE

This condition is hereditary, with onset in childhood or adolescence.[36, 44] In rare cases, which are presumed to be the same disease, the onset occurs in middle life. It is twice as common in males as in females, and presents with proximal weakness in the upper and lower limbs, which may or may not be accompanied by atrophy in the early stages of the disease. Later on, the distal muscles are involved, but the disability is not usually severe and affected individuals continue to be able to get about for many years. The cranial nerves are usually spared. Fasciculation is often present spontaneously, and can be brought out by injecting 1 mg. of neostigmine. The proximal weakness may suggest a myopathy, but biopsy shows neurogenic atrophy, and electromyography exhibits the changes typical of denervation.

PERONEAL MUSCULAR ATROPHY (NEURITIC MUSCULAR ATROPHY, CHARCOT-MARIE-TOOTH DISEASE)

This hereditary disease is characterized by slowly progressive wasting and weakness, and it usually begins in the legs below the knee, in the peroneal muscles. Both clinically and pathologically, the typical case resembles a very slowly progressive peripheral neuropathy, but in some instances additional features are present—pes cavus, scoliosis, ataxia, intention tremor—which link them with the hereditary ataxias.[36] Inheritance is usually dominant, but both recessive and sex-linked modes of transmission have been described.

Pathology. Degeneration of both axons and their myelin sheaths occurs in the distal portions of the peripheral nerves. There is a slight excess of interstitial connective tissue in the affected areas, but the larger nerves may appear normal. In some cases, there is slight degeneration of the posterior columns in association with loss of neurons in the dorsal root ganglion. The muscles show evidence of neurogenic degeneration, together with the secondary myopathic changes which occur in muscles in long-standing cases of neurogenic atrophy.

Clinical Features. The disease is more common in males than in females. It usually starts between the ages of 10 and 20, but it can begin in early childhood or as late as the fifth decade. A feature of the "late starters" is that they seldom notice their incapacity at first, and only seek advice when the disease is well established.

Weakness and wasting usually appear symmetrically in the peronei, followed by the anterior tibial group and the small muscles of the feet. Exceptionally, the disease starts in the hands and lower arms and forearms, or the upper and lower limbs may be affected together. Motor capacity is often retained in the presence of severe wasting. Pes cavus and foot drop develop, and wasting spreads to involve the distal third of the thigh; the muscles above this level are preserved. Fasciculation is seen occasionally. The hands and the distal half of the forearm are affected, but it may take many years before this becomes obvious. Muscles of the head and neck almost invariably escape, but wasting of the spinati and pectoralis major has been described.

Peripheral sensation is slightly reduced in some cases, and impairment of vibration sense in the feet is common. Position sense can be affected in the toes as well, but sensation usually remains normal in the hands. The ankle jerks disappear early, followed much later by the knee jerks. The reflexes in the arms are usually unaffected even in the presence of atrophy. The plantar responses are either flexor or absent, depending on the degree of peripheral paralysis.

Generally speaking, the nutrition of the feet is well preserved, although vasomotor changes may be present. Perforating ulcers can occur, in the presence of an associated sensory polyneuropathy. The sphincters are unaffected.

Some members of families affected by this disease display nothing more than clawfoot and absence of the tendon reflexes in the legs, and slowing of motor nerve conduction is sometimes found in apparently unaffected members of the family.

The course of the disease is slow, extending over many years, and very few of the affected individuals ever become seriously incapacitated. Sometimes spontaneous arrest is seen.

Laboratory Aids. The cerebrospinal fluid is usually normal. Electromyography shows signs of denervation in the affected muscles, and there is marked slowing of motor nerve conduction.

Diagnosis. The muscular dystrophies affect predominantly the *proximal* muscles, hypertrophy is common, and the progress of the disease is more rapid. The wasting of peripheral portions of individual muscles is characteristic of peroneal muscular atrophy. Amyotrophic lateral sclerosis is much more rapid in its course, fasciculation is prominent, pyramidal signs are often present, and sensory loss is absent. Familial hypertrophic polyneuritis is distinguished by palpable thickening of the peripheral nerves and a more marked degree of peripheral sensory impairment.

Treatment. Orthopedic measures to correct deformities in the feet should be deferred as long as possible. Surgical shoes and a light support to prevent foot drop are helpful.

REFERENCES

1. Andrade, C.: A peculiar form of peripheral neuropathy: Familial atypical generalized amyloidosis with special involvement of the peripheral nerves. *Brain* 75:408, 1952.
2. Appenzeller, O., and Richardson, E. P.: The sympathetic chain in patients with diabetic and alcoholic polyneuropathy. *Neurology* 16:1205, 1966.
3. Arnason, B. G. W., and Chelmicka-Szorc, E.: The effect of hydrocortisone on nerve conduction in experimental peripheral nerve segmental demyelination. *Neurology* 20: 390, 1970.
4. Asbury, A. K., Victor, M., and Adams, R. D.: Uremic polyneuropathy. *Arch. Neurol.* 8: 413, 1963.
5. Blanchard, B. M.: Case report: Peripheral neuropathy (non-invasive) associated with lymphoma. *Ann. Int. Med.* 56:774, 1962.
6. Brain, R. L., and Norris, F. H.: *The Remote Effects of Cancer on the Nervous System.* Grune and Stratton, New York, 1965.
7. Brandt, S.: Course and symptoms of progressive infantile muscular atrophy. *Arch. Neurol. Psychiat.* 63:218, 1950.
8. Camermeyer, J.: Neuropathological change in hereditary neuropathies: Manifestations of the syndrome heredopathia atactica polyneuritiformis in the presence of interstitial hypertrophic polyneuropathy. *J. Neuropath. Exp. Neurol.* 15:340, 1956.
9. Croft, P. B., and Wilkinson, M.: The course and prognosis in some types of carcinomatous neuromyopathy. *Brain* 92:1, 1969.
9a. Curley, A., Sedlack, V. A., Girling, E. F., and Hawk, R. E.: Organic mercury identified as the cause of poisoning in humans and hogs. *Science* 172:65, 1971.
10. Davies, D. M.: Recurrent peripheral nerve palsies in a family. *Lancet* 2:226, 1954.
11. Dayan, A. D., and Williams, R.: Demyelinating peripheral neuropathy and liver disease. *Lancet* 2:133, 1967.
12. Denny-Brown, D.: Hereditary sensory radicular neuropathy. *J. Neurol. Neurosurg. Psychiat.* 14:237, 1951.
13. Denny-Brown, D., and Sciarra, D.: Changes in the nervous system in acute porphyria. *Brain* 68:1, 1948.
14. DeVivo, D. C., and Engel, W. K.: Remarkable recovery of a steroid-responsive recurrent polyneuropathy. *J. Neurol. Neurosurg. Psychiat.* 33:62, 1970.
15. Dolman, C. L.: The morbid anatomy of diabetic neuropathy. *Neurology* 13:135, 1963.
16. Garland, H.: The neurological complications

of diabetes. *Proc. Roy. Soc. Med.* 53:137, 1960.

17. Gilliatt, R. W.: Disorders of peripheral nerves. *J. Roy. Coll. Phys.* 1:50, 1966.
18. Goldberg, A., and Rimington, C.: *Diseases of Porphyrin Metabolism.* Charles C Thomas, Springfield, Ill., 1962.
19. Hamilton, C. R., Dobson, H. L., and Marshall, J. A.: Diabetic amyotrophy: Clinical and electronmicroscopic studies in 6 patients. *Amer. J. Med. Sci.* 256:81, 1968.
20. Hart, F. D., and Golding, J. R.: Rheumatoid neuropathy. *Brit. Med. J.* 1:1594, 1960.
21. Haymaker, W., and Kernohan, J. W.: The Landry-Guillain-Barré syndrome. *Medicine* 28:59, 1949.
22. Joiner, C. L., McArdle, B., and Thompson, R. H. S.: Blood pyruvate estimations in the diagnosis and treatment of polyneuritis. *Brain* 73:431, 1950.
23. Kernohan, J. W., and Woltman, H. W.: Amyloid neuritis. *Arch. Neurol. Psychiat.* 47:132, 1942.
24. Khan, M. A., Wakefield, G. S., and Pugh, D. W.: Vitamin B_{12} deficiency in diabetic neuropathy. *Lancet* 2:768, 1969.
25. Kibler, R. F., and Rose, F. C.: Peripheral neuropathy in the "collagen diseases." *Brit. Med. J.* 1:1781, 1960.
26. Locke, S., Lawrence, D. G., and Legg, M. A.: Diabetic amyotrophy. *Amer. J. Med.* 34:775, 1963.
27. Mancall, E. L., and Rosales, R. K.: Necrotizing myelopathy associated with visceral carcinoma. *Brain* 87:639, 1964.
28. Marin, O. S., and Tyler, H. R.: Hereditary interstitial nephritis associated with polyneuropathy. *Neurology* 11:999, 1961.
29. Melby, J. C., and Watson, C. J.: Disorders of porphyria metabolism. *Med. Sci.* 7:821, 1960.
30. Michon, P., Larcan, A., and Streiff, F.: Neuropathies dysglobulinemiques. *Rev. Neurol.* 100:27, 1959.
31. Miller, H. G., and Daley, R.: Clinical aspects of polyarteritis nodosa. *Quart. J. Med.* 15:225, 1946.
32. Miller, H. G., and Stanton, J. B.: Neurological sequelae of prophylactic inoculation. *Quart. J. Med.* 23:1, 1954.
33. Parsonage, M. J., and Turner, J. W. A.: Neuralgic amyotrophy: The shoulder-girdle syndrome. *Lancet* 1:973, 1948.
34. Patten, B. M.: Neuropathy induced by hemorrhage. *Arch. Neurol.* 21:381, 1969.
35. Peters, H. A., Eichman, P. L., and Reese, H. H.: Therapy of acute, chronic, and mixed hepatic

porphyria patients with chelating agents. *Neurol.* 8:621, 1958.
36. Pratt, R. T. C.: *The Genetics of Neurological Disorders.* Oxford University Press, New York, 1967.
37. Raff, M. C., Sangalang, V., and Asbury, A. K.: Ischemic mononeuropathy multiplex associated with diabetes mellitus. *Arch. Neurol.* 18:487, 1968.
38. Refsum, S.: Heredopathia atactica polyneuritiformis. *Acta Scand. Neurol.*, Suppl. 38, 1946.
39. Richards, F. F., and Brinton, D.: Peripheral neuropathy and the diagnosis of acute porphyria. *Brain* 85:657, 1962.
40. Richards, F. F., and Scott, J.: Glycine metabolism in acute porphyria. *Clin. Sci.* 20:387, 1961.
41. Ridley, A.: The neuropathy of acute intermittent porphyria. *Quart. J. Med.* 38:307, 1969.
42. Rundles, R. W.: Diabetic neuropathy. *Medicine* 24:111, 1945.
43. Silverstein, A.: Hemorrhage into nerves. *J.A.M.A.* 190:554, 1964.
44. Smith, J. B., and Patel, A.: The Wohlfart-Kugelberg-Welander Disease. *Neurology* 15:469, 1965.
45. Steinberg, V. L.: Neuropathy in rheumatoid disease. *Brit. Med. J.* 1:1600, 1960.
46. Symmers, W. St. C.: Primary amyloidosis: A review. *J. Clin. Path.* 9:187, 1956.
47. Taylor, R. A.: Heredofamilial mononeuritis multiplex with brachial predilection. *Brain* 83:113, 1960.
48. Tenckhoff, H. A., et al.: Polyneuropathy in chronic renal insufficiency. *J.A.M.A.* 192:1121, 1965.
49. Thomas, P. K., Lascelles, R. G., Hallpike, J. F., and Hewer, R. L.: Recurrent and chronic relapsing Guillain-Barré polyneuritis. *Brain* 92:589, 1969.
50. Trojaborg, W., Frantzen, E., and Andersen, I.: Peripheral neuropathy and myopathy associated with carcinoma of the lung. *Brain* 92:71, 1969.
51. Wallis, W. E., Van Poznak, A., and Plum, F.: Generalized muscular stiffness, fasciculations, and myokymia of peripheral nerve origin. *Arch. Neurol.* 22:430, 1970.
52. Williams, H. M., Diamond, H. D., Craver, L. F., and Parsons, H.: *Neurological Complications of Lymphomas and Leukemias.* Charles C Thomas, Springfield, Ill., 1959.
53. Wisniewski, H., Terry, R. D., Whitaker, J. N., Cook, S. D., and Dowling, P. C.: Landry-Guillain-Barré syndrome. *Arch. Neurol.* 21:269, 1969.

CHAPTER TWENTY-ONE

Intoxications of the Nervous System

ALCOHOL

The effects of alcohol on the nervous system[65] may be divided into four groups: (1) acute intoxication from its direct and immediate depressant action on the nervous system; (2) acute symptoms due to sudden withdrawal in chronic alcoholics —acute tremulousness, hallucinations, delirium tremens, seizures; (3) nutritional disorders—polyneuropathy, Wernicke's syndrome, Korsakoff's syndrome, retrobulbar neuropathy, Marchiafava disease, cerebellar degeneration, and central pontine myelinolysis (Chap. 17); (4) acute and chronic hepatic encephalopathy.

Etiology. Addiction to ethyl alcohol, whether in the form of spirits, beer, or wine, has the same psychological origins as other addictions, but it is more easily acquired because alcohol is so widely accepted as a social lubricant and a refuge from the difficulties of life. Overindulgence bespeaks an underlying neurosis, and is often familial. *It can also be symptomatic of primary depression, schizophrenia, or organic dementia.*

Acute Intoxication

Acute intoxication occurs with blood alcohol levels of 30 to 150 mg. per cent, depending upon the individual's degree of habituation and on the rate of absorption; if the concentration is raised slowly, symptoms are less likely to appear, even at quite high levels. Tolerance is usually reduced in the presence of organic brain damage (e.g., head injury, cerebrovascular disease, tumors, senility), and small doses of alcohol taken on top of barbiturates or tranquilizers (e.g., Doriden) may have a profoundly intoxicating effect. Since drinkers absorb alcohol faster than abstainers and metabolize it at the same rate, habituation seems to indicate that the nervous system acquires a tolerance to the drug; the underlying chemistry of such tolerance is not understood.

The higher centers are usually affected first, so that disorders of thought and conduct are commonly the first to appear. Exceptionally, dysequilibrium occurs before obvious involvement of the higher centers. The subject becomes voluble, raises his voice, and displays euphoria and lack of judgment. Loss of normal inhibition may lead to aggressive behavior and unusual sexual activity. Some people become aggressive and others become depressed. Memory for recent events is impaired. Coordination is affected, with consequent dysarthria, clumsiness of hand movements, and staggering. Difficulty in focusing the eyes and diplopia are common. The pupils are dilated and the reflexes are brisk. At a deeper stage of intoxication (blood alcohol level, 0.25 to 0.4 per cent), the skin is pale and moist, the pupils are dilated, and all reflexes are depressed. The level of consciousness becomes progressively lower. In profound alcoholic poisoning, cardiac and respiratory stimulants are necessary, and peripheral vascular collapse may have to be treated.

It is hardly necessary to state that a smell of alcohol on the breath of an unconscious patient does not prove that the unconsciousness is due to alcohol.

Withdrawal Syndromes

Withdrawal syndromes can be classified under six headings: acute alcoholic tremulousness, tremulousness with transient hallucinations, acute auditory hallucinosis, typical delirium tremens, atypical delusional-hallucinatory states, and seizures.[65] These may occur singly or in combination, and one may follow another. They occur from one to four days after cessation of drinking, although in some cases there may be premonitory symptoms toward the end of a drinking bout. They are commonly seen in periodic or "spree" drinkers but are also apt to occur when a persistent drinker is denied alcohol as a result of intercurrent injury, disease, or operation.

The cause of withdrawal symptoms is unknown: They cannot be due to alcohol per se since they can be mitigated by the administration of alcohol, and they are not nutritional in origin.

ACUTE ALCOHOLIC TREMULOUSNESS ("THE SHAKES"). This is first noticed on the morning after a drinking bout and can be banished by the first drink, but it becomes more violent after complete withdrawal. The patient is alert, agitated, rude, disinclined for food, and sleepless. A coarse tremor is seen on attempted movement; the voice becomes tremulous, the hands unsteady, and the patient may be unable to stand or walk. The pulse is fast and the face flushed. The mind is usually clear, but in some cases there are transient visual or auditory hallucinations, together with nightmares and disordered sensory perceptions. The patient

requires sedation, thiamine, and a graduated return to a normal intake of fluid and food. Suitable sedatives include Librium, chloral hydrate, and paraldehyde. Alcohol can be given to tide the patient over until treatment can be started.

ACUTE AUDITORY HALLUCINOSIS. This is marked by the presence of persistent hallucinations, often of a threatening character, to which the patient may respond in appropriate fashion. Unlike the case in delirium tremens, he is well oriented, and the hallucinations are auditory rather than visual. The condition may continue in a modified form for weeks or even months, and it is therefore thought that some of these relatively uncommon cases may have a schizophrenic basis.

DELIRIUM TREMENS. This is the gravest of the withdrawal syndromes. It may follow a period of tremulousness and hallucination, and usually occurs one to four days after cessation of drinking. It is marked by agitation, extreme restlessness, tremulousness, volubility, confusion of thought and speech, disorientation for time and place, inability to recognize familiar faces and objects, distractibility, and inattention. In mild cases, symptoms occur only at night. Delusions, illusions, and hallucinations determine much of the patient's behavior: Believing himself to be on the street, the patient hails a nonexistent taxi; seeing a helicopter flying through the room, he ducks his head to avoid it. Yet there may be brief episodes of lucidity and clear insight, and for this reason the physician should be guarded in his remarks at the bedside, since such comments may be remembered afterward, though in general the events of the illness are forgotten. A somewhat similar hallucinatory state, but without the tremulousness, may be induced by intoxication with LSD.

The treatment of delirium tremens is the same as for acute tremulousness with hallucinations, but added care is needed to detect and treat intercurrent infections, notably pneumonia, which may themselves trigger the condition in alcoholics. Hypoglycemia should be looked for and treated. At present, the value of intravenous hypertonic solutions (fructose, mannitol) is being evaluated.

SEIZURES IN ALCOHOLICS. Sudden withdrawal of alcohol in a chronic alcoholic may precipitate seizures ("rum fits") just as it may induce delirium tremens, and not infrequently the two occur together. *The patient is sometimes found to be hypoglycemic.* The seizures must be distinguished from the seizures which occasionally occur within a few hours of a sporadic drinking party in nonalcoholics; the latter variety is important in that the precipitation of one or more seizures in this way may be the first indication of idiopathic epilepsy or of structural disease of the brain. Alcohol sometimes precipitates seizures in persons who have had a head injury, recent or remote. Rum fits are treated in the same way as other seizures, and if hypoglycemia is present, intravenous dextrose should be given.

Chronic Mental Deterioration

Chronic alcoholic deterioration is characterized by a gradual dilapidation of the moral and ethical values of the individual, who becomes careless of social graces and increasingly unreliable. There is a general disturbance of intellectual function, based primarily on memory defects, and the situation is further complicated by quarrelsomeness and irritability. The combination of intellectual deterioration and affective disturbances, coupled with a decline in social adaptation, poses considerable domestic and professional problems, and even though the patient stops drinking, the condition may remain irreversible. Permanent commitment to a mental hospital sometimes becomes necessary. This situation, a true organic dementia, is distinct from neurotic and psychotic reactions which excessive indulgence in alcohol sometimes seems to uncover or aggravate, as well as from the dementia of chronic hepatic encephalopathy.

Methyl Alcohol

Methyl alcohol is used as a solvent in industry and as a fuel (methylated spirits, Sterno); it is sometimes resorted to by alcoholics when other sources fail. Methanol is oxidized to formaldehyde and formic acid, which are poisonous to the nervous system and produce acidemia. Methyl alcohol is particularly toxic to the optic nerve and respiratory center.

The symptoms of intoxication are those of drunkenness plus nausea, abdominal cramps, headache, and more blurring of vision than is caused by intoxication with ethyl alcohol. As the patient passes into unconsciousness, there is an initial hyperpnea from acidemia, followed by respiratory depression and cyanosis. This may occur in one to three days; some survivors are left with bilateral visual loss and optic atrophy; there is a universal depression of the visual fields, with particular emphasis on central vision. Methyl alcohol does not cause polyneuropathy or other deficiency syndromes, but since it is usually taken by chronic alcoholics, there may be signs of neuropathy.

If the patient is seen in time, the stomache should be washed out. To combat acidemia, 15 gm. of sodium bicarbonate or sodium lactate are given in 1000 ml. of 5 per cent glucose saline. An oxygen-carbon dioxide mixture should be given if respiration is depressed.

HEPATIC ENCEPHALOPATHY (HEPATIC PRECOMA AND COMA; PORTAL SYSTEMIC ENCEPHALOPATHY)

DEFINITION. "Hepatic encephalopathy" refers to the disorders of cerebral function resulting from severe hepatocellular disease and (less commonly) portacaval shunts.[1, 54, 58, 65]

Etiology. Hepatic encephalopathy commonly occurs in cirrhosis of the liver, but has also been recorded as the result of portacaval anastomosis, portal vein thrombosis, viral hepatitis, and chronic schistosomiasis japonica. In the presence of cirrhosis, the encephalopathy can be precipitated by gastrointestinal hemorrhage, surgical operation, low-output cardiac failure, pneumonia, and the administration of substances with a high nitrogenous content (protein diet, urea, ammonium chloride, methionine).

Despite the apparent link between the symptoms of this condition and the absorption of nitrogenous compounds, the level of arterial ammonia does not always parallel the clinical features. It is thought that some substance or substances normally metabolized by the liver are either incompletely metabolized, owing to hepatocellular failure, or are shunted by new anastomotic channels into the systemic circulation and thus reach the brain. It seems that the toxic factor(s) can be produced by bacterial action on protein in the intestine since wide-spectrum antibiotics and the restriction of dietary protein are beneficial in treatment. Cerebral oxygen consumption is reduced in hepatic insufficiency, and this is apparent even before neurological symptoms appear.[24]

Pathology. There is a characteristic swelling and proliferation of the protoplasmic astrocytes, some of which contain PAS-positive inclusions. The change is found in the gray matter of the cerebrum and cerebellum. The neurons show minor patchy degeneration in acute cases, but in the smaller, chronic group described below, the outfall may be considerable. These pathological changes start to develop within a few days of the onset of symptoms.

Clinical Features. There are two forms of the disease. The first and by far the more common type is a subacute disorder with an intermittent course characterized by disturbances of consciousness and of the motor system.[54, 58] In the second and much smaller group, there are mental, pyramidal, extrapyramidal, and cerebellar disturbances, which pursue a slowly progressive course over a number of years.

In the subacute form, the early symptoms are characteristically intermittent, and individual attacks may consist of anything from slight impairment of thought and disturbances of behavior to gross confusion and stupor. Changes of personality are frequent, the patient becoming childish, irritable, and apt to behave inappropriately. Apathy may be prominent. There may be hypersomnia or an inversion of sleep rhythm, and the level of consciousness may alternate rapidly between lucidity and stupor.

Sometimes focal neurological deficit occurs in a setting of clear consciousness. There may be visual agnosia, and constructional apraxia is common. Calligraphy is disturbed. Speech may be slow and slurred, and aphasia may occur. There is usually a coarse involuntary tremor of the fingers and hands (flapping tremor) which consists of rapid flexion and extension movements at the wrist and adduction-abduction movements of the fingers. These movements are usually reduced by voluntary activity but are aggravated by sustained posture; sometimes there is both a postural tremor and an intention tremor. Muscle tone may be decreased or increased, and the deep tendon reflexes are usually exaggerated; when coma supervenes, the plantar responses become extensor. The breath has an unpleasant, sickly smell. The palmar aspect of the hands is pink, with slight cyanosis; the soles of the feet may be similarly affected.

In severe cases, the spinal fluid contains an excess of protein, glutamine, ammonia, and bilirubin, and the arterial ammonia is usually in excess of 120 μg./ 100 ml. of blood. The electroencephalogram shows characteristic changes which wax and wane with the level of consciousness (Fig. 21–1). There are diffuse 2 to 3 c./sec. slow waves, some in triphasic form.[9] This abnormality can be brought out by administering ammonium chloride by mouth in doses of 0.05 gm./kg. body weight; apparently no dan-

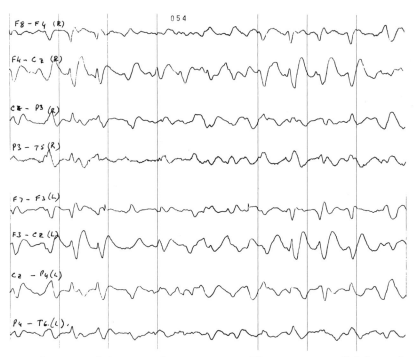

Figure 21-1. Electroencephalogram in hepatic precoma. The patient was slightly confused and disoriented.

gerous side effects have been noted when this test is carried out for diagnostic purposes in suspected (and therefore mild) cases of hepatic encephalopathy.[62] There may be a disturbance of electrolyte levels.[2]

Prognosis. The best outlook is in chronic cirrhotics who have relatively good liver function and extensive collateral circulation, and in those with increased intestinal nitrogen production. It is poor when ascites, jaundice, and a low serum albumin level are present. Even the apparently moribund patient in profound coma may recover, a fact to be remembered in giving a prognosis.

Differential Diagnosis. It is evident that the clinical features of liver failure include a wide and confusing variety of mental and neurological symptoms and that the term "coma" is too restricted in its implications.[58] So protean are its manifestations that limitations of space preclude detailed discussion here; suffice it that hepatic failure should always be remembered as a possible cause of unexplained disturbances of brain function.

The presence of cirrhosis does not by itself prove that the liver condition is responsible for mental or neurological symptoms, however. For example, the apathy, nausea, headache, and episodes of hypotension which occur in cirrhotic individuals with ascites may be the result of hyponatremia produced by diuretics, paracentesis, and restricted sodium intake. Another pitfall is to ascribe to hepatic failure the symptoms of a subdural hematoma, to which cirrhotics are particularly prone because of their tendency to bleed.

Treatment. The patient in coma or precoma should be put on a protein-free diet, and all nitrogen-containing drugs should be stopped. Purges and enemas should be administered to remove nitrogen-containing material from the bowel. A wide-spectrum antibiotic should be given by mouth for a week to inhibit intestinal bacterial activity. Precipitating factors such as infection, alcoholism, gastrointestinal hemorrhage, or barbiturate overdosage must be looked for. Fluid intake and the electrolyte balance should be adjusted. In chronic cases, nitrogen-containing drugs should be avoided, and protein intake should not exceed 50 gm. a day. Free bowel movements should be maintained in all cases.

Chronic Hepatic Encephalopathy

Chronic hepatic encephalopathy is uncommon. The pathological findings are qualitatively the same as in the subacute cases. Clinically, the disorder usually starts with attacks of hepatic coma or stupor, between which the patient appears neurologically intact. After a number of such incidents, other symptoms appear, notably dementia, cerebellar ataxia, parkinsonism, pyramidal signs, dysarthria, and choreoathetosis. These occur in varying combinations, and although they may fluctuate in degree, they tend to progress slowly over a period of several years.

The degree of intellectual deterioration varies from mild impairment of intellectual acuity to dementia. Cerebellar features appear in the form of ataxia of gait and intention tremor of the arms. Choreoathetosis and flapping tremor have been observed, the former simulating the involuntary movements of Huntington's chorea. There may also be evidence of pyramidal tract disorders and extrapyramidal rigidity. Seizures may appear. The EEG abnormality characteristic of subacute cases occurs during bouts of stupor, but it is less obvious in periods of mental clarity. The spinal fluid is normal.

Neuropsychiatric disturbances may also appear following portal systemic shunt procedures in cases of chronic liver disease.[54] Immediately following the shunt, there may be an acute organic brain syndrome; the EEG is abnormal, but it does not display the characteristic pattern associated with hepatic coma. In other cases, the symptoms do not appear for three or more months following the shunt. They include parkinsonian tremor, seizures, myoclonic spasm in combination with either dementia and ataxia, or dementia with spastic paraplegia or tetraplegia. The tremor which occurs as a late event in patients with cirrhosis is parkinsonian in type, in contradistinction to the flapping tremor of acute and subacute hepatic failure. In some cases, there are complaints of "heaviness of the legs" without much weakness but with brisk knee and ankle reflexes and extensor plantar responses.

A recent review of treatment for chronic hepatic encephalopathy reports that neuropsychiatric symptoms are often relieved by the administration of Lactulose, which increases the acidity of the stool and increases ammonia excretion from the blood into the colon.[73]

HEAVY METALS

Lead

Despite advances in industrial hygiene, lead poisoning is comparatively common, especially in slums. In infants and children, it usually causes encephalopathy, and if neuropathy occurs, it is likely to be generalized. In adults, localized neuropathy is commoner than the generalized form, and encephalopathy is rare.[4, 10, 12, 25, 59, 63, 70]

Etiology. In children, the incidence is highest in those from poor neighborhoods, particularly in areas in which houses are being torn down or built, since these activities provide a fine collection of materials for toddlers to chew—putty, painted wood, chips of paint, and the like.[25] Licking of painted toys is less often responsible. In adults, industrial exposure to lead (including tetraethyl lead in the gasoline industry) accounts for most cases; poisoning from the use of lead abortifacients is rare nowadays.

The lead is carried by the red cells to all tissues and is stored in the bones in the form of an insoluble tertiary phosphate. Any event bringing on acidosis in children—such as an infection—releases lead from the bones, and may precipitate symptoms.

Pathology. Lead encephalopathy is marked by swelling of the brain, which is probably due to interference with cellular respiratory enzymes. There is swelling and chromatolysis of the ganglion cells of the cortex and cerebellum; punctate hemorrhages may be present.[10] Demyelination of the corticospinal and posterior columns has been seen. The peripheral nerves show patchy segmental demyelination and degeneration of distal axons in experimental lead poisoning.

Clinical Features. In both children and adults, the neurological effects are usually preceded by symptoms of systemic poisoning—anorexia, loss of weight, colic, and constipation. There may be moderate hypertension, albuminuria, and hypochromic anemia with punctate basophilia. In adults, a "lead line" appears on the gums unless the patient is edentulous.

In children, the onset of encephalopathy is sudden, with generalized or focal seizures and stupor. Focal neurological signs include hemiplegia, monoplegia, cerebellar ataxia, diplopia, and facial palsy. Papilledema is not uncommon. The mortality is in the region of 25 per cent, and survivors show a high incidence of mental retardation,[70] liability to seizures, optic atrophy, and residual paralyses. Peripheral neuropathy in older children is not exclusively motor, and it tends to be more generalized than in adults.

In adults, the onset of neurological symptoms is often preceded by malaise, anorexia, lethargy, lead colic, constipation, a rise of blood pressure, and ill-defined pains in the joints. The neuropathy is usually localized and commonly causes wrist drop or foot drop; less often there is weakness of the shoulder girdle and upper arm. It is thought that localization of the neuropathy depends on which groups of muscles the patient uses most in the course of his daily occupation. Sensory loss does not occur, as a rule. Encephalopathy is uncommon in adults; it is ushered in by headache, memory impairment, and disorientation. Seizures are common. Diplopia, impairment of vision, monoparesis or hemi-

plegia, and ataxia may be seen. Occasionally the onset is fulminating, with convulsions, delirium, and coma.

Laboratory Aids. Laboratory aids include the demonstration of a serum lead level in excess of 0.06 μg./100 ml. whole blood, and a urinary excretion exceeding 60 μg. per liter. The presence of hypochromic anemia with basophilic stippling of the red cells is suggestive. An early sign is an increase in urinary coproporphyrin in excess of 500 μg. in 24 hours. In severe poisoning, there may be 20 to 50 lymphocytes per cubic millimeter in the spinal fluid and a rise of protein. Intracranial pressure is raised in lead encephalopathy.

Treatment.[59] In mild cases, it suffices to remove the source of intoxication. More severe examples have to be treated by measures designed to remove lead from the soft tissues and blood, and this is most efficiently done by the administration of Versene, a chelating agent which inactivates both divalent and trivalent metals.[59] The result is a non-ionized, water-soluble complex, which is nontoxic and is readily excreted in the urine. The daily dosage of 25 mg./kg. body weight/24 hours is divided into two parts, each of which is administered intravenously in 250 cc. of 5 per cent glucose or normal saline over a period of two hours. This procedure is repeated daily for five to six days. The oral dose is 30 mg./kg. of body weight, twice daily. Relapses may occur in patients who have been exposed to lead for prolonged periods because lead is stored in the bones and cannot be eliminated quickly. The seizures of lead encephalopathy are treated on the same lines as status epilepticus. If intracranial pressure is high, it may be necessary to carry out bilateral subtemporal decompression as an emergency measure. Water intake should be restricted, and steroids should be administered.

Arsenic

Arsenical poisoning can give rise to peripheral neuropathy, acute encephalopathy, and (rarely) diffuse myelopathy, in addition to cutaneous, gastrointestinal, hematological, hepatic, and renal disturbances.[4, 26, 63]

Etiology. Intoxication can occur as the result of a single large dose, or from long-continued ingestion of small amounts, as for instance during the mining and smelting of arsenical ores; in the preparation of dyes, paints, and glass; in the manufacture of insecticides, weed killers, and flypapers; in the practices of embalming and taxidermy; and from abuse of arsenic-containing medicines. Intoxication can occur through the use of organic arsenical compounds in the treatment of syphilis and yaws. It is supposed that arsenic (or the arsenate into which it is converted in vivo) produces its effects by inactivating coenzymes concerned in the oxidation of pyruvate.

Pathology. In subjects dying from arsenical encephalopathy, the brain is slightly swollen, and the cut surface may show numerous punctate perivascular hemorrhages (hemorrhagic encephalitis), but not all cases are hemorrhagic. There are disseminated foci of demyelinization and widespread degeneration of ganglion cells with mild swelling and proliferation of astrocytes. In the rare cases of arsenical myelopathy, there are multifocal parenchymatous lesions throughout the spinal cord.

Not all cases of arsenical poisoning develop neurological symptoms, and the toxic dose varies greatly, so personal idiosyncrasy appears to be involved.

Clinical Features. A large single dose gives rise to vomiting and diarrhea, and the symptoms of polyneuropathy develop after four to eight weeks. In chronic poisoning, on the other hand, gastrointestinal symptoms are usually absent or slight, and the polyneuropathy is more insidious in its onset. The patient exhibits weakness, wasting, tenderness of the muscles, sensory impairment, and loss of peripheral tendon reflexes. The skin of the palms and soles may be thickened, and there is often a fine brownish pigmentation of the skin of the covered parts of the body and in the flexures. Conjunctivitis, lacrimation, and hoarseness bear witness to the effect of the poison on the mucous membranes, and purpura, aplastic anemia, and agranulocytosis can occur. Albuminuria and toxic hepatitis are not uncommon.

Bilateral optic neuropathy may develop following the administration of pentavalent arsenicals, notably tryparsamide; impairment of sight develops within 12 hours of the administration of the drug. Visual acuity is reduced, and the peripheral field is grossly restricted. Complete recovery may occur, but more often there is persistence of central depression and restriction of the peripheral fields.

A few cases of myelopathy have been reported following the administration of arsenicals, both in adults and in children. The symptoms and signs are appropriate to multiple focal lesions throughout the length of the spinal cord, with muscular weakness, sensory impairment, sphincter disturbances, and extensor plantar responses.

Laboratory Aids. In arsenical encephalopathy, the electroencephalogram shows slow high voltage activity, which becomes less marked as recovery occurs. In all forms of chronic poisoning there is excess arsenic in the hair, nails, and urine, but caution has to be exercised in interpreting such findings, because figures may be above normal in patients who have been receiving arsenic by mouth and whose symptoms are due to other causes.

Treatment. Chelating agents are used for elimination of arsenic. Versene is preferable to BAL; it is administered in the same way as for lead poisoning (p. 576).

Gold

Intoxication can arise suddenly during the administration of gold salts for tuberculosis, rheumatoid arthritis, and other diseases, even when the dosage falls within the range usually considered safe.[4, 67] Symptoms arise suddenly. They often take the form of psychological disturbances, the patient becoming excited, confused, and hallucinated. In others, there is marked apathy and withdrawal. At this stage, there may be no abnormal neurological signs, but the mental symptoms may be combined with one or more of the following: albuminuria, nausea, diarrhea, mild jaundice, depression of platelets, anemia, agranulocytosis, scaly dermatitis, conjunctivitis, and polyneuropathy. Sometimes irritability and confusion are rapidly followed by blurring of vision, headache, diplopia, incoordination of the hands, staggering gait, and convulsions. Evidence of focal dysfunction in the nervous system may be present or absent, and there may be signs of meningeal irritation. Improvement may occur either spontaneously or following the use of chelating agents. Occasionally peripheral neuropathy is the dominating feature of the intoxication.[67]

Mercury

Poisoning by *inorganic* mercury compounds can occur as a result of the excessive use of mercurial diuretics, ointments, or local antiseptics (e.g., mercuric chloride). It also occurs in workers exposed to the metal; mercury volatilizes at room temperature and can therefore be absorbed from the skin and mucous membranes. In acute poisoning, there is stomatitis with salivation, a metallic taste in the mouth, abdominal pain, chronic diarrhea, and mental symptoms of varying intensity, which range from irritability and mild confusion to delirium with hallucinations. In chronic poisoning, the earliest symptoms are fatigue, depression, and emotional instability (sometimes called erethism). There is tremor of the tongue and hands, which is present during sustained posture and is aggravated by movement. Treatment is by chelating agents.

Poisoning by *organic* mercurial compounds takes a different form. It occurs as a result of eating grain which has been treated by fungicidal agents, by eating the flesh of animals fed on such grain, or—as in Minamata disease[38]—from eating shellfish from waters contaminated by industrial effluents. These organic mercurials cause degeneration of the cortical cells of the cerebrum and cerebellum,[34] and degeneration of peripheral nerves. Clinically, the condition is characterized by the progressive development of cerebellar ataxia of the limbs, dysarthria, dysphagia, constriction of the visual fields (from degeneration of the striate cortex), deafness, and varying degrees of spasticity. Intellectual impairment gives place to stupor and coma in the more seriously affected individuals. Seizures may occur.

Manganese

Manganese poisoning[43a] is due to the inhalation of manganese dust in mining and industry, the metal being absorbed from the lungs and the gastrointestinal tract. The pathological defects differ from those produced by other heavy metals in that there is a striking degree of damage to the ganglion cells of the pallidum, with less marked changes in the other basal nuclei, the cortex, the cerebellum, and the hypothalamus. Cirrhosis of the liver occurs in both man and experimental animals, but cerebral degeneration can occur in the absence of hepatic damage.

The period of exposure necessary before the appearance of the clinical symptoms is inconstant. Mena and his colleagues[43a] report that in 45 cases, the shortest exposure was 5 months, the longest 25 years, with an average of 9 years. The earliest symptoms are physical and mental fatigability, which may be associated with psychological disturbances ("manganese madness") in the form of depression, irritability, confusion, impairment of memory, and aberrations of conduct. The outstanding neurological results of manganese poisoning are slowly progressive parkinsonism, with cogwheel rigidity and tremor of the hands, lower jaw, and head.[13] Oculogyric crises, clonic bilateral spasm of the facial muscles, and spasmodic torticollis have been described. Sialorrhea and facial seborrhea are not uncommon. Insomnia, hypersomnia, and inverted sleep rhythm are not uncommon. Peripheral neuropathy is not a feature of the condition, but symmetrical distal paresthesias may occur. Sphincter disturbances have not been described.

The prognosis is poor. Psychological symptoms sometimes regress when exposure to manganese is stopped, but the neurological disability tends to progress. Chelating agents are not effective.

Thallium

Thallium poisoning usually results from the accidental ingestion of the metal, which is found in rat poison, ointments for the treatment of ringworm, and depilatory creams.[14] Acute poisoning gives rise to abdominal pain, vomiting, and diarrhea, followed by weakness and sensory loss in the limbs, seizures, delirium, blindness, cranial nerve palsies, and death. If the patient survives long enough, the hair falls out, purpura develops, and renal failure occurs.

In chronic poisoning, the hair falls out, and blurring of vision occurs as the result of retrobulbar neuritis. There is loss of central vision and constriction of the peripheral fields, with subsequent optic atrophy. Generalized polyneuritis may occur; it starts with paresthesias and weakness in the legs and then spreads to involve the periphery of the upper limbs. Despite the paresthesias, sensory loss does not usually occur. Choreiform movements and myoclonic jerks of the extremities and neck have been recorded. There may be mental symptoms in the form of restlessness, irritability, confusion, or extreme lethargy. Recovery is slow, and there may be persistent emotional instability, visual impairment, or weakness resulting from polyneuropathy.

Treatment consists of the withdrawal of medication containing thallium and the administration of Versene or other chelating agents.

BROMIDES

Bromides were at one time a common source of chronic intoxication, but they have been replaced in clinical practice by other sedatives, notably the barbiturates and a wide spectrum of tranquilizers. Acute poisoning is rare because large doses irritate the stomach and therefore cause immediate vomiting. Symptoms of chronic intoxication usually occur when the blood bromide level exceeds 150 mg. per cent, but some patients remain free from symptoms when the level is considerably higher.[57]

An acneiform bromide rash is present in many cases, but it may be absent. At first the patient is dull, drowsy, and slow in thought, and has difficulty in concentrating. In bromide delirium there is restlessness, irritability, disorientation, disorderly conduct, and hallucinosis. This toxic psychosis may be accompanied by conjunctivitis and increased secretions of mucus from the upper respiratory tract and bronchi. The electroencephalogram is abnormal in most cases, and the cerebrospinal fluid may contain an excess of protein.

Recovery usually occurs in two to three weeks following withdrawal of bromides and the administration of sodium chloride by mouth (10 to 20 gm. three times a day), or intravenously (4 liters of normal saline daily). If sedation is necessary, paraldehyde and chloral hydrate may be used. Acute poisoning can be treated by dialysis.

BARBITURATES

The wide use of barbituric acid derivatives in medicine makes them readily available, with the result that they are often responsible for both suicide and addiction.

With long-continued use, as in epilepsy, considerable degrees of tolerance can be established; on the other hand, personal idiosyncrasies are marked, and

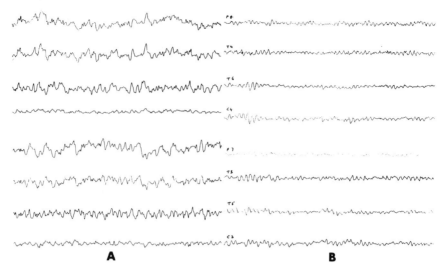

Figure 21–2. Barbiturate intoxication. *A,* At the height of intoxication. The patient showed nystagmus, dysarthria, and staggering gait. *B,* Normal record following disappearance of symptoms 48 hours later.

quite small doses may be followed by signs of intoxication in susceptible persons. Barbiturates and alcohol have a synergistic action so that severe intoxication can occur when they are taken together in doses which would not cause symptoms if they were taken separately.

Chronic barbiturate intoxication causes lethargy, slowing of thought, irritability, outbursts of violence, delusions, and aberrations of social and sexual conduct. It also gives rise to dysarthria, nystagmus, diplopia, ataxia of gait, and intention tremor. Sudden withdrawal may provoke convulsions, whether or not the patient has been subject to seizures. Idiosyncrasy to barbiturates can result in scarlatiniform rashes or urticaria, sometimes associated with pyrexia, and these symptoms can occur with doses which are well within the therapeutic range.

Acute poisoning causes over 1500 suicides in the United States every year. The lethal dose is variable, ranging from 2 to 60 gm. The initial symptoms—headache, ataxia, and confusion—give place rapidly to delirium and then coma. There is progressive depression of the deep reflexes and of the corneal and pupillary reflexes, and the plantar responses become extensor. Respiration is slow, and cyanosis soon appears. The pulse is slow, and the blood pressure falls; consequently, urinary output is reduced. Death is usually due to respiratory failure. In severe intoxications, the electroencephalogram shows bilateral slow waves upon which is superimposed fast activity of 12 to 15 or 18 to 24 c./sec. (Fig. 21–2). In patients who survive, recovery is usually complete, provided that respiration has been maintained, even if the EEG has been completely flat.

Treatment of Acute Barbiturate Intoxication. Gastric lavage is useful if carried out within 12 hours or so of ingestion.[53] The airway must be kept clear by endotracheal intubation or tracheostomy, and in either case repeated suction is essential. Failing respiration may require the use of a respirator. It is important to maintain blood pressure by vasopressor agents and the administration of intravenous saline containing 20 to 40 mEq. of potassium chloride. The patient should be turned every half hour. Analeptic drugs such as picrotoxin and Megimide have not proved useful, and caffeine and amphetamine may be harmful because of their tendency to produce ventricular arrhythmias. Hemodialysis should be used if it is available.

DRUG-INDUCED EXTRAPYRAMIDAL SYNDROMES

The use of phenothiazine tranquilizers is attended by a significant risk of inducing extrapyramidal syndromes, most of which are transient.[6] They usually occur with use of drugs of the piperazine group (Permitil, Stelazine, Compazine, Dartal, Trilafon). The danger is less with the promazine group (Sparine, Thorazine, Tentone, and Vesprin) and is least with the piperidine group (mepazine). Individual susceptibility varies greatly, and women are more affected than men. The syndrome can occur at any age. Symptoms appear between three days and three months from the start of therapy, and fall into four main groups. First, there is a constant awareness of fatigue, which is often accompanied by complaints of aching pain in the muscles, and which may lead to a reduction of voluntary activity. Second, dystonic reactions occur (Fig. 21–3). They include torticollis, facial grimacing, dysarthria, opisthotonos, tortipelvis, and oculogyric crises. Sometimes these are combined, as, for instance, protrusion of the tongue and

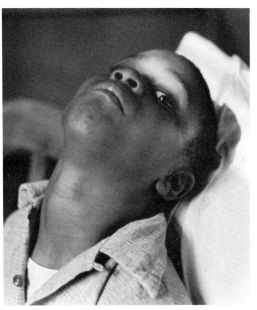

Figure 21–3. Retrocolic spasm induced by phenothiazine. (Courtesy of Dr. Douglas Goldman.)

backward tilting of the head. The involuntary movements are intermittent and bizarre; most of them have also been seen as a part of the extrapyramidal disorders produced by encephalitis lethargica. Third, motor restlessness may be prominent. The patient feels compelled to walk about, and cannot sit still. He may feel impelled to rock the body to and fro when sitting, and at the same time there may be chewing movements of the jaw, smacking of the tongue, and persistent twisting of the fingers. Fourth, there may be a typical parkinsonian syndrome, with generalized cogwheel rigidity, tremors, fixity of expression, poverty of movement, loss of associated movements, and drooling.

It is important to recognize the origin of these bizarre symptoms, which may be misdiagnosed as those of encephalitis, tetanus, epilepsy, or hysteria. Parkinsonism usually subsides when the tranquilizer is withdrawn, but improvement can be expedited by the administration of antiparkinsonian drugs such as biperiden hydrochloride (Akineton), which can be given by mouth, intramuscularly, or intravenously. An oral dose of 3 to 6 mg. a day is usually sufficient, but larger amounts may be required. Two to 5 mg. by intramuscular injection will usually produce relief within 12 to 24 hours; for a quicker effect, the same dose may be given intravenously. Cogentin is sometimes effective. With the more potent phenothiazine drugs such as Fluphenazine, it may be more difficult to control the extrapyramidal symptoms; large doses of the antiparkinsonian drugs are not always satisfactory since they themselves exert psychotropic effects. In this event, the method of choice is the simultaneous administration of small doses of an antiparkinsonian drug plus a barbiturate and gradual reduction of the dose of tranquilizers.

Facial and oral movements, such as grimacing, protrusion of the tongue, and chewing may last for many months[23] after the drug has been withdrawn, and in some cases they are irreversible. Facial dyskinesis can occur from the administration of L-dopa in parkinsonism.

TRIORTHOCRESYL PHOSPHATE POLYNEUROPATHY

The condition, also known as "Jake palsy," was first seen between 1929 and 1930 in the United States as a result of the drinking of alcoholic beverages contaminated with triorthocresyl phosphate. Cases have also occurred following the use of apiol as an abortifacient, and outbreaks have occurred in Algeria and India as a result of cooking food in lubricating oils containing this agent. In mild cases, the disease is limited to degeneration of both the axons and the myelin sheaths of the peripheral nerves, with retrograde alterations in the motor cells of the spinal cord and medulla; patients dying years later have shown fibrosis of the smaller arteries and capillaries in muscles and nerves and degenerative changes in the lateral and dorsal tracts of the spinal cord.[3]

Ingestion usually causes nausea, vomiting, and diarrhea, followed by symmetrical polyneuropathy, which develops some 14 days later. Paresthesias and pain appear in the legs, together with progressive weakness; in severe cases, there is paralysis of the legs and weakness of the upper limbs. There is usually a mild impairment of cutaneous sensibility distally, with loss of the peripheral tendon reflexes. Extensor plantar responses are seen in a minority of cases.

TICK PARALYSIS

Tick paralysis[56] is caused by the bite of the wood tick, *Dermacentor andersoni,* and some species of *Ixodes.* The tick is prevalent in the United States, British Columbia, Southern Africa, and Australia, but it is rare in Europe. It is dangerous to children and to domestic animals, but is seldom so to adults. The tick adheres to the skin; if it is removed quickly, nothing untoward happens, but if it is left for a day or two, the patient's legs become weak, and paralysis rapidly spreads to the arms, trunk, and bulbar nuclei, with a fatal result in a matter of days. Con-

sciousness and sensation are unaffected. If the tick is removed as soon as symptoms appear, recovery can occur.

CARBON MONOXIDE POISONING

Carbon monoxide poisoning may be accidental, homicidal, or suicidal.[19, 28, 52] It sometimes occurs as the result of exposure to charcoal, coal, or gas fires under conditions of poor ventilation. Inhalation of 1 per cent of the gas is fatal in 30 minutes in a resting adult and in 10 minutes if the subject is physically active.

Pathogenesis and Pathology. The affinity of hemoglobin for carbon monoxide is much greater than its affinity for oxygen. The resulting carboxyhemoglobin is stable, and prevents gaseous exchange between blood and cells. The gas also has an affinity for cytochrome oxidase. Cell respiration is interfered with, and it is usually considered that all the results of carbon monoxide poisoning are due to this, though it has also been suggested that the gas has an additional toxic action.

The common pathological result in fatal cases is widespread damage to ganglion cells, especially of the cerebral cortex, hippocampus, cerebellum, and striatum; changes in the white matter are not usually conspicuous, although several authors have described cases of fatal poisoning in which there is severe change in the white matter—a diffuse hemispheric demyelination without significant damage to the ganglion cells. It has usually been seen in cases of delayed neurological deterioration after anoxia from various causes, including carbon monoxide poisoning.[52] The small blood vessels are affected; there is marked venous and capillary dilatation, and many petechial hemorrhages are present, especially in the white matter and corpus callosum; massive hemorrhages can also occur, and arterial thrombosis is sometimes seen.

The considerable case-to-case variability in the extent and distribution of the lesions resulting from anoxia is reflected in its protean clinical manifestations.

Clinical Features. The patient complains of slight headache and the face is flushed and pink. This is followed by a sense of weakness, dizziness, dimness of vision, and nausea. When the blood saturation with carbon monoxide approaches 50 per cent, convulsions may occur, and coma supervenes. In the majority of survivors, there are no after-effects of carbon monoxide poisoning, but in a small percentage the patient emerges from unconsciousness with evidence of both generalized and focal damage to the nervous system. Consonant with the effect of anoxia on the cerebral cortex, organic dementia of varying degree is often a conspicuous feature, but it may be so mild as to be mistaken for a psychoneurosis. Memory suffers, and in some cases this has involved an almost complete obliteration of all of life's experiences for many years, suggesting bilateral damage to the hippocampus. Focal symptoms include aphasia, dysarthria, cortical blindness, hemianopia, hemiparesis, paraplegia, choreoathetosis, parkinsonism, and peripheral neuropathy.[71] The symptoms and signs may fluctuate widely from day to day.

Sometimes there is a severe relapse within 48 hours after apparent recovery from the acute phase.

Diagnosis. The skin and mucous membranes are flushed and bright red owing to the presence of carboxyhemoglobin, and the cherry-red color is particularly marked in areas of skin constricted by clothing, a belt, or other source of pressure. Spectroscopic examination of the blood will confirm the diagnosis.

Treatment. In the acute phase of poisoning, an oxygen-carbon dioxide mixture should be administered. Hyperbaric oxygen is very effective in this emergency, but it is not generally available. It is reported that the intravenous administration of procaine hydrochloride in doses of 0.5 to 1 gm. in 500 to 1000 ml. of normal saline over two hours relieves symptoms.

Chronic Carbon Monoxide Poisoning

The condition occurs in persons exposed to low concentrations of carbon monoxide over a prolonged period.[28] It is seen in garage workers, welders working in enclosed tanks, traffic policemen, and people confined to badly ventilated rooms which are heated by open gas or coal fires. The patient becomes aware of headache, lightheadedness, general lack of strength and energy, irritability, palpitations, and coldness of the hands and feet. The diagnosis is assisted by demonstrating carboxyhemoglobin in the blood; it is usually associated with secondary polycythemia.

HYPOGLYCEMIA

Hypoglycemia is usually the result of insulin overdosage, but it also occurs from endogenous hyperinsulinism and from functional disturbances of the vegetative nervous system associated with emotional instability.[11, 15, 22] Less common causes include: adrenocortical insufficiency, pituitary tumors, lesions of the hypothalamus and brainstem, acute and chronic hepatic disease, large fibromas and fibrosarcomas in the thorax and abdomen,[41, 46] hypothyroidism, gastrectomy and gastroenterostomy, prolonged diarrhea, renal glycosuria, glycogen storage disease, and both familial and sporadic spontaneous hypoglycemia in infants.[21, 43]

Pathology. Severe and prolonged hypoglycemia causes changes in the cells of the nervous system which closely resemble those produced by anoxia because without glucose, its primary source of energy, the ganglion cell cannot use oxygen. Experimental work indicates that the pathological effects are reversible in mild cases, and this explains why, in man, complete clinical recovery is possible even after profound coma. In fatal cases, however, almost all the cells of the central nervous system are affected to some degree, but the most severely affected are those of the cortex, followed in order by the striatum, Ammon's horn, the Purkinje cells of the cerebellum, and the anterior horn cells of the spinal cord.[39] There is both focal and lamina necrosis of the gray matter, with minor changes in the white matter. There is some proliferation of astrocytes and microglia. Massive infarcts occasionally occur in the absence of demonstrable thrombosis or embolism, and this is of interest in view of the fact that lowering the blood sugar in the presence of arterial stenosis can give rise to focal neurological dysfunction.[45] Even in the absence of arterial insufficiency, the symptoms of hypoglycemia are more closely related to the cerebral arteriovenous difference than to the actual level of the blood sugar.

Clinical Features. Individual susceptibility to the effects of hypoglycemia varies considerably.[11, 15, 22] Some patients experience symptoms with a glucose level in the neighborhood of 50 mg. per cent, while others remain asymptomatic at 30 mg. per cent. In untreated diabetics, who are accustomed to a high blood sugar level, symptoms are apt to appear when the serum glucose level is within the range of low normal. Moreover, susceptibility varies from time to time in the same patient, and a rapid fall is more likely to precipitate symptoms than a slow one.

Symptoms fall into two classes: those due to epinephrine secretion triggered by the hypoglycemia and those due to the hypoglycemia itself.

The epinephrine response is most obvious when the decline in blood sugar is rapid. Symptoms include tremulousness, lightheadedness, sweating, apprehension, slowness of thought, irritability, circumoral and peripheral paresthesias, and either nausea or hunger. There is pallor, dilatation of the pupils, and a moderate elevation of the pulse and blood pressure. These symptoms and signs disappear shortly after ingestion of carbohydrates. When hypoglycemia develops slowly, the epinephrine response may be absent because there is time for adaptive mechanisms to operate.

The first symptoms of hypoglycemia per se may be psychological, neurological, or mixed.[11] Mental symptoms vary from slight to severe. In the earliest stages, the patient is usually irritable and confused, and may be negativistic. Loss of judgment and impairment of insight may prevent him from realizing that he needs treatment, and he may reject the notion that there is anything wrong with him. These minor symptoms merge rapidly into a more serious condition of disorientation for time and place, false perception, restlessness, and even maniacal outbursts. Focal or generalized tonic convulsions may occur, and "narcoleptic" attacks have been recorded. Simple loss of consciousness without convulsive movements is common. Evidence of focal neurological dysfunction may be slight or severe, and it takes many forms. These include dysarthria, aphasia, visual disturbances in the form of diplopia, hemianopia, or amaurosis, ataxia of the hands and legs, and myoclonic twitching of muscles, or hemiparesis. It is possible that localized arterial insufficiency may play a part in determining the localization of focal dysfunction.[46]

If hypoglycemia continues, the patient sinks into coma; it should be noted, however, that although the functional type of hypoglycemia can give rise to syncope or even tonic convulsions, it does not cause prolonged coma, spontaneous recovery of consciousness being the rule. In the "organic" group, the face remains pale, the pulse quickens, respirations are shallow, and there is a terminal fall of blood pressure.

Severe and prolonged hypoglycemia, especially if repeated episodes occur, can give rise to permanent mental retardation and ataxia in infants[35] and to mild dementia in adults; however, mental changes after a single attack usually clear up completely. Peripheral neuropathy can occur as the result of repeated attacks, and it may be attended by a considerable degree of muscular wasting.

Laboratory Aids. In functional hypoglycemia, the fasting blood sugar is normal between attacks, but it may be low in organically determined cases. In both groups, the blood sugar is low during an actual attack. In order to arrive at a conclusion as to whether episodes are due to functional or organic hypoglycemia, a five-hour glucose tolerance test is useful. In the functional type, the fasting sugar is normal, and there is a moderate rise of blood glucose in the first and second hours, but this is followed by a hypoglycemic phase, with a return to pretest levels by the fifth hour. In organic hyperinsulinism, the curve remains rather flat, and there is no recovery to pretest levels by the fifth hour. A low-carbohydrate, 1200-calorie diet maintained for three days will usually produce hypoglycemic symptoms in organic hyperinsulinism, and a complete fast for 72 hours will certainly do so. This does not occur in the functional type.

Treatment. Treatment depends upon correction of the underlying cause.[15] In the functional type, which is the variety most commonly encountered by neurologists and psychiatrists, attacks may be prevented by frequent small meals with a high protein content.

DISTURBANCES OF WATER BALANCE AND ELECTROLYTES

That disturbances of serum electrolyte levels should be able to cause psychological and neurological symptoms is not surprising, since cell function is partly dependent on the movement of electrolytes. As the result of the equilibria which govern the distribution and relative concentration of ions in intra- and extracellular fluid, changes in the concentration of one ion often produce changes in other ions. Therefore, it is not always possible to attribute a particular clinical symptom to a specific ionic disturbance, and although the following sections adhere to the conventional method of dealing with each electrolyte separately, it must be remembered that in practice the disturbance is seldom confined to one ion. The situation is further complicated by the fact that although abnormalities of water and electrolyte metabolism are usually caused by non-neurological diseases, and affect the nervous system secondarily, head injuries and cerebral disease can also bring about disturbances of electrolytes and water balance.[17, 18, 29] Such neurogenic disturbances can then have a boomerang effect on the functions of the nervous system. A familiar sequence, for instance, is: head injury — diabetes insipidus — consequent dehydration and hypernatremia — deepening coma.

Water Intoxication

Water intoxication results from excessive intake of water without adequate sodium intake. It is most commonly seen as the result of the administration of simple dextrose solutions postoperatively in amounts exceeding 3 liters/m.^{2} body surface/24 hours; as little as 1 liter/m.^{2} can be harmful if morphine or barbiturates have been used, or if the patient has been subjected for some time to a low-sodium intake. Apart from postoperative cases, water intoxication can occur in compulsive water drinking in mental patients, retention of enemas, hypopituitarism, anuria, from a water diuresis test in the presence of adrenal cortical insufficiency, and from the administration of antidiuretic hormone.

The brain cells appear to be sensitive to dilution of extracellular fluid, which leads to a reduction of both intra- and extracellular ionic concentrations. Recovery can follow the administration of sodium alone, even if the serum potassium remains low, suggesting that the restoration of function may be due to reestablishment of normal osmolarity.

In its mildest form, water intoxication can give rise to lethargy, nausea, vomiting, and mild mental aberration in the form of odd behavior, inattentiveness, and slight confusion. In more severe cases, there may be convulsions, aphasia, hemiplegia, stupor, or coma. It may mimic a subdural hematoma. The symptoms clear up within hours or days if appropriate treatment is given.

Water intoxication is to be suspected

when mental or neurological symptoms appear in a person whose water intake markedly exceeds his urinary output, and it is confirmed by a blood sodium level below 130 mEq. It is only too easy to attribute mental symptoms, hemiplegia, stupor, or coma to a vascular accident after an operation, and when such symptoms arise either postoperatively or under the other circumstances described, the patient's water balance and the levels of his serum sodium and serum potassium should be examined.

The condition can be avoided by ordinary prudence and conservatism in the administration of dextrose solutions containing no salt. In mild cases, no water at all should be given for 24 hours. In more severe cases, the patient should receive 300 ml. of 3 to 5 per cent sodium chloride, followed by isotonic saline until the blood chemistry and the patient's condition are satisfactory.[60, 61] If blood potassium is low, potassium chloride may be added to the infusion.

Hyponatremia

Hyponatremia is usually due to water intoxication resulting from excessive intake of fluid, either by mouth or parenterally, without a corresponding intake of sodium. However, it can also happen, in the absence of overhydration, as a result of inappropriate secretion of antidiuretic hormone.[8, 29, 36] The latter occurs as a result of the production of an antidiuretic substance by oat-cell carcinoma of the lung and carcinoma of the pancreas, and from the release of antidiuretic hormone (ADH) in head injuries, meningitis, brain abscess, cerebral hemorrhage, brain tumor, Guillain-Barré syndrome, and acute intermittent porphyria. It also can occur for reasons which are not fully understood in pulmonary disease, such as advanced tuberculosis, aspergillosis, pneumonia, and lung abscess. Inappropriate release of ADH can accompany Addison's disease, myxedema, and hypopituitarism, and it may be present in cardiac failure, in cirrhosis with ascites, and after surgical operations.

Chemically, the syndrome is characterized by hyponatremia, hypotonicity of the extracellular fluid, and a hypertonic urine.

The symptoms of severe hyponatremia are closely akin to the symptoms of water intoxication. It is desirable to recognize that they can mimic the symptoms of subdural hematoma, among other things, and that they can complicate and obscure the signs of the primary disease.

In mild cases, restriction of water is all that is required, but if the symptoms are acute, hypertonic saline (e.g., 500 ml. of 5 per cent saline) should be infused slowly. If water intake is not limited, the sodium chloride is rapidly lost in the urine and serum sodium concentration may fall to the initial level in a single day. For persons with cardiac failure, the use of hypertonic saline is contraindicated.

Hypernatremia

A rise in serum sodium level is usually the result of dehydration without a corresponding loss of sodium. It occurs as the result of vomiting and diarrhea in infants,[42] inadequate intake of water in unconscious patients (which is particularly dangerous in the presence of excessive sweating and hyperventilation); excessive intravenous administration of saline in patients with renal tubular disease; diabetes insipidus in unconscious patients (e.g., following head injury) who cannot report their thirst and are allowed insufficient fluid; head injuries and brain surgery *in the absence of dehydration*[72]; and in some cases of the Guillain-Barré syndrome.

The hyperosmolarity induced by dehydration and hypernatremia can cause severe brain damage in the form of hemorrhagic encephalopathy, and this is especially likely to occur in the case of infants and young children, in whom it can give rise to thrombosis of the dural sinuses, hemorrhagic infarcts, and swelling of the brain. Experimental work on cats led Luttrell and his associates to conclude that hypernatremia is itself deleterious apart from the effect of hyperosmolarity.[42] Hypernatremia can occur without a corresponding degree of dehydration, as a *result* of brain damage, but hyponatremia due to renal salt-wasting is more usual under these circumstances.

In infants and children, hypernatremia gives rise to irritability and restlessness, hypertonicity, irregular muscular twitchings, occasional seizures, and nystagmus, and these ultimately give place to stupor, coma, and death.[42] Survivors are sometimes left with mental retardation and seizures.[47] Electroencephalography reveals high-voltage slow waves and occasional sharp spikes during the acute phase.

In adults, the conditions under which hypernatremia occurs—head injuries, cranial surgery, strokes[72]—make it almost impossible to discern what symptoms are due, respectively, to hypernatremia, hyperosmolarity, and the primary disease.

The presence of hypernatremia is to be suspected when there is clinical evidence of dehydration—lackluster eyes, sunken cheeks, dry tongue, inelastic skin, and a small output of highly concentrated urine—but these signs are not entirely reliable, and serum sodium estimation is necessary. Hyperkalemia can occur in the same group of patients, and is a far greater threat to survival, so the serum potassium must be measured as well.

Hyperkalemia

Pure hyperkalemia is seen only in familial periodic paralysis (adynamia episodica hereditaria) and as a result of the administration of excessive amounts of potassium salts. More often it occurs in association with other biochemical disorders as a result of the following: (1) Acute renal failure,[37, 40] whether it be prerenal (crush injuries, intravenous hemolysis, acute acidosis) or renal in origin (in chronic nephritis, potassium is usually low or normal unless and until terminal oliguria sets in); (2) dehydration—a relative rise; (3) some severe

head injuries[18]; (4) Addison's disease; (5) hyponatremia; (6) untreated diabetic acidosis.

If large doses of potassium salts are given by mouth, the patient experiences paresthesias in the extremities, followed by weakness and difficulty in walking.[20] When it comes on more gradually, in disease, paresthesias are less evident and may be absent, and paralysis comes on quickly, often without warning. It is a flaccid paralysis with loss of tendon reflexes and depression of muscle excitability. Sometimes there is impairment of position sense and vibration. When the serum potassium reaches the neighborhood of 10 mEq./liter (normal: 4.1 to 5.6 mEq.) cardiac standstill is likely to occur, but before this happens, changes appear in the EKG. The T waves become high and peaked, followed by widening of the QRS complex and finally disappearance of the T wave. Both cardiac and skeletal paralyses are usually attributed to the effects of the ion on muscle rather than on nerve, but the occasional appearance of paresthesias and sensory impairment throws some doubt on this rather restricted view.

The administration of insulin and glucose is the most effective method of treatment. (Insulin should not be given when hyperkalemia is the result of Addison's disease.) Hemodialysis can be used, if available, to prevent the paralysis in cases in which EKG changes and biochemical assays give warning of impending danger, but once paralysis has occurred, treatment with insulin and glucose is quicker than dialysis. Since hyponatremia and acidosis may compound the effects of hyperkalemia, the administration of sodium and dextrose is desirable.

Hypokalemia

Hypokalemia is more common and less serious than hyperkalemia. It occurs in a variety of disorders, which fall into four groups. (1) Potassium loss via the kidneys is seen in potassium-losing nephritis, Fanconi's syndrome, primary aldosteronism,[16] excessive administration of adrenocortical steroids, abuse of mercury diuretics and chlorothiazide, and bilateral ureterocolostomy.[20] (2) Excessive loss from the gastrointestinal tract is seen in chronic diarrheas, excessive use of laxatives and bowel washout,[51] colonic fistulas, prolonged vomiting, and villous adenoma of the rectum. An important practical point is that in paraplegic patients, bowel washouts extract a greater quantity of potassium than in normal persons, and this can lead to serious and even fatal hypokalemia.[51] (3) Deficient intake of potassium is seen in patients who are kept too long on parenteral fluids without the addition of potassium, and as a result of prolonged vomiting. (4) Hypokalemia can also occur during recovery from diabetic coma and is present in the hypokalemic type of familial periodic paralysis.

Symptoms. Potassium deficiency gives rise to weakness of the arms and legs, sometimes spreading to the trunk, but usually sparing the cranial nerves.[20] These symptoms may be obscured by the primary disease, whatever it may be. The electrocardiogram shows flattening or inversion of T waves, prolongation of the QT interval, and a broad or diphasic U wave.

The muscular weakness of hypokalemia is less severe than the weakness of hyperkalemic familial periodic paralysis, and it does not display the periodicity of the latter condition. Myasthenia gravis is not easily mistaken for potassium deficiency since in the former cranial nerve palsies and a clear relationship to effort are usually present.

Hypokalemia can be prevented by the provision of an adequate intake of the ion, whether by parenteral solutions or by mouth. When the condition has developed, it is safer to give potassium by mouth than by intravenous injection, because absorption through the gastrointestinal tract is sufficiently slow to avoid allowing the patient to pass into the more dangerous condition of potassium intoxication. If it has to be given intravenously, the rate of administration should not exceed 20 mEq./hour, and the process should be monitored by serial estimations of serum potassium.

HYPERCALCEMIA

The range of corrected plasma calcium in normal fasting adults is 9.0 to 10.3 mg./100 ml. Quite small deviations from this normal narrow range may produce symptoms.[7, 30, 32, 55, 68] Hypercalcemia can give rise to (1) psychiatric symptoms, (2) delirium progressing to coma if the condition is unrelieved, (3) profound muscular weakness, and (4) gastrointestinal symptoms.

Etiology. The principal function of the parathyroid glands is to maintain a normal plasma calcium level by regulating the balance of calcium between bones and bloodstream. The level of plasma calcium, in turn, determines parathyroid activity, and hypocalcemia is the common stimulus for parathyroid secretion.[68] The possible role of calcitonin, a hormone which is extractable from the thyroid, is still being evaluated; it appears to be effective in the treatment of Paget's disease. Excessive secretion of parathormone raises blood calcium. Rarely, carcinomas, sarcomas, and reticuloses elaborate a parathormone-like substance which acts in a similar manner. Hypercalcemia can also be induced by excessive administration of vitamin D or calcium or both, whether from self-medication, excessive ingestion of milk and alkali, or accidental overdosage in the treatment of hypocalcemia. Increased sensitivity to small doses of vitamin D, which regulates the absorption of calcium, leads to hypercalcemia in some cases of sarcoidosis and occasional cases of idiopathic hypercalcemia of infancy.

The blood calcium may also be elevated when the bones are involved by carcinoma, multiple myeloma, the reticuloses, rapidly advancing Paget's disease, and the osteoporosis which follows prolonged immobilization in childhood. Untreated thyrotoxicosis can act similarly.

Rarely, hypercalcemia occurs in Addison's disease and following adrenalectomy.

Clinical Features. Hypercalcemia gives rise to headache, anorexia, nausea, vomiting, thirst, dry mouth, constipation, and lassitude.

Mental symptoms are relatively common in primary hyperparathyroidism.[32] They vary widely in type and severity in patients with comparable biochemical abnormalities, and it is probable that the previous personality of the patient plays a role. Acute symptoms occur when the serum calcium reading is above 17 mg. per cent. There is progressive lethargy, drowsiness, confusion, and impairment of intellect. There is profound muscular weakness. Delirium and hallucinations may occur, and if the condition is unrelieved, coma supervenes, the blood pressure drops, and death occurs. Osteitis fibrosa cystica may be present or absent. The cerebrospinal fluid protein is often increased, a circumstance which makes it only too easy to attribute the organic brain syndrome to structural intracranial disease. This mistake is particularly likely to occur when the hyperglycemia is caused by the secretion of a parathormone-like substance by a visceral carcinoma, in which event the cerebral symptoms can be mistaken for evidence of intracranial metastases.

Proximal muscular weakness and wasting, hypotonia, discomfort on movement, and—an unusual finding in myopathy—exaggerated tendon reflexes are present in some cases. Dysphagia occasionally occurs. Electromyography reveals no evidence of denervation, but there are polyphasic potentials of short duration. The differentiation from polymyositis is made by the brisk tendon reflexes and the elevation of serum calcium. When nephrocalcinosis complicates hyperparathyroidism, episodic muscular weakness may occur, owing to potassium depletion, but the muscular weakness is intermittent, and the tendon reflexes are reduced or abolished.

Treatment. If the hypercalcemia can be relieved, there is rapid improvement in the cerebral and muscular symptoms. This is best seen following the removal of a parathyroid adenoma. However, when hypercalcemia has been present for a long time, full recovery of mental function is not always achieved, especially in older patients, whereas chronicity of muscular symptoms is no barrier to complete recovery.

The treatment of hypercalcemia depends on its cause and is beyond the scope of this book.

HYPOCALCEMIA

Hypocalcemia exists when the serum level of total calcium is below 9 mg./100 ml. At this level, symptoms may occur, but they are seldom acute until the level approaches 6 or 7 mg./100 ml.[55, 68] The symptoms include tetany, seizures, parkinsonism, psychological disturbances, and raised intracranial pressure with papilledema.[55]

Etiology. The most common cause of hypocalcemia is hypoparathyroidism caused by the inadvertent removal of parathyroid tissue during thyroid surgery. Rarely, in "idiopathic" hypoparathyroidism, the parathyroid glands have been found to be completely replaced by fat. Other causes of hypocalcemia include low calcium intake, defective calcium absorption from the intestine (vitamin D deficiency, sprue, diarrhea), high calcium loss from the urinary tract in essential hypercalciuria and renal tubular failure, and as a result of elevated serum phosphorus in glomerular insufficiency and excessive ingestion of phosphates (as in infants fed on cow's milk).

Clinical Features. The outstanding feature of hypocalcemia is tetany, but it should be noted that tetany can also occur as the result of alkalosis, without a fall of serum calcium, e.g., following hyperventilation, loss of chlorides from vomiting, excessive ingestion of alkali, and in hypomagnesemia.[66] The tetany of hypocalcemia usually starts with paresthesias around the lips and in the fingers and toes, accompanied by cramps in the muscles and followed by carpopedal spasms. These phenomena are related to the fact that with a decrease of ambient calcium ions, there is an increase in the mechanical and electrical excitability of somatic nerves, and increased irritability of sympathetic ganglion cells. In some cases, only fragments of carpopedal spasm are seen. Thus, a foot may drag for a second or two, or there may be sudden transient immobility of the legs, causing the patient to fall. Carpopedal spasms may be associated with cramps in the jaw and respiratory muscles, producing dyspnea and inability to talk; if the spasms are very severe, they lead to choking and cyanosis which, in turn, can lead to unconsciousness. Spasm involving the external ocular muscles have been described.

Seizures are not uncommon, especially in children. They usually take the form of grand mal, in which event the EEG shows the symmetrical spike and wave discharges appropriate to that condition, and it is likely that in such cases, the hypocalcemia uncovers "idiopathic" epilepsy. Atypical attacks, sometimes very bizarre, are also seen, and in these, the EEG commonly shows bursts of 2 to 5 c./sec. waves.[48]

Psychological symptoms are not infrequent and may be severe, especially in the period immediately following parathyroidectomy.[7, 30] There may be delirium, paranoid psychoses, hallucinations, psychoneurotic behavior patterns or simple mental slowing. In children, spontaneous hypoparathyroidism can cause mental retardation. In chronic hypoparathyroidism, fatigue, listlessness, anxiety, and tension are not uncommon.

Symptoms attributable to basal ganglia disease have been described[55]—chorea, choreoathetosis, dystonia, and parkinsonism—and in this connection, it is significant that punctate calcification is sometimes seen in the basal ganglia, although it is not always associated with extrapyramidal symptoms or with disordered calcium metabolism.

A rise of intracranial pressure associated with papilledema may occur in parathyroid deficiency following thyroidectomy, and in the "spontaneous" variety of hypoparathyroidism. Headache may be severe, and the combination of headaches, seizures, and papilledema may falsely suggest the presence of a cerebral tumor; the danger of misdiagnosis is increased by the fact that tetany may be absent in some cases. Conversely, hypocalcemia can lower the epileptic threshold and bring to light evidence of a cerebral lesion previously unrecognized.

Cortical cataracts are common. When hypoparathyroidism occurs before the permanent teeth mature, they may show malformation of the enamel, and shortening of the roots. The nails may be malformed and brittle, and may be infected with candidiasis. The skin is coarse and dry, and there is defective growth of the hair on the head and body.

Latent tetany can be demonstrated by Chvostek's and Trousseau's signs, which depend on the hypersensitivity of nerves to percussion and ischemia, respectively. However, both signs may be absent in hypocalcemia, and both may be positive in the presence of a normal serum calcium.[55]

The serum calcium is depressed and serum phosphate is elevated. Calcium is absent from the urine. The electrocardiogram shows an increase in the QT interval, which is restored to normal when the blood calcium is brought up to a normal level.

Treatment. Acute episodes require prompt intravenous injection of 10 ml. of 20 per cent calcium gluconate, or 10 to 30 ml. of 10 per cent calcium lactate in 1000 ml. of normal saline. This must be given as often as is necessary to control the symptoms. At the same time, 4 gm. of calcium lactate should be given orally 6 times a day, together with vitamin D.

Chronic hypoparathyroidism can be treated effectively by parathormone but the effect diminishes with prolonged administration. A simpler method of treatment is to administer dihydrotachysterol (AT-10), a substance related to vitamin D, which aids the absorption of calcium and increases the excretion of urinary phosphorus. It is given by mouth in doses of 1.25 mg. twice daily until the blood calcium is normal, and the dose is then adjusted in accordance with the results of serial estimations of serum calcium.

Magnesium Deficiency

Fall of the serum magnesium below the normal 1 to 7 mEq./liter can occur as the result of the prolonged administration of magnesium-deficient fluids parenterally, persistent vomiting, intestinal malabsorption, prolonged alcoholic bouts, renal tubular acidosis, and hepatic disease. A variety of symptoms have been attributed to hypomagnesemia, including tetany (which is clinically indistinguishable from hypocalcemic tetany), convulsive seizures, tremor, muscular twitching, weakness, choreic and athetoid movements, mental confusion, and hallucinations.[31, 50] It is often difficult to estimate the effects of a deficiency of the magnesium ion because of the existence of other metabolic disturbances in the conditions referred to above, and a direct relationship between individual symptoms and hypomagnesemia can be established only when the symptoms disappear following in-the symptoms disappear following intramuscular administration of 2 gm. of magnesium sulfate. The maximum intravenous dose should not exceed 5 gm. in 100 ml. in three hours; larger amounts can cause muscular weakness, respiratory depression, a fall of blood pressure, and diarrhea.

NEUROLOGICAL EFFECTS OF UREMIA

Renal failure is associated with a wide spectrum of mental and neurological symptoms, not all of which are due to the uremia per se.[37, 40, 44, 49, 64] Some of them may be due, for instance, to hypertensive cerebrovascular disease or to the condition which has caused the renal failure, or to side effects of uremia such as anemia and cardiac failure. Perhaps the clearest view of the results of uremia is obtained in acute renal failure with oliguria or anuria occurring as the result of shock, hemorrhage, crush injuries, infections, transfusion reactions, and renal poisons. However, even in these cases, it is difficult if not impossible to see a clear correlation between individual chemical disturbances and specific neuropsychiatric symptoms (potassium intoxication excepted), and the only thing which is certain is that a raised blood urea is not wholly responsible for the effects of uremia on the central nervous system, although it does serve as index of renal function. The blood-brain barrier is breached in uremia, allowing the passage into the brain and spinal fluid of substances which are normally kept out, and this contributes to the intoxication.[27]

Clinical Features. During the oliguric phase of acute renal failure, the symptoms and signs are predominantly those of cardiovascular, gastrointestinal, and neurological dysfunction.[40, 44] Cardiovascular effects occur in two forms—cardiac failure with pulmonary edema, and cardiac standstill due to hyperkalemia. Gastrointestinal symptoms take the form of anorexia, nausea, vomiting, diarrhea, and abdominal distention. There may also be slight fever, severe anemia, and gross loss of weight due to increased protein catabolism.

Mental and neurological features are often prominent and sometimes severe. Early mental symptoms are those of a mild toxic psychosis with lethargy, poor memory, short attention span, disorientation, and slowing of thought. These often fluctuate from hour to hour. Later on, the symptoms are more marked, and the patient may be delirious, noisy, and uncooperative. If untreated, the disease ends in somnolence, convulsions, coma, and death.

Neurological dysfunction is usually elusive and transient. Cranial nerve disturbances which may come and go include amaurosis, hemianopia, diplopia, nystagmus, slight facial weakness, and dysarthria. The most prominent motor disability is profound generalized muscular weakness associated with fasciculation. In some cases, myoclonic twitches occur, especially when the cerebrospinal fluid phosphate is increased.[27] The tendon reflexes are often hyperactive, but become depressed as intoxication deepens. In patients who live long enough, the muscles waste rapidly, and may be tender. Neck stiffness and a positive Kernig sign may appear, the result of chemical meningitis; in such cases, the spinal fluid shows pleocytosis and elevation of protein. In other cases, there is generalized hypertonicity of the muscles, and this may also cause stiffness of the neck. There may be transient monoplegia or hemiplegia, cerebellar ataxia, or generalized rigidity. Sensory symptoms and signs are not obvious in acute renal failure, but peripheral neuropathy can occur in chronic nephritis and may become severe during the early stages of dialysis (p. 564).

Generalized or jacksonian seizures are not uncommon, and the electroencephalogram may show a replacement of background alpha by bilateral slow waves and spikes. Not all patients with an abnormal EEG have seizures. The electroencephalographic changes—which do not correlate with any single alteration in blood chemistry—show a marked tendency to follow photic driving, and photic stimulation can evoke both seizures and myoclonus.[49]

In the oliguric or anuric phase, the serum sodium and chlorides fall, and the potassium rises. There is a reduction of CO_2 combining power, reflecting a metabolic acidosis. Serum calcium falls, phosphate increases in the blood and spinal fluid, and the rise correlates with the presence of muscle twitching. The lowered calcium and raised phosphorus are reminiscent of hypoparathyroidism, in which tetany and convulsions can also occur. There is marked azotemia. Electrocardiography occasionally shows changes typical of hyperkalemia (p. 587).

The treatment of acute renal failure is beyond the scope of this book; dialysis, if available, is life-saving, but if carried out too quickly, it may cause a subdural hematoma or hemorrhagic encephalopathy with cerebral edema and uncal herniation.

ORAL CONTRACEPTIVE HORMONES

There is statistical evidence of a slightly increased tendency toward venous thrombosis in women taking oral contraceptive hormones. The most important complication is pulmonary embolism, but fortunately this is rare. Arterial thrombosis has been recorded.

The evidence as to whether these agents predispose to stroke in young women is less certain. A study in Minnesota disclosed that there had been no increase in number of recorded cases of stroke in women of child-bearing age since the introduction of these agents, but many neurologists dispute this evidence in the light of their own experience. Leaving aside cases of acute cerebral vascular incidents which can be attributed to embolism from cardiac disease, syphilitic thrombosis, intracranial hemangiomatous malformations, collagen disease, and so on, there are a few cases in which it seems reasonable to incriminate oral contraceptives. The clinical features are often unusual and sometimes bizarre. Cases seen by the author include a girl of 19 who took oral contraceptives for two periods of time (separated by a year) and on both occasions presented with symptoms and signs consistent with a cerebral infarction. Another woman, aged 38, developed spontaneous thrombosis of the left internal carotid artery. A woman of 23 suffered an abrupt infarction of the left occipital lobe, with consequent right homonymous hemianopia. Mandel has reported bilateral thrombotic occlusion of the carotid arteries in a healthy young woman, and a report from Sweden tells of death from thrombotic occlusion of the celiac artery. There have been several deaths from intracranial venous thrombosis, including the superior sagittal sinus.[5]

The administration of these drugs is accompanied by alterations in the clotting time, increased plasma triglyceride levels, a decrease of postheparin lipolytic activity, and increased platelet sensitivity to adenosine diphosphate. Moreover, there is usually an increase in the agglutination of circulating red cells.

Further work is needed to establish whether these factors play a significant role in the vascular complications of contraceptive therapy.

The severity and frequency of migraine attacks are often increased by oral contraceptives, and certain cases of benign intracranial hypertension (pseudotumor cerebri) have been attributed to their use.

On present evidence, it would seem prudent for women who experience symptoms and signs related to the vascular system while on oral contraceptive agents to adopt some other method of contraception.

HEROIN ADDICTION

Heroin addiction has become a major problem in many parts of the world; it is the leading cause of death in the 15 to 25 year age group in Harlem, New York City. A number of fatal and nonfatal neurological sequelae have been defined, but their pathology is not fully understood. Quinine, which is often mixed with heroin in potentially toxic doses, may play a part (e.g., in producing optic atrophy), and the effects of hypoxia have to be taken into account in subjects coming to autopsy after prolonged unconsciousness and respiratory depression. The effects of infection at injection sites, including phlebitis and myositis, have to be considered. Paralysis of a single peripheral nerve may be due to an incorrectly placed injection. Malnutrition, with especial reference to the vitamin B complex, may also contribute to the neurological symptoms in some cases.

Clinical effects include (1) acute and chronic organic brain syndromes, with coma, convulsions, stroke, and parkinsonian disorders; (2) optic atrophy; (3) acute transverse myelitis;[54a] (4) mononeuropathy and polyneuropathy; (5) acute myopathy with myoglobinuria; (6) infections — tetanus, hepatitis, bacterial, tuberculous, and fungal meningitis, epidural spinal abscess, acute endocarditis with cerebral embolism, cerebral abscess, and malaria.

MARIJUANA (CANNABIS)

Weil[69] has classified adverse reactions to marijuana under four headings. Many persons who smoke marijuana experience no subjective effects, and those who do get "high" find the experience pleasurable. On the other hand, the drug may precipitate brief but acute depression in neophytes, possibly from a sense of guilt. Second, a panic reaction may occur when the smoker misinterprets the physical and psychological effects of the drug and thinks that he is "losing his mind." Here, too, guilt may contribute to the panic. Weil points out that if the doctor approaches the patient as a psychiatric emergency and administers tranquilizers or urges hospitalization, he will often prolong the panic by inadvertently confirming the patient's fears of a mental breakdown. All that is needed is reassurance that nothing is radically wrong. A third reaction takes the form of a toxic psychosis, which occurs when the cannabis is ingested orally. The patient is disoriented, confused, hallucinated, and often prostrated. It should be noted in this context that individuals who have had hallucinations as a result of taking other hallucinogenic drugs, notably LSD, may have a recurrence of hallucinations when they smoke marijuana; in addition, delayed psychotic reactions may follow several months after the last use of hallucinogens, even without smoking marijuana.

Psychotic patients, notably schizophrenics, often find the effects of marijuana unpleasant. There have been reports of psychosis precipitated or triggered by marijuana.

REFERENCES

1. Adams, R. D., and Foley, J. M.: The neurological disorders associated with liver disease. *Res. Pub. Ass. Res. Nerv. Ment. Dis.* 32:198, 1953.
2. Amatuzio, D. S., Stutzman, F., Shrifter, N., and Nesbitt, S.: A study of serum electrolytes (Na, K, Ca, P) in patients with severely decompensated portal cirrhosis of the liver. *J. Lab. Clin. Med.* 39:26, 1952.
3. Aring, C. D.: The systemic nervous affinity of

triorthocresylphosphate (Jamaica ginger palsy). *Brain* 65:34, 1942.

4. Aring, C. D., and Trufant, S. A.: The effect of heavy metals on the nervous system. *Res. Pub. Ass. Res. Nerv. Ment. Dis.* 32:463, 1953.

5. Atkinson, E. A., Fairburn, B., and Heathfield, K. W.: Intracranial venous thrombosis as complication of oral contraception. *Lancet* 1:914, 1970.

6. Ayd, F. J.: A survey of drug induced extrapyramidal reactions. *J.A.M.A.* 175:1054, 1961.

7. Bartter, F. C.: The parathyroid gland and its relationship to diseases of the nervous system. *Res. Pub. Ass. Res. Nerv. Ment. Dis.* 32: 1, 1953.

8. Bartter, F. C.: The syndrome of inappropriate secretion of antidiuretic hormone. *J. Roy. Coll. Phys.* 4:264, 1970.

9. Bickford, R. G., and Butt, H. R.: Hepatic coma: The electroencephalographic pattern. *J. Clin. Invest.* 34:790, 1955.

10. Blackman, S. S.: Lesions of lead encephalitis in children. *Bull. Johns Hopkins Hosp.* 61: 1, 1937.

11. Boudin, G., Lamas, A., and Labet, R.: Les encephalopathies hypoglycemies spontaniés. *World Neurol.* 2:849, 1961.

12. Byers, R. K.: Lead poisoning. Review of the literature and report of 45 cases. *Pediatrics* 23:585, 1959.

13. Canavan, M. M., Cobb, S., and Drinker, C. K.: Chronic manganese poisoning. *Arch. Neurol. Psychiat.* 32:502, 1934.

14. Chamberlain, P. H., Stavinoah, W. B., Davis, H., Kniker, W. T., and Panos, T. C.: Thallium poisoning. *Pediatrics* 22:1170, 1958.

15. Conn. J. W.: Spontaneous hypoglycemia. *Amer. J. Med.* 19:460, 1955.

16. Conn, J. W., Louis, L. H., Fajans, S. S., Streeten, D. H. P., and Johnson, R. D.: Intermittent aldosteronism in periodic paralysis. *Lancet* 1:802, 1957.

17. Cooper, I. S.: Disorders of electrolyte and water metabolism following brain surgery. *J. Neurosurg.* 10:389, 1953.

18. Cooper, I. S., and MacCarty, C. S.: Unusual electrolyte abnormalities associated with cerebral lesions. *Proc. Mayo Clin.* 26:354, 1951.

19. Courville, C. B.: Anoxia incident to carbon monoxide poisoning. *Clinical Neurology.* Edited by Baker, A. B., Paul B. Hoeber Div., Harper and Row, New York, 1962, p. 651.

20. Danowski, T. S., and Tarail, R.: Potassium metabolism and dysfunction of the nervous system. *Res. Pub. Ass. Res. Nerv. Ment. Dis.* 32:372, 1953.

21. Dekaban, A., Field, J. B., and Stevens, H.: Familial idiopathic hypoglycemia. *Arch. Neurol.* 7:529, 1962.

22. Duncan, G. G.: Spontaneous hypoglycemia. *Diseases of Metabolism: Detailed Methods of Diagnosis and Treatment.* W. B. Saunders Co., Philadelphia, 1964, Chap. 12.

23. Evans, J. H.: Persistent oral dyskinesia in treatment with phenothiazine derivatives. *Lancet* 1:458, 1965.

24. Fazekas, J. F., Ticktin, H. E., Ehrmantraut, W. R., and Alman, R. W.: Cerebral metabolism in hepatic insufficiency. *Amer. J. Med.* 21:843, 1956.

25. Ford, F. R.: Lead poisoning. *Diseases of the Nervous System in Childhood and Adolescence.* 4th Ed. Charles C Thomas, Springfield, Ill., 1960, pp. 724–730.

26. Ford, F. R.: Arsenic poisoning. *Diseases of the Nervous System in Childhood and Adolescence.* 4th Ed. Charles C Thomas, Springfield, Ill., 1960, pp. 730–734.

27. Freeman, R. B., Sheff, M. F., Maher, J. F., and Schreiner, G. E.: The blood-cerebrospinal fluid barrier in uremia. *Ann. Int. Med.* 56: 233, 1962.

28. Gilbert, G. J., and Glaser, G. H.: Neurologic manifestations of chronic carbon monoxide poisoning. *New Eng. J. Med.* 261:1217, 1959.

29. Goldberg, M., and Handler, J. S.: Hyponatremia and renal wasting of sodium in patients with malfunction of the central nervous system. *New Eng. J. Med.* 263:1037, 1960.

30. Greene, J. A., and Swanson, L. W.: Psychosis in hypoparathyroidism with report of five cases. *Ann. Int. Med.* 14:1233, 1941.

31. Hanna, S., Harrison, M., MacIntyre, I., and Fraser, R.: The syndrome of magnesium deficiency in man. *Lancet* 2:172, 1960.

32. Henson, R. A.: The neurological aspects of hypercalcemia with especial reference to hyperparathyroidism. *J. Roy. Coll. Phys.* 1: 41, 1966.

33. Higgins, G., Lewin, W., O'Brien, J. R., and Taylor, W. V.: Metabolic disorders in head injury. *Lancet* 1:61, 1954.

34. Hunter, D., and Russell, D. S.: Focal cerebral and cerebellar atrophy in a human subject due to organic mercury compounds. *J. Neurol. Neurosurg. Psychiat.* 17:235, 1954.

35. Ingram, T. S., Stark, G. D., and Blackburn, I.: Ataxia and other neurological disorders as sequels of severe hypoglycemia in childhood. *Brain* 90:851, 1967.

36. Keeler, R.: Effect of hypothalamic lesions on renal excretion of sodium. *Amer. J. Physiol.* 197:847, 1959.

37. Knutson, J., and Baker, A. B.: The central nervous system in uremia. A clinicopathologic study. *Arch. Neurol. Psychiat.* 54:130, 1945.

38. Kurland, L. T., Faro, S. N., and Siedler, H.: Minamata disease. *World Neurol.* 1:370, 1960.

39. Lawrence, R. D., Meyer, A., and Nevin, S.: The pathological changes in the brain in fatal hypoglycemia. *Quart. J. Med.* 11:181, 1942.

40. Locke, S., Merrill, J. P., and Tyler, H. R.: Neurologic complications of acute uremia. *Arch. Int. Med.* 108:519, 1961.

41. Lowbeer, L.: Hypoglycemia-producing extrapancreatic neoplasms. A review. *Amer. J. Clin. Path.* 35:233, 1961.

42. Luttrell, C. N., and Finberg, L.: Hemorrhagic encephalopathy induced by hypernatremia.

Arch. Neurol. Psychiat. 81:424, 1959; *Arch. Neurol.* 1:153, 1959.

43. McQuarrie, I.: Idiopathic spontaneously occurring hypoglycemia in infants; clinical significance of problem, and treatment. *Amer. J. Dis. Child.* 87:399, 1954.

43a. Mema, I., Marvin, O., Fuenzalida, S., and Cotzias, G.: Chronic manganese poisoning. *Neurology,* 17:128, 1967

44. Merrill, J. P., and Hampers, C. L.: Uremia. *New Eng. J. Med.* 282:953, 1019, 1970.

45. Meyer, J. S., and Portnoy, H. D.: Localized cerebral hypoglycemia simulating a stroke. A clinical and experimental study. *Neurology* 8:601, 1958.

46. Miller, D. R., Bolinger, R. E., Janigan, D., Crockett, J. E., and Friesen, S. R.: Hypoglycemia due to nonpancreatic mesodermal tumors: Report of 2 cases. *Ann. Surg.* 150: 684, 1959.

47. Morris-Jones, P. H., *et al.*: Prognosis of the neurological complications of acute hypernatremia. *Lancet* 2:1385, 1967.

48. Odoriz, J. B., DelCastillo, E. B., Manfredi, J. F., and DeLaBalze, F. A.: Parathyroid insufficiency and the human electroencephalogram. *J. Clin. Endocr.* 4:493, 1944.

49. Olsen, S.: The brain in uremia. *Acta Psych. Neurol. Scand.*, Suppl. 156, Vol. 36, 1961.

50. Petersen, V. P.: Metabolic studies in magnesium deficiency. *Acta Med. Scand.* 173: 285, 1963.

51. Plum, F., and Dunning, M. F.: Enema-induced potassium loss in patients with disease of the spinal cord and cauda equina. *Amer. J. Med. Sci.* 233:387, 1957.

52. Plum, F., Posner, J. B., and Hain, R. F.: Delayed neurological deterioration after anoxia. *Arch. Int. Med.* 110:18, 1962.

53. Plum, F., and Swanson, A. G.: Barbiturate poisoning treated by physiological methods, with observations of the effects of B-B-methylglutarimide and electrical stimulation. *J.A.M.A.* 163:827, 1957.

54. Read, A. E., Sherlock, S., Laidlaw, J., and Walker, J. G.: Neuropsychiatric syndromes associated with chronic liver disease and extensive portal-systemic collateral circulation. *Quart. J. Med.* 36:13, 1967.

54a. Richter, R. W., and Rosenberg, R. N.: Transverse myelitis associated with heroin addiction. *J.A.M.A.* 206:1255, 1968.

55. Robinson, P. K.: The clinical effects of hypo-calcemia in the nervous system. *J. Roy. Coll. Phys.* 1:36, 1966.

56. Rose, I.: A review of tick paralysis. *J. Canad. Med. Ass.* 70:175, 1954.

57. Sensenbach, W.: Bromide intoxication. *J.A.M.A.* 125:769, 1944.

58. Sherlock, S.: *Diseases of the Liver and Biliary System.* 2nd Ed. Charles C Thomas, Springfield, Ill., 1958.

59. Sidbury, J. B., Jr.: Lead poisoning. *Amer. J. Med.* 17:932, 1955.

60. Stern, W. E.: Problems in fluid replacement and cerebral edema in the management of surgical lesions of the central nervous system. *Amer. J. Surg.* 100:303, 1960.

61. Talbot, N. B., Crawford, J. D., and Butler, A. M.: Homeostatic limits to safe parenteral fluid therapy. *New Eng. J. Med.* 248:1100, 1953.

62. Tsukiyama, K., Omura, I., Kobayashi, Y., Kuga, C., Sekihara, T., and Shimo, O.: A new provocative test by oral ammonium for abnormal electroencephalogram in hepatic encephalopathy. *Med. J. Osaka Univ.* 12:95, 1961.

63. Turner, J. W. A.: Metallic poisons and the nervous system. *Lancet* 1:661, 1955.

64. Tyler, H. R.: Neurologic disorders in renal failure. *Amer. J. Med.* 44:734, 1968.

65. Victor, M.: Alcoholism. *Clinical Neurology.* 2nd Ed. Edited by Baker, A. B., Paul B. Hoeber Div., Harper and Row, New York, 1962, Chap. 22.

66. Walker, W. E. C., Moore, F. D., Ulmer, D. D., and Vallee, B. L.: Normocalcemic magnesium deficiency tetany. *J.A.M.A.* 180:161, 1962.

67. Walsh, J. C.: Gold Neuropathy. *Neurology* 20: 455, 1970.

68. Watson, L.: Calcium metabolism and neurology. *J. Roy. Coll. Phys.* 1:28, 1966.

69. Weil, A. T.: Adverse reactions to marijuana. *New Eng. J. Med.* 282:997, 1970.

70. White, H. H., and Fowler, F. D.: Chronic lead encephalopathy; a diagnostic consideration in mental retardation. *Pediatrics* 25:309, 1960.

71. Wilson, G., and Winkelman, N. W.: Multiple neuritis following CO poisoning. A clinicopathologic study. *J.A.M.A.* 82:1407, 1924.

72. Wise, B. L.: Neurogenic hyper-osmolarity (hypernatremia). *Neurology* 12:453, 1962.

73. Treatment of chronic hepatic encephalopathy [editorial]. *Lancet* 2:449, 1970.

CHAPTER TWENTY-TWO

Disorders Produced by Electric Shock, Heat, Cold, and Radiotherapy

ELECTRICAL INJURIES

Electrical injuries may be received from lightning and from contact with a high tension conductor. The effects depend on the nature and voltage of the current, the duration of exposure, the resistance of the skin at the point of contact, the grounding, and the part of the body traversed by the current—a list of variables sufficient to explain the apparently capricious behavior of electrical shocks.[1, 3, 13]

Pathology. The current takes the shortest route from entrance to exit, and may jump the flexures, thereby causing local burns. Its effects are threefold: the production of heat, with consequent coagulation necrosis; the electrolytic production of gas in the tissues, especially the brain; and gross physical disruption of the tissues, causing fissuring in the brain and fractures of bones, as a result of electrostatic forces which are especially liable to accumulate if the patient is partly insulated from the ground. The immediate cause of death can be either ventricular fibrillation or respiratory arrest. Late pathological effects in non-fatal cases are slight. Permanent changes in the walls of blood vessels can be caused by the heat generated by the electrical current, but there is no evidence that progressive symptoms result therefrom.

Clinical Features.[1, 3, 6, 13] Mild shocks cause painful paresthesias and a violent tetanus of muscle; the latter may prevent the victim from releasing an object such as a wire or an electric kettle, thereby converting an unpleasant experience into a fatality. More severe shocks cause immediate loss of consciousness, with convulsions and protracted coma, which may end in death or complete recovery. In many cases, death is virtually instantaneous, from ventricular fibrillation, while in others it occurs rapidly because of respiratory arrest; the latter is common enough to justify prolonged artificial respiration in every case. Most investigators agree that if death does not occur, complete recovery usually occurs. In the first few weeks there may be complaints of headache, drowsiness, impairment of memory and concentration, or paresthesias and weakness of the limbs through which the current passed, but these usually pass off completely. The limbs may be cold and blue, suggesting vasomotor paralysis, but this clears up in a matter of hours. Traumatic neurosis is common, especially when there is a question of compensation.

Ocular complications are not infrequent. Immediate reactions, which include amaurosis, unformed visual hallucinations, clouding of the cornea and lens, and retinal edema, usually pass off in hours or days. Cataract formation is not unknown, and is probably due to electrical burns. It may become apparent within two weeks to two years of the injury. Optic atrophy has been recorded.[1]

It is important to distinguish between the effects of electrical injuries and injuries sustained as a result of falls incidental to the shock. A workman may fall off a scaffold as a result of a slight shock and fracture his skull or injure his spinal cord. Persons struck by lightning are often thrown a considerable distance if they happen to be standing close to some other object, owing to the mechanical repulsion which is exerted between similarly charged bodies. The injuries sustained in this way can be severe, but there will usually be superficial abrasions to indicate their origin. This repulsion explains why lightning can strip the victim of his clothes, burst his boots, and scatter objects in all directions.

ACUTE EFFECTS OF HEAT

The capacity to withstand extreme heat and humidity varies from person to person and from race to race. It is reduced in the very young and the very old, by general ill-health, and by lack of acclimatization. The effects of heat are varied, a fact which is mirrored in a chaotic terminology, but for practical purposes it will suffice to define four conditions, with the proviso that mixed and transitional syndromes are common.[2, 9, 10, 15, 16]

HEAT EXHAUSTION. This is marked by weakness, headache, lightheadedness, unsteady gait, irritability, pallor, and clammy sweating. Aggressive and irresponsible behavior may occur. The pulse is weak and rapid, and the temperature is usually low. Syncope is not uncommon. The condition is largely the result of loss of fluid and salt in the sweat, and is likely to occur as a result of prolonged overexertion in hot atmospheres, but cardiovascular disease can be a pre-

disposing cause. The patient should be rested in a cool atmosphere and given plenty of salinized fluids. The incidence of heat exhaustion in troops newly arrived in the tropics in World War II was much reduced by insistence on the addition of 0.1 per cent salt to drinking water. After acclimatization, the loss of sweat and chlorides in response to heat is much reduced, and preventive measures are less important.

HEAT CRAMPS. These develop in persons doing hard physical work in hot, humid atmospheres, e.g., stokeholds, blast furnaces, mines. They consist of repetitive painful muscular cramps in the extremities, and are due to loss of sodium chloride and water in the sweat. Vomiting may occur. Treatment is by administration of saline, either by mouth or intravenously. People engaged in this type of work should take a liberal quantity of salt with their food, and the drinking water provided should contain 0.1 per cent of salt.

HEAT SHOCK. This is usually caused by exposure to a hot sun, and is one form of so-called sunstroke. It is not uncommon in temperate climates on an unusually hot day. It starts with nausea and a feeling of faintness, which speedily progresses to unconsciousness and a condition of shock, with a low blood pressure, fast thready pulse, clammy skin, subnormal temperature, and irregular respiration. The clammy skin and low temperature distinguish it from heat stroke. Consciousness may return in a minute or two, or the patient may remain in a rousable stupor for hours. Recovery is usually complete, without aftereffects. It must be remembered that not everyone who faints on a hot day is necessarily suffering from heat shock; ordinary syncope is a commoner explanation, while more serious conditions such as subarachnoid hemorrhage or a stroke may be to blame. Moreover, persistent unconsciousness may be due to a head injury sustained when the syncopal patient falls to the ground. The treatment of heat shock is recumbency, rest, and warmth.

Heat stroke and heat hyperpy-rexia. This is a medical emergency which requires prompt treatment if death or serious sequelae are to be avoided. It occurs after long exposure to high humidity and is especially likely to arise in persons who perspire little or who are in a poor state of health.[2, 5, 9, 15, 16] Unsuitable clothing and heavy physical exercise are important predisposing causes (as in players of American football).

The effect of high temperatures on the nervous system is to diminish its activity, so sweating—among other functions—may be diminished or lost. This leads to a sharp rise of body temperature. At the same time, catabolism is increased and excretion is diminished, so that toxic catabolites accumulate in excessive quantities. In fatal cases, the kidneys are congested and swollen, and renal function may be severely impaired. Liver damage is prominent, as is shown by raised serum levels of bilirubin, iron, and glutamic oxaloacetic transaminase, and by a fall in prothrombin and fibrinogen. Thrombocytopenia and a prolonged bleeding time are common and are probably responsible for the widespread hemorrhages found in those dying late in the disease.[9, 16] A polymorphonuclear leukocytosis is usually present in severe cases, and this may make it difficult to identify a superimposed infection.

The onset of heat stroke may be abrupt, or it may be preceded by heat exhaustion over a period of hours or even days. Depression of sweating may occur as much as 48 hours in advance of the attack, but Shibolet and his colleagues[16] have emphasized that sweating may be present in the case of healthy men engaged in strenuous physical activity during hot weather; in such cases, heat stroke results from overloading rather than from breakdown of the thermoregulatory mechanism.

There is a rapid rise of temperature to 105°F. or more, coupled with varying degrees of cerebral dysfunction. Convulsions are common. At the onset, there is confusion and delirium, but coma rapidly supervenes, and death may occur within a few hours. The pulse is rapid and blood pressure falls[18]; the hypotension is resistant to therapy in fatal cases. The urine is scanty, concentrated, and contains albumin. The chloride content is markedly reduced. The cerebrospinal fluid is clear, but the pressure may be raised.

Course and Prognosis. In patients who are to recover, the temperature falls, the pulse improves, the coma lightens and sweating returns, if it has been absent, but *the condition may recur within a few hours.* A second danger to life is bronchial pneumonia following the pulmonary congestion that is part of the circulatory failure induced by heat stroke.[18] Aftereffects vary.[10] Capacity to sweat adequately may remain in abeyance for weeks, and evidence of renal and liver damage may persist for months. Headache, photophobia, vertigo, and varying degrees of mental impairment are common, but they usually pass off in a few months. Transient cerebellar ataxia may occur, as may persistent peripheral neuropathy.[18] In one case, the patient developed polyuria, narcoplexy, obesity, and sexual dystrophy immediately after a nearly fatal episode of heat stroke.

Treatment. The first essential is the reduction of the pyrexia. How this is to be done depends on the facilities which are available. Ideally, the patient should be cooled in an air-conditioned room with numerous ice-filled plastic bags applied to the skin; an electric cooling blanket is an additional advantage. If these are not available, the patient should be immersed in an ice bath, or covered by a wet sheet and placed under a fan. The rectal temperature is taken every five minutes, and the cooling process is stopped when the temperature falls to 102°F. Shivering, which is harmful, can be prevented by the intravenous administration of 100 mg. each of chlorpromazine and promethazine in 200 ml. of 5 per cent glucose. Oxygen should be given to combat tissue anoxia and acidosis. Dehydration must be corrected, but in view of the possible presence of renal damage, overhydration must be avoided. Serial serum potassium and pH determinations should be made, and potassium should be administered if the serum level is reduced. If there is renal engorgement and pulmonary congestion, venesection is indicated. If malaria is present, quinine should be given by intramuscular injection; intravenous injection is dangerous in these cases because it can aggravate the existing hypotension.

THE EFFECTS OF COLD

GENERAL EFFECTS. The response of the body to a fall of environmental temperature is an increase of the metabolic rate, accompanied by shivering. If the temperature falls still further, there is a shift of water from the blood to the tissues, with consequent hemoconcentration, slowing of the peripheral circulation, depression of the dissociation rate of oxyhemoglobin, and depression of metabolism. The result is a general retardation of movement and thought, and an overpowering desire for sleep. The body temperature begins to fall, and coma sets in when it reaches about 27°C. Fatigue, lack of food, and—in the case of climbers and aviators—oxygen lack accelerate the process.

VASOMOTOR DISORDERS FROM THE LOCAL EFFECTS OF COLD. Certain persons possess a digital arteriolar system which is unduly sensitive to cold, as is evidenced by the fact that their fingers become blanched, numb, and eventually cyanotic on exposure to cold—Raynaud's phenomenon. In other cases, similar symptoms are initiated by a single exposure to extreme cold, and subsequently recur in cold weather which formerly would not have had any effect. Raynaud's phenomenon can also appear as a symptom of the cervical rib syndrome, polycythemia vera, syphilitic arteritis and scleroderma, and from the use of vibrating tools. The syphilitic form is very rare, but it is of interest that it can be associated with hemoglobinuria in response to cold, and may give rise to persistent ischemia and consequent necrosis of the finger tips.

FROSTBITE. In this condition, there is actual freezing of the tissues; with total stoppage of the local circulation and death of cells. The affected part is completely anesthetic and analgesic. In minor cases, there may be persistent sensory loss for months afterward.

IMMERSION FOOT.[7, 8, 17] This term was coined during World War II to describe the effect on the feet of prolonged exposure to cold sea water, and has been retained, although the condition can occur in the hands as well. It is not, in fact, a new syndrome, having been recognized as far back as 1727, and is almost certainly identical with the "trench foot" of World War I. It is the result of chilling rather than freezing, and moisture (or water) appears to be an essential factor. Most cases arise as a result of being in cold sea water for many hours.

During exposure, the affected limbs gradually become numb and powerless. Cramps, paresthesias, and pain are either slight or absent. At this stage, the legs are bright red if the water is near freezing point, and a mottled blue or yellow if it is less cold. After many hours of exposure, the feet and legs begin to swell, and examination shows edema, absence of arterial pulsation, severe peripheral sensory loss, and weakness or paralysis of the distal muscles. Within two to five hours after the patient is rescued, the skin becomes hot and flushed, and the pulse returns to the ankle (or wrist, as the case may be). This phase is intensely painful, but the worst of the discomfort abates in a day or two, and the patient is left with paresthesias and occasional stabbing pain. The former are aggravated by warmth and reduced by cold, so the patient usually prefers to keep the limbs exposed to the air. There may be small areas of superficial necrosis, and the skin of the whole area is friable and easily injured. Sensory recovery usually starts within 24 hours, and proceeds rapidly for a few days, leaving impairment of both superficial and deep sensation, which may take months to disappear. Atrophy and weakness of the peripheral muscles usually improves, but permanent contractures may occur in severe cases.

There is usually loss of sweating peripherally, but as time goes on, this is replaced by hyperhidrosis. The cutaneous hyperemia takes months to subside, and does so spasmodically rather than uniformly, so that it varies in degree from day to day. The feet remain extremely sensitive to low temperatures and warm up very slowly after exposure to quite moderate cold; they may also become unpleasantly hot as a result of exercise, a hot bath, or too warm a room.

The clinical features of immersion hand are generally similar to those seen in the foot, but there seems to be more muscular involvement and less sensory loss than in the latter.

The pathology of the immersion syndrome has been studied in patients who died from exposure.[17] The peripheral nerves undergo patchy Wallerian degeneration, which affects the fine fibers more than the large. The muscles are edematous and friable, and may contain hemorrhages. The vascular tree is normal, surprisingly enough, and thromboses are not seen.

TREATMENT. Prophylactic measures include the removal of gloves or footwear which might restrict the circulation when the limb swells, and the generous use of oils or silicone ointment as a protective covering, should such substances be available by some miracle of foresight.

Treatment is still a matter of debate. The affected limbs are easily injured, and must therefore be protected. The patient must not be allowed to walk, and massage is contraindicated. The limb is elevated, exposed to the air, and kept dry. Most authorities recommend that the limbs be kept cool, rapid warming after exposure being condemned. Sympathectomy should not be resorted to in the stage of recovery, but may have a place in the later stage of hyperhidrosis and increased sensitivity to cold.

"PADDY FOOT." A warm-water version of the condition, "paddy foot," was encountered in the South Pacific during World War II and in the Vietnam war. It occurs when the booted feet are sub-merged in water for a long time. The foot swells, the superficial layers of the skin desquamate, and in severe cases there are persistent paresthesias during recovery. Application of a silicone ointment to the skin before immersion reduces the incidence and severity of the condition.

X-RAY THERAPY

The Brain. Therapeutic irradiation for intracranial tumors or for rodent ulcer of the scalp can result in damage to the brain.[4, 11] Fortunately this is very rare.

In man,[11] neurons disappear from the cortex, and the astrocytes are swollen. The small vessels show fibrinoid necrosis, and some are thrombosed. Fibrinous exudate is present in some parts of the cortex and subjacent white matter. In rabbits, exposure to a single dose of 2850 r. (roentgens) produces no symptoms until about the one-hundredth day. The earliest lesions are small ring and ball hemorrhages around capillaries, followed by fibrinoid necrosis of some arterioles. Swelling of astrocytes and gliosis occurs, but cortical changes are slight and are usually confined to patchy loss of the Purkinje cells of the cerebellum.

The symptoms may appear for the first time at any time between five months and five years after the treatment.[11] In some cases, the symptoms come on suddenly, progress to a point, and then become arrested. In other cases, they come on gradually and lead to death. The symptoms and signs are appropriate to the area of brain which has received the maximum radiation.

RADIATION MYELOPATHY. This commonly affects the cervical cord, and the pathological findings are similar to those present in the brain.[12, 14] In some cases, immediately following irradiation, the patient complains of paresthesias in the feet and hands, and Lhermitte's sign may be positive. However, these symptoms commonly disappear over a period of months, and nothing more happens.[6a] In a very small minority, new symptoms develop five months to five years later. There is an insidious onset of paresthesias in the lower limbs, later spreading to the upper limbs. There may be shooting pains in the neck or across the back. Spastic weakness of the legs follows; it is usually symmetrical and progressive, but a Brown-Séquard syndrome can occur. The arms may become weak and ultimately sphincter symptoms appear. The weakness is complicated by sensory ataxia if, as is sometimes the case, proprioception is more effective than superficial sensation.

Myelography shows nothing amiss. A modest elevation of the cerebrospinal fluid protein is present in some cases.

Prognosis is poor, most patients dying within one to four years of the onset.

There is, perhaps, a place for treatment by steroids in this condition. In one case, the patient's symptoms failed to advance while he was kept on a maintenance dose of steroids but became much more severe when the medication was stopped for three weeks. This was followed by marked improvement in power, sensory responses, and sphincter control when the steroids were resumed.

REFERENCES

1. Bambridge, W.: Optic atrophy with retinal changes caused by high tension current. *Brit. Med. J.* 2:958, 1930.
2. Borden, D. L., Wadill, J. F., and Grier, G. S.: Statistical study of 265 cases of heat disease. *J.A.M.A.* 10:849, 1961.
3. Critchley, M.: Neurological effects of lightning and of electricity. *Lancet* 1:68, 1934.
4. Greenfield, J. G.: *Neuropathology.* 2nd Ed. Williams and Wilkins Co., Baltimore, 1963.
5. *Heatstroke.* Lancet 1:31, 1968.
6. Hyslop, G. H.: The effects of electric shock on the nervous system. *Injuries of the Brain and Spinal Cord and Their Coverings.* Edited by Brock, S., Springer Publishing Co., New York, 1960, Chap. 23.
6a. Jones, A.: Transient radiation myelopathy. *Brit. J. Radiol.* 37:727, 1964.
7. Lange, K., Wiener, D., and Boyd, L. J.: The functional pathology of experimental immersion foot. *Amer. Heart J.* 35:238, 1948.
8. Learmonth, J. R.: Discussion on immersion injuries and vasomotor disorders of the limbs in wartime. *Proc. Roy. Soc. Med.* 36:515, 1943.
9. Malamud, N., Haymaker, W., and Custer, R. P.: Heat stroke. Clinicopathologic study of 125 fatal cases. *Mil. Surg.* 99:397, 1946.
10. Mehta, A. C., and Baker, R. N.: Persistent neurological deficits in heat stroke. *Neurology* 20:336, 1970.
11. Pennybacker, J., and Russell, D. S.: Necrosis of the brain due to radiation therapy. *J. Neurol. Neurosurg. Psychiat.* 11:183, 1948.
12. Pallis, C. A., Louis, S., and Morgan, R. L.: Radiation myelopathy. *Brain* 84:460, 1961.
13. Pritchard, E. A. B.: Changes in the central nervous system due to electrocution. *Lancet* 1:1163, 1934.
14. Reagan, T. J., Thomas, J. E., and Colby, M. Y.: Chronic progressive radiation myelopathy. *J.A.M.A.* 203:128, 1968.
15. Schmidt, G.: Effect of sunstroke on the central nervous system. *J. Indust. Hyg. Tox.* 23:110, 1941.
16. Shibolet, S., Coll, R., and Sohar, E.: Heatstroke. *Quart. J. Med.* 36:525, 1967.
17. Ungley, C. C., and Blackwood, W.: Peripheral vasoneuropathy after chilling. Immersion foot and immersion hand. *Lancet* 2:447, 1942.
18. Wilson, G.: The cardiopathology of heat stroke. *J.A.M.A.* 114:557, 1940.

Index

Page numbers in *italics* indicate pages on which illustrations appear.